HEALTH OF PEOPLE, PLACES AND PLANET

REFLECTIONS BASED ON TONY MCMICHAEL'S FOUR DECADES OF CONTRIBUTION TO EPIDEMIOLOGICAL UNDERSTANDING

HEALTH OF PEOPLE, PLACES AND PLANET

REFLECTIONS BASED ON TONY MCMICHAEL'S FOUR DECADES OF CONTRIBUTION TO EPIDEMIOLOGICAL UNDERSTANDING

EDITED BY COLIN D. BUTLER, JANE DIXON
AND ANTHONY G. CAPON

Australian National University
PRESS

Published by ANU Press
The Australian National University
Acton ACT 2601, Australia
Email: anupress@anu.edu.au
This title is also available online at http://press.anu.edu.au

National Library of Australia Cataloguing-in-Publication entry

Title: Health of people, places and planet : reflections based on Tony McMichael's four decades of contribution to epidemiological understanding / edited by Colin Butler, Jane Dixon, Anthony Capon.

ISBN: 9781925022407 (paperback) 9781925022414 (ebook)

Subjects: Epidemiology.
Epidemiology--History.
Public health.
Public health surveillance.
Social change--Health aspects.

Other Creators/Contributors:
Butler, Colin D., 1955- editor.
Dixon, Jane, 1951- editor.
Capon, Anthony G., 1960- editor.

Dewey Number: 614.4

Cover design and layout by ANU Press using artwork by Kerry Shepherdson.

CONTENTS

Part 3: Environmental and Social Epidemiology

Part 4: Nutrition and Food Systems

Part 5: Climate Change and Health

Part 6: Ecosystem Change, Infectious Diseases and Well-being

Part 7: Transformation

LIST OF FIGURES

LIST OF TABLES

LIST OF ACRONYMS

AAS	Australian Academy of Science
ABLV	Australian bat lyssavirus
ABARE	Australian Bureau of Agricultural and Resource Economics
ABLV	Australian bat lyssavirus
ACT	Australian Capital Territory
AFCO	Australian Federation of Consumer Organisations
AIHW	Australian Institute of Health and Welfare
AMR	antimicrobial resistant (resistance)
ANU	Australian National University
API	American Petroleum Institute
ARC	Australian Research Council
ASEAN	Association of Southeast Asian Nations
ASH	Action on Smoking and Health
AusUVI	Australian Ultraviolet Radiation and Immunity
BMI	body mass index
Bt	billion tonnes
CAF	content analysis framework
CAFO	concentrated animal feeding operations
CBD	Convention on Biological Diversity
CDD	Canadian Disaster Database
CE	Common Era
CFE	carbon fertilisation effect
CJD	Creutzfeldt–Jakob disease
CNS	central nervous system
COP	conference of the parties
CRC	Centre for Research Excellence
CSIRO	Commonwealth Scientific and Industrial Research Organisation
CVD	cardiovascular disease
DCCEE	Department of Climate Change and Energy Efficiency
DDT	dichlorodiphenyl-trichloroethane
DNA	deoxyribonucleic acid
DRC	Democratic Republic of Congo

EBV	Epstein–Barr virus
ECOHOST	European Centre on Health of Societies in Transition
EID	emerging infectious disease
EMS	Environmental Mutagen Society
ENSO	El Niño Southern Oscillation
FAO	Food and Agricultural Organization
GDP	gross domestic product
GFC	global financial crisis
GHG	greenhouse gas(es)
GM	genetically modified
Hectare	ha
HFCS	high-fructose corn syrup
HIA	health impact assessment
HiAP	health in all policies
HIV	human immunodeficiency virus
HIV/AIDS	human immunodeficiency virus/acquired immunodeficiency syndrome
IARC	International Agency for Research on Cancer
ICCIDDs	International Council for the Control of Iodine Deficiency Disorders
ICIS	International Centre for Integrated Assessment and Sustainable Development
ICONICS	International Committee on New Integrated Climate Change Assessment Scenarios
ICSU	International Council for Science
IDD	iodine deficiency disorders
IEA	International Epidemiology Association
IGT	impaired glucose tolerance
IHD	ischaemic heart disease
ILO	International Labour Organization
I = PAT	impact (I) = a function of population (P), affluence (A) and technology (T)
IPCC	Intergovernmental Panel on Climate Change
IRM	Indigenous research methods
ISEE	International Society for Environmental Epidemiology
ISSC	International Social Science Council

IUCN	International Union for the Conservation of Nature
JCU	James Cook University
JDC	job demands–control
JNAP	Joint National Action Plan
KSHV	Kaposi sarcoma-associated virus
KLH	keyhole limpet haemocyanin
LDCs	less-developed countries; least-developed countries
LEB	life expectancy at birth
LPI	Living Planet Index
LSH&TM	London School of Hygiene and Tropical Medicine
MD	doctor of medicine
MPH	master of public health
MDG(s)	Millennium Development Goal(s)
MEA	Millennium Ecosystem Assessment
miRNA	micro-RNA
MJ	megajoule
MS	multiple sclerosis
MUST	Maastricht University Graduate School of Sustainability Science
NCCARF	National Climate Change Adaptation Research Facility
NCCHAP	National Climate Change and Health Action Plans
NCDs	non-communicable diseases
NCEPH	National Centre for Epidemiology and Population Health
NCI	National Cancer Institute
NDCs	now-developed countries
NDP	National Development Plan
NGO	non-governmental organisation
NIH	National Institutes of Health
NH&MRC	National Health and Medical Research Council
NUAUS	National Union of Australian University Students
OECD	Organisation for Economic Co-operation and Development
OPEC	Organization of Petroleum Exporting Countries
OR	odds ratio
OSHA	Occupational Safety and Health Administration
PATH	personality and total health
PIC	Pacific island country
PPCS	The Port Pirie cohort study

PPM	parts per million
PRSPs	poverty reduction strategy papers
PVC	polyvinylchloride
RACGP	Royal Australian College of General Practitioners
RMIT	Royal Melbourne Institute of Technology
RNA	ribonucleic acid
RRV	Ross River virus
SARS	severe acute respiratory syndrome
SDGs	Sustainable Development Goals
SECA	South-East Coast Adaptation
SEIFA	Socio-economic Indexes for Areas
SGS	Sydney Gallery School
SIG	special interest group
SHWB	science for health and well-being
SIV	simian immunodeficiency virus
SLAPP	strategic lawsuit against public participation
SOFI	state of food insecurity (in the world)
spp.	species
SRES	Special Report on Emission Scenarios
STOU	Sukhothai Thammathirat Open University
TAFE	technical and further education
T2D	type 2 diabetes
TB	tuberculosis
TBE	tick-borne encephalitis
TEEB	The Economics of Ecosystems and Biodiversity
TIA	Tobacco Industry of Australia
TDR	Special Programme for Tropical Diseases Research (also known as the Special Programme for Research and Training in Tropical Diseases)
UB	urban bias
UC	University of Canberra
UN	United Nations
UNCSD	United Nations Commission on Sustainable Development
UNEP	United Nations Environment Programme
UNESCO	United Nations Educational, Social and Cultural Organization
UNICEF	United Nations Children's Rights and Emergency Relief Fund

UNFCCC	United Nations Framework Convention on Climate Change
UNSW	University of New South Wales
UNU	United Nations University
UNU-IIGH	UNU International Institute for Global Health
UQ	University of Queensland
UV	ultraviolet
UWA	University of Western Australia
WBGT	wet bulb globe temperature
WHO	World Health Organization
WMO	World Meteorological Organization
WTO	World Trade Organization

DEDICATION

This book is dedicated to those who work to protect and advance public health, particularly from an academic position. It is not always easy to challenge powerful views, as Tony's life work exemplifies, but it is made easier by the collegial spirit revealed through assembling this book. It is also dedicated to the late Susan Starr Woldenberg Butler (1948–2014), who died on 4 October, the day following what would have been Tony McMichael's 72nd birthday. Tony (1942–2014) had died only one week beforehand. They are very sadly missed. Both played valuable roles in the creation of this book. Tony's career, of course, inspired the whole volume. But Tony also contributed to its design, co-authored a chapter, reviewed another and wrote or co-wrote the nine papers or book extracts that form the frame on which the book is constructed. Susan helped to edit many chapters, also contributed to the book design and nurtured and supported this book's senior editor, Colin.

ACKNOWLEDGEMENTS

This book, three years in preparation, has involved numerous people in its various stages from conception to completion.

We start by thanking Professor Gabriele Bammer, then Director of the National Centre for Epidemiology and Population Health (NCEPH) at The Australian National University (ANU), who in 2011 conceived the holding of a conference in honour of Professor Tony McMichael, who was to retire at the end of 2012. ANU and NCEPH, with others, provided funding for the conference, held in November 2012. NCEPH then made further financial and in kind contributions to the production of this book, which completes Tony's festschrift.[1]

We thank ANU Press, and especially Dr Farid Rahimi (from the ANU Press Colleges of Science Committee) and Emily Tinker, who respectively shepherded the manuscript through the review and production processes.

During the process of compiling the book, Colin Butler moved to the University of Canberra (UC), which graciously supported the task of finishing it. We also particularly thank Emeritus Professor Colin Soskolne at the University of Alberta, Canada, and an adjunct professor at UC. Finally, we thank all reviewers, all authors and the many well-wishers.

1 Traditionally, festschrifts are books. 'Fest' conveys celebration, 'schrift' denotes text. In this case, we assert both the conference and this book were part of Tony's festschrift with an Australian flavour.

ABOUT THE REVIEWERS

Many reviews were double blind. In alphabetical order (with permission), reviewers were Glenn Albrecht, Bruce Armstrong, Bianca Brijnath, Adam Bumpus, Gemma Carey, Archie Clements, Doug Cocks, Angus Cook, Steve Cork, Carlos Corvalán, Phyll Dance, Keith Dear, Steve Dovers, John Glover, Simon Hales, Trevor Hancock, Alana Hansen, Adrian Hayes, Jane Heyworth, Paul Komaresoff, Nancy Krieger, John Last, David Legge, Gweneth Leigh, Claus Leitzmann, Mariann Lloyd-Smith, Robyn Lucas, Lenore Manderson, Geoff Morgan, Jonathan Patz, Anne Louise Ponsonby, John Potter, John Powles, Colin Soskolne, Susan Thompson, Sotiris Vardoulakis, Graham Vimpani, Phil Weinstein, Jennifer Wilkins, Alistair Woodward, and three reviewers who preferred to remain anonymous. We also received formal comments from two anonymous reviewers of the book, as well as useful informal comment from other readers, including Jo Walker.

ABOUT THE REPRINTS

We thank the following publishers. In addition, specific acknowledgements, using wording (if requested) by each publisher, will be included. In alphabetical order, these are the *American Journal of Epidemiology*, *Bulletin of the World Health Organization*, Cambridge University Press, *Journal of the National Cancer Institute*, *Journal of Occupational Medicine*, *Medical Journal of Australia*, *New England Journal of Medicine*, *Nature Medicine* and Penguin Australia.

ABOUT THE CONTRIBUTORS

Zahide Ceren Atli

Zahide Ceren Atli was born in Istanbul, Turkey. She has lived in California, USA, for more than 12 years. Ms Atli completed her licence education at the University of California, Berkeley, in the Department of Rhetoric. Her area of interest involves public health and public policy. Ms Atli has multiple papers in these areas and is continuing research. She is also actively involved in translating scholarly articles between Turkish and English. Ms Atli is currently living in San Francisco, California, and in her spare time enjoys contributing to public enrichment projects in her locale.

Hilary Bambrick

Hilary Bambrick is Professor and chair of Population Health at the University of Western Sydney, Australia. She is an environmental epidemiologist and bioanthropologist whose principal research area is health impacts assessment and adaptation planning associated with climate variability and change, especially in more vulnerable populations. Her work is largely based in Australia, the Pacific and Africa, focusing on vector-borne, respiratory and gastrointestinal disease and malnutrition and child health. She consults on climate impacts and adaptation planning for governments in Australia and overseas. In 2011, she received a NSW Young Tall Poppy Award for outstanding achievements in scientific research and communication.

Melanie Bannister Tyrrell

Melanie completed a Bachelor of Philosophy with first class Honours and won the University Medal at The Australian National University in 2010. Her Honours thesis examined the association between weather variation and dengue virus outbreaks in far North Queensland. Subsequently, Melanie worked as a research assistant for Tony McMichael, exploring the impact of climate change on infectious diseases. Melanie was awarded a John Monash scholarship to attend the London School of Hygiene and Tropical Medicine in 2011 and graduated with a Master of Science (Epidemiology) with Distinction in 2012. Melanie is currently completing a PhD at the Institute of Tropical Medicine, Antwerp, through the Erasmus Mundus Trans Global Health PhD fellowship.

Cathy Banwell

Dr Cathy Banwell is an Associate Professor at NCEPH, ANU. She has drawn on her background in social anthropology and public health to conduct research on the sociocultural contexts and health risks associated with the consumption of alcohol, other drugs and poor diets. With others, she has recently authored a book examining the social and cultural trends contributing to rising levels of obesity in Australia (*The Weight of Modernity*, 2013) and has jointly edited a book *When Culture Impacts Health* (2013), which provides exemplars of research approaches to the interrelationship between culture and health in Australasian and Asian settings.

Michael Bentley

Michael Bentley is a health services researcher at the University of Tasmania and Adjunct Research Fellow in the Southgate Institute for Health, Society and Equity at Flinders University, South Australia. He focuses on research and evaluation in public and community health that is grounded in a broader social, economic and environmental context. Michael holds a Doctor of Public Health degree from Flinders University. His research interests are in the social complexity of and ecological approaches to health, equity and the environment. Michael is a member of the Public Health Association of Australia and the Tasmanian Social Determinants of Health Advocacy Network.

Carijn Beumer

Carijn Beumer is a PhD researcher at Maastricht University (The Netherlands), assessing cultural perspectives on biodiversity conservation in a changing world and exploring the potential role of urban greening for the conservation of nature. How do citizens perceive and contribute to urban greening? Special attention is given to the role of domestic gardening: how can home gardens best contribute to larger green infrastructures, biodiversity and ecosystem services? Between 2009 and 2012, Carijn was involved as a researcher in the Interreg IV SUN project (Sustainable Urban Neighbourhoods). Next to her research projects, Carijn is coordinating and teaching MA and BA courses on Sustainable Development and Global Dynamics at Maastricht University.

Peng Bi

Professor Peng Bi is Professor of Public Health at the University of Adelaide, Australia. His expertise falls in the fields of environmental and infectious disease epidemiology. He has wide research experience in identifying and managing environmental health problems, including the impact of heatwaves on population health and relevant adaptation strategies. Professor Bi has been successful in winning many research grants. He has worked in collaboration with relevant government organisations and NGOs and has provided evidence to inform policy decisions. He was Node Leader of Heat and Health of the National Climate Change Adaptation Research Facility (NCCARF) and helped redevelop National Climate Change and Population Health Research Strategies and Directions.

Kathryn Bowen

Kathryn's area of expertise is climate change and health. She has been at NCEPH since 2008. Kathryn has worked in global health research and policy since 1999, across public, private and university sectors. She is a Research Fellow within the Earth System Governance project and Fellow of the Adaptation College and the Centre for Sustainability Leadership. Kathryn is co-founder of Just Change, a climate change and equity organisation, and sits on an environment advisory committee for the City of Melbourne. Currently, her main work is a range of consultancies for the World Health Organization (WHO) (country/regional offices) on climate change and health.

Devin C. Bowles

Devin Bowles is a PhD student at the National Centre for Epidemiology and Population Health at The Australian National University. Devin's research topic, initially inspired by one of Tony McMichael's presentations, is the socially mediated health effects of climate change, with a focus on conflict, migration, undernutrition and health inequity. Devin has an ongoing interest in the psychological and social barriers to climate change mitigation. He obtained Honours degrees in anthropology and psychology and a Master of Arts in anthropology. Previous publication topics include religious change, Aboriginal health, prosopagnosia (face blindness) and the intersection of conflict prevention and health care.

Stephen V. Boyden, *AM*

Stephen Boyden FAA is qualified in Veterinary Science (London, 1947). From 1949 to 1965, he performed research in immunology in Cambridge, New York, Paris, Copenhagen and Canberra. From 1965, he pioneered human ecology and biohistory at ANU. In the 1970s, he directed the Hong Kong Human Ecology Programme. After retirement (1991), he formed and worked with the *Nature and Society Forum* – a community-based organisation concerned with the well-being of humankind and the environment. He has published books on biohistory. At present, he is actively involved in the *Frank Fenner Foundation for Healthy People on a Healthy Planet*, of which he is Patron.

Colin D. Butler

Professor Colin Butler is based at the University of Canberra, and is also a Visiting Fellow at NCEPH at the ANU. In 1989, he and his late wife, Susan co-founded BODHI (Benevolent Organisation for Development, Health & Insight). In 2014, he co-founded Health-Earth (www.canberra.edu.au/centres/ceraph/H-earth). Colin has published widely, including on health, sustainability, justice, conflict and engaged Buddhism. He was a co-ordinating lead author for the Millennium Ecosystem Assessment. In 2009, he was named one of '100 doctors for the planet' by the French Environmental Health Association. Butler edited *Climate Change and Global Health* (CABI, 2014). His collaboration with Tony McMichael started in 1993.

Anthony G. Capon

Professor Capon directs the International Institute for Global Health at United Nations University, based in Kuala Lumpur. Tony is a public health physician and an authority on environmental health and health promotion. Since 2008, he has been working with the International Council for Science to develop the global interdisciplinary science programme on health and well-being in the changing urban environment using systems approaches. Tony has held National Health and Medical Research Council and World Health Organization fellowships, as well as leadership roles with the Australasian Faculty of Public Health Medicine and the International Society for Urban Health.

Kaila-Lea Clarke

Kaila-Lea Clarke, BSc, MA, is a geographer and senior policy analyst for Canada's federal ministry of health. Her career and research contributions relate to climate change and human health, health systems and Aboriginal health and wellness. Her research examines risk perception and human health vulnerabilities to extreme heat, and other climate-related health impacts and emergencies in urban and rural settings. She has co-authored several national studies to advance the understanding of climate change impacts, adaptation and actions to enhance climate change resilience. Email: kaila-lea.clarke@hc-sc.gc.ca.

Devra Davis

Dr Davis, MA, MPH, PhD, has a long and distinguished career has spanned academia, public policy and scientific research. She has written several award-winning books, including *The Secret History of the War on Cancer*, a top pick by *Newsweek*, and over 190 other publications in books, journals and blogs. She has received many awards, including for breaking the paradigms of how women are perceived and the Artemis Award, for outstanding contributions to science and public health policy. In 2007, she founded the non-profit Environmental Health Trust, which provides basic research, education and policy advice about environmental health hazards. She is currently working on two new books.

Keith Dear

Keith Dear is Research Professor of Global Health (Environmental Health) at Duke Global Health Institute (USA) and Director of Graduate Studies in Global Health at Duke Kunshan University in China. He was, until 2013, Senior Fellow in Biostatistics at The Australian National University, where he worked closely with Tony McMichael. He has worked in cancer clinical trials, meta-analysis, psychiatric epidemiology and environmental epidemiology. He contributed to the 2008 Garnaut Review of Climate Change in Australia, is a contributing author to the 5th IPCC report and a coordinating lead author for the Urban Climate Change Research Network's second assessment report.

Jane Dixon

Jane Dixon is Senior Fellow at the National Centre for Epidemiology and Population Health, The Australian National University. Her research takes place at the intersection of sociology and public health and focuses on transformations within national food systems and the sociocultural determinants of health transitions. She has advised numerous bodies on adopting a food system perspective, including the International Union on Health Promotion and Education and the Western Pacific Regional Office of WHO. Recent books include *When Culture Impacts Health* (Elsevier) and *Weight of Modernity* (Springer). She is currently researching for a new book, *The Culinary Footprint* (Bloomsbury).

Bob Douglas

Bob Douglas retired from the post of Foundation Director of NCEPH at ANU in 2001 after a 40-year medical career, which included work as specialist physician in Papua New Guinea, as an epidemiologist working on the development of a pneumonia vaccine in the USA, as a community medicine academic and General Practitioner at the Adelaide Medical School and as Dean of the Adelaide Medical School. Following his retirement in 2001, with five colleagues from various walks of Australian life, he established a new body, Australia21, the board of which he chaired from 2001 to 2011.

Kristie L. Ebi

Kristie L. Ebi is a professor at the University of Washington and Guest Professor at Umea University, Sweden. She conducts research on the impacts of and adaptation to climate change, including extreme events, food-borne safety and security and vector-borne diseases. Work as an independent consultant (ClimAdapt, LLC) in the USA, Central America, Europe, Africa, Asia and the Pacific focused on understanding sources of vulnerability and designing adaptation policies and measures to reduce the risks of climate change in a multi-stressor environment. She co-chairs the International Committee on New Integrated Climate Change Assessment Scenarios (ICONICS), facilitating development of new climate change scenarios.

Ferne Edwards

Ferne Edwards has a background in cultural anthropology, specialising in sustainable cities, food systems and social movements. She has published widely on topics of food waste, freeganism, food mapping, climate change and beekeeping. For her doctorate, Ferne conducted research on alternative food networks in Sydney and the food sovereignty movement in Venezuela. Ferne spoke at the 2008 World Economic Forum in South Korea and was appointed a World Social Science Fellow by the International Social Science Council (ISSC) in 2013. Ferne is currently coordinating a book with ISSC and is a researcher at RMIT University investigating ethical consumption in Australia.

Donna Green

Donna Green is a Senior Lecturer and Researcher at the Climate Change Research Centre and Associate Investigator for the ARC Centre of Excellence for Climate Systems Science at the University of New South Wales, Australia. Her research interests include taking an interdisciplinary approach to understanding and explaining climate impacts on Indigenous communities in northern Australia. She also teaches and conducts research on the connections between climate change and energy policy. She was a contributing author to the fourth and fifth Intergovernmental Panel on Climate Change (IPCC) reports and has advised on climate policy around the world.

Hülya Gül

Professor Dr Hülya Gül graduated from Istanbul University (Turkey). She has been working in the Department of Public Health in the Medical Faculty, Istanbul University. She got her PhD degrees in preventive oncology and public health from Istanbul University Medical Faculty in 1995 and 2002, respectively. She studied at the Occupational Studies Section of the National Cancer Institute,

NIH, in the USA for one year in 1992. She has been actively involved in research on environmental and occupational health. She is the author of more than 100 papers in national and international scientific journals and conference proceedings.

Andy Haines

Sir Andy Haines is the Professor of Public Health and Primary Care, London School of Hygiene & Tropical Medicine. He was Director of the London School of Hygiene & Tropical Medicine (LSH&TM) from 2001 to October 2010. He has worked internationally, including in Nepal and the USA. and chaired the Scientific Advisory Panel for the 2013 World Health Report. He was a member of the UN Intergovernmental Panel on Climate Change for the 2nd and 3rd assessment exercises and is review editor of the health chapter in the 5th assessment. He has published many papers in high-impact journals on topics such as primary care, health systems research and the relationship between environmental change and health.

Trevor Hancock

Professor Trevor Hancock is a public health physician, currently at the University of Victoria, British Columbia, Canada. He is a founder of the (now global) Healthy Cities and Communities movement and originated the term 'healthy public policy'. His public health interests include health promotion, environment and health, healthy and 'green' hospitals and health futurism. He has been called 'one of the 10 best health futurists in the world'. In the 1980s, he was the first leader of the Canadian Green Party and later co-founded the Canadian Association of Physicians for the Environment and the Canadian Coalition for Green Health Care.

Elizabeth Hanna

Dr Hanna is a Fellow at Australia's National Centre for Epidemiology and Population Health, The Australian National University, and President of the Climate and Health Alliance. She convened Australia's National Climate Change Adaptation Research Network for Human Health and she continues to represent public health and environmental health interests on various State and Federal Government committees. Through 2002–09, Liz also convened the Environmental Health special interest group (SIG) for the Public Health Association of Australia. Her research addresses the environmental determinants of health, nowadays primarily climate change; the factors (exposures, knowledge, attitudes, behaviour, policy and health infrastructure) that elicit protective responses adopted by individuals, communities and governments.

David Harley

David Harley is a zoologist, medical doctor, epidemiologist and public health physician. He is currently Associate Professor of Epidemiology at the National Centre for Epidemiology and Population Health and The Medical School at The Australian National University. He has a major interest in infectious disease epidemiology, and particularly in vector-borne diseases. Ross River virus, Australia's most important climate-sensitive arbovirus, is a long-standing interest. He has published on tuberculosis, adenovirus, meningococcus, malaria and dengue. He currently leads a major research project on climate and the epidemiology of dengue in North Queensland, for which Professor Tony McMichael was a co-investigator.

Basil S. Hetzel, *AC*

Dr Basil Hetzel graduated in medicine from the University of Adelaide in 1944. After postgraduate study in Adelaide, New York and London, he became Professor of Medicine at the University of Adelaide (1956–68), Foundation Professor of Social and Preventive Medicine, Monash University Melbourne (1968–75) and Chief, CSIRO Division of Human Nutrition (1975–85). He has made a significant contribution to public health in Australia and to world health through his work on the elimination of iodine deficiency as a cause of brain damage – with an at-risk population of two billion from 130 countries. He remains Chairman Emeritus of the International Council for Control of Iodine Deficiency Disorders, an expert group that works closely with WHO, the United Nations Children's Rights and Emergency Relief Fund (UNICEF) and other agencies.

Graeme Hugo

Graeme Hugo, who died in January 2015, was an ARC Australian Professorial Fellow, Professor of Geography, Environment and Population and Director of the Australian Population and Migration Research Centre at the University of Adelaide. His research interests centred on population issues in Australia and Southeast Asia, especially migration. He authored over 400 books, articles and chapters, as well as many conference papers and reports. His recent research focused on migration and development, environment and migration and migration policy. In 2012, he was named an Officer of the Order of Australia (AO), for service to population research for his leadership roles with national and international organisations.

Gian S. Jhangri

Gian S. Jhangri is a double Masters-level biostatistician. He holds an Associate Professorship in the School of Public Health at the University of Alberta, Edmonton, Canada. As an applied biostatistician, most of his research is collaborative. Professor Jhangri has authored/co-authored 104 peer-reviewed publications, including 74 in the past 10 years (2004–13). He has been involved in different research projects across many of the health sciences disciplines. His experience makes him uniquely multi- and interdisciplinary. As an award-winning teacher and service-oriented colleague, he holds an administrative position of Director of Graduate Education in the School of Public Health. Email: gian.jhangri@ualberta.ca.

Tord Kjellstrom

Tord Kjellstrom has researched and taught environmental and occupational epidemiology for 40 years at universities in New Zealand, Australia and Sweden. He worked for 12 years at WHO on global project management in his field and directed the new office responsible for the analysis of and guidance on climate change and health. His research interests have included the health effects of heavy metals, asbestos, air pollution, road transport crashes, urban health, globalisation and sustainable development. This work has generated more than 400 publications (68 on climate, health and productivity issues between 2000 and 2014). Tord knew Tony McMichael from the early 1970s, and they collaborated many times.

Justine D. A. Klaver-Kibria

Justine D. A. Klaver-Kibria received her MSc (Epidemiology) in 2001 from the University of Alberta, Edmonton, Canada. Ms Klaver-Kibria focused her research on climate change and health in the Canadian Prairies. Post-MSc, she was the research associate and coordinator for the study reported in this festschrift. Currently, she has an environmental health consulting company focusing on healthy home environments. Email: jkibria@telus.net.

Su Mon Kyaw-Myint

Su Mon Kyaw-Myint was originally trained as a medical scientist. Since 2005, she has been involved in various occupational health and safety research projects, with a main focus on occupational exposures. She completed her PhD (at NCEPH, at ANU) in occupational health in 2012 and works at Safe Work Australia, the National Occupational Health and Safety agency. Her work involves providing research and data for the development and evaluation of national occupational health and safety policy.

Tim Lang

Tim Lang has been Professor of Food Policy at the Centre for Food Policy at City University, London, since 2002. He was a hill farmer in Lancashire, England, in the 1970s. This formed his interest in the politics of the relationship between food, health, the environment and culture, and he has been engaged in public and academic research and debate about food policy ever since. He was a Commissioner on the UK Government's Sustainable Development Commission (2006–11). He is co-author with Geof Rayner of *Ecological Public* (2012) and with David Barling and Martin Caraher of *Food Policy* (OUP, 2009). Email: t.lang@city.ac.uk. Postal address: Centre for Food Policy, City University, Northampton Square, London EC1V 0HB, UK. Telephone: +44 (0)20 7040 8798.

Robyn Lucas

Professor Robyn Lucas is Head of the National Centre for Epidemiology and Population Health at The Australian National University, and leads the Environment, Climate and Health research group. She is a medical epidemiologist and public health physician whose research focuses on the risks and benefits of sun exposure, particularly through modulation of immune function. She led the WHO Global Burden of Disease due to Ultraviolet Radiation assessment and leads the health chapter of the United Nations Environment Programme (UNEP) Environmental Effects Assessment Panel for the Montreal Protocol on Ozone Depletion.

Pim Martens

Pim Martens holds the chair 'Sustainable Development' at Maastricht (the Netherlands) and Leuphana (Germany) University, and is a Professor extraordinary at Stellenbosch University, South Africa. He is the (founding) Director of the Maastricht University Graduate School of Sustainability Science (MUST) and has been Director of the International Centre for Integrated Assessment and Sustainable Development (ICIS) from 2004 to 2013. Apart from his scientific work, Pim Martens is also a scientivist, intending to contribute to a better, more sustainable society.

Karen M. McDonald

Karen M. McDonald, PhD, is Professor and Director of the Department of Public Health at Concordia University College of Alberta, Edmonton, Canada. Her research focuses on atmospheric chemistry, including the assessment of exposure to ambient air contaminants through monitoring and modelling experiments. A primary goal of this research is to test fundamental concepts of chemical transformations under conditions found in northern climates and to apply these to atmospheric models for use in air quality regulatory decision making. Email: karen.mcdonald@concordia.ab.ca.

Ro McFarlane

Ro McFarlane trained as a veterinarian and worked in zoos and agriculture before focusing on One Health, natural resource management and community conservation. She has worked in the western deserts of Australia with traditional owners, developing Indigenous Protected Areas; in Antarctica, researching biosecurity risks to humans and wildlife, and with farmers, to develop ecologically connected landscapes that nurture biodiversity, agriculture and people. In 2013, she completed her doctorate on the impact of biodiversity loss and land-use change on changing infectious disease patterns of humans and animals in Australasia, supervised by Professors Tony McMichael and Adrian Sleigh at NCEPH, ANU.

Lachlan McIver

Lachlan McIver is a medical doctor specialising in remote and tropical medicine and public health. Lachlan spent two years working for the World Health Organization South Pacific office supporting Pacific island countries with climate change and health vulnerability assessments and adaptation planning. He now works as a climate change and health consultant for WHO in the South Pacific and Cambodia, while also pursuing his passion for rural and remote primary health-care development in Australia and the Asia Pacific region.

Martin McKee

Martin McKee is Professor of European Public Health at the London School of Hygiene and Tropical Medicine (LSH&TM), where he founded the European Centre on Health of Societies in Transition (ECOHOST), a WHO Collaborating Centre. He is also Research Director of the European Observatory on Health Systems and Policies, a unique partnership of universities, national and regional governments and international agencies, and is President of the European Public Health Association. He trained in medicine and public health and has written extensively on health and health policy, with a particular focus on countries undergoing political and social transition.

Philip McMichael

Philip McMichael is a Professor and Chair of Development Sociology, Cornell University, Ithaca, New York, USA and is an active member of the Civil Society Mechanism in the FAO's Committee on World Food Security. Current research is on agrarian movements, land questions and food regimes. He is the author of *Settlers and the Agrarian Question: Foundations of Capitalism in Colonial Australia* (Cambridge, 1984), *Development and Social Change: A Global Perspective* (Sage, 2012, 5th edn) and *Food Regimes and Agrarian Questions* (Fernwood, 2013), and editor of *Contesting Development: Critical Struggles for Social Change* (Routledge, 2010).

Stefano Moncada

Stefano Moncada is an assistant lecturer at the Institute for European Studies of the University of Malta. His background is in development economics and political science, with the main areas of research being climate change adaptation and development, focusing on adaptive capacity in least-developed countries. He has worked on several development projects based in Eastern Europe, South America and Africa, mainly in relation to poverty reduction and environmental management. He is currently in the final phases of his PhD with the Economics Department in the field of climate change adaptation and development. Email: stefano.moncada@um.edu.mt.

John D. Potter

John D. Potter, MBBS, PhD, is Senior Advisor to the Fred Hutchinson Cancer Research Center and Professor Emeritus of Epidemiology, University of Washington, both in Seattle, USA. He worked with Tony McMichael at the Commonwealth Scientific and Industrial Research Organisation (CSIRO) Division of Human Nutrition from 1977 to 1986. He chaired and edited *Food, Nutrition, and the Prevention of Cancer: A Global Perspective*, a seminal 1997 report. His research has focused on understanding the causes and intermediate biology of colorectal, breast and pancreatic cancers. His international awards include the 2012 Medal of Honour of the International Agency for Research on Cancer, Lyon, France. He has written or co-authored more than 600 scientific papers, chapters and books.

Geof Rayner

Geof Rayner, PhD, was born on Merseyside, UK, moving to Australia in the 1950s. After working with his builder father, he took a degree at London University, where he was later hired as a research officer. Engaged in health activism, he left university for local authority health promotion and voluntary sector campaigning. In the 1980s, he managed the launch conference of the Public Health Alliance and became chair of its successor organisation, the UK Public Health Association. Geof is joint author of *Ecological Public Health* (Routledge, 2012), with Tim Lang, and *The Metabolic Landscape* (Black Dog, 2014), with Gina Glover and Jessica Rayner.

John Reid

John Reid is an Emeritus Fellow of The Australian National University (ANU); Visiting Artist, ANU School of Art; and Visiting Fellow, ANU Fenner School for Environment and Society. As a visual artist, he addresses issues of human rights and the visualisation of landscape as a construction of regional identity. He collaborates with scientists and activists to communicate aesthetically about ecologically significant landscapes. A nationally awarded visual art educator, he instigated the ANU School of Art Field Study programme in 1966, which has been action research into a best practice educational procedure for artist and community engagement about the environment (www.engagingvisions.com.au).

J. Peter Rothe

J. Peter Rothe, PhD, is an Adjunct Professor at the School of Public Health, University of Alberta, Canada. Before retiring, he was an Associate Professor in the same school, as well as research scientist at the Alberta Centre for Injury Control and Research. His research interests were centred on the phenomenological analysis of driver behaviour, risk taking, intentional and unintentional injury and cultural patterns of safety. He is presently involved in several studies on pain and expectations of injury recovery. Email: prothe@ualberta.ca.

Sam-ang Seubsman

Dr Sam-ang Seubsman, PhD, is a community nutritionist at the Faculty of Human Ecology in Thailand's Sukhothai Thammathirat Open University. She has trained in nutritional epidemiology and has worked extensively on both pre-transitional nutritional problems (childhood malnutrition) and post-transitional nutritional problems (obesity and diabetes). For the past 10 years, she has led the Thai Health-Risk Transition Project, funded by the Wellcome Trust and the National Health and Medical Research Council (NH&MRC). This project collaborates with Australian counterparts from ANU, Monash University and the University of Queensland. Her research in Thailand is very productive and includes a nationwide community cohort of nearly 90,000 people under observation since 2005.

Adrian Sleigh

Adrian Sleigh, MD, is Professor of Epidemiology at NCEPH, ANU. He is a medical graduate with postgraduate training in tropical health and epidemiology. His work has included long periods in Los Angeles, Brazil, China, Thailand and Papua New Guinea. For several decades, he has worked on health and development projects as a health service leader (remote Aboriginal services) or as a health researcher. His early research was on schistosomiasis and Chagas disease. For the past 10 years, he has concentrated on emerging infections (TB in China, SARS in Hong Kong, avian flu in Thailand), as well as instituting long-term studies on the population-wide transition from infection–malnutrition to injury–chronic disease.

Kirk R. Smith

Kirk Smith, MPH, PhD, is Professor of Global Environmental Health at the University of California Berkeley. Professor Smith serves on a number of national and international scientific advisory committees, including the Global Energy Assessment, National Research Council's Board on Atmospheric Science and Climate, the Executive Committee for WHO Air Quality Guidelines, the International Comparative Risk Assessment and the Intergovernmental Panel on Climate Change. He holds visiting professorships in India and China and bachelor's, master's and doctoral degrees from UC Berkeley and is a member of the US National Academy of Sciences. In 2009, he received the Heinz Prize in Environment and in 2012 was awarded the Tyler Prize for Environmental Achievement.

Colin L. Soskolne

Colin L. Soskolne, PhD, Professor Emeritus, was based at the University of Alberta, Edmonton, Canada, between 1985 and 2013. He built epidemiology and biostatistics in its now accredited School of Public Health and, most recently, he established the academic arm of the University's Office of Sustainability in the Provost's Office. His focus is on the global ecological determinants of health. Currently, he is Adjunct Professor, University of Canberra. He was two-term President of the Canadian Society for Epidemiology and Biostatistics (2007–11) and is current Chair of the International Joint Policy Committee of the Societies of Epidemiology. Website: www.colinsoskolne.com. Email: colin.soskolne@ualberta.ca.

Donald W. Spady

Donald W. Spady, MD, MSc, FRCP(C), holds two Adjunct Professorships at the University of Alberta, Edmonton, Canada; one of Paediatrics in the Faculty of Medicine and Dentistry and one in the School of Public Health. He is Chair of the Advisory Board of the Children's Environmental Health Centre, based in Edmonton, which is the only health centre in Canada specifically addressing issues of children's environmental health. His current professional interests include children's environmental health, ecological integrity, climate change and resource depletion – particularly energy – and how these will affect human health, especially public health and health-care delivery. Email: dspady@ualberta.ca.

Lyndall Strazdins

Lyndall Strazdins is a Clinical Psychologist and Associate Professor (PhD Psychology, M Clinical Psych) at the National Centre for Epidemiology and Population Health, The Australian National University. Lyndall has been awarded an Australian Research Council Future Fellowship investigating time as a resource for health and she leads the work and family component of the federally funded Longitudinal Study of Australian Children, a study of 10,000 families. Lyndall is also a consultant to the Paid Parental Leave Evaluation and an advisor on the ACT Healthy Workplaces, Health Promotion panel and to the Department of Veterans Affairs.

Ashwin Swaminathan

Dr Ashwin Swaminathan completed his doctoral studies in the field of environmental epidemiology at The Australian National University under the supervision of Professors McMichael, Lucas and Dear. His research interests include the health effects of solar ultraviolet radiation exposure, vitamin D status and climate change. He also practices as a Consultant Physician at the Canberra Hospital, specialising in infectious diseases and internal medicine.

Peter Tait

Peter Tait has been a General Practitioner for 32 years, 29 in Aboriginal health in Central Australia. He was the 2007 RACGP GP of the Year. Since moving to Canberra in 2011, he has continued work in general practice. He is an Adjunct Senior Lecturer at ANU Medical School. He is involved in climate change research at UNSW and ANU, where he achieved a Masters of Climate Change in 2010. Peter believes a person's health is grounded in a healthy society, and a healthy society on a healthy ecosystem. He is active in the Public Health Association Australia, Doctors for the Environment Australia, Frank Fenner Foundation and other environment groups.

Karen Smoyer Tomic

Karen Smoyer Tomic holds a PhD in geography from the University of Minnesota, with a focus on health geography. She is based in the greater Philadelphia area, USA, and leads the US Value Demonstration Practice of Oxford PharmaGenesis™, a global medical communications consultancy. Previously, Dr Tomic was tenured Associate Professor in Earth and Atmospheric Sciences at the University of Alberta, Edmonton, Canada. Among Dr Tomic's areas of expertise is the use of real-world data to study health resource utilisation, pharmaco-epidemiology and health outcomes. Email: ketomic@gmail.com.

Shilu Tong

Professor Tong has over 200 refereed publications, including in highly prestigious journals such as *NEJM*, *The Lancet*, *JAMA*, *BMJ*, *Nature Climate Change*, *Environmental Health Perspectives*, *American Journal of Epidemiology* (*AJE*), *International Journal of Epidemiology* and *Epidemiology*. He serves on several Journal Editorial Boards, including *AJE*, *Environmental Research* and *PLoS ONE*. As the principal investigator, Professor Tong has been awarded seven ARC and four NH&MRC grants and a number of other internal/external research grants. Professor Tong has supervised/mentored 21 postgraduate students (including 10 PhD) to completion, most of whom are now flourishing in research, teaching and clinical positions at universities, government agencies and hospitals.

Paolo Vineis

Professor Paolo Vineis, MD, MPH, FFPH, is Chair of Environmental Epidemiology at Imperial College, London. His research focuses on cancer epidemiology and in particular, the environmental causes of cancer, the use of laboratory methods (epigenetics, adducts, mutations) applied to the study of cancer aetiology in populations and gene–environment interactions. He has led methods development in the field of molecular epidemiology. He is Head of the Genetic and Molecular Epidemiology Unit at the HuGeF (Human Genetics) Foundation in Torino, Italy, and Course Director of the BSc in Global Health at Imperial College, London. (See www.environment-health.ac.uk/our-research/exposome-and-health, www1.imperial.ac.uk/publichealth/education/undergrad/bscglobalhealth/.)

Mark L. Wahlqvist, *AO*

Mark L. Wahlqvist, educated in Adelaide (MD) and Uppsala, Sweden (MD), is a consultant physician with deep connections to universities and research institutes in Melbourne (Monash and Deakin), Taiwan (National Health Research Institute) and China. He was President of the International Union of Nutritional Sciences from 2001 to 2005 and has been Editor-in-Chief of the *Asia Pacific Journal of Clinical Nutrition* for most of its 23-year history. Since 2013, he has directed the Fuli Institute of Food Science and Nutrition at Zhejiang University in Hangzhou, China. His ongoing research interests include eco-nutrition and food systems, migration and cross-cultural health, population health and ageing.

Janet Wall

Janet Wall is a Senior Research Officer in the Department of Geography, Environment and Population at the University of Adelaide. Since 1982 she has worked closely with Professor Graeme Hugo on all of his research projects and publications, including the *Atlas of the Australian People* based on the 1986, 1991 and 1996 censuses and funded by the former Department of Immigration and Multicultural Affairs, his ARC Federation Fellowship on 'The New Paradigm of International Migration To and From Australia: Dimensions, Causes and Implications' (2002–06) and his ARC Australian Professorial Fellowship on 'Circular Migration in Asia, the Pacific and Australia: Empirical, Theoretical and Policy Dimensions' (2010–14).

Leanne Webb

Dr Leanne Webb has worked in the climate impacts field with CSIRO, University of Melbourne and at the University of New South Wales over the past decade. Her work has focused on the use of spatial tools to link biophysical metrics with climate data. She has explored the impact of projected climate change in many sectors, particularly the wine industry, agriculture and health. More recently, she has been involved with examining the impact of climate change on the health of Indigenous Australians.

Philip Weinstein

Professor Philip Weinstein is Head of School of Biological Sciences at the University of Adelaide. He holds dual qualifications in ecology (PhD Entomology) and public health (MBBS, FAFPHM). Phil was formerly Professor of Public and Environmental Health at UQ and at UWA, and has also lectured zoology at JCU. He has over 250 publications on the environmental determinants of water-borne and mosquito-borne disease, and also led a major research programme on air quality and respiratory health through the Asthma CRC. He was a member of the Board of Review Editors for the Millennium Ecosystem Assessment, served as Co-Chair of the International Medical Geology Association, and remains an enthusiastic teacher. Email: philip.weinstein@adelaide.edu.au.

Robin A. Weiss

Robin Weiss, PhD, is Emeritus Professor of Viral Oncology at University College, London. Born in London in 1940, Weiss worked in India, Czechoslovakia and the USA before returning to London in 1972. He was Director of Research at the Institute of Cancer Research from 1980 to 1998. He is noted for the discovery of retroviruses inherited as host Mendelian traits, that CD4 is the HIV receptor and for HIV vaccine research. Weiss was President of the Society for General Microbiology from 2006 to 2009. He is a Fellow of the Royal Society and a Foreign Associate of the US National Academy of Sciences.

Alistair Woodward

Alistair Woodward is Professor of Epidemiology and Biostatistics at the University of Auckland, New Zealand. Since his PhD (on passive smoking and acute respiratory illness in children), he has been interested in the environment and health. He has worked on radon and lung cancer, mobile phones and brain tumours, the causes of bicycle crashes, health-promoting transport policies, consequences of smoke-free laws, climate and vector-borne diseases, the effects of heat and adaptations to climate change, for instance. His book *A Healthy Country? A History of Life and Death in New Zealand*, co-authored by Tony Blakely, was published in September 2014.

FOREWORD

STEPHEN V. BOYDEN

This remarkable collection of papers bears witness to the breadth, depth and originality of Tony McMichael's outstanding contribution to the health sciences over the past four decades. Appropriately, contributions range from discussions of the results of epidemiological studies on specific health issues, many of which McMichael worked on himself, to the importance of a systems approach to epidemiology, and even to some philosophical issues such as how important the future really is. Many papers refer to or focus on an area that was of special interest to McMichael over recent decades – the impacts of climate change on human health.

McMichael's quantitative epidemiological studies on the relationships between life conditions, environmental factors and patterns of health and disease are highly regarded for their rigour and innovativeness. However, his contribution and influence extend well beyond this, and lie especially in what I will call his panoramic approach.

There are two facets to McMichael's panoramic framework. First, he discussed human health against the background of the story of life on Earth and our own evolutionary history. The medical profession, and even that part of the health sector which specialises in public health and epidemiology, has been slow to wake up to the fact that this biohistorical perspective is essential for the proper understanding of issues of human health in the modern world.

The second characteristic of McMichael's panoramic approach was his transdisciplinarity. The evolution of the culture of academia over the past century or so has led to a situation in which different groups of scholars focus on different aspects of the total situation – giving rise to the various so-called academic disciplines. Attempts to study the system as a whole are typically met with indifference, and even disdain, from specialists in conventional disciplines; and yet, in reality, human situations always involve a constant and highly significant interplay between elements in the different parts of the total system – biological, physical, cultural, economic, sociological, and so on.

McMichael defied this academic tradition. He recognised that the kind of understanding we need for making wise decisions in public health, and in society in general, requires knowledge of this interplay between these different parts of the total system.

He drew our attention to the fact that the health and well-being of human populations was linked inexorably with the health of the living systems around us. Climate change is at present the most critical illustration of this, although there are many other examples, past and present.

McMichael also highlighted the recent explosive increase in the scale and intensity of human activities on Earth and the fact that they were unsustainable ecologically, and thus socially. In other words, the future health and well-being of humankind will require big changes in society that will ensure the health of the ecosystems which underpin our existence.

In fact, McMichael advocated a shift to what has been called elsewhere a 'biosensitive society' – that is, a society that is in tune with, sensitive to and respectful of the processes of life within us and around us (Boyden, 2004).

In a biosensitive society, the dominant culture (e.g. world-view, priorities), societal arrangements (e.g. economic system, governmental regulations) and human activities (e.g. resource and energy use) would promote the health of both humans and the ecosystems of which they are a part.

The notion of biosensitivity is encapsulated in the 'triangle of biosensitivity' in Figure 1.

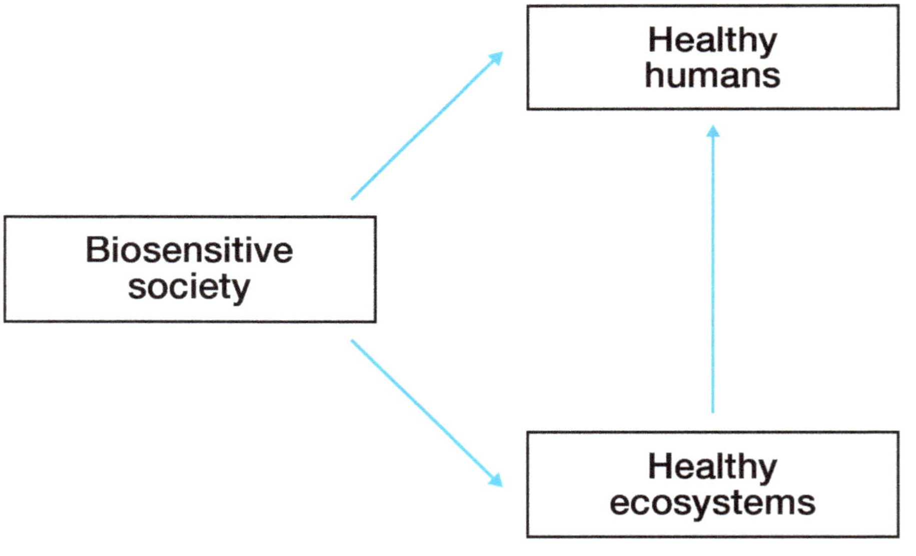

Figure 1 The 'triangle of biosensitivity'.
Source: Author's work.

Certainly, for ecological reasons, the future well-being of humankind will depend on big changes in the patterns of human activity on Earth. However, these changes will not come about unless and until McMichael's panoramic vision spreads well beyond the epidemiological and medical fraternity. The survival of civilisation needs this vision to become centrally embedded in the dominant cultures of human society all over the world.

References

Boyden, S. 2004. *The Biology of Civilisation: Understanding Human Culture as a Force in Nature*. UNSW Press, Sydney, Australia.

PART 1

INTRODUCTION

REPRINT A

Preface to 'Planetary Overload: Global Environmental Change and the Health of the Human Species'

ANTHONY J. MCMICHAEL

McMichael, A.J. 1993. Preface. *Planetary Overload: Global Environmental Change and the Health of the Human Species*. Cambridge University Press, Cambridge, UK. pp. xiii–xvi.

Pages: 3 to 10

Preface

The most serious potential consequence of global environmental change is the erosion of Earth's life-support systems. Yet, curiously, the nature of this threat to the health and survival of the world's living species – including our own – has received little attention.

Over aeons, the evolution of life has gradually transformed the environment that clothes the planet's surface. The lower atmosphere's composition has changed; stratospheric ozone has formed from oxygen emitted by plants; soil has been created by oxidation, plants and microbes; and forests speed the recirculation of rainwater. Life's genetic diversity confers a capacity for adaptive change. However, this fabric of life-supporting mechanisms is now starting to unravel, in a brief geological moment, as the cumulative global impact of human activity escalates.

We fret about the more easily understood effects of environmental damage upon national economies, property values, amenities and pristine nature. In its 1992 Report, the World Bank says: 'Soils that are degraded, aquifers that are depleted, and ecosystems that are destroyed in the name of raising incomes today can jeopardize the prospects for earning income tomorrow.'[1] The report also notes, *en passant*, that local environmental pollution by toxic chemicals may impose costs to human health that retard economic development. This exemplifies how we typically overlook the more fundamental fact that Earth's natural systems provide the essential life-support services that enable organisms to remain healthy and to breed. Today's unprecedented global environmental changes – particularly climate change, ozone layer depletion, land degradation and loss of biodiversity – may therefore have profound effects upon the health of human populations.

This is unfamiliar territory. Overloading the biosphere can affect population health in ways that differ fundamentally from the local, direct-acting, toxicity of environmental pollutants such as sulphurous fumes in air and heavy metals in food. Rather, such overload reduces the stability and productivity of the natural systems that support life. We have created environmental agencies to address the familiar type of toxic pollutant problem highlighted at the 1972 UN Environment Conference – such as those due to air pollutants, contaminated drinking water, toxic waste sites and garbage disposal. Today, however, we face environmental problems that reflect ecological disruption, transcend national and regional boundaries, and pose a more profound, albeit longer-term, threat to health.

The political consequences are as complex as the science. For example, we may soon live in a world in which global warming, caused mainly by industrialised and industrialising countries, causes inundation of coastal communities in Bangladesh and increased spread of malaria to highland communities in Latin America and Africa. For such reasons, some governments have begun examining the health impacts of greenhouse-induced climate change and ozone layer depletion. The World Health Organization submitted to the 1992 UN Earth Summit a report on the health impact of current patterns of energy use, urbanisation, industry and agriculture. The UN's Food and Agricultural Organization now acknowledges that the combination of soil erosion, desertification, climate change and population growth portends more food shortages.

Overall, however, our response has been tentative. I think this is largely because we still have a shallow understanding of the ultimate dependence of our health upon the integrity of ecosystems. We talk about 'life-support' systems, but, frankly, the idea that the survival of *Homo sapiens* depends upon the sustaining of ecosystems still seems a bit far-fetched. Most developed countries have cultures characterised by religions with anthropoid gods, where the notion of Man as Master endures. Relatedly, under modern, internationalised, capitalism – now uncontestedly the dominant influence on world trade and national economies – we have conferred upon the market economy a life of its own, and, by defining our social purpose within this framework, we further distance ourselves from the rhythms of natural systems.

Those working in the health sciences, too, have been slow to perceive the significance of ecological disruption for population health. Some aspects seem clear enough – ozone depletion will enhance skin cancer rates and temperature rises will enlarge the habitat of malarial mosquitoes – but those are only the tip of a much bigger iceberg. Below the water-line loom wider-ranging hazards to human health. Meanwhile, despite the many uncertainties, the world's vital signs appear to be generally negative. The ozone layer is thinning faster than we expected. The 1980s was the hottest decade on record, sustained into the early 1990s. After three buoyant decades the world's per-person food output has recently faltered, and land degradation is occurring widely. The extinction of species and loss of genes, many directly useful to our future survival as food and pharmaceuticals, continues to accelerate. The arms race has yielded increasingly dreadful weapons that can destroy whole ecosystems. Underlying all of these, the burgeoning world population and the debilitating burden of Third World poverty and desperate subsistence agriculture weigh heavily on the environment.

These seemingly disparate problems arise from the sheer scale and intensity of human economic activity. If these problems continue, their impact will be geographically uneven. Land degradation, deforestation and climate change will occur mostly in poor countries at low latitude; direct exposure to increased ultraviolet radiation will increase most in rich countries at high latitude. Eventually, however, weather instability, climatic impairment of crop yield, rising seas and loss of genetic resources would affect the health of human populations everywhere. Of course, there is much that scientists do not yet understand about these ecological disturbances and their consequences. But we cannot ignore the probability that these global environmental changes will have various adverse effects upon the health and wellbeing of *Homo sapiens*.

Some of the predicted effects may not become serious for a generation or two. Much of the impact of today's environmental excesses will be to impoverish the environment in which future generations must live. This would be the first time, at a global level, that one generation has conferred a *negative* legacy upon future generations. That poses an unprecedented moral problem, since the usual expectation of human society (in particular, modern western society) has been that each generation will increase, or at least preserve, the store of scientific knowledge, technological skills and the material infrastructure of society for future generations.

Finally, a more personal comment. Writing about environment and health within an ecological framework has required ranging over a wide terrain – further widened by the need to consider political, social and ethical aspects. Although no-one can hope to be fully informed over so wide a terrain, I am reassured by the comment of an Australian philosopher, John Passmore, who, in *Man's Responsibility for Nature*, says: 'Everybody who writes about ecological problems is, in respect to certain of the topics he is discussing, an amateur.'[2] The import of

Passmore's remark is that these problems cannot be meaningfully addressed *unless* they are considered within a multidisciplinary context. Passmore goes on to say: 'So far as the Western tradition discourages communication between specialists, it presents an obstacle to the adequate examination of ecological problems. Inter-disciplinary investigations are in this area not a luxury, but a necessity.'

Accordingly, I have attempted a broad analysis which I hope will provide a useful synthesis, particularly for those who have not previously thought much about human population health within an ecological context. This should inform and strengthen our response to the challenge posed by global environmental overload. Many commentators judge that we may not have long to develop the far-reaching social responses required to solve these problems. If a clearer understanding of the risks to human health facilitates such responses, this book will have achieved something worthwhile.

Acknowledgements

I have sought advice from many colleagues in writing this book. Comments on early drafts were made by Matt Gaughwin, Tony Worsley, David Shearman, Stephen Boyden, Sara Parkin and John Powles. Brian MacDermott and Ken Dyer gave subsequent advice on the ordering of ideas. Comments on particular sections came from John Moss, John Hatch, Michael Manton, Philip McMichael, Richie Gun, Mary Beers, Alistair Woodward, Bruce Armstrong, Andrew Oates, Basil Hetzel, Harvey Marchant, Barrie Pittock, Ernesto Kahan, Philip Weinstein, John Young, Graeme Hugo and Tord Kjellstrom. I discussed the general issues with Andrew Haines and John Last, two health scientists who saw early the importance of this topic. Louise Stafford, in correcting various drafts, ably decoded my tortuous annotations. My wife, Judith, encumbered with writing her doctorate, put up with my elastic working-hours. The enthusiasm of my daughters, Anna and Celia, for the ideas and practice of environmentalism, gave me added impetus.

Adelaide, January, 1993 A. J. McM

References

1. World Bank. *World Development Report* 1992. *Development and Environment*. Oxford: Oxford University Press, 1992.
2. Passmore J. *Man's Responsibility for Nature*. London: Duckworth, 1974 (Second Edition, 1980).

END OF REPRINT A

Preface to 'Planetary Overload: Global Environmental Change and the Health of the Human Species'

ANTHONY J. MCMICHAEL

1

FROM *SILENT SPRING* TO THE THREAT OF A FOUR-DEGREE WORLD

The Context of Tony McMichael's Career

COLIN D. BUTLER AND ALISTAIR WOODWARD

Abstract

This chapter positions the late Tony McMichael's contributions in the social, political and ecological context in which he worked from the early 1970s to the present. We document how his research and writing were shaped by this milieu and explore some of the barriers, challenges and opportunities that shaped his career.

McMichael's work was distinguished in two respects. These are, first, the range of epidemiology subspecialties that he mastered (including occupational health, cancer, nutrition and environmental health), and second, the depth and lasting impact of his research. We provide examples of the work he and his colleagues carried out on lead, smoking, health inequalities and the links between diet and cancer. In recent decades, Tony was probably known best for his focus on the effects of adverse global ecological and environmental changes, and climate change in particular. He contributed to an improved understanding of causality within epidemiology, rejecting an exclusive focus on downstream, 'proximal' determinants of health and disease. He also challenged his discipline to extend its temporal boundaries, both into the past and the future.

There are many challenges ahead for epidemiology and for the broader discipline it endeavours to serve, public health. Tony McMichael's thinking and writing, and the example he set as an epidemiologist advocate for environment and health, will be as relevant and influential in the future as they have been in the past four decades.

Introduction

Two of the greatest 19th-century French health scientists were Claude Bernard and Louis Pasteur. At the end of his life, Pasteur was said to have conceded 'Bernard was right – the microbe is nothing: the milieu is everything' (James, 1982–84; Goldstein, 2008). Clearly, the milieu is not everything – but it certainly matters, for people as well as for microbes. In this chapter, we outline the major political and social events of the past 40 years and consider their influence on Tony McMichael's remarkable career.

'It's Time' – The 1970s

In 1972, smoking in Australian society seemed ubiquitous, and the lighted cigarette was prevalent in restaurants, theatres, public transport, university tutorials and hospitals. Blood lead concentrations of 20 μg/l were unremarkable. Abortion was illegal, abductions of mixed race children by Australian welfare agencies had just ended and the deceptive removal of newborn infants from some unmarried white women for adoption by childless white couples was still practised. The pill, first trialled without informed consent on poor women in Puerto Rico in the mid-1950s (Duster, 2006), was just beginning to alter Australian demography.

Epidemiology was an unusual career choice for medical graduates when Tony, 1967 President of the National Union of Australian University Students, became the first PhD student at the newly established Department of Social and Preventive Medicine at Monash University, in Melbourne. Tony was supervised by the Foundation Professor, Basil Hetzel (see Chapter 2, this volume), with whom Tony published papers on mental health (McMichael and Hetzel, 1974, 1975) and a book, *The LS Factor* (Hetzel and McMichael, 1987) (see Reprint F, Part 4, this volume).

In the early 1970s, the Vietnam War dragged on in the face of vociferous public opposition, inflamed by the conscription of men too young to vote but old enough to fight. Opposition to the war forged networks in civil society, including among student groups and labour unions. These same actors, with Indigenous organisations, were also involved in Aboriginal land rights movements and related civil rights activism. The Aboriginal Tent Embassy was established in Canberra; the Women's Electoral Lobby was created to ensure that women's rights were on the political agenda; and in 1972, Gough Whitlam was elected to government on a mandate for change (his campaign slogan was 'It's time').

Non-violent protests continued against the building of the three dams that drowned Lake Pedder, Tasmania; these led to the founding of the world's first ecological political party, also in 1972.

Vegetarianism was becoming fashionable; *Diet for a Small Planet* (Lappé and Collins, 1971) sold in large numbers. It was the heyday of The Club of Rome: one of its reports, *The Limits to Growth* (Meadows et al., 1972), sold millions of copies. The 1972 Stockholm Conference on Environment and Development ('Rio minus twenty') was championed by the microbiologist turned planetary ecologist, René Dubos (1980; Piel and Segerberg Jr, 1990) and two years later, Karim Singh, representing Indian Prime Minister, Indira Gandhi, at the 1974 Bucharest meeting on population, famously declared that 'development is the best contraceptive' (Sinding, 2000). Demographic and development issues were to become an enduring theme in McMichael's work (see Chapters 9, 10, 14, 17, 22, this volume; and McMichael, 1995).

The publisher, Richard Walsh, spotted Tony's writing gifts, and for a while his Spaceship Earth columns were a regular feature in *Nation Review* (see Box 1.1). Reading these columns today brings to mind Tony's prescience. He wrote about issues such as global pollution, resource scarcity and human population pressure, which are familiar today (Ehrlich and Ehrlich, 2013) but which scarcely registered on the agenda of public health in the 1970s. There were rare exceptions, such as a paper in the *Medical Journal of Australia* by the ecologist, Stephen Boyden (1972), who later became a close colleague of Tony's (Foreword, this volume). The orthodox scientific literature then included no outlets such as *Ecosystem Health* or *Global Change and Human Health* (both of which McMichael was an editor). While neither journal still exists, their legacy continues in *EcoHealth*.

Box 1.1 This is bigger than the sanitary movement*

TONY McMICHAEL

CYNICS have said that the ecology movement is just a passing bandwagon; an artificial and ephemeral conscience-salving exercise for idle middle class minds. Well, middle class minds (among all radical *Review* readers there must be a few middle class minds) if the cap fits ...

However, a recently published Gallup poll reports that 62 percent of Australians think that the world will be unliveable in twenty years without prompt curbs on population and pollution. You can't tell me that ecology bandwagoning has become a widespread indulgence of the silent majority. Rather, it suggests that the current upsurge of concern reflects genuine doubt about the world's future if today's trends continue.

Indeed, the prevailing mood has a clear precedent in the sanitary movement of the nineteenth century. The preceding burst of affluence; the subsequent quickening of social conscience towards deprived minorities (industrial slum dwellers then – racial minorities, women, and homosexuals now); the broad social and political base of dismay over a deteriorating quality of life; and the recognition that the laisser-faire ethic is inadequate (economic theory then – industrial technology now). These are the common themes in the environmental revolutions of then and now.

The English suddenly realised 130 years ago that, in the words of one historian, they were "living on a dungheap". The early years of the industrial revolution had spawned a new and comfortable middle class, and had extruded overcrowded industrial slums where poverty and disease were rife.

In the first flush of steam powered laisser-faire economics, the bourgeoisie dreamed of progress unlimited. Government was best that governed least. There were lots of unprecedented treasure at the end of the industrial rainbow. Outside these middle class dreams, the newly migrated urban working class festered in fetid slums, their fevered infants dying of infection, their children working in pits, their adults exposed to disease and industrial injury.

Then the rainbow tarnished. Social reality intruded into men's consciousness. Middle class optimism was tempered with awareness of the accumulating squalor amongst the working class. A few consciences were pricked, and, in the 1840s, social reform movements gathered momentum.

Equally important in the rude awakening, however, was the realisation that the shoddiness of the slums was impinging on the general quality of urban life. Infectious disease spilled over the whole community - cholera, typhoid and "consumption" (tuberculosis). Water supplies became contaminated, rivers turned foul, the air turned black, and (because of the high sulphur content of British coal) the acidic air started eating holes in domestic middle class masonry.

* Spaceship Earth. *THE REVIEW*, April 8–14, 1972, 708.

People were perturbed. Their future was turning sour. They expected remedial action by the government – but the government, accustomed to being seen but not heard during the first flowering of laisser-faire capitalism, was slow to act against the mounting urban squalor. People became disenchanted. A mood of dismay and dissent stirred the nation, forging strange alliances between church and industrialist, Whig and Tory, worker and gentleman.

In this emerging field of public health, sir Edwin Chadwick, a Benthamite utilitarian, propounded the empirical connection between disease and urban squalor. Traditional mystical interpretations of disease (especially infectious disease) were replaced by an empiricist working theory: "All smell is disease." And so, even though the germ theory of infectious disease had not yet been discovered, the sanitary movement was launched.

Ultimately, as public health polemic became self-evident truth, the fundamental importance of sanitation became enshrined in the culture. Notwithstanding the fact that they only bath once a week, it is fair to say that, for the last hundred years, the British have regarded soap, sewers and sanitation as prerequisites for civilisation.

Now, in the 1970s, our society is confronted by another environmental threat to health and welfare. Postwar affluence is being tempered with the realisation that unrestrained modern technology is unleashing new agents of biological damage – radioactive wastes, noxious fumes, persistent pesticides, heavy metal contaminants, and so on.

Technological wastes and side effects are the modern equivalent of last century's urban excreta. The effects on health may be less dramatic – but they are no less real. Chronic respiratory disease is now on the increase in the cities of the developed world (after allowing for the effects of cigarette smoking). Likewise, premature deafness, and the road toll. Similar fears exist for the effects of mercury lead and cadmium on brain function, pesticide residues on liver and brain function, and carbon monoxide on heart disease.

As in the 1840s, it is being realised (in America, if not here) that certain deprived groups are the most exposed to some sorts of pollution. Lead poisoning is prominent among ghetto children, chronic respiratory disease is prominent in working class suburbs beneath the shadow of industrial smoke-shacks. Consciences are again being pricked.

They are becoming the immediate spurs to action – concern over human physical health and welfare. Related, but less immediate concerns are with the soul-destroying competitive anonymity of life in megalopolis, and the destruction of esthetic and recreational assets.

The sanitary movement changed the world because it changed men's understanding of disease. In today's era of recent affluence and current social uneasiness and dissent, the ecology movement may yet change the world for the better. But the changes required are more fundamental and urgent than those of last century.

Twenty-one years after McMichael's doctoral graduation, the development of niche journals on global environmental change and health was foreshadowed by keynote addresses delivered at the 1993 congress of the International Epidemiological Association, held in Sydney, by two University of Adelaide medical graduates. One was Tony McMichael (1993a), the other John Last (1994), editor of the *Dictionary of Epidemiology*. Both addresses led to papers in the *International Journal of Epidemiology* (Last, 1994; McMichael, 1993a).

In the same year, and of even greater significance, McMichael (1993b) published *Planetary Overload* (see Reprint A, Part 1, this volume). Never before had an epidemiologist written in depth about the questions that had been raised so strongly by leading ecologists in earlier decades (Carson, 1962; Ehrlich, 1968; Shepard and McKinley, 1969). For example, the miracle of the Green Revolution brought relief from abysmal hunger from the 1960s (Tribe, 1994), but Tony and others pointed out that there were still serious obstacles in the way of sustainable production and equitable distribution of global food supplies (see Chapter 14, this volume). McMichael's influential book linked the concerns of ecologists and environmental scientists to the health of the human population, worldwide.

Environmental Contaminants, Ecology and Health

The public debate on the effects of chemical contamination and exogenous hormones on human and animal health, and the environment more broadly, had been launched in 1962 by Rachel Carson's book, *Silent Spring* (Carson, 1962). These recurred as a theme throughout Tony's career (McMichael and Potter, 1980; Potter and McMichael, 1983), especially in the time he was involved with the Commonwealth Scientific and Industrial Research Organisation (CSIRO) (1976–83), the International Agency for Research on Cancer (IARC) (Chair of the Scientific Committee, 1989–92) and the International Society for Environmental Epidemiology (ISEE), where he was president from 2008 to 2009. Many chapters in this volume (3, 5–8, 11–14, 18, 20, 21, 24, 33 and 34) by colleagues from these organisations[1] are included in this book; one (Chapter 11) focuses on overlapping material – epigenetics. Another influence on Tony's work was Shepard and McKinley's (1969) book, *The Subversive Science, Essays Towards an Ecology of Man*. The use of the word 'subversive' dates to a short but influential paper from 1964, which argued that ecology might be 'taken seriously as an instrument for the long-run welfare of mankind' (Sears, 1964). *Subversive Science* included chapters by René Dubos, Lynn White, Alan Watts and Aldo Leopold.

1 Not necessarily contemporaneous.

Diet and Cancer

When one of the authors of this chapter started medical school in 1980, he was told that diet had virtually nothing to do with health, quite contrary to the position often taken even then by journalists, countercultural activists, members of new religions and complementary and alternative medical practitioners. Much of what was known at that time about diet and health was not in quantitative form and could not be judged against the famous Bradford Hill (1965) criteria to assess causality. In the 1980s, McMichael and his colleagues at the CSIRO Division of Human Nutrition published extensively on the links between nutrition and cancer (and other conditions), but more importantly, they demonstrated the general principle: diet indeed matters to health. McMichael was a member of the international panel that produced *Food, Nutrition, and the Prevention of Cancer: A Global Perspective*, a seminal 1997 report on the feasibility of reducing cancer incidence through diet and other environmental factors (World Cancer Research Fund Panel (Potter J.D. Chair), 1997). Several chapters of this volume (11, 13–16) concern diet, health and nutrition.

Lead

McMichael and colleagues are well-known for a large cohort study of child development carried out at Port Pirie, South Australia, the site of what is still the world's third largest lead–zinc smelter. The study showed that levels of lead once thought to be quite acceptable had caused neurological harm, including impaired cognitive development (see Chapter 7 in this book and Reprint D in Part 3). These findings had an important impact on policies, including the withdrawal of lead from petrol.

In 1970, in the USA, an occupational exposure to lead that resulted in a concentration of 70–80 µg/dl was considered acceptable (Ambrose et al., 2000). Today, there is good evidence that lead levels as low as 2.4 µg/l are associated with loss of IQ points (Lanphear et al., 2005), but contamination of the environment by lead continues. Despite considerable effort, lead levels in children in Port Pirie remain elevated, with about 25 per cent of children aged five having levels above 10 µg/dl, due to the persistence of lead-carrying dust from the smelter (Taylor et al., 2013). Tony's best-known contribution to occupational health on 'the healthy worker effect' is reprinted in Part 2, this volume (see Reprint C), but he made other contributions in this field, including a study of cancer mortality among rubber workers in Brazil (McMichael et al., 1976). Chapters 4–6 in this book relate especially to occupational health.

Climate Change and Health

The long-term effects of the accumulation of greenhouse gases were first described in the 19th century, and were the subject of a seminal paper (Callendar, 1957) in the International Geophysical Year, published when McMichael was still at high school. His 'Spaceship Earth' papers did not refer to climate change. However, the topic became more prominent in the late 1980s, an era leading up to the Ottawa Charter for Health Promotion, the Brundtland Report, the Montreal Protocol and, in 1992, the Earth Summit itself – an extravaganza held in Rio de Janeiro that was attended by 103 heads of state.[2]

About this time, papers linking climate change and health appeared in the *New England Journal of Medicine* (Leaf, 1989), *The Lancet* (Editorial, 1989) and, soon after, in an editorial written by McMichael in the *Medical Journal of Australia* (see Reprint G, Part 5, this volume). This was the first such publication by a public health or medical worker in the Australian scientific literature (McMichael, 1991). McMichael then had the vision, persistence, leadership qualities and opportunity to bring together a co-edited book, *Climate Change and Human Health*, probably the first in the world (authored or edited) on this topic, published by the World Health Organization (WHO) in 1996 (McMichael et al., 1996).

McMichael had noted that the first Intergovernmental Panel on Climate Change (IPCC) assessment (1990) contained no chapter on health and said very little about the subject throughout. This deficit was remedied in the second and third assessments, when McMichael served as coordinating lead author, a task shared by Alistair Woodward and Kirk Smith in the fifth assessment (see Chapters 12 and 34, this volume). Several other IPCC contributors to the health chapter have also written in this book (Chapters 14, 20 and 33). Many other chapters of this volume (including 10, 11, 13–15, 17–24 and 30–38) also discuss climate change.

Today, the field of climate change and human health has expanded enormously, but still policymakers and the general public do not have a full understanding of its significance. Already, temperature anomalies of 20 degrees C have been reported in the Arctic.[3] Ice melt is accelerating, not only from Greenland but also from large parts of Antarctica (Shepherd et al., 2012). There are concerns that the polar jet stream has been deformed, delivering blasts of frigid air to mid-latitudes.[4] Sea level rise from melting land ice is increasing and remains on track with the most pessimistic IPCC projections (Rahmstorf et al., 2012).

---

2 www.un.org/geninfo/bp/enviro.html, accessed 10 April 2015.

3 arctic-news.blogspot.com.au/2012/12/arctic-anomalies-linked-to-extreme-weather.html, accessed 10 April 2015.

4 arctic-news.blogspot.com.au/2012/12/polar-jet-stream-appears-hugely-deformed.html, accessed 10 April 2015.

Emissions of carbon dioxide are tracking high-end warming projections and the chance of a 'two-degree world' appears to be fading (Peters et al., 2012). There are reports of greenhouse gas emissions, especially methane, arising from the Arctic, from expanding wetlands, melting tundra and possibly even melting deposits of methane hydrate (Shakhova et al., 2010; Graef et al., 2011). The possibility of positive (amplifying) feedbacks to climate change has been recognised for several decades (Cicerone, 1988), and becomes more serious as the rate of environmental change increases.

Some extreme weather events are more common than in previous decades (Chapter 21), and climate change may be an amplifying factor through, for instance, increased sea surface temperatures and higher sea levels (Trenberth, 2011). Collectively, these changes are eroding the environmental foundations of population health. The climate scientist, Hans Schellnhuber, has warned that the difference between two degrees and four degrees of warming may be civilisation itself. We are playing, he warns, 'Earth roulette' (Schellnhuber, 2010). Several chapters contemplate civilisation decline and how we might transform it so that humanity continues to prosper (Chapters 30 and 37, this volume).

Inequality and Health

As McMichael's career was warming up, social opportunities for many were starting to narrow, driven by what the economist, Jeffrey Sachs, called libertarianism (Sachs, 2012), an extreme form of what others label neoliberalism, economic rationalism, economism, marketism, and in the USA, Reaganomics, and in New Zealand, Rogernomics. Factors that contributed to this political shift included the cyclic nature of economics and steep rises in the cost of living, brought about by the first significant spike in oil prices (Szreter, 1997). Although the 1972 oil squeeze was typically presented in a negative light, money paid to the Organization of the Petroleum Exporting Countries (OPEC) for its oil was, in fact, helping to redistribute global income. It perhaps improved global social justice by redistributing funds from petrol pumps in the West, not just to sheiks and oil barons but also, in some cases, to the citizens of oil-rich nations.

By the 1980s, as libertarianism strengthened, it was less propitious to speak against other forms of injustice, whether in the West or globally. This decade saw little of the aspiration and idealism of individuals such as Albert Schweitzer, Martin Luther King, Lester Pearson and WHO Director, General Halfdan Mahler, who had endorsed calls for 'Health for All by 2000' (Werner and Sanders, 1997; Butler, 2008).

In association with this shift to the political right, McMichael suggested that many epidemiologists were retreating from large-scale aspirations, essentially political, to focus on narrower, more 'downstream' positions (McMichael, 1999). (See 'Prisoners of the Proximate: Loosening the Constraints on Epidemiology in an Age of Change'; Reprint B, Part 1, this volume.) In this, he was undoubtedly stimulated by Gary Taubes' paper, 'Epidemiology faces its limits' (Taubes, 1995), an article recommended for students studying 'emerging themes in epidemiology' at the London School of Hygiene and Tropical Medicine (LSH&TM) in 1996, as one of the authors of this chapter recalls. Taubes argued that the easy questions in epidemiology (e.g. the causes of cholera or lung cancer) had been answered, and that epidemiologists were now spending most of their time in blind alleys searching for increasingly trivial causal cofactors. In response, McMichael argued for a closer investigation of broader 'upstream' determinants, following a path explored by his predecessor at the LSH&TM, the influential British epidemiologist, Geoffrey Rose. Rose famously had pointed out that causes had causes (Rose, 1992), a point also highlighted in *The LS Factor* (Part 4, this volume).

One colleague from the LSH&TM has written a chapter in this book (31); another chapter (22) is by Andy Haines, appointed as Dean soon after Tony had returned to Australia.[5] Another contribution (Chapter 37) is from Bob Douglas, who recruited Tony as foundation professor of environmental health at the University of Adelaide. Later, Tony succeeded Bob as Director of the National Centre for Epidemiology and Population Health (NCEPH).

The 'Epidemiological Wars' Concerning Poverty and Disease

In the late 1990s, there was a well-publicised clash of opinions on the nature and scope of epidemiology. This debate was later described (with a touch of hyperbole) as 'the epidemiology wars'. On one side was Ken Rothman, famous and highly esteemed as editor of *Modern Epidemiology* and the journal, *Epidemiology*. Despite stating explicitly that 'all poverty is unacceptable', Rothman and his colleagues argued that epidemiologists should not and could not try to alter the fundamental determinants of health, especially poverty and disadvantage:

> Is poverty eradication a public health programme? How exactly should it be accomplished? ... Perhaps the critics believe that epidemiologists should second-guess economists and attempt to eradicate poverty using

5 Haines had a minor role in the publication of *Planetary Overload* by suggesting McMichael approach Cambridge University Press.

> their own epidemiological model. Given the scope of the task, sympathy might go to the epidemiologists who prefer to focus on a comparatively simple problem, such as the causes of cancer. (Rothman et al., 1998, p. 812)

But, what is left? Remedies – polypills or magic bullets – that cost-effectively would relieve suffering and extend life? The suggestion that epidemiologists should focus on 'comparatively simple' problems, such as the causes of cancer, suggests aetiological frameworks that exclude social phenomena such as poverty, and is, incidentally, dismissive of Rose's challenge to seek the 'causes of the causes'. For instance, smoking is a cause of cancer, a fact established by epidemiologists. But to change the frequency and harmfulness of smoking, one needs to know of its association with poverty (among other things) (Graham, 1987). Some might say that it is the task of other public health professionals to grapple with questions related to social policy, but others argue that epidemiologists can play an important role; for example, by advising policymakers as to whether poverty is a major or minor causal factor.

McMichael (1998) agreed that eradicating poverty was 'beyond the capacity of epidemiology', but disputed that this task should be left to economists, or any other single discipline or professional group. Others took a similar position, including Woodward and Kawachi (2000), who suggested a variety of reasons for tackling health inequalities. Apart from the matter of justice or fairness, there are frequently 'spillover effects' (such as poverty-related infectious diseases and violence) that should motivate the better off. In some instances, well demonstrated, cost-effective means of reducing the burden of ill health due to social disadvantage are at hand. But interventions for systemic problems such as poverty generally require 'upstream' solutions (McMichael, 1999). Proximal actions, such as food supplements delivered directly to poor children, or screening and immunisation services targeted to high-needs groups, have to be embedded in a population-wide approach to be effective.

Consciously or not, Rothman and his colleagues (1998) appeared to be reflecting their own, North American milieu, in a time when neoliberalism predominated. A similar political climate applied elsewhere. In the UK, a long period of Conservative rule (1979–97) had entrenched the view that social problems were primarily a result of harmful personal behaviours, despite persistent evidence of the importance of context (Graham, 1987). It was at this level, the level of individuals and families, Margaret Thatcher and her contemporaries argued, that interventions were most likely to succeed. In New Zealand, a country with a strong collectivist tradition and high levels of social welfare, it was a Labour administration that was responsible in 1984 for radical government disinvestment and corporate deregulation. The mindset of the Labour reformers

(Roger Douglas and colleagues), which assumed that public benefits were maximised by promoting private wealth, dominated all policy debates in New Zealand in health, education and welfare until the early 2000s.

Debates between conservative and more liberal thinkers in health have deep roots. For example, in the late 19th century, arguments about the importance of the milieu versus the microbe involved not only Bernard and Pasteur (as mentioned above) but also the two most eminent contemporary figures of German medical science – Rudolf Virchow[6] and Robert Koch. In his preface to Thomas Brock's book, *Robert Koch: A Life in Medicine and Bacteriology*, Strick writes:

> More extreme liberals, such as ... Virchow, insisted that social reforms for those living in destitute, unclean, underfed, overworked conditions were the only real cure for epidemic diseases. Virchow and his supporters would always be highly suspicious of germs as any kind of true causative agents, recognizing that the easiest way for a conservative government to avoid expensive and democratizing social reforms was to blame epidemics entirely upon a germ from without, and so to avoid issues of poverty and inequality altogether and insist that all that was needed was quarantine and disinfection. (Strick, 1998)

This argument can be broadened beyond infectious diseases: poorer people smoke more, eat less healthily and have numerous other behaviours that increase their risk of many non-infectious diseases. Virchow's distrust of a 'germs only' explanation of disease has implications for the epidemiological skirmishes of the late 20th century. Since the papers by Rothman and his like-minded colleagues, the pendulum has swung some way 'upstream'. Many epidemiologists have pointed out that the microscopic view of disease causation, on its own, is inadequate (Blakely and Woodward, 2000; Mackenbach, 2009). There has been a growing interest in systems thinking, recognising that the health of populations is more than the sum of the individual components and increasing application of techniques such as systems dynamic modelling to investigate the emergence and spread of modern outbreaks (Galea et al., 2010).

The WHO Commission for the Social Determinants of Health (2008) has modernised the argument that social inequality is a root cause of ill health. Its work culminated in the 2011 Rio Political Declaration, endorsed subsequently by the World Health Assembly, committing national governments to improve public health by eradicating poverty and improving daily living conditions. Even so, in most countries, there are still substantial inequalities in health, and in some instances the gap between the most and the least advantaged groups in society has increased, suggesting the wider battle is being lost (OECD, 2011).

---

6 Virchow is reported to have opposed the revolutionary hygienic insights of Ignaz Semmelweiss.

Infectious Diseases

McMichael also engaged in infectious diseases epidemiology (Weiss and McMichael, 2004) (Reprint H, Part 6, this volume). As his career started, some leading US figures were reported as pronouncing the demise of infectious diseases (though perhaps not US Surgeon General William Stewart, as has been widely reported) (Spellberg and Taylor-Blake, 2013). But in Philadelphia in 1976, an epidemic occurred that came to be called Legionnaires disease, raising concerns that infections could make a comeback. This was followed by initially mysterious but disturbing reports from Africa (later associated with Haiti and then among gay men, especially in the USA) of what was sometimes called slim disease, but is now known as HIV/AIDS. McMichael's contribution was not in these areas of new and emerging diseases, but rather in furthering our understanding of the implications of climate and other forms of global environmental change for familiar and re-emerging infectious diseases. His research drew attention to the role of social and economic factors in shaping the epidemiological distribution and persistence of 'old' infectious diseases such as malaria and schistosomiasis, and the importance of an integrated approach to ecological change, environmental change and infectious diseases. The association between environment, vector and host has been the domain of particular concern to the Special Programme for Research and Training in Tropical Diseases (TDR), and in the preparation of the Global Report for Research on Infectious Diseases of Poverty (TDR 2012). McMichael co-chaired a multidisciplinary group into Environment, Agriculture and Infectious Diseases of Poverty, published as a WHO Technical Report in 2013 (McMichael et al., 2013). Several chapters (24–27, this volume) focus on infectious diseases and their relationship to environmental change. Other chapters in this volume discuss different aspects of environmental change and non-infectious disease (Chapters 8, 28–29, 31).

Conclusion

McMichael's contributions are numerous and distinguished. The academic contributions mentioned above and amplified in this book demonstrate his innovation and leadership. This book, extensive as it is, is far from comprehensive. Many colleagues who could not write chapters for this book have contributed by reviewing them, others have sent photographs (see Figure 1.1) and tributes. Many attended the conference, held in late 2012, that marked Tony's formal retirement, including several from overseas.

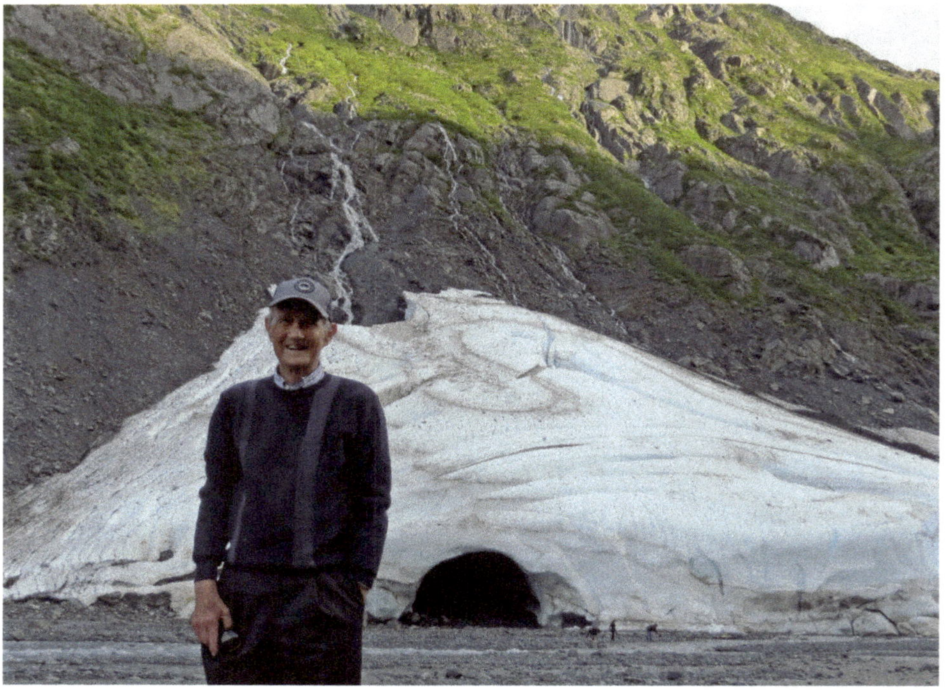

Figure 1.1 Tony McMichael in Anchorage, Alaska, where he spoke at the 20th International Epidemiological Association congress.
Source: Kristie Ebi.

McMichael nurtured and supported the career of many early-career researchers. His career demanded prodigious energy and remarkable attention to detail. He was blessed by the support of his wife, Associate Professor Judith Healy, two talented daughters and his musical skill and appreciation, especially of the piano. Several of his immediate family shared his musical and/or academic talents and interests, including his brother Philip (Chapter 16, this volume). Other forms of art also have a place in this book (Chapter 3, this volume).

And while McMichael consistently stressed the importance of quantitative work, he was open also to qualitative issues and recognised the importance of social science to public health (e.g. Chapters 16 and 20, this volume). His ability to focus on detail was combined with an ability to look at the big picture, and to encourage others to do the same. He also had considerable diplomatic skills, perhaps most evident in the chairing of scientific groups, including for the IARC, the National Health and Medical Research Council (NH&MRC), the UK's Medical Research Council, WHO, the Millennium Ecosystem Assessment, the IPCC, the TDR and the Earth System Science Partnership. He nurtured many students and early-career researches. Several students whom Tony recently supervised or helped in other ways have contributed here (Chapters 4, 8, 17, 20, 23, 25, 26 and 32, this volume). Other authors in this book were students of Tony in the past (Chapters 7 and 12–14, this volume).

McMichael also made important contributions to non-government organisations, including The Australia Institute (Director 2002–10)[7], The Climate Institute (Board member 2005–14) and the Frank Fenner Foundation (also until his passing in 2014). As well as his presidency of the ISEE, McMichael was president of the Public Health Association of Australia from 1988 to 1990. He also made substantial contributions to policy development, including for Doctors for the Environment Australia.

McMichael displayed persistent courage. Tony's testing interactions with tobacco companies over passive smoking are described in Chapter 12, this volume (see also Everingham and Woodward, 1991). The work in Port Pirie challenged the lead industry, and Tony also faced concerns in the community that there would be unemployment and economic hardship if controls on emissions caused the smelter to close. Later, his work challenged even more powerful commercial interests, those of the fossil fuel and meat industries (McMichael et al., 2007). He showed academic fortitude, repeatedly raising topics considered to be outside the disciplinary mainstream, such as ecology and population.

Trapped in time, it can be hard to discern the shift of the continually evolving milieu in which we are embedded. When we wrote the first draft of this chapter, a prolonged heatwave of unprecedented severity and extent had affected most of Australia. While younger people may be assuming there is nothing unusual in ever more extreme weather, the then Australian Prime Minister, Julia Gillard, linked this extended heatwave to climate change,[8] an opportunity missed during the severe Australian east coast floods of 2011 and 2013.

It is not clear what lies ahead. For example, will the Australian Government join with others to call for emergency action to phase out fossil fuels rapidly? In any case, McMichael's heirs and successors face a plethora of challenges. Some (population growth, for instance) were visible in 1972; others, such as climate change, are only now taking full shape. There are opportunities to meet these challenges, such as new technologies to harness renewable energy sources, but many obstacles remain, including those of vested interest and denial. Other chapters in this volume describe the agenda for 21st-century epidemiology in more detail. We hope this book will introduce McMichael's work to a new audience, and that some of those readers will feel inspired to follow in his path.

7 He served on the research committee for The Australia Institute until his death.

8 www.theage.com.au/environment/weather/prepare-for-more-scorchers-gillard-warns-20130107-2ccve.html, accessed 10 April 2015.

References

Ambrose, T.M., Al-Lozi, M. & Scott, M.G. 2000. Bone lead concentrations assessed by *in vivo* X-ray fluorescence. *Clinical Chemistry* 46, 1171–8.

Blakely, T. & Woodward, A. 2000. Ecological effects in multi-level studies. *Journal of Epidemiology and Community Health* 54, 367–74.

Boyden, S. 1972. The environment and human health. *The Medical Journal of Australia* 116, 1229–34.

Butler, C.D. 2008. Sustainable health for all by the year 2100? *International Journal of Public Health* 53, 223–4.

Callendar, G.S. 1957. On the amount of carbon dioxide in the atmosphere. *Tellus* 9, 421.

Carson, R. 1962. *Silent Spring*. Houghton Mifflin, Boston, Massachusetts, USA.

Cicerone, R.J. 1988. Methane linked to warming. *Nature* 334, 198.

Commission for the Social Determinants of Health, 2008. *Closing the Gap in a Generation. Health equity through action on the social determinants of health.* World Health Organization, Geneva.

Dubos, R. 1980. *The Wooing of Earth*. Charles Scribner's Sons, New York, USA.

Duster, T. 2006. Lessons from history: why race and ethnicity have played a major role in biomedical research. *The Journal of Law, Medicine & Ethics* 34, 487–96.

Editorial 1989. Health in the greenhouse. *The Lancet* 333, 819–20.

Ehrlich, P.R. 1968. *The Population Bomb*. Ballantyne, London, UK.

Ehrlich, P.R. & Ehrlich, A.H. 2013. Can a collapse of global civilization be avoided? *Proceedings of the Royal Society B: Biological Sciences* 280. DOI: 10.1098/rspb.2012.2845.

Everingham, S. & Woodward, S. 1991. *Tobacco Litigation. The Case Against Passive Smoking AFCO v TIA*. Legal Books, Sydney, New South Wales, Australia.

Galea, S., Riddle, M. & Kaplan, G. 2010. Causal thinking and complex system approaches in epidemiology. *International Journal of Epidemiology* 39, 97–106.

Goldstein, D.S. 2008. Computer models of stress, allostasis, and acute and chronic diseases. *Annals of the New York Academy of Sciences* 1148, 223–31.

Graef, C., Hestnes, A.G., Svenning, M.M. & Frenzel, P. 2011. The active methanotrophic community in a wetland from the High Arctic. *Environmental Microbiology Reports* 3, 466–72.

Graham, H. 1987. Women's smoking and family health. *Social Science & Medicine* 25, 47–56.

Hetzel, B.S. & McMichael, A.J. 1987. *The LS Factor: Lifestyle and Health.* Penguin, Melbourne, Victoria, Australia.

Hill, A.B. 1965. The environment and disease; association or causation? *Proceedings of the Royal Society of Medicine* 58, 295–300.

James, D.G. 1982–84. The Hunterian oration on Louis Pasteur's final judgement. Host reaction, soil or terrain. *Transactions of the Medical Society of London* 99–100, 131–47.

Lanphear, B.P., Hornung, R., Khoury, J., Yolton, K., Baghurst, P., Bellinger, D.C., et al. 2005. Low-level environmental lead exposure and children's intellectual function: an international pooled analysis. *Environmental Health Perspectives* 113, 894–9.

Lappé, F.M. & Collins, J. 1971. *Diet for a Small Planet*. Institute for Food and Development Policy, San Francisco, California, USA.

Last, J.M. 1994. New pathways in an age of ecological and ethical concerns. *International Journal of Epidemiology* 23, 1–4.

Leaf, A. 1989. Potential health effects of global climatic and environmental changes. *The New England Journal of Medicine* 321, 1577–83.

Mackenbach, J. 2009. Politics is nothing but medicine at a larger scale: reflections on public health's biggest idea. *Journal of Epidemiology and Community Health* 63, 181–4.

McMichael, A. 1991. Global warming, ecological disruption and human health: the penny drops [editorial]. *Medical Journal of Australia* 154, 499–501.

McMichael, A.J. 1993a. Global environmental change and human population health: a conceptual and scientific challenge for epidemiology. *International Journal of Epidemiology* 22, 1–8.

McMichael, A.J. 1993b. *Planetary Overload. Global Environmental Change and the Health of the Human Species*. Cambridge University Press, Cambridge, UK.

McMichael, A.J. 1995. Contemplating a one child world. Falling grain stocks and rising population spell disaster and demand debate. *BMJ* 311, 1651–2.

McMichael, A.J. 1998. The role of epidemiologists in eradicability of poverty. *The Lancet* 352, 1627.

McMichael, A.J. 1999. Prisoners of the proximate: Loosening the constraints on epidemiology in an age of change. *American Journal of Epidemiology* 149, 887–97.

McMichael, A.J. & Hetzel, B.S. 1974. An epidemiological study of the mental health of Australian university students. *International Journal of Epidemiology* 3, 125–34.

McMichael, A.J. & Hetzel, B.S. 1975. Mental health problems among university students, and their relationship to academic failure and withdrawal. *The Medical Journal of Australia* 1, 499–504.

McMichael, A.J. & Potter, J.D. 1980. Reproduction, endogenous and exogenous sex hormones and colon cancer: a review and hypothesis. *Journal of the National Cancer Institute* 65, 1201–7.

McMichael, A.J., Andjelkovic, D.A. & Tyroler, H.A. 1976. Cancer mortality among rubber workers: an epidemiologic study. *Annals of the New York Academy of Sciences* 271, 125–37.

McMichael, A.J., Haines, A., Slooff, R. & Kovats, S. (eds) 1996. *Climate Change and Human Health*. World Health Organization, Geneva, Switzerland.

McMichael, A.J., Powles, J., Butler, C.D. & Uauy, R. 2007. Food, livestock production, energy, climate change and health. *The Lancet* 370, 1253–63.

McMichael, A.J., Zhou, Z.-N., Blignaut, J., Bradshaw, C., Butler, C.D., Gillespie, S., et al. 2013. *Research Priorities for the Environment, Agriculture and Infectious Diseases of Poverty*. World Health Organization, Geneva, Switzerland.

Meadows, D., Meadows, D., Randers., J. & Behrens III, W. 1972. *The Limits to Growth*. Universe Books, New York, USA.

OECD 2011. *Divided We Stand. Why Inequality Keeps Rising. An Overview of Growing Income Inequalities in OECD Countries: Main Findings*. OECD, Paris France. www.oecd.org/els/soc/dividedwestandwhyinequalitykeepsrising.htm, accessed 19 February 2015.

Peters, G.P., Andrew, R.M., Boden, T., Canadell, J.G., Ciais, P., Quéré, C.L., et al. 2012. The challenge to keep global warming below 2°C. *Nature Climate Change* 3, 4–6.

Piel, G. & Segerberg, O. Jr (eds) 1990. *The World of René Dubos: A Collection from His Writings*. Henry Holt and Company, New York, USA.

Potter, J.D. & McMichael, A.J. 1983. Large bowel cancer in women in relation to reproductive and hormonal factors: a case-control study. *Journal of the National Cancer Institute* 71, 703–9.

Rahmstorf, S., Foster, G. & Cazenave, A. 2012. Comparing climate projections to observations up to 2011. *Environmental Research Letters* 7, 044035 (5 pp.).

Rose, G. 1992. *The Strategy of Preventive Medicine*. Oxford University Press, Oxford, UK, New York, USA.

Rothman, K.J., Adami, H.-O. & Trichopoulos, D. 1998. Should the mission of epidemiology include the eradication of poverty? *The Lancet* 352, 810–4.

Sachs, J. 2012. *The Price of Civilization*. Vintage Books, London, UK.

Schellnhuber, H. 2010. Tragic triumph. *Climatic Change* 100, 229–38.

Sears, P.B. 1964. Ecology – a subversive subject. *Bioscience* 14, 11–3.

Shakhova, N., Semiletov, I., Salyuk, A., Yusupov, V., Kosmach, D. & Gustafsso, Ö. 2010. Extensive methane venting to the atmosphere from sediments of the East Siberian Arctic shelf. *Science* 327, 1246–50.

Shepard, P. & McKinley, D. 1969. *The Subversive Science: Essays Towards an Ecology of Man*. Houghton Miflin, Boston, Massachusetts, USA.

Shepherd, A., Ivins, E.R., Geruo, A., Barletta, V.R., Bentley, M.J., Bettadpur, S., et al. 2012. A reconciled estimate of ice-sheet mass balance. *Science* 338, 1183–9.

Sinding, T.S.W. 2000. The great population debates: how relevant are they for the 21st century? *American Journal of Public Health* 90, 1841–5.

Spellberg, B. & Taylor-Blake, B. 2013. On the exoneration of Dr William H. Stewart: debunking an urban legend. *Infectious Diseases of Poverty* 2, 3. doi:10.1186/2049-9957-2-3 www.idpjournal.com/content/2/1/3, accessed 19 February 2015.

Strick, J. 1998. Preface. *Robert Koch: A Life in Medicine and Bacteriology (Thomas D Brock)*. Springer, Berlin, Germany. 202.114.65.51/fzjx/wsw/newindex/wswfzjs/pdf/koch.pdf, accessed 1 July 2015.

Szreter, S. 1997. Economic growth, disruption, deprivation, disease and death: on the importance of the politics of public health. *Population and Development Review* 23, 693–728.

Taubes, G. 1995. Epidemiology faces its limits. *Science* 269, 164–9.

Taylor, M.P., Camenzuli, D., Kristensen, L.J., Forbes, M. & Zahran, S. 2013. Environmental lead exposure risks associated with children's outdoor playgrounds. *Environmental Pollution* 178, 447–54.

TDR, 2012. Global Report for Research on Infectious Diseases of Poverty. TDR, Geneva, Switzerland.

Trenberth, K.E. 2011. Attribution of climate variations and trends to human influences and natural variability. *WIREs Climate Change* 2, 925–30.

Tribe, D. 1994. *Feeding and Greening the World*. CAB International in association with the Crawford Fund for International Agricultural Research, Wallingford, UK.

Weiss, R.A. & McMichael, A.J. 2004. Social and environmental risk factors in the emergence of infectious diseases. *Nature Medicine* 10, S70–6.

Werner, D. & Sanders, D. 1997. *Questioning the Solution: the Politics of Primary Health Care and Child Survival*. HealthWrights, Palo Alto, California, USA.

Woodward, A. & Kawachi, I. 2000. Why reduce health inequalities? *Journal of Epidemiology and Community Health* 54, 923–9.

World Cancer Research Fund Panel (Potter J.D. Chair) 1997. *Food, Nutrition, and the Prevention of Cancer: A Global Perspective*. American Institute for Cancer Research, Washington, DC, USA.

2

A LONG COLLABORATION

Professors Basil Hetzel and Tony McMichael

BASIL S. HETZEL

Abstract

This short essay reflects on the diverse and distinguished career of Tony McMichael from a unique perspective, that of his doctoral supervisor, when I was the Foundation Professor of Social and Preventive Medicine at Monash University (Melbourne) in 1968.

The Foundation: Politics and Preventive Medicine at the Universities of Adelaide and Monash

In the late 1960s, the National Health and Medical Research Council (NH&MRC) was beginning to encourage academic development in the field of epidemiology and public health. In 1968, the NH&MRC awarded me two NH&MRC Fellowships as a newly appointed Foundation Professor of Social and Preventive Medicine at Monash University for this purpose. I was thus able to offer Tony a PhD Fellowship, and in the following year he joined my newly established Department of Social and Preventive Medicine to train in epidemiology and public health. Tony was the first student and was to become the first graduate.

Prior to this, Tony had graduated with distinction in Medicine at the University of Adelaide, where I had taught as Michell Reader and then Michell Professor of Medicine (1956–68), after returning from study in New York (1951–55) as a Fulbright Research Scholar. I also had contact with Tony as a medical student, including arranging a placement for him in India at the Christian Medical College at Vellore (near Madras, now Chennai) in South India. This medical school has been recognised as second only to the All India Institute of Medical Sciences in Delhi.

During his undergraduate course, Tony became interested in politics, serving as President of the National Union of Australian University Students (NUAUS) following his final year. But Tony was then uncertain about his course; a mutual friend – Mark Wahlqvist – suggested he might consult me, which he did. Later, Mark became Professor of Nutrition at Deakin University, Geelong (see Chapter 15, this volume).

Keen to develop the discipline of epidemiology, I was able to recruit Dr Tony Ryan, another Adelaide graduate, who had just completed his Masters of Public Health (MPH) in epidemiology at the Harvard School of Public Health. He had earlier carried out a major pioneering study of traffic accidents in the Department of Pathology at the University of Adelaide, for which he received an MD (Doctor of Medicine).

I had recently supervised a study by Dr Bob Heddle, Director of Student Health at the University of Adelaide, which had led to his MD degree. This was a time of increasing international student turbulence, emanating from centres such as Paris and Berkeley, California. Australian students were part of this upheaval; Monash was no exception. I suggested to Tony that he studied the health of Monash University students. He took up this challenge with enthusiasm – his recent political experience was useful! We also benefited from recently published studies of student health from Harvard and Edinburgh Universities. This led to several papers (McMichael and Hetzel, 1974, 1975), as well as a successful PhD thesis. At that time, I was also developing my interest in the global problem of iodine deficiency (Pharoah et al., 1971; McMichael, 2012a; see Box 2.1).

This experience encouraged me to push for greater attention to be given to the discipline of epidemiology. I was able to become a member of the International Epidemiology Association (IEA), and then a member of the IEA Council at an early stage of its development. This facilitated enjoyable contact with colleagues all over the world, especially from the UK and the USA, and was of considerable value not only to my department at Monash but also to other academic public health departments in Australia.

In Australia, we were able to make good use of the national data sets on coronary heart disease and cancer mortality then becoming available from work by the health economists, John Deeble (later one of Colin Butler's PhD supervisors) and Dick Scotton, in their preparation of the case for National Health Insurance. Their analysis of these data was very useful for our work, including teaching.

Box 2.1 Commentary: Epidemiology, iodine deficiency and the power of multidisciplinary sufficiency[1]

Anthony J McMichael

This commentary is based on my recollections during the development of what became a multidisciplinary research-and-intervention odyssey. Around 1970, Basil Hetzel clearly saw the need and opportunity to pursue a programme of research for which this classic article (see Box 2.1) is the prime foundation. The programme sought, via epidemiological research and then animal experimental studies, a fuller understanding of the developmental and health consequences of lifelong iodine deficiency.

Though goitre had been known for many centuries, its usual causation by iodine deficiency was not fully understood; neither was its linkage with a wider range of neurological disabilities. Hence the importance of research to elaborate the full spectrum of iodine deficiency disorders (IDD) and to mobilize international agency support for large-scale population intervention and evaluation.

Following Hetzel's clarification of the syndrome of IDD in the early 1980s (Hetzel 1983), IDD prevention became part of modern global public health architecture. This 'translational' step is where the really hard work often begins. How to actually prevent disorders and diseases for which there is now clear empirical evidence of major risk factors? Hetzel and colleagues saw it was necessary to create an authoritative body to deal with international agencies and national governments. In 1985, they established an international NGO, the International Council for Control of Iodine Deficiency Disorders (ICCIDD), with Hetzel as Executive Director. With help from WHO and UNICEF in particular, the ICCIDD was then able to assist in the development of a global programme of elimination of IDD.

From Cobalt to Lead at the CSIRO Division of Human Nutrition

After graduation in 1971, I was pleased that Tony had five years of further training and experience at the well-known University of North Carolina School of Public Health, before returning to Australia in late 1976. By that time, I had returned to Adelaide as Chief of a newly established CSIRO Division of Human Nutrition. This had been created from a former Division of Animal Nutrition, which had made its name by identifying animal health-harming deficiencies of

1 Adapted from McMichael, 2012a.

copper and cobalt in the south-eastern desert area of South Australia. This was one of the big CSIRO success stories. It was decided to switch from animal to human nutrition!

I had funds to create three Research Fellowships; these were filled quickly by three epidemiology students, supervised by Tony and myself. All completed doctorates: John Potter (bowel cancer) (see Reprint E and Chapter 13, this volume), Terry Dwyer (heart disease) and Robert Scragg (gallstone disease). Tony also made good use of available data, steadily producing papers on gastrointestinal cancer, smoking and cholesterol. He also collaborated with our biostatistician, Peter Baghurst, in the long-term study of lead exposure in Port Pirie (Reprint D, Part 3, this volume), and then with his student, Dr (now Professor) Shilu Tong (Chapter 7, this volume). This has become a leading global study.

In 1987, Tony and I published a Penguin book, *The LS Factor: Lifestyle and Health*, which summarised the available evidence (excerpted in Reprint F, Part 4, this volume). This book has continued to sell and it has also been translated into Chinese.

From London to the US National Academy of Sciences

After 10 years at CSIRO, Tony moved back to the University of Adelaide, becoming the First Professor of Occupational and Environmental Health. There, he was able to develop his interest in climate change and health. I was then very pleased by Tony's appointment in 1994 to the prestigious Chair of Epidemiology at the London School of Hygiene and Tropical Medicine, where he stayed until late 2000. There, he was able to pursue his interest in climate and environmental change, including by several major joint publications in *The Lancet*. In 2001, he returned to Australia as Director of the National Centre for Epidemiology and Population Health at the Australian National University. Between 1993 and 2006, Tony played a leading role in the health risk assessment of the Intergovernmental Panel on Climate Change, which shared the Nobel Prize in 2007.

I was again gratified when Tony was elected in 2011 to the National Academy of Sciences in the USA. This was indeed a notable event and well deserved. His paper published at the time of his election to the Academy is a major contribution and will become a classical reference (McMichael, 2012b). This is a remarkable achievement for an Australian; we can all be proud of this.

In summary, I was fortunate to have known Tony from his student days, to supervise his doctoral work and then to work with him as a staff member.

He became a global figure in public health, as indicated by the range of papers in this book. This range includes his own studies and extensive collaborative work.

He had a very good sense of humour and we were, and I am still, both passionate about the piano, he as a practitioner and I as a listener!

References

Hetzel, B.S. 1983. Iodine deficiency disorders (IDD) and their eradication. *The Lancet* 322, 1126–29.

Hetzel, B.S. & McMichael, A.J. *The LS Factor: Lifestyle and Health*. Penguin, Melbourne, Australia.

McMichael, A.J. 2012a. Commentary: Epidemiology, iodine deficiency and the power of multidisciplinary sufficiency. *International Journal of Epidemiology* 41, 599–600.

McMichael, A.J. 2012b. Insights from past millennia into climatic impacts on human health and survival. *Proceedings of the National Academy of Sciences (USA)* 109, 4730–7.

McMichael, A.J. & Hetzel, B.S. 1974. An epidemiological study of the mental health of Australian university students. *International Journal of Epidemiology* 3, 125–34.

McMichael, A.J. & Hetzel, B.S. 1975. Mental health problems among university students, and their relationship to academic failure and withdrawal. *The Medical Journal of Australia* 1, 499–504.

McMichael, A.J., Baghurst, P.A., Wigg, N.R., Vimpani, G.V., Robertson, E.F. & Roberts, R.J., 1988. Port Pirie cohort study: environmental exposure to lead and children's abilities at the age of four years. *New England Journal of Medicine* 319, 468–75.

Pharoah, P.O.D., Buttfield, I.H. & Hetzel, B.S. 1971. Neurological damage to the fetus resulting from severe iodine deficiency during pregnancy. *The Lancet* 297, 308–10.

3

MUCH SAID, MUCH TO BE DONE

A Field Collaboration between Scientists and Visual Artists about Contested Landscapes in Western Sydney

JOHN REID, ANTHONY G. CAPON AND JANE DIXON

Abstract

The Australian National University (ANU) School of Art Field Study programme is a well-researched and pedagogically awarded procedure for artist engagement with community for the production of visual art about the environment. In 2009, researchers from the ANU National Centre for Epidemiology and Population Health, then under the aegis of Professor Tony McMichael, collaborated with a field study programme to inform artists who were inspired to produce visual aesthetic imagery to raise community awareness about the contested landscapes of Western Sydney. Unexpectedly, awareness was also raised about the scholarly relationships that evolved between the artists and the scientists. This chapter recounts these developments, leading to the conclusion that the artists opened the minds of the scientists to a more nuanced, and yet in some ways more disturbing, contestation.

The Merits of the Idea

Professor Tony McMichael, Director of the National Centre for Epidemiology and Population Health (NCEPH) at ANU, took his seat at the Centre's Lunchtime Seminar, as he had done many times. On this occasion, 15 September 2011, the speakers were John Reid, ANU School of Art, and Tony Capon and Jane Dixon, both from NCEPH. The seminar, titled 'The Artist, the Scientist, a Basin and a Recipe', outlined a collaboration between scientists and visual artists to raise community awareness about the contested landscapes in the western part of the Sydney basin, and the implications of these contests for the health and well-being of both people and planet.

The event pulled together several threads of activity. One of them was Tony McMichael's support for collaborative relationships between NCEPH and the creative arts. Also discernable in the collaborative fabric was the touch of Allen Kearns from the Commonwealth Scientific and Industrial Research Organisation (CSIRO), who facilitated the financial viability of the enterprise through a CSIRO Flagship Collaboration Fund grant.

The collaboration itself had its origins in May 2009 at an ANU forum for academics from NCEPH and the ANU Fenner School for Environment and Society to explore further potential for environmental research initiatives. Tony Capon and Jane Dixon were there, as was John Reid – brought into the orbit of Fenner School academic life by its then Director, Professor Will Steffen. At the forum, Reid outlined a programme that he had developed at the ANU School of Art called 'Field Studies', which facilitated student artist contact in field locations with scientists and community informants, to inspire the production of visual aesthetic imagery in response to prevailing environmental issues. The art folios generated by the programme meet both the curriculum requirements of the artists involved and, through the public exhibition of the folios, a community appetite for a cultural response to the environmental issues that they faced. 'Might a Field Study', Tony Capon enquired, 'focus on the contests across Western Sydney between housing, agriculture, roads and industry?' The merits of the idea were immediately apparent.

ANU School of Art *ArtForum*

In October 2009, an ANU School of Art *ArtForum* was held to canvas the appeal of this potential study with the school community. Capon and Dixon were joined by David Mason, NSW Department of Primary Industries, to expound the theme for a 2010 Field Study based on their current research activity in Western Sydney. This would provide scholarly reference material to inform artist field observations and assist visual interpretation. All three gave a passionate account of the contested landscapes of Western Sydney.

Tony Capon outlined the broader context of urban agriculture, and its relevance to cities like Sydney.

> Historically, Australia has been a food-rich country – a net food exporter. We currently export up to 80% of our production of two commodities, wheat and meat, and, until recently, Australia was self-sufficient

in almost all nutritionally important food groups. However, free trade and other market 'forces' (rather than lack of sufficient fertile areas or climatic suitability) have seen the increasing loss of this capacity, so that today, we import a significant quantity of foods which are important for dietary diversity, including fruit, vegetables and fish.

Australian agriculture will be hit early and hard by climate change. The Australian Bureau of Agricultural and Resource Economics (ABARE) estimates agricultural production could decline by up to 10% by 2030 and 19% by 2050, due to climate change. Some researchers, such as Julian Cribb (2010), are now asking a new question: could a combination of vulnerabilities – climate change, population growth and the loss of niche agricultural production –make Australia a comparatively food-poor country in the future?

We tend to think there is plenty of space to grow food in Australia; however, only 6% of the continent is suitable for intensive agricultural production. Most cities develop in places that have been relatively fertile and watered. As cities grow, much of this arable land has been built on; the little that remains is at risk from further urban development, driven in part by Australia's population growth. one of the highest in the Organisation for Economic Co-operation and Development (OECD). Urban planners are beginning to highlight the value of planning for food security, noting that once land is lost to urban development, it is almost impossible to regain for food growing purposes (Noble 2008).

Urban agriculture – both commercial and civic agriculture – has a health and social value (Mason and Docking, 2005). Civic agriculture includes growing food in community gardens, backyards, on verandas and in the street. Its health benefits can include nutrition, exercise, social interaction, cultural exchange and mental well-being.

The future of Australia's eastern seaboard is a case in point. The coastal strip from Nowra to Noosa, between the Great Dividing Range and the Pacific Ocean, is a rapidly urbanising landscape. Already, 40% of the Australian population lives along this coastal strip – more than 8 million people. By 2050, it is likely that 15 million or more will live there. This narrow strip of land – about 1000 km in length – contains some of Australia's best agricultural land and (currently) has reasonably good and reliable rainfall. And, it is home to a rich diversity of natural fauna and flora.

In the interest of future food security and health, we should think strategically about land use along this strip. How can we house, feed and

> move people in healthy and sustainable ways? International experience is instructive. Urban growth boundaries have been used to protect agricultural land in Canada and the USA.
>
> The experience of Cuba during its 'special period' – 1989–2000, after the collapse of the socialist bloc – is also particularly interesting from a health perspective. During this time, a large number of urban food gardens emerged in Cuban cities in response to reduced food imports. Daily per capita food energy intake reduced. Levels of physical activity increased because there was less oil available to power machines and motorised transport. In 2007, measurable health benefits were reported in the *American Journal of Epidemiology*. Obesity rates declined by 50%, and total deaths fell by 18% (Franco et al., 2007). Of course, we would not wish for such a trade and economic crisis here in Australia; however, there are lessons for a resource-constrained future.
>
> Our future food security and health depends on wise land-use planning. It is good to see land-use contests on the city fringe are prominent in the recent review of Sydney's metropolitan plan. The precautionary principle would have us protect our limited supply of agricultural land from further urban expansion.

Tony then introduced the background to the scientific study:

> In order to more thoroughly examine these issues, one of seven CSIRO-funded projects will adopt a case study approach based in Western Sydney, the fastest growing urban region in Australia during the 1990s. The project team is to concentrate its efforts on identifying the present and near-term threats (20 years) to foods being produced and processed in the Sydney Basin.

The students were provided with a description of the scientific team's background research, which revealed how much land had been re-zoned away from agricultural purposes toward housing development and services, including extensive road networks[1] (Edwards et al., 2011; Mason et al., 2011), with significant implications for farmer/grower numbers and locally produced fruit and vegetable yields in particular (Malcolm and Fahd, 2009).

David Mason followed by providing insights, not only as a public servant working in primary industries over several decades but also as a chronicler of the region's agricultural history, possibly preceding European settlement

1 Early on, NCEPH PhD student, Ferne Edwards, was appointed as Research Associate to provide the team with background materials, and these were presented to the field studies students once they began in the field. The 2011 reference (Edwards et al., 2011) represents the final version of this work.

(Mason and Docking, 2005; Mason and Knowd, 2010). Importantly, he detailed major changes in land use post-World War II, which were attributed to the planning profession's view that the agricultural lands were 'awaiting higher economic development' (namely, residential and commercial developments).

At the conclusion of the *ArtForum*, 42 artists entered their contact details to an expression-of-interest list. Planning for the 2010 Field Study began in earnest.

The Field Study Programme

The pedagogic attributes of Field Study programmes have developed as field procedures and have been progressively researched. The programme had its origins with backpacking trips into remote locations in south-east New South Wales in the early 1980s, which demonstrated the pedagogic value of instigating creative art production in locations that afforded inspirational, high-quality sensory experiences. This provided a much-needed option to the prevailing curricula focus on highly culturally processed material as starting points for creative expression, such as artwork in galleries, visual and literary references found in libraries and on the emerging Internet. Student feedback regarding this alternative was extremely positive.[2]

By the mid-1990s, the programme was more comprehensive and embraced rural and suburban field locations with their resident populations. An emphasis on community consultation emerged and opened up the prospect of long-term, genuine engagement. Expert informants such as local scientists, Indigenous leaders, landholders, shire officials, community activists and local artists interpreted pertinent, observable subject matter as creative stimuli for participating artists. By way of reciprocation to this community generosity, exhibitions of artwork generated by Field Study programmes (more than 30 of them) have been held in the field locations that inspired them. Communities invariably responded with great enthusiasm, pointing out how much they appreciated viewing, in their regional centres, meaningful, aesthetic visual imagery about where they lived and worked. The art exhibitions also renewed their appreciation of the lifestyle values to which they subscribed and often forgot under the stresses of everyday life. Inspiration to act on pressing environmental issues transferred from artist to community. Collaborations with public and private environmental agencies flourished.

2 Later, as the programme continued to consolidate, the October 2003 ANU CEDAM Student Evaluation for the Enhancement of Teaching at the School of Art revealed that 35 students from the 254 respondents had undertaken Field Study programmes. On a rating scale from 1 to 5, the minimum score was 3, maximum was 5, mean was 4.7 and standard deviation was 0.79.

Following on from teaching awards (ANU 1998–99) and national pedagogic citations (Reid, 2006) for innovative practice, the Field Study programme, and the environmental issues it was addressing in the Murray–Darling Basin from 2003 to 2007, became the focus of an Australian Research Council (ARC) Linkage project called 'Engaging Visions' (2007–10), with the Murray–Darling Basin Commission (now Authority) as industry partner. The outcome was a refined field procedure based on scholarly evidence gathered from participating artists and the communities with whom they consulted (Reid et al., 2010). The Contested Landscapes of Western Sydney Field Study was the first beneficiary of this effort.

The Contested Landscapes of Western Sydney Field Study

The first of three five-day field trips to the north-western part of the Sydney Basin commenced on Wednesday, 3 March 2010, with 18 participating artists. Keynote briefings were delivered at various field locations by community activists, landholders, council officials and academics, including Tony Capon and Jane Dixon. The desirability of involving student artists who lived in Sydney and working with them as partners in the Field Study was acknowledged from the very beginning. The Sydney Gallery School (SGS), Meadowbank College of Technical and Further Education, which had undertaken a very successful Field Study jointly with the ANU School of Art a few years earlier, was an obvious choice. The Sydney-based artists scheduled their own fieldwork, but both artist groups came together for a series of exhibitions that extended into 2013.

Exhibition venues included galleries in Sydney and Canberra. The Canberra exhibition coincided with the 2010 Australian Academy of Science Fenner Conference, 'Healthy Climate, Planet and People. Co-Benefits for Health from Action on Climate Change'. The exhibition in Sydney was at the See Street Gallery, Meadowbank College, TAFE NSW. The exhibitions in Western Sydney — at the Purple Noon Art Gallery, Freemans Reach; and The Sassafras Creek Gallery, Kurrajong Village — resonated with the communities in which they were mounted by delivering aesthetic visual statements about issues of local significance. The research knowledge that Tony Capon and Jane Dixon (and the scientific team that came with them) shared with artists in the field made a major contribution to the conceptual foundations and pertinence of the work that the artists produced. The benefits that the scientist delivered to the artist were very apparent.

Extensions to the Field Study

An exhibition of selected works from the Contested Landscapes of Western Sydney Field Study was mounted in the NCEPH corridors leading to the very lecture theatre in which the NCEPH Lunchtime Seminar, referred to at the beginning of the chapter, would take place – another thread, although this one continued to spin. Just over a year later, in November 2012, a compilation of Western Sydney contested landscape artwork was mounted at the Shine Dome, Canberra, ACT, for Tony McMichael's Festschrift, *From Healthy Workers to a Healthy Planet*. Supplemented by a major body of new artwork, produced from a second Field Study in Western Sydney in the second half of 2012, the repository of visual imagery about Western Sydney's contested landscapes enabled another substantial exhibition, 'Biting the Carpet. Food Security and the Lay of the Land', ANU School of Art Foyer Gallery, curated and mounted for the XIX International Conference of the Society for Human Ecology held at ANU in February 2013.

Scientist–Artist Partnerships

None of the Field Study programmes delivered in the period prior to the 2010 Field Study had been informed by a current scientific research project; and certainly none of the scientists participating in previous Field Study programmes, who had briefed artists in the field, had reflected openly on the interaction itself and how it might deliver benefits for *their* research. At least, no one had done it quite like Jane Dixon did; and here we acknowledge anthropologist Bronwyn Isaacs who along with Jane conducted and analysed interviews with all of the ANU Field Study participants as they were putting the final touches to their works. The interviews were semi-structured and aimed to elicit artist motivations for involvement in the Field Study, their understanding of what they observed, and how they incorporated this understanding in their art work.

In her contribution to the NCEPH Lunchtime Seminar, Dixon began to thread her thoughts about her involvement in the 2010 Field Study into a tentative hypothesis about artist–scientist partnerships. Dixon had prior experience with Australia Council and local government funded community artists and their role in community building. She was aware that community arts had become a vibrant aspect to mental health and health promotion programmes (see www.artsandhealth.org.au). However, the Field Study did not fit that mould.

Unlike community art, where the focus is on excellence in process, a Field Study is founded on fine art, which aspires to excellence in output. Trained to perceive and conceptualise meaningful relationships by looking, the visual fine artists involved in the 2010 Field Study responded by formulating aesthetic visual propositions. Consequently, the Field Study did not equate to being a science communication exercise either. Unlike science communication, where the focus is on comprehension, works of fine art, informed by science, invoke a more comprehensive human experience by synthesising reliable knowledge and personal opinion with aesthetic appeal intended to instigate emotional investment. Immersion in a Field Study, with its fine art objectives, stimulates the intellect, which leads inevitably to critical reflection of the overall research agenda – scientific or otherwise. All works of fine art are aesthetic evaluations (Reid, 2011).

Jane Dixon articulated her experience as follows:

'Public health researchers have a strong commitment to bridging the research–policy divide so that the rhetoric of evidence-based policy is reflected in practical actions. At NCEPH, the attempt to forge links with policymakers takes multiple forms:

1. Industry partnership grants: ARC Linkage grants and NH&MRC Partnership grants, CSIRO Flagship grants, CRC involvements.
2. Sitting on high-level advisory committees and briefing government committees.
3. Undertaking consultancies for government.
4. Writing for 'applied' journals, e.g. *New South Wales Public Health Bulletin*, read by more than 14,000 people on a regular basis.
5. Making submissions to parliamentary enquiries.
6. Writing op eds for newspapers.
7. Posting policy briefs on websites.

A less direct way to inform policy, but one that has a proud track record in public health, is to work with civil society or communities on issues of concern to them. What might be termed 'grass roots engagement' is undertaken in the hope that better-briefed citizens will demand more of their politicians, and that bottom-up pressure will advance policy options. Empowered health citizens can also teach health scientists about their experience of their environments and why they believe that they are in poor health. The public's understanding of the causes of ill health (referred to as 'lay epidemiology') can be a powerful influence on everyday behaviours (as has happened with smoking cessation, AIDS prevention, SIDS prevention; see Banwell et al., 2013).

It is this philosophy regarding the important role of civil society in policy change and behavioural change that encouraged my participation in The Contested Landscape project. Initially, I believed that the artists could help the scientists better communicate the science regarding the relationship between sprawling urban housing development and diminishing urban agricultural production. However, my year-long involvement broadened my assumptions about what a partnership between scientists and artists could achieve. In particular, I now regard artists as lay scientists, and as a result, they make an invaluable contribution to the scientific endeavour.

First, the artists involved in this project sharpened our fundamental hypothesis. We began by arguing that urban housing development was consuming food-producing lands. However, owing to their educated eye and evaluative approach, the artists brought an observational acuity to their own deliberations. They noted, for example, the proliferation of non-residential uses that were overtaking the landscape: equestrian-related enterprises, turf farms and flower farms, plus areas dedicated to water sports and to other sports. They challenged us to broaden the hypothesis about the nature of land-use changes and the nature of the inequitable changes from land that was once affordable for small farms to lands with higher-value uses.

Renowned Australian anthropologist, Gillian Cowlishaw, who has also worked in the Sydney area, defined ethnography, a fundamental research approach adopted in anthropology, in the terms that reflected my observations of the way the artists went about their work. She says, 'Ethnographers provide evidence of amazing variation in the social worlds human beings have created, encompassing dramatic differences in everyday habits, material creations, systems of knowledge and belief' (Cowlishaw, 2009, p. x11). They do this by going 'among people' and relating 'to them as far as possible on their own terms' (Cowlishaw, 2009, pp. 6–7). In this project, the artists went into the natural and built environment and tried to relate to that in its own terms, yielding enormous variation in perspective but some common threads, as I describe below.

Second, they did not shy away from judging the aesthetic qualities of what they observed – ugliness, impoverished landscapes because of monocultural activity – including housing estates. For many social scientists, the very notion of aesthetics is to be avoided because of its highly subjective nature. It is hard to measure and to assess. I was confronted by my own adoption of cultural relativism which denied any group the right to claim a more authentic, correct or judgemental position. While this could be an egalitarian position to adopt, it was also akin to fence sitting, thereby making it difficult to recommend directions for change, which was an important aim of the CSIRO research.

However, when you have a nearly unanimous position being advanced on matters of environmental qualities by a group of 40 artists, the argument becomes more compelling. Thus, in assessing land-use changes, the scientists could add the more ephemeral aesthetic consequences to the existing list of economic, social and environmental consequences gathered in the background research.

For example, Marzena Wasikowska's photographs of massive investment in suburban housing on reclaimed agricultural land visually and compellingly complement the evidence that it is almost impossible to regain land, lost to urban development, for food growing purposes. Jo Donnelly's mixed media work addresses the western Sydney 'contest' as cultural heritage in a sweeping landscape where the opposing forces of food producers and urban housing developers strategically manoeuvre like armed forces on age-old tapestries. Judith Ringger renders a desolate future. Aria Stone, in dialogue with both Donnelly and Ringger, paints a solitary, spaced-out cow standing on a desolate patch of ground bulldozed for cul-de-sacs and turf. Sue Downes in her screen-printed, precautionary principle tee shirts graphically advocates a 'cool' solution to restraining urban growth and expected urban overheating by drafting zones for food production just as we allocate national parks to preserve biodiversity. An A.G. Stokes canvas of freshly picked veggies descending from the sky on inner Sydney could have sold ten times over in cultural support of city dwellers fertilising asphalt footpaths with the seeds of edible plants. John Reid's photograph documents a threatened landscape extending from an orchard near Kurrajong Village to the Grose Valley that painter Leo Robba also renders in accord with a future scenario. And, in one masterly work in acrylic on canvas, titled *Branching Out*, Kerry Shepherdson articulates the complexity of the Field Study theme. (See reproductions of these artworks at the end of the chapter and on the front cover).

Third, the individual and collected works can become props for action research. This is a form of research that places a premium on inspiring reflection about social phenomena, which in turn may lead to actions to change circumstances (Wadsworth, 2011). As participating student Leo Robba remarked on his involvement in the project:

> As a landscape painter, the way I would usually work would be to move through the landscape and choose scenes that would carry their own message. Looking for a landscape that conveys a message that is often ambiguous but one that can be heightened by the way I choose to frame

> what I see. The 'human' content embedded in the view. My hope is that the viewer can share the artist's experience and if very successfully can actually sense time, place and meaning.
>
> With the work for Contested Landscape I found it quite difficult to work in my usual way. One panel was painted en plein air and the other (night scene) in the studio. This more conceptual approach is not so familiar to me but I felt the need for a more overt political statement.

The man who inspired several of the powerful images was described by Leo in these terms:

> John Maguire [an orchardist who briefed the artists] was inspiring and the view from the balcony of his coffee shop/produce shed grew in importance the more I heard his story: the family history and his passion for the farming culture and the culture that his land represents. On listening to John it felt like he had decided it was up to him to make what could be the last stand.

The travelling exhibition, along with the catalogue, provided material to generate responses from residents in the Sydney Basin. One of our research associates, Ferne Edwards, has used the catalogue as a discussion starter with the Sydney Basin's amateur bee-keepers, and gives the catalogue as a present.

The catalogue is essentially a document that reminds readers that the landscape has been crafted by human activity and will continue to be so. The images can create alternative visions for the landscape and a desire by viewers to exert pressure on important decision makers. Indeed, we had instances where the artists themselves became active politically, as Fran Ifould recounts:

> I'm also extremely concerned about the standard of the urban sprawl ... We went to Orin Park and we have written the [developers] a letter about our concern that there were no provisions for community gardens or anything like that ... The first display house that we walked into, we walked through a foyer into a kitchen, open plan, into a living room, architecturally designed with all these down-lights. That house had sixty ceiling down-lights in the foyer, the kitchen and the living room; I mean, it's not sustainable. Where are we going here?

Fourth, the artists are a repository of data. A majority of the artists had a prior or present connection to the area under study, which added an emotional and educated quality to their responses. We interviewed them all, and three themes emerged:

1. *Nostalgia and sense of loss at how the landscape was being transformed.*

   Shirley Dunn expressed a sentiment common to the other participating artists:

   > I have been working in ceramics and ... for me the rectangular platters I have used symbolize the Hawkesbury-Nepean River valley. In the work, 'Only for Houses', the symbolic housing estates on small plates are like rafts drifting into the landscape of the river. In the second work, 'The Last Fruit', the valley is covered with small housing blocks that replace the apple orchards and the farms ...
   >
   > I found the field trips very inspirational, I had not visited this area for a number of years and to see first-hand the changes was important to me. The river and its surrounds are very beautiful but are being destroyed with the increase of housing estates.
   >
   > My mother retired to live at McGraths Hill and I often took her for drives around the area until her death in 1995. She knew her family had once lived and farmed in the area. Her father was born at Castlereagh Road near Penrith. His father and grandfather built the old slab cottage called 'Puddledock', and I suspect he was born there in 1864. My mother's family have researched our background and I am descended from the Herberts, the Purcells, the Howells, the Kennedys, the Burns and the Marshes, all neighbours who had small farms along the river from as early as 1803.
   >
   > While it is easy for me to be sentimental about my ancestors, their farms would have destroyed the rich natural environment that once supported the Aboriginal population along the river. I have very negative feelings about the gravel mining companies at Penrith. I am unimpressed with what ... they have taken to support building developments in wider Sydney.

2. *Concern for loss of control over the food system.*

   Miriam Cullen's account of her work *Fruitless* similarly resonated with what we heard from a majority of participating student artists:

   > It's a sculpture of two fruit branches, with some of the fruit transformed into suburban streets – they are covered with the maps of Sydney suburbs. It communicates a blight or affliction across the landscape, in the same way the suburbs are a blight across Western Sydney. The piece also suggests that attempts to halt the spread are 'fruitless'. The farm land has been lost under concrete and McMansions. I was inspired by a re-release of the first 'Gregory's' Sydney's maps from

1934. It illustrates a very different Sydney, a Sydney not mapped further west than Blacktown. The maps themselves have spread and over-ridden the landscape. The contrast to today illustrates how the sprawl is intractable, unstoppable.

3. *The emergence of an ugly aesthetic.*

   Rosina Wainwright echoed the views of many when she said:

> I recently read that Western Sydney had the 'biggest houses in the world', so I went and visited the new housing developments. We can't afford it, it's appalling; it's taking no account of climate change. I photographed the 'biggest houses in the world' and used it in my work – cardboard fruit boxes with rows of houses – all squashed in. I work with assemblage, which is like poetry and metaphor. My father was a builder and valuer – from the age of about eight years old he taught me to look at houses. In the developments we saw in Sydney, I was struck by the facades – no detailing, they are like warehouses. They display very little wood. I think people are being manipulated, they have all that open plan which is very hard to heat. It's driven by the market.

In conclusion, I have experienced first-hand the process of science-into-art and also art-into-science. Cowlishaw's definition of ethnography encompasses a researcher's insistence on experiencing particular social conditions and specific social relationships. This type of practice, she says, 'is a close up experience of people who are likely to change your mind' (Cowlishaw, 2009, p. xvi). This is how the artists have made their mark on the project: they have not only produced powerfully provocative artworks, through close encounters with local people in their natural and built environments they have opened the minds of the scientists to a more nuanced, and yet in some ways more disturbing, contestation beyond land zoning to who gets to decide how the dynamics between nature and society and between the past and the future will play out.'[3]

The Legacy

Since the 2013 contribution to the XIX International Conference of the Society for Human Ecology, the Field Study programme has moved its attention to the far south coast of New South Wales, where it collaborated with the National

3 The research assistant, Ferne Edwards, went on to recast her PhD topic to reflect multiple land-use contestations and food security. Edwards and Dixon embarked on research, which is ongoing, regarding bee-keeping in the suburbs: a marked point of contestation; and Dixon and Capon took their new understanding into the article led by Proust (2012).

Climate Change Adaptation Research Facility (NCCARF)-funded South-East Coast Adaptation (SECA) Research Project. The SECA Project, led by Professor Barbara Norman, University of Canberra (UC), with researchers from the University of Wollongong, UC and ANU, investigated the profile of climate-adapted coastal settlements in 2030. In November 2013, as part of the SECA Research Project's communication strategy, the SECA Field Study programme mounted an exhibition of visual art titled, 'Now & When' in Eden, New South Wales. About 300 people and 120 schoolchildren viewed the show. The Planning Institute of Australia has recently acknowledged this initiative in its 2014 National Awards in the category of Cutting Edge Research and Teaching.

The momentum continues with research projects currently being drafted to address climate change with Griffith University's College of Art and the Griffith Climate Change Response Program; and healthy and sustainable cities in partnership with Tony Capon. Both projects incorporate the communicative talents of creative artists building on Tony McMichael's legacy and Jane Dixon's reflective thinking. It is the intension of these projects to investigate the efficacy of integrating Field Study-inspired fine artwork into social science methodologies as data in its own right; and as intellectual and emotional stimulus for quality data collection from communities via subsequent focus groups, interview, and survey.

References

Banwell, C., Ulijaszek, S. & Dixon, J. (eds) 2013. *When Culture Impacts Health: Global Lessons for Effective Health Research*. Elsevier Science, Amsterdam, The Netherlands.

Cowlishaw, G. 2009. *The City's Outback*. UNSW Press, Sydney, New South Wales, Australia.

Cribb, J. 2010. *The Coming Famine. The Global Food Crisis and What We Can Do to Avoid It*. CSIRO Publishing, Collingwood, Victoria, Australia.

Edwards, F., Dixon, J., Friel, S., Hall, G., Larsen, K., Lockie, S., et al. 2011. Food systems, climate change adaptation and human health in Australia. Discussion Paper for the Human Health Adaptation Research Network, NCEPH, ANU, Canberra, ACT, Australia.

Franco, M., Orduñez, P., Caballero, B., Granados, J.A.T., Lazo, M., Bernal, J.L., et al. 2007. Impact of energy intake, physical activity, and population-wide weight loss on cardiovascular disease and diabetes mortality in Cuba, 1980–2005. *American Journal of Epidemiology* 166, 1374–80.

Malcolm, P. & Fahd, R. 2009. Ground truthing of the Sydney vegetable industry in 2008. Report prepared for HAL by NSW DPI (HAL Report/Project No VG07073), Australia.

Mason, D. & Docking, A. 2005. *Agriculture in Urbanising Landscapes – A Creative Planning Opportunity*. Planning Institute of Australia Congress, Melbourne, Australia.

Mason, D. & Knowd, I. 2010. The emergence of urban agriculture: Sydney, Australia. *International Journal of Agricultural Sustainability* 8, 62–71.

Mason, D., Dixon, J., Isaacs, B., Edwards, F. & Hall, G. 2011. Briefing Paper: The dynamic situation of urban agriculture in the Sydney Basin. Report for the Urbanism, Climate Change and Health CSIRO Climate Adaptation Flagship, National Centre for Epidemiology and Population Health. Available at: climatehealthcluster.org/wp-content/uploads/2011/03/Mason-et-al-2011-BRIEFING-PAPER.pdf, accessed 1 March 2015.

Noble, M. 2008. Gastronomic Planning Policy: Planning for Food in Sydney, Honours Thesis. University of New South Wales. www.be.unsw.edu.au/sites/default/files/upload/pdf/cf/hbep/research/Theses/MNoble_Thesis.pdf, accessed 15 February 2014.

Proust, K., Newell, B., Capon, A., Brown, H., Browne, C., Burton, A., et al. 2012. Taking a systems approach to human health and climate change in urban environments, *International Journal of Environmental Research and Public Health* 9(6), 2134–58.

Reid, J. 2006. Carrick Award Citation. Available at: engagingvisions.com.au/history/carrick-award-2006, accessed 26 April 2014.

Reid, J. 2011. Cape York Peninsula World Heritage Program Criterion (VII): The Aesthetic Point of View ANU Enterprise/Queensland Government Commission, Australia.

Reid, J., Lamberts, R., Young, C. & Tambiah, C. 2010. Engaging visions: engaging artists with the community about the environment. ANU, Canberra, ACT, Australia. Available at: www.engagingvisions.com.au.

Wadsworth, Y. 2011. *Building in Research and Evaluation. Human Enquiry for Living Systems*. Allen & Unwin, Sydney, New South Wales, Australia.

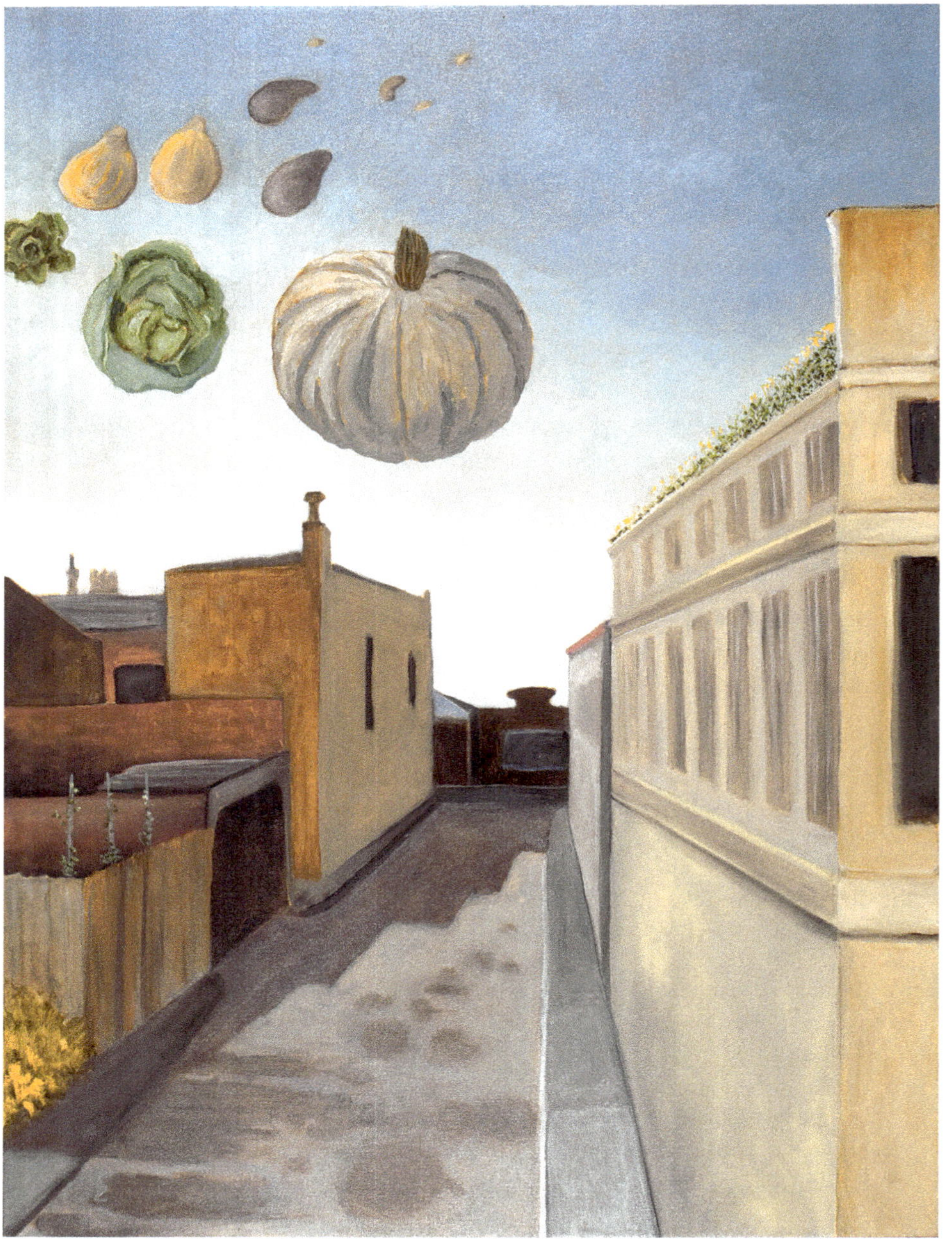

Figure 3.1 A.G. Stokes, *Veggies in the sky*, 2010, 111.2 cm x 82.0 cm, oil on canvas.

Dislodged from their shrinking traditional home in outer Western Sydney, the vegetables fly over the inner suburbs where there is a burgeoning mood for growing things.

Source: The Contested Landscapes of Western Sydney Field Study catalogue. Edition 1. 2010.

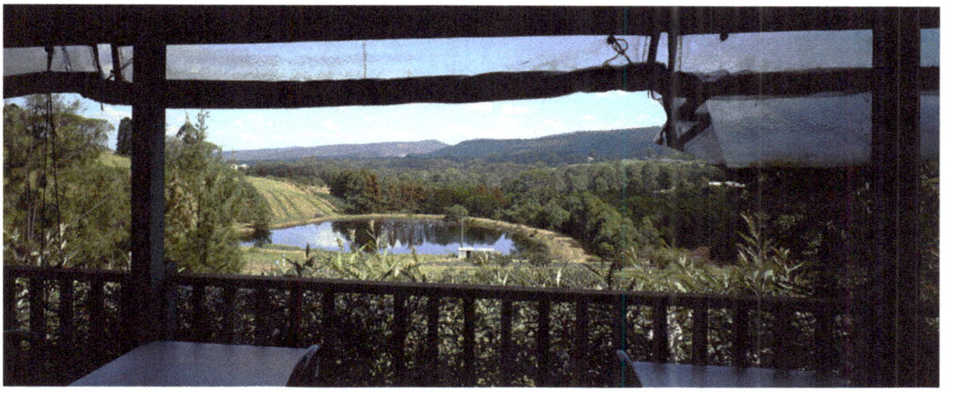

Figure 3.2 John Reid, *View to Grose Valley from Enniskillen Orchard Stall*, 2010, 40.0 cm x 90.0 cm, digital print on rag paper.

This panorama documents contested land in Western Sydney. Current landholders, many of whom are food producers, are under tremendous stress from a political climate that favours re-zoning for intensive residential development. The landscape in this photograph is depicted in the scenario painting by Leo Robba.

Source: The Contested Landscapes of Western Sydney Field Study catalogue. Edition 1. 2010.

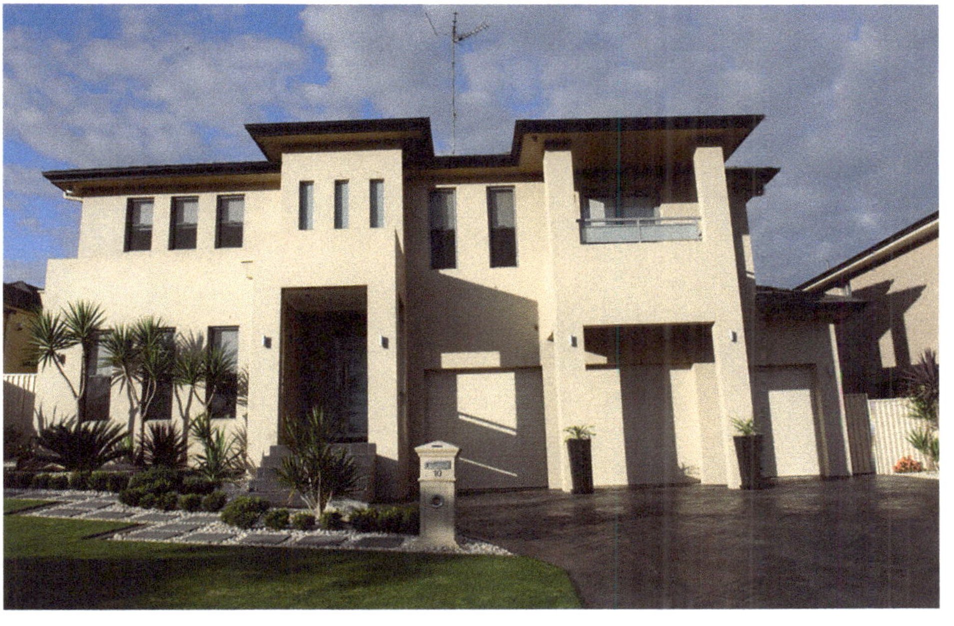

Figure 3.3 Marzena Wasikowska, *Western Sydney Landscape Contestants 1–4* (detail: *1 Intensive Real Estate*), 2010, 65.0 cm x 95.0 cm x 4, digital photographs on rag paper.

This image is one of a series of photographs documenting types of residential land in Western Sydney. Other images include life-style blocks, quarter-acre blocks and orchards.

Source: The Contested Landscapes of Western Sydney Field Study catalogue. Edition 1. 2010.

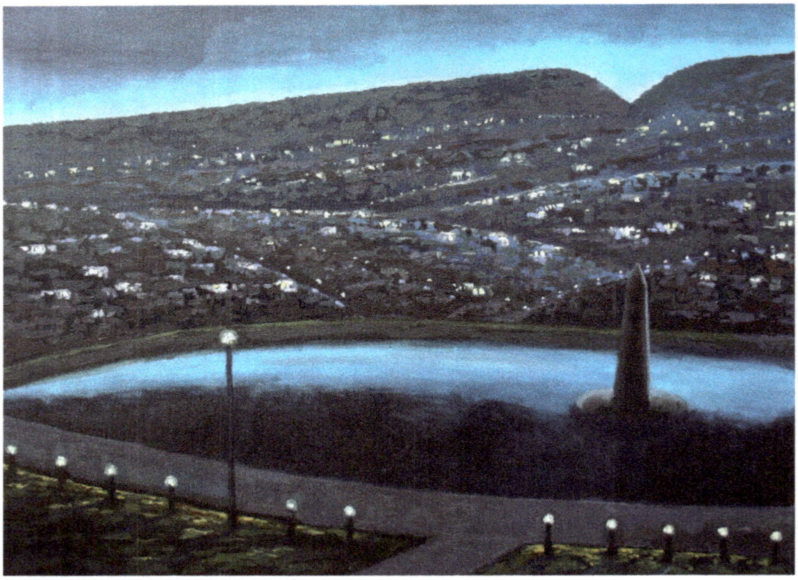

Figure 3.4 Leo Robba, *Contested Landscapes: Split Views* (detail), 2010, 128.0 cm x 80.0 cm in two panels, acrylic on canvas.

The landscape in this panel is the view to Grose Valley from Enniskillen Orchard (as documented in John Reid's panoramic photograph), rendered as sprawling suburbia.

Source: The Contested Landscapes of Western Sydney Field Study catalogue. Edition 1. 2010.

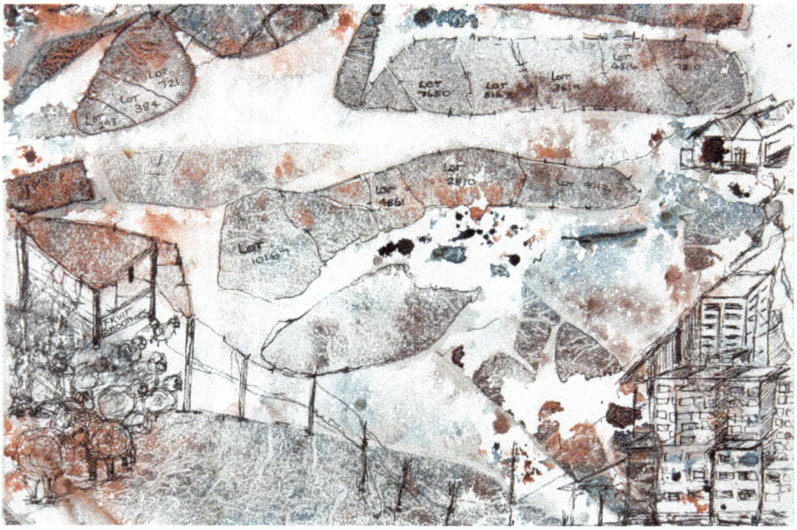

Figure 3.5 Jo Donnelly, *Populate and Perish!*, 2010, 58.0 cm x 41.5 cm, mixed media on paper.

Urban sprawl is an ever-increasing problem as our cities try to accommodate our growing population. Planning and protecting the fertile land of Sydney's food basin seems fundamental to a sustainable future.

Source: The Contested Landscapes of Western Sydney Field Study catalogue. Edition 1. 2010.

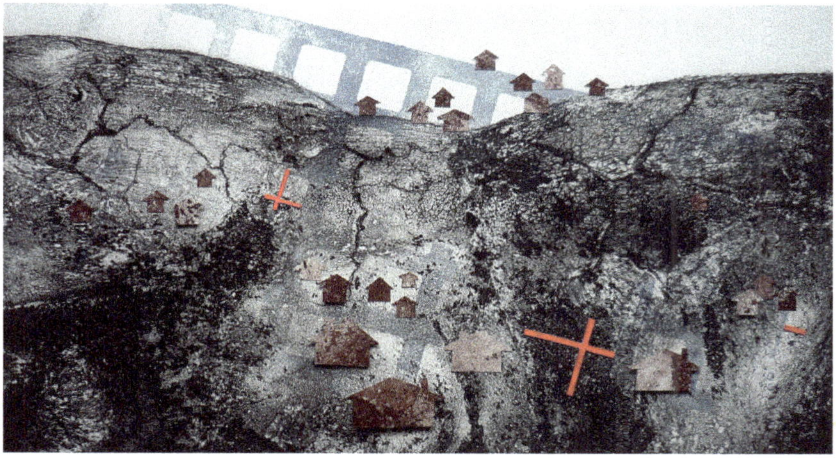

Figure 3.6 Judith Ringger, *'cheque' burial*, 2010, 22.6 cm x 37.4 cm, etching with monoprint.

Don't be the clown, don't allow for folly and foolishness. Act against the greedy developer, the ringmaster who calls the shots. In the spotlight is the dwindling arable food producing land in the Sydney Basin, so the apathetic shouldn't grizzle, 'what can you do, it will be done anyway!' Instead create a huge embarrassing political spectacle. Yell louder than the ringmaster, show up his conniving ways and point fingers at his chums who gloat over the spoils in the wings. Don't lie down in the rich soil and allow little houses to be built all over you, wearing a 'cheque' burial shawl, dead in your own paddock of apathy and malaise.

Source: The Contested Landscapes of Western Sydney Field Study catalogue. Edition 1. 2010.

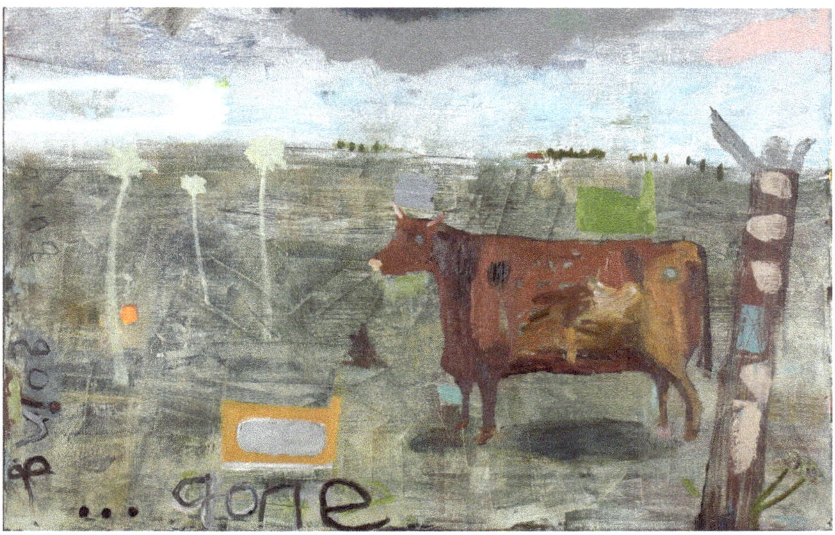

Figure 3.7 Aria Stone, *Going ... Going ... Gone*, 2010, 80.0 cm x 120.0 cm, acrylic, oil and wax medium on canvas.

This painting speaks about our precious history of small farming in the fertile basin of Sydney's Western outer suburbs. It is all too common to realise the value of things once they are gone. Let's prevent the loss of this precious food recourse to housing development.

Source: The Contested Landscapes of Western Sydney Field Study catalogue. Edition 1. 2010.

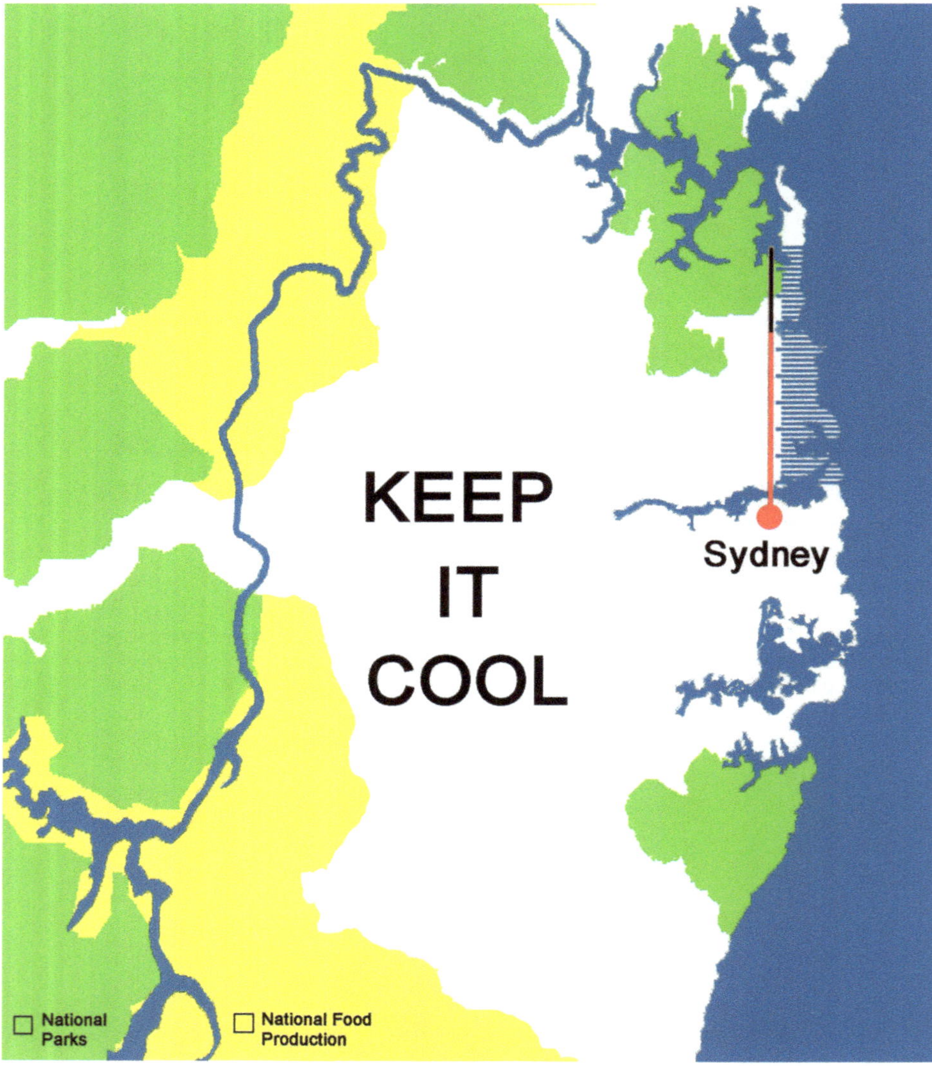

Figure 3.8 Sue Downes, *Keep it cool*, 2010, 22.7 cm x 19.4 cm, silkscreen print, tee shirt.

Growing food in Western Sydney will help to keep Sydney cool by having green areas and by reducing the need for transport. The National preservation of food growing areas, similar to National Parks, would have its benefits: a lower limit for the subdivision of land, e.g. a minimum of 10 acres and; local councils, who might have vested interests in development, would be stopped from rezoning fertile farm land.

Source: The Contested Landscapes of Western Sydney Field Study catalogue. Edition 1. 2010.

REPRINT B

Prisoners of the Proximate: Loosening the Constraints on Epidemiology in an Age of Change

ANTHONY J. MCMICHAEL

McMichael, A.J. 1999. Prisoners of the Proximate: Loosening the Constraints on Epidemiology in an Age of Change. *American Journal of Epidemiology* 149, 887–97.

Pages: 57 to 70

American Journal of
EPIDEMIOLOGY

Volume 149
Number 10
May 15, 1999

Sponsored by the Society for Epidemiologic Research

COMMENTARY

Prisoners of the Proximate: Loosening the Constraints on Epidemiology in an Age of Change

A. J. McMichael

"Modern epidemiology" has a primary orientation to the study of multiple risk factors for chronic noncommunicable diseases. If epidemiologists are to understand the determinants of population health in terms that extend beyond proximate, individual-level risk factors (and their biological mediators), they must learn to apply a social-ecologic systems perspective. The mind-set and methods of modern epidemiology entail the following four main constraints that limit engagement in issues of wider context: 1) a preoccupation with proximate risk factors; 2) a focus on individual-level versus population-level influences on health; 3) a typically modular (time-windowed) view of how individuals undergo changes in risk status (i.e., a life-stage vs. a life-course model of risk acquisition); and 4) the, as yet, unfamiliar challenge of scenario-based forecasting of health consequences of future, large-scale social and environmental changes. The evolution of the content and methods of epidemiology continues. Epidemiologists are gaining insights into the complex social and environmental systems that are the context for health and disease; thinking about population health in increasingly ecologic terms; developing dynamic, interactive, life-course models of disease risk acquisition; and extending their spatial-temporal frame of reference as they perceive the health risks posed by escalating human pressures on the wider environment. The constraints of "the proximate" upon epidemiology are thus loosening as the end of the century approaches. *Am J Epidemiol* 1999;149:887–97.

epidemiology; history; methods; population; social environmental

The past 3 decades have witnessed the methodological consolidation of "modern epidemiology," with its particular orientation to studying the multiple risk factors for chronic noncommunicable diseases. That conceptual and methodological orientation arose from midcentury as epidemiologists formally engaged in the study of diseases of long latency, multiple causality, and apparently noninfectious etiology (1). (I will refer to such diseases as "chronic diseases," while also noting the likely involvement of infectious agents in the etiology of some of them.)

It is axiomatic that the theoretic framework within which we formulate our research questions determines the scope, content, and social relevance of our answers. The question of context has excited much recent debate about the mission, models, and methods of modern epidemiology (2). To understand the determinants of population health in terms beyond proximate, individual-level risk factors (and their biological mediators) requires a social-ecologic systems perspective. Yet, modern epidemiology has largely ignored these issues of wider context. We have typically assumed that populations are merely aggregates of free-range individuals and that methodologically correct local studies can estimate presumed universal individual-level risk relations. Such an approach, however, forfeits understanding of the causes and distribution of disease within populations and thus restricts the social usefulness of the research, particularly in a rapidly changing world.

That familiar word, "understanding," has great epistemologic significance. It refers to the intellectual framework within which we gather and interpret our

Received for publication August 20, 1998, and accepted for publication December 16, 1998.

Abbreviation: CHD, coronary heart disease.

Department of Epidemiology and Population Health, London School of Hygiene and Tropical Medicine, London, England.

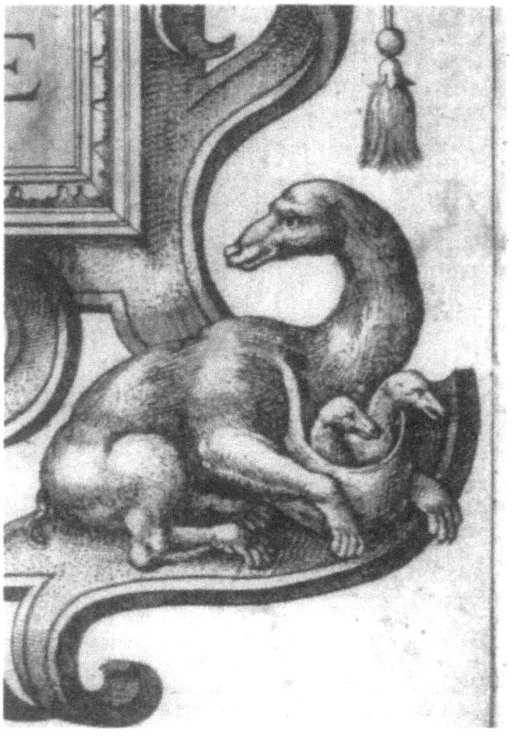

FIGURE 1. The power of the prevailing paradigm: drawing of an Australian kangaroo by a sixteenth-century Dutch artist (Cornelis de Jode), based on descriptions by early explorers.

observations. Figure 1 shows how a Dutch artist of the sixteenth century, Cornelis de Jode, visualized an Australian kangaroo from early explorers' reports. Presumably, he was told that the mother kangaroo carried the young in a sort of a bag at the front of the body. The paradigmatic carry-bag, for European city dwellers, is something hanging from a shoulder strap. Hence, this bizarre artistic rendition.

Likewise, our understanding of disease causation reflects the theoretic paradigm, the epistemologic framework, within which we do our research. Has epidemiology become predominantly a discipline of *technique* rather than of *substantive understanding* (3)? Krieger and Zierler argue that modern epidemiology has theories of causal modeling and of errors, but lacks a theory of "what shapes population patterns of disease" (4, p. 107). Pearce states: "Epidemiology has largely ceased to function as part of a multidisciplinary approach to understanding the causation of disease in populations and has become a set of generic methods for measuring associations of exposure and disease in individuals" (5, p. 678). Rothman et al. (6) have responded, expressing misgivings about the capacity of epidemiology to "eradicate poverty" by studying its sedimentary role in disease causation and preferring instead to concentrate on poverty-associated, measurable, proximate risk factors for which clear-cut answers can be gleaned. Meanwhile, on another front, the elucidation of proximate "risk factor" relations has been enjoying newly forged links with the microepidemiologic world of molecular biology (1, 7).

PHASES IN THE HISTORY OF EPIDEMIOLOGY

Was there a time when epidemiologists took a more deliberate interest in the social patterning of disease? Table 1 summarizes the historical ebb and flow of epidemiologic ideas about the determinants of population health and disease over recent centuries.

The first stirrings of formal epidemiology were in John Graunt's descriptive analysis of London's bills of mortality in the 1660s (8). At that time, the classical-rationalist approach to the causes of *illness* was being challenged by the ontologic notion of specific *diseases* (9). The idea arose that empirical observations could usefully be made about disease causation (such as in Ramazzini's linking of particular occupations with particular diseases (10)).

In the late 1700s, epidemiologic enquiry in Britain began to address several specific problems. Thomas Lind carried out his miniaturized controlled trials of the dietary prevention of seaboard scurvy. Case series of unusual diseases—such as scrotal cancer in chimney sweeps and colic in Devon cider drinkers—indicated particular environmental causes. However, analyses of differential mortality and disease causation were still principally framed in terms of geography, relative wealth, and occupation. Epidemiologic concepts remained broad; methods of inquiry were, by today's standards, extremely crude.

In early nineteenth-century industrializing Europe, a more humane, egalitarian, post-Enlightenment interest emerged in public health problems associated with urban squalor, deprivation, and crowding. The observations of Villermé in France and Virchow in Germany emphasized the association of diseases with urban conditions, poverty, and hazardous occupations (11, 12). In 1845, Engels described Manchester's factory-working masses as "pale, lank, narrow chested, hollow-eyed ghosts" (13, p. 128) afflicted with ricketts and scrofula. He documented a doubling in death rates between families living in the best and the worst housing.

Throughout the first half of the nineteenth century, the miasma theory of disease causation prevailed, tempered by minority support for the alternative idea of "contagion," first mooted in the sixteenth century (14).

TABLE 1. Four centuries of epidemiologic research: evolution of ideas about the causes of disease in populations

Period	Protagonists	Perspective
1600s	Graunt and Ramazzini	Basic description of patterns of disease mortality
1700s	Casal, Lind, Pott, and Baker	Specific causation of diseases
Early 1800s	Villermé, Virchow, Farr, Chadwick, and Engels	Social-environmental etiology Holistic ideas of the sanitationists
Mid–1800s	Semmelweiss, Snow, Holmes, Panum, and Budd	Transmissible "particulate" agents
1880s	Pasteur and Koch	Germ theory: specific etiology (Henle-Koch postulates)
Late 1800s–early 1900s	Takaki, Goldberger, and Funk	Micronutrient deficiencies as specific causes
	Rehn et al.	Specific causes of occupational diseases
	Galton and Pearson	Ideas of specific "genes" (and eugenics) appear
1920s–1930s	Frost, Greenwood, and Sydenstricker	Broader causal model: host, environment, agent; "crowd diseases"
1950s–1960s	Doll, Hill, Wynder, Kannel, Keys, et al.	Specific, multiple causes of chronic (noncommunicable) diseases
1980s–1990s	Susser, Rose, Pearce, Krieger, et al.	Emphasis on social causation of disease, population perspective

The manifest tendency of certain diseases such as influenza, cholera, and yellow fever to sweep over entire populations seemed to confirm that nonspecific miasmatic emanations from decaying organic matter were the cause. Accordingly, William Farr explained the marked district variations in cholera mortality within London in terms of housing quality, residential height above sea level, and general air quality (15). This was epidemiologic research that moved easily between population, neighborhood, and individual levels (1). Overall, a social and environmental holism in public health characterized the early 1800s.

Then, from midcentury in Britain, the application of Chadwick's "Sanitary Idea" foreshadowed a narrower, technical stratagem to banish miasmas by purifying the water and air. Hamlin (16) described this rise of sanitary engineering as the "degreening" of nineteenth century public health. Meanwhile, the accruing evidence of contagion, especially from Semmelweiss' studies of puerperal fever (17) and Snow's studies of cholera (18), challenged the miasma theory. Eventually, in the 1880s, the germ theory reoriented epidemiology toward the idea of specific causation: Diseases could each be understood in terms of a single causal infectious agent.

This powerful idea was reinforced by the discovery of certain occupational exposures as causes of cancer and by the implication of specific vitamin deficiencies in nutritional disorders. Meanwhile, early crude ideas about the human genetic determinants of individual constitutional "fitness" were boosted by the rediscovery of Mendel's work on particulate genetics in peas (19). So, here, in the early twentieth century was a world in which disease was caused by germs, carcinogens, vitamin deficiencies, and genes. Disease causation could now be interpreted in terms of proximate personal exposures and attributes.

However, epidemiologists (like humans everywhere) keep returning to the search for wider meaning and understanding. In the second quarter of this century, the triumphant germ theory was broadened to accommodate the interactive roles of environmental conditions and host susceptibility. In the United States in 1927, Wade Hampton Frost sought to "establish a theory" to explain the distribution of disease within populations (20). Greenwood (21) in England and Sydenstricker (22) in the United States wrote of "crowd diseases," the social environment, and social inequalities in health.

Since the 1950s, as infectious diseases receded, epidemiologists in developed countries have been preoccupied with chronic diseases of complex etiology. Faced with this diversity of diseases and risk factors, they adopted an essentially empirical approach. Numeric reasoning, based on statistical modeling, has been central to the effort. A growing preoccupation with the role of multiple proximate risk factors largely eclipsed ideas of social causation of disease. We have thus evolved a modern epidemiology that is adept at determining which individuals are at increased risk, but not at understanding disease distribution within and between populations. We have been busy reacting to our consumer society's procession of new, potentially hazardous exposures: mobile telephones, replacement estrogens, vitamin supplements, mad cows, photochemical smog, and endless new chemicals and drugs.

The explanation goes deeper, however. As also followed the rise of the germ theory, modern epidemiology's search for specific proximate causes has deflected us from social-contextual models of disease causation. It has changed the conceptual framework. Hence, the recent calls for restoring the population perspective, for recognizing that population history, culture, and social structure determine the level and internal distribution of disease risk (4, 5, 23, 24). Some argue that a theoretical "black box" positivist epidemiology should be recast within an "ecologic" paradigm attuned to population processes, interdependencies, and multilevel causality (1, 3). This proposed systems perspective is being reinforced by emerging ideas about the life-course evolution of chronic disease risk (25).

So epidemiology is edging, again, toward a more integrative view of the sources and distribution of disease. This time, we are countenancing a more ecologic view of how the social and environmental conditions of life influence population health. (Epidemiologists have long misused this word "ecologic," borrowed from sociology (26). Ecology is the formal study of the interrelations between groups of organisms, populations, and species and their surroundings. I here use the word liberally to refer to contexts characterized by interdependencies between individuals and groups of humans and their environments.) In seeking an epidemiology that integrates across macro-, meso-, and microlevels of causal analysis and deals with complex social and ecologic relations, we must understand the constraints that currently confine us.

"PROXIMATE" CONSTRAINTS ON MODERN EPIDEMIOLOGY

The mind-set and methods of modern epidemiology entail four types of proximate constraints upon our research agenda. They are:

1. Our preoccupation with proximate risk factors
2. Our focus on individual-level versus population-level influences on health
3. Our typically modular (time-windowed) view of how individuals undergo changes in risk status
4. The, as yet, unfamiliar challenge of scenario-based forecasting of health consequences of future, large-scale, social and environmental changes.

Figure 2 represents these four interrelated constraints. Epidemiology, shown as a little orb, is "imprisoned" at bottom left. Let us consider these four constraints in more detail.

Preoccupation with proximate risk factors

Most contemporary epidemiologic research focuses on proximate risk factors, that is, specific exposures, circumstances, or behaviors that are measurable at the individual level. During 5 decades, this has yielded many important new insights into chronic disease causation. With seemingly fewer large effects remaining to be discovered, however, such research is becoming less informative (1, 27, 28). Nevertheless, important findings continue to be made (29), in part reflecting improved measurement methods and the use of very large studies or meta-analyses (8, 30).

The preoccupation with seeking specific proximate risk factors has been disdainfully referred to as "risk factorology" (28, 31). The criticism is misleading; the fault is not in doing such studies, but in *only* doing

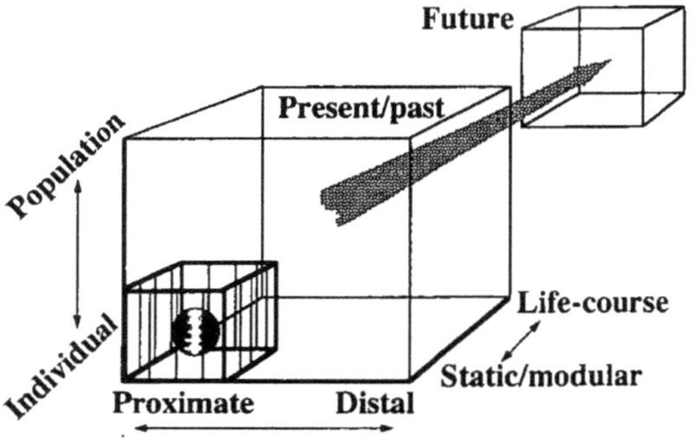

FIGURE 2. Epidemiology as "prisoner of the proximate": schematic representation of the four axes, along each of which much of modern epidemiology is constrained by its current concepts and methods.

such studies. We should also be looking upstream for a fuller account of disease causation within a population context; we must extend our focal length. Consider alcohol consumption and liver cirrhosis. The proximate "cause" of liver cirrhosis is the individual's drinking behavior—or the ethanol itself. However, we also wish to account for the within-population distribution of alcohol-related liver cirrhosis. Are there differences between generations, social classes, ethnic groups, or occupations? Are those differences due to subculture, peer pressure, commercial advertising, opportunity, or employment status?

How epidemiologists relate to that upstream category of question is influenced by whether we perceive the distal determination of disease as being part of either a linear causal chain or a systems-based causal web. The former model may tempt us to argue that, while it is the epidemiologist's task to define the downstream relation between alcohol consumption and disease, it is the separate task of social scientists working upstream to elucidate the determinants of drinking behavior and why it differs between population subgroups (32). The latter, systems-based, approach envisions a causal web that extends inward, via multiple paths, from the encircling realms of the population's history, culture, and socioeconomic relations, through residential conditions and subpopulation attitudes, to the inner proximate factors of individual behaviors and exposures and their biomedical manifestations (33). Causal processes within this web are not necessarily linear and sequential, but may involve interactions and feedbacks. We may not, as epidemiologists, like this complexity, but life is like that; it comprises complex systems.

Attuning epidemiologic methods to social complexity. Kaufman and Cooper argue that "the traditional epidemiologic method is ill-suited for considering social quantities as risk factors" (34). We should be seeking a systems-based model of the observable world, they say, and not statistically estimating risks by reference to what, in this context, entails an untenable (unobservable) "counterfactual." For example, we can consider a smoker who, we can imagine, does not smoke (i.e., the idealized unexposed "counterfactual") as being otherwise still the same person (thereby guiding our selection of an appropriate unexposed comparison group). However, we cannot consider that a socially disadvantaged person, if no longer socially disadvantaged, would otherwise be the same person, since many other complex determinants and concomitants of socioeconomic status would also be changed.

With race and gender, they argue, the counterfactuals become even more meaningless. If we seek to explain the differences in health status between Black and White Americans in proximate biomedical terms, then we might choose to treat socioeconomic status as a potential confounder that requires routine adjustment, like age and sex. However, this naively assumes that the "risk" attributes of socioeconomic status are independent of those associated with race, including the experience of racism at individual, institutional, and societal levels (35). Kaufman et al. (35) therefore advocate more creative approaches to causal explanation in social epidemiology, drawing on the concepts of infectious disease epidemiology and systems analysis. Using multilevel or pathway modeling, and collaborating with other disciplines, epidemiologists can then develop quantitative and structural analyses of how social variables affect health outcomes.

Consider the widening social class gradient in coronary heart disease (CHD) mortality in Britain over the past 2 decades (36, 37). This divergence reflects a much sharper decline in CHD deaths in the upper classes than in the lower classes. The principal challenge is to understand why, in terms of material circumstances, social relations, knowledge, and behaviors, this class-related gap in the risk of dying from CHD has widened (38). Why is the class-related CHD gradient evident in northern European countries but not in France, Switzerland, and Mediterranean-Europe countries, where, instead, the class gradient is most evident for cancers and gastrointestinal diseases (39)? Explanations for such patterns cannot come from exclusively downstream research. From the experience of social epidemiology, we need to learn how to conceptualize and analyze this complex of proximal and distal influences on health outcomes (1, 33).

Epidemiologists must, of course, continue to study proximate causes. Further important causal relations will be revealed at that level. However, if that is *all* we do, ignoring wider social-environmental causes, then we risk reinforcing inefficient programs of local "health promotion" accessible only to the better-educated, better-resourced stratum of society (40). Effective and equitable social interventions require an understanding of the contextual determinants of health risk distribution within the population.

Rose's "sick population" perspective. There is another, related issue. We may wish to distinguish between factors that explain the occurrence of disease in individuals within a specific population and those that account for the overall population rate of the disease. Geoffrey Rose (41) pointed out that a factor that is an important cause of disease in *individuals* within a population may differ from one that primarily determines the disease rate within the *whole population*.

Rose illustrated his argument with risk factors from the familiar downstream catalogue, each of which could be meaningfully measured at either the individual or the population level. Consider an example in which population A has a higher rate of CHD than does population B. Within each population, individuals who smoke have twice the CHD risk of nonsmokers. Nevertheless, the prevalence of smoking is identical in each population and, hence, cannot account for the between-population difference in CHD rates. However, population A has a generalized higher consumption of saturated fat than does population B. Hence, the between-population difference in CHD rates is explained by differences in diet, not smoking, even though smoking is the dominant risk factor at the individual level.

That example would be equally plausible if we interchanged smoking and dietary fat. Often, however, the factors that operate at individual and group levels are not interchangeable, being of qualitatively different scale and content. This brings us to the second category of constraint.

Levels of causal analysis: individual versus population

Implicit in the focus on proximate risk factors is an assumption that the individual is the site of etiologic action. We thus assume that, while social and environmental influences may originate on a broader front upstream, they ultimately become manifest, as risk factors, at the level of the individual. The individual, therefore, is viewed as the natural unit of epidemiologic observation. Larger-scale variables that affect whole groups or populations, such as poverty and cultural disruption, are only important because they translate into individual-level risk factors. Poverty affects diet, cultural disruption breeds alcoholism, and so on.

This population/individual distinction, however, needs careful consideration. Are we, as in the previous section, merely distinguishing between upstream social contexts and their downstream proximate manifestations? Or is there a category of risk factor that, in some collective way, influences the health of the population at large via processes that have no direct downstream manifestation? Further, complex entities such as poverty, for example, can have very different meanings and can measure qualitatively different constructs at the individual and population levels (42).

Susser has recently reminded us that the subject matter of epidemiologic research is "ecological in the original biological sense of organisms in a multilevel interactive environment" (1, p. 609). The sociologist Émile Durkheim, in the late nineteenth century, was one of the first to argue that society's characteristics at large can affect a health outcome (43). The suicide rate, he said, was not simply the aggregate of individual suicidal tendencies. Rather, it reflected properties of the population: the underlying social values, the pattern of social relations, and the moral significance accorded to the act of suicide. The usual individualistic accounts, he said, were therefore deficient.

Consider the well-known example of herd immunity in relation to infectious disease (44). If, within a population, sufficient of the potential contacts of a primary infectious case are immune, then the average number of secondary cases will be too few for the infection to spread. By definition, it is only a population that can have herd immunity; it has no direct, corresponding representation at the individual level. It is this constitutional property of the population that determines whether the infectious disease can be sustained within the population. Therefore, there is an interdependence of risk between the unit members of the population, reflecting the prior experience of that population as a whole.

Indeed, infectious disease epidemiologists well understand that the individual-level risk of infectious disease often reflects population-level characteristics (45). For example, the sexual spread of human immunodeficiency virus within a population is strongly determined by the *pattern* of sexual activity within the population, which, in turn, reflects economic relations, demographic mobility, and cultural traditions. An individual's risk, for a given number of sex partners, depends on who is having sex with whom and on the prevalence of the infection within that contact network. Individuals have sex; populations have patterns of sex. Both are risk factors, but at different levels.

The distribution of income within a population is another interesting population characteristic: Individuals have a personal income; populations have an income distribution. At the individual level, income has a well-known relation to health: Poor individuals die younger. Davey-Smith et al. (46, 47) have recently demonstrated a clear gradient in mortality across 14 income classes in US Blacks and Whites separately. Low absolute personal income, we presume, affects individual health principally via material deprivation.

At the population level, however, the relation between wealth and health is different. Wilkinson (48) and others have demonstrated, in developed countries, that differences in average life expectancy *between* countries show little correlation with average income. Rather, average life expectancy correlates inversely with the extent of within-population income inequality. This relation reflects health experiences across the income scale and is not a simple arithmetic consequence of extremely poor health in a deprived minority. Nor is it explained by interpopulation differences in levels of public expenditure on health and welfare (49).

At a subnational scale, Kaplan et al. (49) have shown for the US states that the inverse correlation between average state income and mortality is entirely accounted for by differences in within-state income inequality.

Something about a population's internal income relativities thus appears to affect overall population health independently of any effect of average personal income. Recently, in a study in 39 US states, Kawachi et al. (50) showed that, in states where income differences are greater, people experience their social environment as more hostile; they are less likely to join community organizations and more likely to mistrust other people. Those researchers conclude that the gap between rich and poor affects social organization and that the resulting loss of "social capital" may impair the population's health.

How is this effect mediated? Some of these investigators invoke individual-level physiologically based explanations via the neuroendocrine response to status deprivation, insecurity, and chronic stress. Studies in primate colonies indicate that individual-level measures of status-related stress, cortisol levels, and atherogenesis are positively associated (51, 52). Recent epidemiologic evidence suggests that the rate of progression of atherosclerosis is inversely proportional to socioeconomic status (53) and occupational reward:effort ratio (54).

So, is this search for individual-level explanation merely biological realism? Or does it reflect the hegemonic power of individual-based biomedical thinking? Might it be that lessened income inequality reduces rates of alienation, violent crime, and infectious disease risk behaviors in ways that confer protection on everyone? Perhaps the generalized relative paucity of material assets (including health care facilities) in unequal societies (55) and, indeed, the legacies of social, cultural, and political history of those unequal societies impair their health prospects (56). We are not well placed to answer these questions because we have not yet undertaken the types of multilevel analysis that could elucidate coexistent and interactive influences at the population and individual levels (33). Perhaps part of the widely reported individual-level inverse association between income and mortality actually results from the group-level experiences of subpopulations experiencing relative deprivation. The debate continues.

The bleak mortality experience of central and eastern Europe in recent decades raises other population-level questions. During the 1970s and 1980s, as life expectancies increased in western Europe, central and eastern European countries experienced increasing mortality from many causes, including heart disease, stroke, respiratory infections, accidents, and violence, all especially in men (57). The striking east-west divergence in death rates during those decades cannot be explained simply in terms of individual-level risk behaviors (such as smoking and drinking) or exposure to environmental pollutants (58). Watson (58) postulates that the generalized state control of daily life, poverty of community networks, and suppression of individual initiative induced a collective learned helplessness and community disengagement, while reinforcing inward-looking traditional family values (59). This loss of social capital eroded the traditional role of men more than that of women and created conditions that jeopardized health. In post-Soviet Russia, social frustration and disintegration appear to have underlain the dramatic surge in premature male mortality attributable to excessive alcohol consumption during 1990–1995 (60). Regional analysis shows that the local decline in life expectancy was clearly correlated with local labor turnover, recorded crime rates, and unequally distributed income (61). Rapid social and economic change apparently disrupts stabilizing social-behavioral patterns, leading to self-destructive behaviors.

There is other historical evidence that social, cultural, and political characteristics of a society influence susceptibility to disease. After European settlement, the emergence of CHD in indigenous Amerindian, Maori, and Australian Aboriginal populations reflected the social structures of both the indigenes and the settler populations (62). More generally, changes in the life expectancy of the native population was influenced by the social and political structures of settler populations and by the form of interaction between populations.

These examples underscore the importance of studying the role of population-level influences on health. Such factors, intrinsically difficult to characterize, are neither the mere aggregation of individual risk factors nor the directly connected upstream determinants of proximate factors. Rather, there appear to be constitutional properties of populations, such as herd immunity, income inequality, and social morale, that affect health processes at a supra-individual level, in addition to any manifestations of risk that they might induce at the individual level.

Life-stage versus life-course models of risk acquisition

A third constraint on our thinking is that much epidemiologic research implies a static, modular view of the acquisition of risk. In caricature, we take 1,000 healthy adults, add 10 cigarettes per day or a regular dose of air pollution, and then see by how much the health status changes. This approach is not necessarily wrong, but it often gives incomplete or misleading answers. Much risk of disease, especially noninfectious disease, evolves over a lifetime via cumulative and interactive processes.

An intriguing example comes from research done in a rural population in The Gambia, West Africa. Survey data show that the average weight of adult women in that population fluctuates seasonally, being 5–7 percent greater in the harvest season. An historical survival analysis of children born around midcentury revealed that those children born during the harvest season experienced distinctly better survival in adulthood than did those born in the nonharvest season. By the fifth decade of life and with no survival difference apparent before age 15 years, survival in the two groups was approximately 65 and 45 percent, respectively (63). Something to do with perinatal nutrition has profoundly affected long-term biological robustness.

Asthma offers another example. For several decades, we have sought immediate environmental causes: air pollutants, environmental tobacco smoke, and aeroallergens. Yes, many of these exposures probably trigger attacks in susceptible persons. However, why has the disease increased severalfold in western populations over the last 25 years? Why, in ecologic terms, are we producing successive generations of children with increasing susceptibility to asthma? Perhaps early childhood experiences (infections, contact with environmental bacteria, vaccinations, etc.) affect immune system programming along allergic or nonallergic pathways (64).

Over the past decade, considerable evidence has accrued that biological processes and experiences in early life, especially fetal life, affect lifelong susceptibilities to various adult disease processes: cardiovascular disease, diabetes, immune disorders, respiratory diseases, and others. Research along these lines in Britain, especially by Barker (65) and others, has greatly extended Forsdahl's work in Norway in the 1970s and, indeed, that of certain British nutritional scientists in the 1930s (66, 67). These ideas need to be subjected to critical tests of replication (68) and require biological corroboration from laboratory and clinical sciences. Further, the public health ("attributable risk") significance of these potentially important early-life influences on adult disease risks should also be assessed.

Inevitably, many of these dynamic causal models are complex. The relative importance of early-life and adult-life influences varies between categories of disease outcome. A cohort study of Scottish men found that the risk of stroke and stomach cancer mortality depended primarily on childhood socioeconomic conditions, whereas heart disease mortality was influenced by conditions in both childhood and adulthood (69). Early-life experiences may critically affect some heart disease risk factors, such as triglyceride levels, while cholesterol level and blood pressure are affected by both early and adult lives (70). Further, the combination of being a small baby and a large adult—a combination that maximizes the metabolic mismatch between life stages—markedly elevates the risk of hypertension (figure 3) and of cardiovascular disease mortality (71, 72).

A life-course model of disease etiology is thus evolving, distinct from the static "adult lifestyle" model. It posits coexistent, often interactive, chains of biological and social influences that underpin the development of adult disease risk (73). These life course-based insights, intrinsically scientifically interesting, also have important implications for disease prevention, of course. This line of research will require various new data-analytic techniques, such as repeated-measures techniques, multistate modeling, and adaptive genetic algorithms.

Forecasting health risks under conditions of global change

The fourth constraint is our confinement, as essentially empirical scientists, to working in the present and recent past tenses. We are not yet well attuned to forecasting future health risks in relation to potentially important future "exposures." Indeed, the possibility of major adverse systemic environmental change has not previously pressed upon us.

Because of the combined weight of human numbers, economic activity, and technology, we are starting to change the conditions of life on Earth. Such a change will affect the global patterns of human health and disease (1, 74). For the past 2 centuries, epidemiologists have lived and worked in a world in which large-scale, natural life-support systems have not been perceptibly perturbed and weakened. We no longer live in such a world. We must therefore now think beyond the traditional striving for incremental health gains within populations; we must also address the issue of the *sustainability* of population health against the prospect of a deteriorating natural environment.

The two best-known global environmental changes are the accumulation of heat-trapping greenhouse gases in the lower atmosphere (troposphere) and the depletion of stratospheric ozone caused by ozone-destroying gases. Authoritative international scientific reviews have semiquantitatively characterized the anticipated, mostly adverse health consequences of these global change processes (75, 76). These, however, are only part of a longer list of newly recognized, global and worldwide environmental changes (77). Other major changes include losses of biodiversity, depletion of supplies of freshwater, degradation of food-producing systems on land and at sea, and the worldwide dissemination of persistent organic chemicals, each entailing potentially great risks to human health (78).

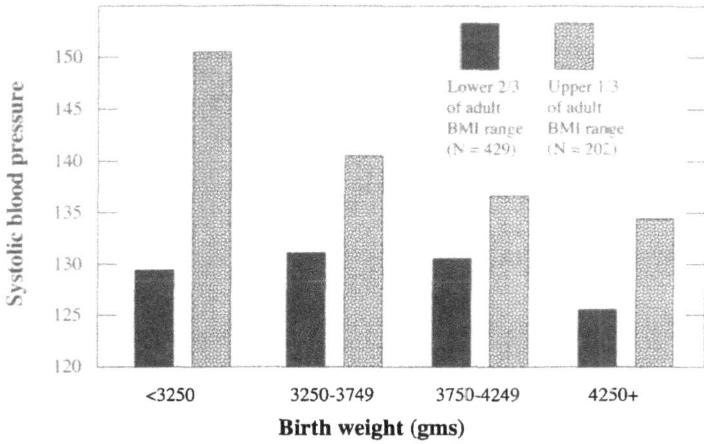

FIGURE 3. Relation of systolic blood pressure at age 50 years in Swedish men to, jointly, birth weight and adult relative body weight (71). The relation is similar for diastolic blood pressure.

Is the role of epidemiology essentially reactive? Is it limited to helping society understand and tidy up its public health messes after they occur and, thus, to reducing the likelihood of recurrence? Hopefully not. Rather, as the scale of humankind's impact on large biophysical systems increases, triggering unfamiliar global-scale environmental changes, epidemiologists should acquire new skills in anticipatory, scenario-based, health risk assessment (79). The role of such assessment is primarily to assist human society to foresee and understand the range of likely consequences of current and emerging economic, social, and environmental trends (80). Only by entering the rapidly developing arena of "futures studies" (81), rich in interdisciplinary challenge, can epidemiologists engage in health risk assessment that can guide the development of proactive policies to constrain these large-scale environmental changes.

Research into how future changes in world climate, in ambient ultraviolet radiation exposure, and in other large-scale environmental changes are likely to influence health risks is still in an early developmental phase. There are two major categories of research needs:

1. Empirical studies into the relation between relevant environmental variations (e.g., meteorologic variables and ultraviolet radiation levels) and human health outcomes. Such studies can serve two purposes: the extension of knowledge about these causal relations and the detection of early health impacts of these environmental changes. As time passes, the relevance of the latter use increases.
2. Integrated mathematical modeling of the future health outcomes in relation to the forecast scenarios of environmental change (i.e., scenario-based health risk assessment).

A balance is needed between empirical and predictive research. The latter, relying substantially on integrated mathematical modeling, is important for assessing the range of plausible outcomes (for example, geographic shifts in the potential transmissibility of vector-borne infections, changes in regional food security and levels of malnutrition, and increases in skin cancer incidence rates) and also for revealing gaps in knowledge about relations and processes (79). The former, empirical research will fill those gaps and enhance our capacity to forecast future scenario-based health impacts. Empirical studies of the health consequences of recent variations in exposure—for example, El Niño climatic episodes (82)—will yield further understanding of these environment-health relations.

The advent of these macroscale environmental risks to human health means that a future-oriented interdisciplinary research effort is required in which epidemiologists play a substantive role.

CONCLUSIONS

As we enter a new century, we epidemiologists must broaden our causal models and recognize the important ecologic dimensions of social-environmental influences on health and disease. Last century, epidemiologists recognized that the unhygienic conditions and socioeconomic disparities of urban-industrial life were the major cause of disease. Our modern preoccupation has been to understand disease occurrence in individuals in terms of consumer behaviors, individual exposures, metabolic factors, and genes. The advent, early next century, of "bar-coded" individual genotypes on microchips may yet further distract us from the task of managing our social and natural environments.

The landscape is changing, however. Infectious diseases continue their apparent reemergence (83). There are increasing pressures on the wider environment from burgeoning human numbers and economic activity. We are gaining new insights into the complex social and environmental systems that are the context for human health, thinking more about population health in ecologic terms, and extending our spatial-temporal frame of reference. The constraints of "the proximate" upon epidemiology are thus being loosened as we approach century's end.

ACKNOWLEDGMENTS

Keynote paper presented to the Annual Conference of the Society for Epidemiologic Research, Chicago, Illinois, June 1998.

Many of the ideas in this paper have evolved from discussions with David Leon, with whom the author teaches a Masters-level unit entitled "Emerging Themes in Epidemiology." We have each benefited from discussions with our student classes. Helpful comments were also received from George Davey-Smith, Alistair Woodward, and John Lynch.

REFERENCES

1. Susser M. Does risk factor epidemiology put epidemiology at risk? Peering into the future. J Epidemiol Community Health 1998;52:608–11.
2. Rothman KJ, Poole C. Our conscientious objection to the epidemiology wars. J Epidemiol Community Health 1998;52:1–2.
3. Susser M, Susser E. Choosing a future for epidemiology. I. Eras and paradigms. Am J Public Health 1996;86:668–73.
4. Krieger N, Zierler S. What explains the public's health? A call for epidemiologic theory. Epidemiology 1996;7:107–9.
5. Pearce N. Traditional epidemiology, modern epidemiology, and public health. Am J Public Health 1996;86:678–83.
6. Rothman KJ, Adami H-O, Trichopoulos D. Should the mission of epidemiology include the eradication of poverty? Lancet 1998;352:810–12.
7. McMichael AJ. "Molecular epidemiology": new pathway or new travelling companion? Am J Epidemiol 1994;140:1–11.
8. Graunt J. Natural and political observations mentioned in a following index, and made upon the Bills of Mortality. London, England: Printed by T. Rycroft for John Martin, J. Allestry, and T. Dicas, 1662. Reprinted by Wilcox WF, ed. Baltimore, MD: Johns Hopkins University Press, 1939.
9. Hudson RP. Concepts of disease in the West. In: Kiple KF, ed. The Cambridge world history of human disease. Cambridge, England: Cambridge University Press, 1993:45–52.
10. Ramazzini B. De morbis artificum. On the diseases of workers. Published in 1700.
11. Coleman W. Death is a social disease: public health and political economy in early industrial France. Madison, WI: University of Wisconsin Press, 1982.
12. Ackernecht EH. Rudolf Virchow: doctor, statesman, anthropologist. Madison, WI: University of Wisconsin Press, 1953.
13. Engels F. The condition of the working class in England. (First edition, 1845). Harmondsworth, England: Penguin, 1987.
14. Fracastor, Hieronymus. De Contagione et Contagiosis Morbis et Eorum Curatione. (Originally published in Venice in 1546.) Wright WC, translator. New York, NY: G. P. Putnam's Sons, 1930.
15. Farr W. Vital statistics: a memorial volume of selections from the reports and writing of William Farr. Humphreys NA, ed. London, England: Office of the Sanitary Institute, 1885.
16. Hamlin C. Public health and social justice in the age of Chadwick, Britain, 1800–1864. Cambridge, England: Cambridge University Press, 1998.
17. Semmelweiss IP. The etiology, the concept and prophylaxis of childbed fever. Published in 1861. Translated and republished in Medical Classics 1941;5:350-773.
18. Snow J. On the mode of communication of cholera. 2nd ed. London, England: Churchill, 1855. Reproduced in Snow on cholera. New York, NY: Commonwealth Fund, 1936.
19. Pearson K. The intensity of natural selection in man. Proc Roy Soc B 1912;85:469–76.
20. Frost WH. Epidemiology. In: Maxcy KF, ed. Papers of Wade Hampton Frost, MD: a contribution to epidemiologic method. New York, NY: Commonwealth Fund, 1941:439–542.
21. Greenwood M. Epidemics and crowd diseases: an introduction to the study of epidemiology. London, England: Williams & Northgate, Ltd., 1935.
22. Sydenstricker E. Health and environment. New York, NY: McGraw Hill Co., 1933.
23. Loomis D, Wing S. Is molecular epidemiology a germ theory for the end of the twentieth century? Int J Epidemiol 1990;19:1–3.
24. Beaglehole R, Bonita R. Public health at the crossroads. Cambridge, England: Cambridge University Press, 1997.
25. Kuh D, Ben-Shlomo Y. A life course approach to chronic disease epidemiology. Oxford, England: Oxford University Press, 1997.
26. Goodman LA. Ecological regressions and the behaviour of individuals. Am Soc Rev 1953;18:663–4.
27. Taubes G. Epidemiology faces its limits. Science 1995; 269:164–9.
28. Pearce N, McKinlay J. Back to the future in epidemiology and public health. J Clin Epidemiol 1998;51:643–6.
29. Trichopoulos D. The future of epidemiology. BMJ 1996; 313:436–7.
30. Doll R. Weak associations in epidemiology: importance, detection, and interpretation. J Epidemiol 1996;6:S11–S20.
31. Skrabanek P. The emptiness of the black box. Epidemiology 1994;5:553–5.
32. Mackenbach JP. Multilevel ecoepidemiology and parsimony. J Epidemiol Community Health 1998;52:614–15.
33. Krieger N. Epidemiology and the web of causation: has anyone seen the spider? Soc Sci Med 1994;39:887–903.
34. Kaufman JS, Cooper RS. Seeking causal explanations in social epidemiology. Am J Epidemiol (in press).
35. Kaufman JS, Cooper RS, McGee DL. Socioeconomic status and health in Blacks and Whites: The problem of residual confounding and the resiliency of race. Epidemiology 1997;8:621–8.
36. Marmot M. Improvement of social environment to improve health. Lancet 1998;351:57–60.
37. Phillimore P, Beattie A, Townsend O. Widening inequality of

health in northern England, 1981–91. BMJ 1994;308:1125–8.
38. Vandenbroucke JP. New public health and old rhetoric. BMJ 1994;308:994–5.
39. Kunst AE, Groenhoef F, Mackenbach JP, and the EU Working Group on Socioeconomic Inequalities in Health. Occupational class and cause-specific mortality in middle aged men in 11 European countries: comparison of population based studies. BMJ 1998;316:1636–42.
40. Woodward A, Kawachi I. Why should we reduce health inequalities? Reasons for acting on the social, cultural and economic factors that cause ill-health. National Health Committee: health determinants programme background paper 2. Wellington, New Zealand: Ministry of Health, 1998.
41. Rose G. Sick individuals and sick populations? Int J Epidemiol 1985;14:32–8.
42. Schwartz S. The fallacy of the ecological fallacy: the potential misuse of a concept and the consequences. Am J Public Health 1994;84:819–24.
43. Durkheim E. Suicide. A study in sociology. New York, NY: Free Press, 1951.
44. Fine PEM. Herd immunity: history, theory, practice. Epidemiol Rev 1993;15:265–302.
45. Koopman JS, Longini IM Jr. The ecological effects of individual exposures and nonlinear disease dynamics in populations. Am J Public Health 1994;84:836–42.
46. Davey-Smith G, Neaton JD, Wentworth D, et al. Socioeconomic differentials in mortality risk among men screened for the Multiple Risk Factor Intervention Trial. Part I. Results for 300,685 white men. Am J Public Health 1996;86:486–96.
47. Davey-Smith G, Neaton JD, Wentworth D, et al. Socioeconomic differentials in mortality risk among men screened for the Multiple Risk Factor Intervention Trial. Part II. Results for 20,224 black men. Am J Public Health 1996;86:497–504.
48. Wilkinson RG. Income distribution and life expectancy. BMJ 1992;304:165–8.
49. Kaplan GA, Pamuk ER, Lynch JW, et al. Inequality in income and mortality in the United States: analysis of mortality and potential pathways. BMJ 1996;312:999–1003.
50. Kawachi I, Kennedy BP, Lochner K, et al. Social capital, income inequality, and mortality. Am J Public Health 1997;87:1491–8.
51. Sapolsky RM. Endocrinology alfresco: psychoendocrine studies of wild baboons. Recent Prog Horm Res 1993;48:437–68.
52. Shively CA, Laird KL, Anton RF. Behaviour and physiology of social stress and depression in female cynomolgus monkeys. Biol Psychiatry 1997;41:871–82.
53. Lynch J, Kaplan GA, Salonen R, et al. Socioeconomic status and progression of carotid atherosclerosis. Prospective evidence from the Kuopio Ischemic Heart Disease Risk Factor Study. Arterioscler Thromb Vasc Biol 1997;17:513–19.
54. Lynch J, Krause N, Kaplan GA, et al. Workplace demands, economic reward, and progression of carotid atherosclerosis. Circulation 1997;96:302–7.
55. Gough I, Thomas T. Why do levels of human welfare vary among nations? Int J Health Serv 1994;24:715–48.
56. Lynch JW, Kaplan GA. Understanding how inequality in the distribution of income affects health. J Health Psychol 1997;2:297–314.
57. Bobak M, Marmot M. East-West mortality divide and its potential explanations: proposed research agenda. BMJ 1996;312:421–5.
58. Watson P. Explaining rising mortality among men in Eastern Europe. Soc Sci Med 1995;41:923–34.
59. Hertzman C, Kelly S, Bobak M, eds. East-west life expectancy gap in Europe: environmental and non-environmental determinants. *Series 2. Environment—no. 19. Dordrecht*, the Netherlands: Kluwer, 1996.
60. Leon D, Chenet L, Shkolnikov VM, et al. Huge variations in Russian mortality rates 1984–94: artefact, alcohol, or what? Lancet 1997;350:383–8.
61. Walberg P, McKee M, Shkolnikov V, et al. Economic change, crime, and mortality crisis in Russia: regional analysis. BMJ 1998;317:312–18.
62. Kunitz SJ. Disease and social diversity: the European impact on the health of non-Europeans. Oxford, England: Oxford University Press, 1994.
63. Moore SE, Cole TJ, Poskitt EM, et al. Season of birth predicts mortality in rural Gambia. Nature 1997;388:434–6.
64. Holt PG, Sly PD. Allergic respiratory disease: strategic targets for primary prevention during childhood. Thorax 1997;52:1–4.
65. Barker DJP. Mothers, babies and disease in later life. London, England: BMJ Publishing, 1994.
66. Forsdahl A. Living conditions in childhood and subsequent development of risk factors for arteriosclerotic heart disease. J Epidemiol Community Health 1978;32:34–7.
67. Kuh D, Davey-Smith G. When is mortality risk determined? Historical insights into a current debate. Soc Hist Med 1993;6:101–23.
68. Paneth N, Susser M. Early origin of coronary heart disease (the "Barker hypothesis"). BMJ 1995;310:411–12.
69. Smith GD, Hart C, Blane D, et al. Adverse socioeconomic conditions in childhood and cause-specific adult mortality: prospective observational study. BMJ 1998;316:1631–5.
70. Davey-Smith G. Socioeconomic differentials. In: Kuh D, Ben-Shlomo Y, eds. A life course approach to chronic disease epidemiology. Oxford, England: Oxford University Press, 1997:242–73.
71. Leon DA, Koupilova I, Lithell HO, et al. Failure to realise growth potential in utero and adult obesity in relation to blood pressure in 50 year old Swedish men. Br Med J 1996; 312:401–6.
72. Frankel SJ, Elwood P, Sweetnam P, et al. Birth weight, body mass index in middle age and incident coronary heart disease. Lancet 1996;348:1478–80.
73. Kuh D, Ben-Shlomo Y, eds. A life course approach to chronic disease epidemiology. Oxford England: Oxford University Press, 1997.
74. McMichael AJ, Bolin B, Costanza R, et al. Globalization and the sustainability of health: an ecological perspective. BioScience 1999;49:205–10.
75. Intergovernmental Panel on Climate Change (IPCC). Second assessment report. Climate change 1995. Vol. I. New York, NY: Cambridge University Press, 1996.
76. United Nations Environment Programme (Ozone Secretariat). Environmental effects of ozone depletion: 1998 assessment. Nairobi, Kenya: UN Environment Programme, 1998.
77. McMichael AJ. The impact of global environmental change upon human health: a conceptual and scientific challenge. Int J Epidemiol 1993;22:1–8.
78. McMichael AJ. Planetary overload. Global environmental change and the health of the human species. Cambridge, England: Cambridge University Press, 1993.
79. McMichael AJ. Integrated assessment of health risks from global environmental change: prospects and limitations. Environ Modelling Assessment 1997;2:129–37.
80. McMichael AJ, Haines A. Global climate change: the potential effects on health. BMJ 1997;315:805–9.
81. Bell W. Foundations of futures studies. Human science for a new era. Vols. 1 and 2. New Brunswick, NJ: Transaction Publishers, 1997.
82. Bouma MJ, van der Kaay HJ. The El Niño southern oscillation and the historic malaria epidemics on the Indian subcontinent and Sri Lanka: an early warning system for future epidemics? Trop Med Int Health 1996;1:86–96.
83. World Health Organization. The world health report 1996. Fighting disease, fostering development. Geneva, Switzerland: World Health Organization, 1996.

END OF REPRINT B

Prisoners of the Proximate: Loosening the Constraints on Epidemiology in an Age of Change

ANTHONY J. MCMICHAEL

PART 2

HEALTHY WORKERS

REPRINT C

Standardized Mortality Ratios and the 'Healthy Worker Effect': Scratching Beneath the Surface

ANTHONY J. MCMICHAEL

McMichael, A.J. 1976. Standardized mortality ratios and the 'healthy worker effect': scratching beneath the surface. *Journal of Occupational Medicine* 18, 165–8

Pages: 73 to 80

Published with permission of Wolters Kluwer Health.

Standardized Mortality Ratios and the "Healthy Worker Effect": Scratching Beneath the Surface

A. J. McMichael, M.D., Ph.D.

The age-standardized mortality ratio (SMR) is a frequently used summary index of mortality in occupational epidemiologic studies. By expressing the observed mortality experience of the occupational study population relative to the mortality that would otherwise by expected (in the absence of any mortality hazard within that occupational environment), an evaluative measure of the force of mortality is obtained.

Certain basic limitations of the SMR have been discussed elsewhere. Firstly, since the SMR computation involves an indirect age-adjustment procedure,[1] hence SMR's calculated for two or more study populations, although using the same standard population death rates for calculating expected deaths, cannot themselves be directly compared to one another.[2]

Secondly, the acual numeric magnitude of the SMR depends directly on the choice of standard population. Many factors other than the occupational environment influence mortality, and yet only one such factor (albeit a major one) is controlled for in the computation of the SMR, namely, age. This situation is exemplified by the somewhat inappropriate, but convenient, comparison of an industrial working population with the general population. This latter population, which includes sick and disabled persons, is usually at greater mortality risk than a population of active workers healthy enough to have been (and to remain) employable. If working in a safe environment, such a population of active workers has been variously estimated to have a mortality risk 60%-90% that of the general population. This difference in mortality risk, due to selection forces, has been described as the "healthy worker effect".[3] An epidemiologic comparison of a working population with the general community must take account of this effect.

A third limitation of the SMR is that it is a measure of the average relative mortality of what is usually a heterogeneous study population. As a summary index of population mortality it necessarily glosses over differences in the mortality experience of various sub-groups within the population. Now, a primary purpose of occupational epidemiologic studies is to compare the mortality experience of subgroups of workers exposed to different physico-chemical agents, or working in different jobs. However, there may also be major differences in mortality experience between subgroups differentiated by criteria other than work exposure. That is, the healthy worker effect may not apply equally throughout the study population. Therefore, if one attempts to improve the meaningfulness of an SMR by adjusting for the healthy worker effect, allowance must be made for variation in this effect between different age groups, different races, different work-status (active, inactive, retired, etc.) groups, different periods of observation, and different causes of death. Thus, the application of a constant 'adjustment factor (say .90, as recently suggested by Goldsmith[4]) will, in some circumstances, produce misleading results.

This article presents illustrative examples from a variety of occupational epidemiologic studies, to demonstrate the variation in healthy worker effect among different subgroups of workers. In each of the following examples, the standard population, with whose mortality the mortality of the occupational population is compared, is the national United States population.

Discussion

When a population of active and retired workers, embracing a large age-range, is followed for a number of years, the SMR is usually higher in the older age-bands. Figure 1 illustrates this trend, showing the SMR's in four successive age-bands within a population of 6678 male rubber workers, aged 40 or more Jan. 1, 1964 and followed for ten years. (The composition and follow-up of this study population have been described elsewhere.[5])

The SMR for the full age-range studied, 40-84, is 98. For the active employment age-range, 40-64, the SMR is 87; whereas for the older, post-retirement age-range, 65-84, it is 103. Within the 40-64 age-range, the SMR increases from 81 (ages 40-54) to 89 (ages 55-64). Likewise, in the post-retirement years, the SMR continues to increase, from 95 (ages 65-74) to 113 (ages 75-84).

The explanation for this gradient has several facets, partly over-lapping. In terms of pathologic processes, the diseases causing excess mortality in this population are mostly long-term or chronic (e.g. cancers, chronic lung disease) occurring only after a sufficient period of exposure and/or time since first exposure and therefore most evident at older ages.

In terms of the healthy worker effect, younger workers are

Dr. McMichael is associated with the Department of Epidemiology, and Occupational Health Studies Group, School of Public Health, University of North Carolina, Chapel Hill, NC 27514.

Presented at the 60th Annual Meeting of the American Occupational Medical Association, American Industrial Health Conference, San Francisco, April 14-17, 1975.

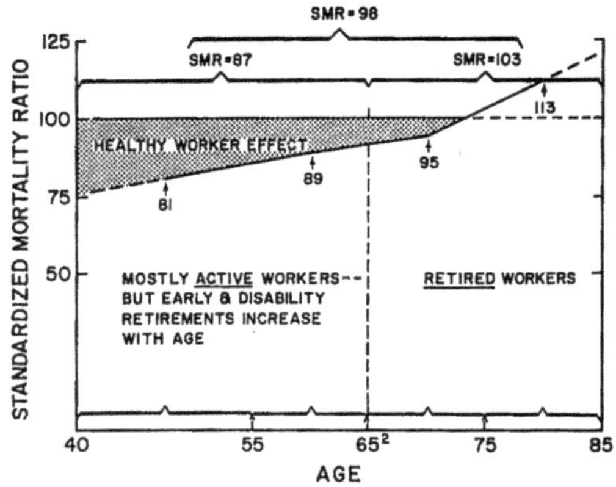

1. Expected deaths calculated from 1968 U.S. male age-specific death rates within 5-year age-bands.
2. Normal retirement occurs at age 65.

Fig 1. — Decline in healthy worker effect with age, male rubber workers.

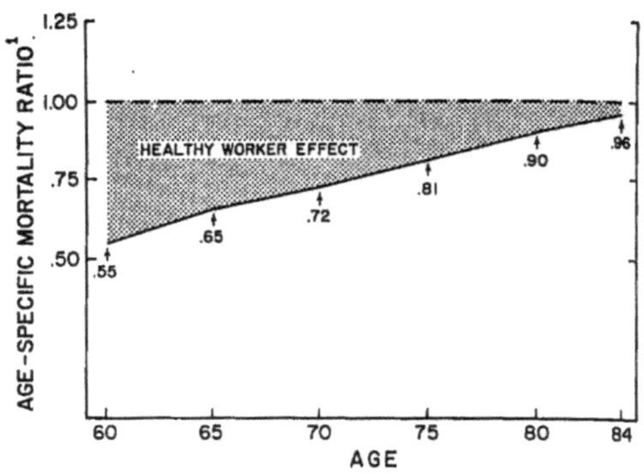

1. Ratio of q_x values for actuarially-defined population of non-disabled industrial retirees, 1968-72, to U.S. males, 1968.

Fig 3. — Further evidence of declining carry-over of the healthy worker effect in post retirement age range.

least distant from the time of initial selection (i.e. hiring on) and are therefore most likely to demonstrate the survival advantage resulting from their initial better-than-community-average health status. In addition, within the age-range 40-64, workers developing discomforting illnesses are most likely to voluntarily extend the selection process by leaving the industry, if still young enough to have the emotional,mental and financial independence necessary to learn a new job or trade. The SMR for the younger years, 40-54, therefore remains low. However, older workers in this 40-64 age-range, if unhealthy, are more likely to either stay on in less demanding jobs (e.g. janitoring) or take an early or disability retirement and thus remain on the company's pension register. The SMR for ages 55-64, in Figure 1, is thus based on a mixture of active and early or disabled retirees. Within the post-retirement age-range, 65-84, the "healthy worker" selection process no longer operates actively. The residual survival advantage it confers declines with age, as the retirees come to increasingly resemble the general population in their health status characteristics. The healthy worker effect disappears by around age 75.

Figure 2 presents the mortality experience of a population of actively employed male workers in the Bell System. Single-year age-specific mortality ratios are plotted for these active male employees, aged 40-64 (from data published previously[3]). The healthy worker effect is greatest at the youngest ages and declines steadily with age until eight years before normal retirement, when, presumably, the out-selection of the less healthy (via early retirement) causes the healthy worker effect to increase among the remaining active workers. (This phenomenon of the increase in healthy worker effect in the later years of working, and the accompanying mortality experience of early and retired workers, is currently under investigation within the rubber industry.[6])

In similar vein, Figure 3 provides further evidence of the declining carry-over of the healthy worker effect in the post-retirement age-range. Life table (q_x) data for an actuarially

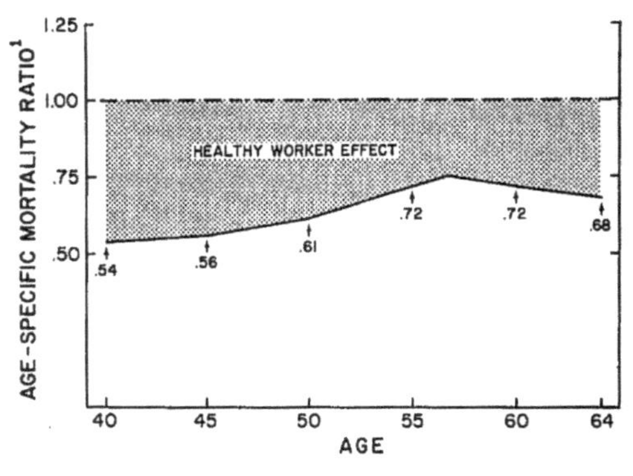

1. Ratio of life-table q_x values in Bell System male employees, 1959-63, to U.S. males, 1960.

Fig 2. — Mortality experience of a population of actively employed male workers.

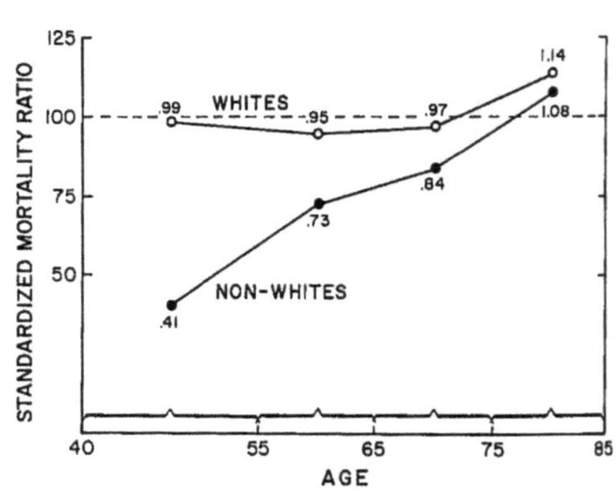

Fig 4. — Healthy worker effect is greater for nonwhites than whites, at all ages.

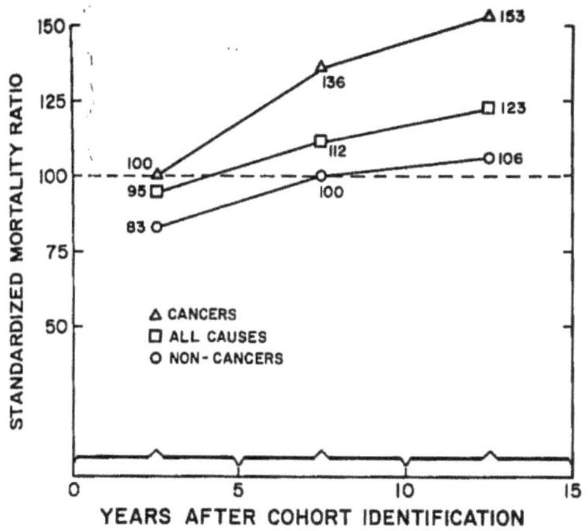

Graph based on tabular data from Enterline, P.E. (1965).

Fig 5. — Decline in the healthy worker effect with passage of time after initial identification of a cohort of active workers (asbestos products).

defined population of nondisabled male, industrial retirees, 1968-72,[7] indicate an initial mortality of only 55% of the general population. This effect declines steadily with age such that, at age 84, the mortality is 96% of the general population.

Figure 4 shows that, within the same rubber worker population of Figure 1, the healthy worker effect is greater for nonwhites than whites, at all ages. In particular, nonwhite male workers in the active employment age-range, 40-64, are at a substantial survival advantage compared to the national nonwhite male population (many of whom are unemployed, indigent, retired due to poor health, or working in hazardous occupations.) That is, the quality of the comparison differs for the two race groups. On the one hand, working-class whites are being compared to the national average "middle-class" white population; on the other hand, working-class nonwhites

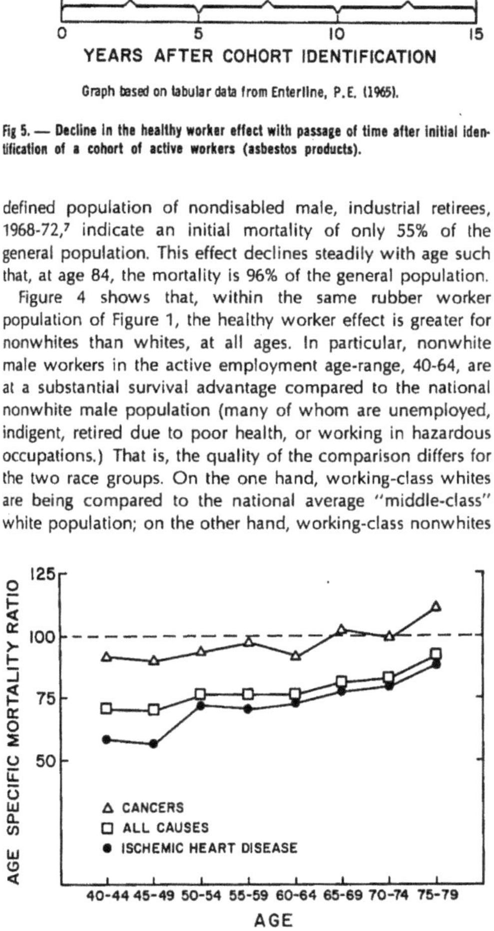

Source: Graph based on tabular data from Milham, S. (1974).

Fig 6. — Considerable difference can occur in the healthy worker effect for different causes of death (carpenters and joiners).

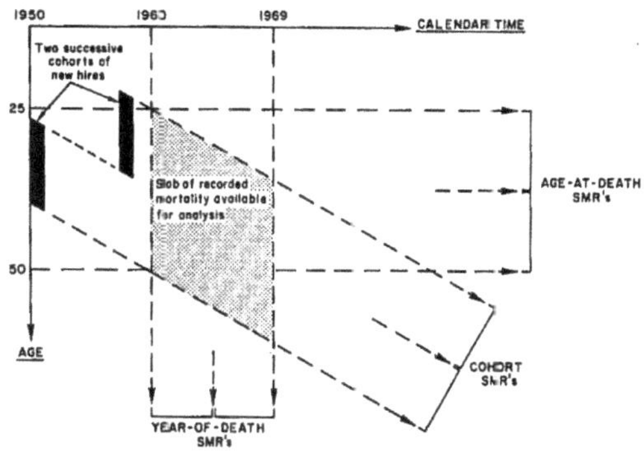

Fig 7. — Three different "directions" that can be followed in calculating SMR's.

are being compared to the national average "lower-class" nonwhite population. The assessment of race-specific healthy worker effects is therefore confounded by class differences. Clearly, the greater the proportion of nonwhites in a working population, the lower the race-standardized SMR's will tend to be and the greater the risk of not perceiving an actual, but small or moderate, excess of mortality.

Figure 5 illustrates the decline in the healthy worker effect with the passage of time after the identification of a cohort of already active workers. The graphs are based on tabular data from a cohort mortality study of asbestos products workers, by Enterline.[8] When follow-up is achieved of a total cohort, including those that quit or retire early for health reasons, then the initial healthy worker effect associated with active employment declines with time, because of the absence of any continued selection process. For total mortality, the effect in this cohort disappeared after five years largely due to the increase in cancer mortality in the second and third quinquennial period of follow-up.

Figure 6 illustrates the considerable difference that can occur in the healthy worker effect for different causes of death. The graphs are based on tabular data from a cross-sectional study of mortality in carpenters and joiners, by Milham.[3] At all ages, there is an obvious mortality deficit of about 25% for ischemic heart disease, whereas for cancers the mortality ratio remains in the vicinity of 100 throughout. Although part of this higher figure for cancer may reflect excess deaths from certain specific cancers for which Milham reports that these workers are at increased risk of death, part of the explanation lies in the cause-specific variation in the healthy worker effect. Where cancer is a "silent" disease, with long-deferred clinical manifestations, ischemic heart disease is a chronic and readily detectable condition. Heart disease is therefore much more likely to be selected against than is cancer, in the recruitment and retention of an active workforce.

Finally, Figure 7 presents, diagrammatically, three different "directions" that can be followed in calculating SMR's. A "slab" of recorded mortality experience within an occupational population (see hatched area, Fig 7) may result in an overall SMR of, say, 85. However, by partitioning the total mortality experience in different directions, significant excursions above and below that figure may be detected. SMR's can be calculated by age at death, by successive cohorts (year of birth, or year of hire cohorts), or by year of death. The choice of one or more of these approaches depends upon one's anticipations of the data.

An example of variation in SMR's by age at death has been given in Figure 1. An example of mortality differences between year-of-hire cohorts is to be found in a recent study of bladder cancer deaths, during 1967-71, in a population of 16,035 British rubber workers.[10] Workers joining the industry before 1950 had a bladder cancer SMR of 130, while for those joining in or after 1950 the SMR was 97. The major presumed bladder carcinogen, beta-naphthylamine, was removed from the British rubber industry in 1949. The third approach, using year-of-death SMR's (i.e. period mortality), would be useful in identifying temporary mortality excesses resulting from some short-term exposure to an agent whose use was subsequently discontinued (for reasons, say, unrelated to health). For example, a chemical with potent respiratory sensitization or irritation properties might precipitate excess deaths among workers with chronic respiratory ailments. Mortality analysis by year-of-death SMR's would best identify this problem.

Summary

The age-standardized mortality ratio (SMR) is a relative index of mortality, expressing the mortality experience of the study population relative to that of a comparison ("standard") population. With the general population as the "standard", the SMR for an occupational population will underestimate the mortality experience of that latter population (since it comprises individuals necessarily healthy enough to be employable — and whose mortality risk is therefore initially lower than the general population average). However, this "healthy worker effect" does not apply equally to all groups within the study population. Therefore, if one attempts to adjust for this effect, the summary nature of the SMR must be recognized, and allowance must be made for variation in the healthy worker effect between different age groups, different races, different work-status groups, different causes of death, and different elapsed-time periods of observation.

References

1. Bradford Hill A: Principles of Medical Statistics: 215-217. Oxford University Press, New York, 1971.

2. Miettinen OS: Standardization of risk ratios. *Amer J Epid* **96**:383-388, 1972.

3. McMichael AJ, Haynes SG, Tyroler HA: Observations on the evaluation of occupational mortality data. *JOM* **17**:128-131, 1975.

4. Goldsmith J: What we expect from an occupational cohort? *JOM* **17**:126-127, 1975.

5. McMichael AJ, Spirtas R, Kupper LL: An epidemiologic study of mortality within a cohort of rubber workers, 1964-72. *JOM* **16**:458-464, 1974.

6. Andjelkovic DA et al. Unpublished data on differential mortality experience of active, early retirees and disability retirees. Paper in preparation.

7. Toussaint RC, Driscoll FT: Note on a New Mortality Table for use in pension plans. Unpublished data from the George B. Buck Consulting Actuaries, 1974.

8. Enterline PE: Mortality among asbestos products workers in the United States. *Ann NY Acad Sciences* **132**:156-165, 1965.

9. Milham S: Mortality Experience of the AFL-CIO United Brotherhood of Carpenters and Joiners of America, 1969-70. DHEW Publication No. (NIOSH) 74-129, 1974.

10. Fox AJ, Lindars DC, Owen R: A survey of occupational cancer in the rubber and cablemaking industries: results of five-year analysis, 1967-71. *Br J Indust Med* **31**:140-151, 1974.

END OF REPRINT C

Standardized Mortality Ratios and the 'Healthy Worker Effect': Scratching Beneath the Surface

ANTHONY J. MCMICHAEL

4

OCCUPATIONAL STRESS

SU MON KYAW-MYINT AND LYNDALL STRAZDINS

Abstract

In 1979, Tony McMichael co-authored a paper showing how occupational stress not only affected mental health; it also exacerbated the effect of chemical and physical hazards on respiratory and skin symptoms. This study was among the first to place occupational stress within the same framework as chemical and physical hazards. It also showed that stress and mental health faced complex assessment challenges, but that these were similar to those faced by the assessment of exposure to chemical and physical hazards, especially in large-scale epidemiological studies.

More recently, occupational stress has been termed a 'psychosocial hazard' by some jurisdictions in an attempt to place it into the existing occupational risk management and risk assessment framework. However, progress has been slow and regulation of occupational stress remains outside standard occupational health and safety practices.

This chapter reviews the current state of the regulation of occupational stress and compares this to the context in which McMichael and colleagues undertook their research over three decades ago. We then trace some of the challenges posed by mainstreaming occupational stress, the role of McMichael and colleagues in laying the foundation for future research and describe recent research undertaken in Australia to achieve this goal.

Occupational Stress

Work, so fundamental to well-being, has its darker and more costly side. Work can adversely affect our health, well beyond the usual counts of injuries that we think of as 'occupational health'. The ways in which work is organized – its pace and intensity, degree of control over the work process, sense of justice, and employment security, among other things – can be as toxic to the health of workers as the chemicals in the air. (Gordon and Schnall, 2009, p. 1)

One of the first to recognise that the organisation of work could impact the mental and physical health of workers was Friedrich Engels. In 1845, he published *The Conditions of the Working Class*, in which he described physical and mental health problems of workers thought to be caused by the organisation of work and its social and physical environments. A few years later, Karl Marx wrote about how capitalism treated workers as commodities and how this led to the alienation of workers (Marx, 1988). Their groundbreaking work informed subsequent research into the health effects of the organisation of work. However, it was not until the 1960s that systematic and scientific research into the impact of occupational stress[1] began in the USA and in Nordic countries.

The origins of research on occupational stress came from a variety of disciplines, such as management, medicine, sociology and psychology. One of the most influential models of occupational stress, the Job Demands–Control (JDC) model, began with an article published in 1979 by Robert Karasek on the effect of job demands and job control on mental health (Karasek, 1979).

Tony McMichael's Contribution to Occupational Stress Research

Around the same time as the publication of the JDC model, Tony McMichael co-authored, with James House and other colleagues, a seminal article on the effect of occupational stress on health among factory workers (House et al., 1979). This research into occupational stress was consistent with Tony's lifelong research interests into social and environmental determinants of health, such as the study on lead exposure in pregnancy and its effect on young children (McMichael et al., 1986), discussed elsewhere in this book.

This important work on occupational stress was among the first to place occupational stress within the same framework as chemical and physical hazards. The paper was a response to the insight that much of the research on blue-collar workers concentrated solely on physical and chemical hazards and had not considered how exposure to occupational stress might influence, and possibly amplify, the effects of concurrent exposure to physical and chemical hazards. In addition, while there was recognition at the time that occupational

1 In this chapter, the term 'occupational stress' is used to describe stressors relating to the way work is organised, such as workload and role conflict, rather than the reaction to stressors.

stress was associated with many diseases in both blue- and white-collar workers, most research focused on a single health outcome, instead of a range of health outcomes. House and colleagues were aware that to understand fully the range of health problems associated with occupational stress and the mechanisms by which these effects occurred, multiple exposures to occupational hazards, including occupational stress, needed to be examined.

By way of review, the three aims of their cross-sectional research (House et al., 1979) were to:

1. Document the impact of occupational stress as well as physical and chemical hazards on the health of blue-collar workers.
2. Consider how these hazards combine either additively or interactively to impact on health.
3. Determine the range of health outcomes affected by occupational stress and how these are brought about.

Their sample comprised 1809 male workers who were not in a supervisory role from a tyre, rubber, plastics and chemicals manufacturing plant in the USA.

Occupational stress was measured as self-reported job pressures (workload, responsibility pressure, role conflict, quality concern, job versus non-job conflict) and job gratification (lack of intrinsic or extrinsic rewards, importance rewards, control rewards, general job satisfaction). A number of health outcomes such as angina pectoris, gastrointestinal ulcers, neurosis, itch and rash on skin, persistent cough and phlegm were assessed using a self-report questionnaire. In addition, a subset of workers (n = 353) was evaluated medically for hypertension, heart disease risk, dermatitis and respiratory symptoms. Type A behaviour pattern was also assessed and was used as a predictor variable. Neurotic symptoms were assessed by the Health Opinion Survey, and this measure captured symptoms associated with depression and anxiety. Exposure to physical and chemical hazards was measured in two ways: the first was the industrial hygienist's assessment of respirable particulates in the broad areas of the plant; the second measure was self-reported exposure to dust, fumes and chemicals, which were then combined into a single exposure index.

Analyses controlled for age, education, self-reported exposure to physical and chemical hazards, obesity and a measure of the physical activity required in the job. House, McMichael and colleagues (1979) found that all occupational stress measures were associated with at least some of the self-reported health outcomes. Neurotic symptoms were associated with all job pressure scales and job gratification scales. Similar findings were observed for cough and phlegm.

Angina and ulcers were also affected by a limited number of occupational stress measures (role conflict, job/non-job conflict, interpersonal tension and self-esteem).

Furthermore, although not as strong, similar findings were also observed for occupational stress measures and medically assessed health outcomes. Work pressure variables were generally significantly associated with hypertension, and job gratification variables showed an association with hypertension and high cardiovascular disease (CVD) risk factors. The results overall showed that occupational stress was associated with increased risk of angina, ulcers, neurosis, high blood pressure and other CVD risk factors. In relation to respiratory and skin symptoms, the authors hypothesised that stress alone might not contribute to these symptoms; rather, stress might interact and exacerbate these symptoms in the presence of exposure to physical and chemical hazards. Subsequent analyses examining interaction effects found that an interaction effect was indeed present for respiratory and skin problems. Where there was no exposure to chemical and physical hazards, there was no statistically significant association between occupational stress and respiratory and skin problems. In contrast, among those workers who were exposed to dusts, fumes and chemicals, there was a consistent synergistic effect.

This work by House, McMichael and colleagues (1979) informed subsequent research on occupational stress, such as studies examining the effect of occupational stress on particular health outcomes such as CVD and depression in blue-collar workers (Kawakami et al., 1992). However, only a few studies continued to examine the relationship between both physical and chemical hazards and occupational stress (e.g. Bromet et al., 1992).

In contrast, since 1979, the majority of research has focused on the impact of stress on particular health outcomes such as mental health. This has enabled the evidence of the health impacts of occupational stress to accumulate, especially with several longitudinal studies being conducted. However, much of this research was occurring without consideration of how occupational health hazards were usually addressed in the workplace.

Occupational Stress: Beginnings and Struggles for Recognition

Tony McMichael's collaboration with James House set the course for the recognition that occupational stress was, indeed, a significant occupational health hazard. Although it was a scientific finding, like many landmark ideas, it had profound political ramifications. Other authors have subsequently acknowledged how this political dimension has shaped the extent to which occupational stress has been viewed as a health risk that workplaces must address (e.g. Dollard and Winefield, 1996).

Much of the earlier research on occupational stress had focused on individual factors, trying to address occupational stress by focusing on the individual by, for example, increasing coping among workers. This in itself placed occupational stress in a framework quite different from other occupational hazards where the usual approach was to modify the work environment so that most workers were protected from unsafe levels of occupational hazards. Similar to House, McMichael and colleagues, another leading researcher in occupational stress, Dean Baker (Baker, 1985), argued that occupational stress needed to be placed in a similar context as other occupational hazards and that efforts should be directed towards those conditions that could be modified to reduce occupational stress. They noted that the focus on individual perception and susceptibility made it seem that stress affected a special group of workers rather than all workers, and thus moved it away from the public health approach for preventing ill health.

The controversy in recognising and addressing occupational stress is not unique to this particular occupational hazard. The history of occupational health and safety is filled with examples of hazards that have taken decades to be legitimised and become mainstream. Some of the early occupational health and safety legislation in countries such as the UK, the USA and Australia came about to address the high rates of occupational accidents in industries, such as mining and factories, by addressing hazards such as machine guarding, ventilation and inspection of machinery and equipment (Quinlan et al., 2010). Similar to the labelling of some workers as particularly susceptible to the effects of occupational stress, occupational injury itself was once controversial, with the term 'accident proneness' coined in the 1920s to attribute the cause of occupational injury to deficiencies in individual workers, rather than to place the onus on employers to provide a safe work environment.

For policy or legislative interventions relating to occupational hazards that cause non-traumatic health outcomes, accumulation of the scientific evidence and the availability of methods to translate scientific evidence into practical tools that can be applied in workplaces are usually required. Workers who became sick from exposure to hazardous substances were once told that they were 'hypersusceptible', or that it was their diet and hygiene causing their health problems (Corn, 1992). This enabled employers to refrain from taking action to reduce exposure to slate dust. For example, for many decades the US cotton industry denied the link between exposure to cotton dust and byssinosis. It was only when British researchers, who found a link between cotton dust exposure and byssinosis in the UK, began conducting studies in the USA that the industry eventually accepted that exposure to cotton dust should be reduced.

So far, occupational stress has followed a similar trend as other occupational disease-causing hazards. Despite the strong evidence linking occupational stress to a number of health outcomes, the political nature of the issue, including the questioning of the scientific evidence by industry, has led to delayed action. Even when occupational stress is widely acknowledged as a hazard to be addressed, it remains difficult to regulate and provide practical advice for workplaces because, so far, it remains outside of regulatory frameworks in most countries.

Policy Approaches to Occupational Stress

At the time of this important research by House, McMichael and colleagues (1979), the focus of occupational health and safety legislation was still primarily on occupational injury and physical ill health. The first health and safety legislation in the UK during the 1800s, and on which initial Australian health and safety legislation was based, dealt with protecting children and women.[2] Later, health and safety legislation dealt with physical hazards such as machine-related injuries. Even in the 1970s and 1980s, the main focus of health and safety legislation in most industrialised countries was on reducing the risk of physical injury, such as machine guarding, lighting and ventilating work rooms (Gunningham, 1984). Most legislation was limited to specific types of workers, places of work or operations.

Although legislative reforms in the late 1970s and later began to incorporate general duties of employers to protect the health and safety of their employees, there was still neglect of the work environment and organisational factors that could cause ill health, even though research into occupational stress was taking off at the time. The Scandinavian countries were one exception where legislation was introduced to regulate work environments, including psychosocial working conditions (Elden, 1986).

However, at the end of the 20th century, occupational stress became an important issue in the occupational health and safety framework in industrialised countries. This was, in part, due to the magnitude and cost of occupational stress (International Labour Office, 2000; Parent-Thirion et al., 2007). There was also mounting evidence of the health effects of occupational stress from longitudinal studies (Johnson et al., 1996; Stansfeld et al., 1999; Virtanen et al., 2013).

2 More recent legislations, such as those limiting lead exposure in workers, also followed on from attempts to protect children's health based on the evidence of the adverse effects of lead on children's neurodevelopment.

Improved understanding of the health effects of occupational stress led to policies aimed at reducing exposure, such as limiting work hours and requirements to consider the design of work (such as workload). Europe has been the leader, with several policy initiatives to address this hazard. The 1989 European Directive on Safety and Health of Workers at Work (89/391/EEC) made reference to the design of work and the organisational context of work, although it did not specifically mention occupational stress (Leka et al., 2010). In the 1990s, occupational stress was again indirectly addressed in two European-level directives on work with display screen equipment and the organisation of working time.

Many countries in Europe now have specific legislation addressing occupational stress. These include the Danish Working Environment Act, which requires the assessment of the psychosocial working environment to address occupational stress, and the Law on Health and Safety in Germany, which defines health and safety risks to include forms of work, the amount of work and working time. More specific mentions and requirements to address occupational stress were seen in Italy, with a mandatory assessment of occupational stress. In the Netherlands, the Working Conditions Act and its associated regulations state that workers must be able to have an influence on the rhythm of work and that very high or low workloads must be avoided. In countries such as the UK, USA and Australia, there are direct or indirect requirements to address occupational stress with many advisory tools and guidance materials. However, occupational stress is still not mentioned specifically in health and safety acts and regulations.

There has been some progress in efforts towards placing occupational stress in the risk management framework used in occupational health and safety (Cox et al., 2000). There was recognition that risk management of occupational stress could follow the typical risk management approach with the first crucial step of risk assessment. The outcomes of the risk assessment process can then inform risk reduction strategies in the workplace to reduce occupational stress. This risk management approach for occupational stress was a major step forward in addressing occupational stress; however, the nature of occupational stress still made it a difficult occupational hazard for which to assess risk by those used to dealing with physical hazards and traumatic injuries.

Consequently, despite the large body of knowledge on the harmful effects of occupational stress, it remains a major challenge. This indicates that there is a failure to translate the existing scientific knowledge into practical action and policy.

Recent Research

Following on from the work of House, McMichael and colleagues (1979), research conducted at The Australian National University has explored ways to place occupational stress in a similar framework as that for physical and chemical hazards. Exposure to occupational health hazards is usually addressed by setting health-based critical exposure levels. Such critical exposure levels are based on dose–response modelling from epidemiological or experimental animal data, providing a quantifiable level of exposure in the workplace that is considered to be adequate to protect most workers. This approach is what Baker (1985) was referring to when he called for a public health approach to occupational stress ... as was in place for chemical exposures. Having critical levels of exposure in the workplace enable both regulatory agencies and employers to determine if workplaces have hazardous levels of exposure and, if so, what actions need to be taken to reduce the level of exposure. An example is an acceptable exposure level for noise, which is 85 dB (A) in Australia.

Even though critical exposure levels provide a common method of regulating occupational health hazards, there have been no formal attempts to identify critical exposure levels for occupational stress. The lack thereof makes it difficult for both regulators and employers to undertake risk assessment. Critical exposure levels could also guide in designing and targeting primary level interventions in the workplace (see Figure 4.1).

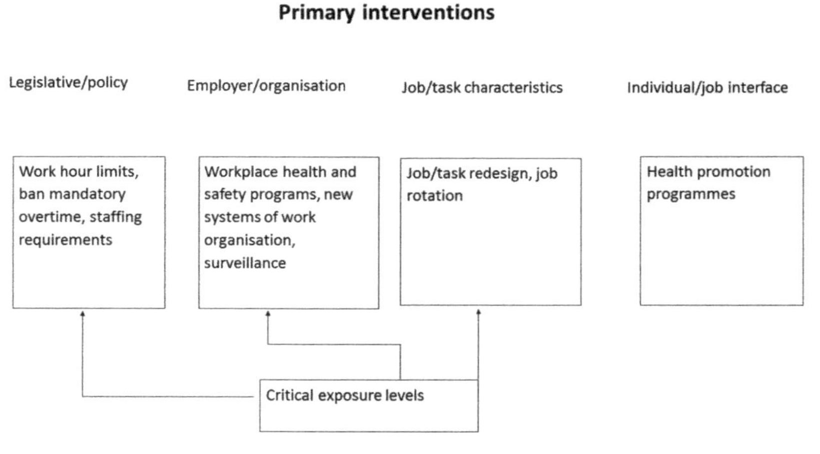

Figure 4.1 Levels of work organisation primary interventions and where critical exposure levels can be used to inform these interventions.

Source: Author's work.

A recent study (Kyaw-Myint, 2012) sought to identify critical exposure levels for two aspects of occupational stress: job control (the amount of decision authority and skill usage a person has in his or her job) and job demands (primarily a measure of quantitative workload). This study involved the analysis of two waves of data from 4,004 workers in a prospective cohort study, the Personality and Total Health (PATH) through Life study in south-eastern Australia. Previous research using this data set demonstrated that occupational stress influenced metal health outcomes using both cross-sectional and longitudinal analyses of the data (D'Souza et al., 2003; Strazdins et al., 2011). Critical exposure levels were identified using the benchmark dose method; namely, a dose–response modelling method used to identify critical exposure levels for chemicals (Filipsson et al., 2003).

In addition to attempting to place the regulation and risk assessment of occupational stressors in the same framework as other occupational hazards, this research addressed individual susceptibility, which has been a cause of controversy in relation to occupational stress. Individual factors such as personality and previous mental health status, age, gender and socio-economic status were included in dose–response modelling. Stressors (job demands and job control) were measured using a self-report questionnaire from the UK Whitehall II study, which was shown to have good predictive validity (Stansfeld et al., 1999). Mental health symptoms were assessed using the Goldberg Depression and Anxiety Scale (Goldberg et al., 1998).

The dose–response modelling undertaken in this study also took into account the shape of the dose–response relationship between each stressor and mental health outcomes. This is important because previous studies have shown that occupational stress can have a curvilinear relationship with a variety of outcomes, such as ill health or job satisfaction (e.g. Karanika-Murray, 2010). Job control was found to have a linear relationship with both depressive symptoms and anxiety symptoms. Job demands had a linear dose–response relationship with depressive symptoms and a curvilinear dose–response relationship with anxiety symptoms. Critical exposure levels for both mental health outcomes for each stressor were first identified. Of the two critical exposure levels identified for each stressor (job demands or job control), the most health-protective critical exposure level was then chosen as the final critical exposure level for each stressor. After taking individual factors into account, the critical exposure level for job control was identified as having nine out of 15 different aspects of job control measured in the PATH through Life study (Kyaw-Myint, 2012). For job demands, the critical exposure level was identified as having two out of four different aspects of job demands measured in the PATH through Life study (Kyaw-Myint, 2012). However, the small number of dose groups for job demands meant that the finding for job demands could be considered only suggestive. Validation of this finding with a more extensive measure of job demands is recommended for future research.

This research was first to adapt the benchmark dose method to identify critical exposure levels for different aspects of occupational stress. It demonstrated that critical exposure levels of job control and job demands could be identified using poor mental health as an outcome measure. These levels can then be used in risk assessment of the work environment, thus addressing the difficulty in managing occupational stress. In addition, it provided a method that could be used in future studies to determine critical exposure levels of other work organisational hazards and other health outcomes. Hence, similar to the seminal work by House, McMichael and colleagues (1979), this study on critical exposure levels for occupational stress legitimised occupational stress as another occupational hazard, enabling the risk of occupational stress to be assessed in the same way as other occupational hazards, such as chemicals.

Where To From Here?

With this 2012 study, risks associated with occupational stress can now be assessed in a similar framework as other occupational hazards. However, the challenge still lies in the acceptance of applying such an approach to occupational stress by employers and policymakers. The main focus for occupational health and safety remains more tangible hazards such as machine guarding and noise. Occupational stress, being invisible, is likely to remain less of a workplace priority.

The issue of addressing occupational stress is even more challenging because effective interventions require interventions at both the individual level and at the organisational level (LaMontagne et al., 2007). In many smaller workplaces and workplaces where occupational health and safety competes with production and supply-chain pressures, the reliance on individual-level interventions, such as personal protective equipment, over engineering or work design solutions is commonly reported (e.g. Lingard and Holmes, 2001). Redesign of work to reduce high levels of job demands or providing workers with more control over different aspects of their job will be harder to achieve than individual-level interventions such as providing counselling for workers.

Employers may argue that the redesign of work may not be economically or technically feasible because of globalisation and recent events such as the Global Financial Crisis (GFC), which have placed greater demands on employers to minimise costs and reduce pay and workplace conditions. At the same time, economic recessions, such as the GFC, have been shown to expose workers to a higher level of occupational stressors than non-recession times (Houdmont et al., 2012). However, as stated previously, the challenge faced by occupational stress is not unique. McMichael raised similar economic and political issues when discussing the importance of the need to address the health effects of climate change, especially when there were no clear-cut links between exposure and health effects, as in the case of multifactorial diseases (McMichael, 2001).

Despite the foregoing, there are encouraging signs that occupational stress and poor mental health are considered important issues in the Australian occupational health and safety environment. Mental health is now included in the definition of health in the model Work Health and Safety Act, which has been adopted by most Australian states and territories. Moreover, the new Australian Work Health and Safety Strategy 2012–2022, which is Australia's guiding document on health and safety priorities, identifies mental disorders as a priority occupational disease. Improvements in health and safety through better work design are also included in the Australian strategy. This shows that efforts to reduce occupational stress are gaining momentum in Australia; there is now general agreement by employers, workers and policymakers that the issue of occupational stress deserves attention. Thus, Tony McMichael, in conducting his research into occupational stress, laid the foundation for the work of future researchers and contributed towards the recognition of occupational stress as a legitimate occupational hazard. His work also contributed towards the compelling evidence on the social determinants of health and helped underpin arguments made to address this issue worldwide (Commission on Social Determinants of Health, 2008).

References

Baker, D.B. 1985. The study of stress at work. *Annual Review of Public Health* 6, 367–81.

Bromet, E.J., Dew, M.A., Parkinson, D.K., Cohen, S. & Schwartz, J.E. 1992. Effects of occupational stress on the physical and psychological health of women in a microelectronics plant. *Social Science and Medicine* 34, 1377–83.

Commission on Social Determinants of Health 2008. *Closing the Gap in a Generation: Health Equity Through Action on the Social Determinants of Health. Final Report of the Commission on Social Determinants of Health.* World Health Organization, Geneva, Switzerland.

Corn, J. 1992. *Response to Occupational Health Hazards: A Historical Perspective.* Van Nostrand Reinhold, New York, USA.

Cox, T., Griffiths, A., Barlowe, C., Randall, R., Thomson, L. & Rial-Gonzalez, E. 2000. *Organisational Interventions for Work Stress: A Risk Management Approach*. Institute of Work, Health and Organisations, University of Nottingham Business School, Nottingham, UK.

Dollard, M. & Winefield, A. 1996. Managing occupational stress: a national and international perspective. *International Journal of Stress Management* 3, 69–83.

D'Souza, R.M., Strazdins, L., Lim, L.L., Broom, D.H. & Rodgers, B. 2003. Work and health in a contemporary society: demands, control, and insecurity. *Journal of Epidemiology and Community Health* 57, 849–54.

Elden, M. 1986. Sociotechnical systems ideas as public policy in Norway: empowering participation through worker-managed change. *The Journal of Applied Behavioral Science* 22, 239–55.

Engels, F. 1845. The *Condition of the Working Class in England*. Oxford University Press, London, UK.

Filipsson, A., Sand, S., Nilsson, J. & Victorin, K. 2003. The benchmark dose method – review of available models, and recommendations for application in health risk assessment. *Critical Reviews in Toxicology* 33, 505–42.

Goldberg, D., Bridges, K., Duncan-Jones, P. & Grayson, D. 1998. Detecting anxiety and depression in general medical settings. *BMJ* 297, 897–9.

Gordon, D.R. & Schnall, P.L. 2009. Beyond the individual: connecting work environment and health. In: Schnall, P.L., Dobson, M. & Rosskam, E. (eds) *Unhealthy Work: Causes, Consequences, Cures*. Baywood Publishing Company, Inc, Amityville, New York, USA, 1–15.

Gunningham, N. 1984. *Safeguarding the Worker: Job Hazards and the Role of the Law*. Law Book Company, Sydney, NSW, Australia.

Houdmont, J., Kerr, R. & Addley, K. 2012. Psychosocial factors and economic recession: the Stormont study. *Occupational Medicine* 62, 98–104.

House, J.S., Wells, J.A., Landerman, L.R., McMichael, A.J. & Berton, H.K. 1979. Occupational stress and health among factory workers. *Journal of Health and Social Behavior* 20, 139–60.

International Labour Office 2000. *Mental Health in the Workplace*. International Labour Organization, Geneva, Switzerland.

Johnson, J.V., Stewart, W., Hall, E.M., Fredlund, P. & Theorell, T. 1996. Long-term psychosocial work environment and cardiovascular mortality among Swedish men. *American Journal of Public Health* 86, 324–31.

Karanika-Murray, M. 2010. Work and health: curvilinearity matters. In: Houdmont, J. & Leka, S. (eds) *Contemporary Occupational Health Psychology: Global Perspectives on Research and Practice*. John Wiley & Sons Ltd, Chichester, UK, 151–68.

Karasek, R. 1979. Job demands, job decision latitude, and mental strain: implications for job redesign. *Administrative Science Quarterly* 24, 285–308.

Kawakami, N., Haratani, T. & Araki, S. 1992. Effects of perceived job stress on depressive symptoms in blue-collar workers of an electrical factory in Japan. *Scandinavian Journal of Work, Environmental and Health* 18, 195–200.

Kyaw-Myint, S.M. 2012. *Mainstreaming Mental Health in Occupational Health and Safety: An Exploration of Benchmark Dose Modelling to Regulate Job Demands and Job Control*. Unpublished doctoral dissertation, PhD, Australian National University, Canberra, ACT, Australia.

LaMontagne, A., Keegel, T., Louie, A.M., Ostry, A. & Landsbergis, P.A. 2007. A systematic review of the job-stress intervention evaluation literature, 1990–2005. *International Journal of Occupational and Environmental Health* 13, 268–80.

Leka, S., Jain, A., Zwetsloot, G. & Cox, T. 2010. Policy-level interventions and work-related psychosocial risk management in the European Union. *Work & Stress* 24, 298–307.

Lingard, H. & Holmes, N. 2001. Understandings of occupational health and safety risk control in small business construction firms: barriers to implementing technological controls. *Construction Management and Economics* 19, 217–26.

McMichael, A.J. 2001. Climate change and health: information to counter the White House Effect. *International Journal of Epidemiology* 30, 655–7.

McMichael, A.J., Vimpani, G.V., Robertson, E.F., Baghurst, P.A. & Clark, P.D. 1986. The Port Pirie cohort study: maternal blood lead and pregnancy outcome. *Journal of Epidemiology and Community Health* 40, 18–25.

Marx, K. 1988. *Economic and Philosophic Manuscripts of 1844 (M. Milligan trans)*. Prometheus Books, Amherst, Massachusetts, USA.

Parent-Thirion, A., Macías, E.F., Hurley, J. & Vermeylen, G. 2007. Fourth European Working Conditions Survey. Office for the Official Publications of the European Communities, Luxembourg.

Quinlan, M., Bohle, P. & Lamm, F. 2010. *Managing Occupational Health and Safety: A Multidisciplinary Approach*. Palgrave Macmillan, Melbourne, VIC, Australia.

Stansfeld, S., Fuhrer, R., Shipley, M.J. & Marmot, M.G. 1999. Work characteristics predict psychiatric disorder: prospective results from the Whitehall II Study. *Occupational and Environmental Medicine* 56, 302–7.

Strazdins, L., D'Souza, R.M., Clements, M., Broom, D.H., Rodgers, B. & Berry., H.L. 2011. Could better jobs improve mental health? A prospective study of change in work conditions and mental health in mid-aged adults. *Journal of Epidemiology and Community Health* 65, 529–34.

Virtanen, M., Nyberg, S.T., Batty, G.D., Jokela, M., Heikkilä, K., Fransson, E.I., et al. 2013. Perceived job insecurity as a risk factor for incident coronary heart disease: systematic review and meta-analysis. *BMJ* 347, f4746.

5

A PUBLIC HEALTH APPROACH TO ENVIRONMENTAL AND OCCUPATIONAL HEALTH PROBLEMS IN DEVELOPING COUNTRIES

HÜLYA GÜL AND ZAHIDE CEREN ATLI

Abstract

The struggle to preserve and improve human and environmental health is meaningful and valuable. The role of public health scientists is to assemble and analyse evidence, leading, if possible, to proof of the health effects of environmental and occupational exposure. At the same time, it is the duty of the political superstructure to replace dangerous agents with substances that are safer, if possible eliminating all health risks entirely. Ideally, it is in this context that epidemiological research of environmental and occupational health problems should be conducted.

The discipline of public health is to investigate, comprehend and, as far as is possible, explain fully the causes, mechanisms and consequences of such hazards, and to develop and implement solutions such as preventive programmes, political initiatives and advocacy. The pursuit of sustainable development requires the construction of necessary social bodies and administrative mechanisms. Policies and academic studies that facilitate minimal environmental damage with maximum efficiency are required.

This chapter describes ways by which workplace and environmental health epidemiology can be used to improve public health and create a more habitable world for future generations. The chapter has a particular focus on Turkey, with a limited discussion of these issues in other developing countries.

Introduction

Despite great scientific and technological advancement, many factors have created serious health problems in low-income, 'developing' countries. Industrialisation, irregular urbanisation and migration are associated with material and psychological distress, including from unemployment and income inequality. This process has been accelerated by the relocation of many polluting industries to less-developed countries, where labour is cheaper, regulation weaker and exploitation more systematic and ruthless.

The characterisation and prioritisation of environmental health problems and their causes through epidemiological and scientific research is needed to guide and advance sustainability. Sustainable development requires social and administrative mechanisms, including regulated policies that reduce environmental harm.

Although the 21st century is regarded as an era of significant scientific and technological development, it will also be recalled as a time scarred by increasing environmental degradation, natural disasters, industrial accidents and climate change (Dixon et al., 2009; Balbus et al., 2013; McMichael, 2013). Insufficient attention is given to the environmental and social pressures that permeate our living systems.

Many factors influence human and environmental health. Humans depend on their environments in every facet of their lives and are vulnerable to a myriad of physical, chemical, psychosocial, biologic, ergonomic and other factors that are either directly environmental or related to the environment. In developed countries, the burden of disease of many classical occupational health problems has been greatly reduced, such as lead poisoning and pneumoconiosis. But these gains are partly offset by newer problems, such as repetitive strain disorders, childhood cancers, multiple chemical sensitivity syndrome and sick building syndrome (McMichael and Butler, 2006; Gül, 2011).

Epidemiological science provides a logical approach to evaluate diseases and their causes, and thus to promote their prevention. Epidemiology can also be used to investigate the efficacy of existing or newly developed health initiatives.

In this chapter, stress is placed on the need to create healthy workplaces both for people and for a healthier planet. Harmful working conditions and practices will be discussed, focusing on environmental conditions and their context in developing countries.

Environmental Determinants

Ecological degradation, pollution, climate change, rapid technological development, rapid population growth, poverty, globalisation and economic crises all affect health (Butler and Weinstein, 2011; Bowen et al., 2012; Kjellstrom and McMichael, 2013). Contemporary public health recognises that humans are not solely biological creatures, but exist within a social and environmental milieu. Public health provides a multidisciplinary means to improve knowledge, competencies and behaviours that protect and enhance human well-being. Public health advocates the cost-effectiveness of studies that aim to prevent diseases and to promote health, rather than their treatment, together with causal enquiry and the development of integrated approaches, including political intervention and advocacy (Butler and McMichael, 2010; Hanlon et al., 2012). Pollution to air, water, food and soil, whether caused by climate change, industry, traffic or human waste, can have direct and indirect unwanted health consequences (Capon and Rissel, 2010; Kjellstrom and McMichael, 2013). Disease causation has fixed and modifiable factors, varying by age, gender, location, workplace, social class, etc. Adverse environmental exposures often begin prenatally. The elderly, children and those with chronic diseases are especially vulnerable to environmental threats. Environmental pollution directly causes some diseases, aggravates others and, in some cases, accelerates their propagation.

Although, in developed countries, some forms of environmental pollution have declined, this is not the case in most developing nations. Furthermore, some kinds of environmental pollution, such as climate change, are not only geographically ubiquitous but also affect all social and economic strata, though at this stage to varying degrees. But some diseases can be prevented and even eradicated if their environmental causes can be removed. Modifiable factors include lifestyle choices (e.g. smoking) and other social habits. Over longer periods, some socio-economic, cultural and environmental conditions can also be altered.

Many diseases and social problems aggravated by climate change are preventable, if we take efficient measures (Huang et al., 2011; McMichael and Lindgren, 2011; Hanlon et al., 2012). However, unaddressed, climate change may prove the worst environmental catastrophe of our time; as such, it should direct attention towards the deterioration of the Earth's ecological balance.

Although the cost of climate change to the global economy is an important though disputed subject, its direct health effects are increasingly understood. Climate change is manifest through alterations to temperature, precipitation, humidity, clouds, wind, air pressure, fog and sea level. Health effects include increasing vector-borne diseases and worsened food and nutritional security. Increased cardiovascular and respiratory diseases due to air pollution interacting with heat waves from climate change are also likely.

The causes of human-made climate change include rising levels of carbon dioxide and other greenhouse gases, especially due to burning of fossil fuels. At the moment, combustion of fuels such as coal and oil are widely viewed as vital for ongoing industrial development, though this is challenged increasingly by the environmental movement. In Turkey, greenhouse gas emissions arise from the energy sector (71 per cent), industrial (13 per cent), waste (9 per cent) and agriculture (7 per cent) (TÜİK, 2013a). One study found a deterioration in lung function, measured by spirometry, for people living within the vicinity of a coal-fired thermal power plant in Kutahya (Karavuş et al., 2002). This is consistent with many other studies that show impaired respiratory health in association with coal particles.

The frequency and severity of diseases such as cancer are also related to many forms of environmental pollution (IARC, 2012). Cancer is the second leading cause of death (after cardiovascular disease) in both developed and developing countries. This pattern also applies in Turkey. In 2012, systemic circulatory diseases caused 37.9 per cent of deaths, followed by malignant neoplasm (21.1 per cent) and respiratory diseases (9.7 per cent) (see Tables 5.1 and 5.2) (TÜİK, 2013b).

Table 5.1 Subgroups of cancer, by year in Turkey (per cent).

Diseases/year	2010 (%)	2011 (%)	2012 (%)
Total	100	100	100
Disease of the circulatory system	39.6	38.8	37.9
Malignant neoplasms	21.3	21.1	21.1
Disease of the respiratory system	8.3	10.1	9.7
Endocrine, nutritional and metabolic diseases	6.4	6.3	6.0
Diseases of the nervous system and the sense organs	3.7	3.7	4.3
External causes of injury and poisoning	4.4	4.1	4.1
Other (infectious and parasitic diseases, mental and behavioural disorders, diseases of the musculoskeletal system/connective tissue, etc.)	16.3	15.9	16.9

Source: TÜİK, 2013b.

Table 5.2 Distribution (per cent) of causes of death by year in Turkey.

Subgroup/year	2010 (%)	2011 (%)	2012 (%)
Larynx and trachea/bronchus/lung	31.2	31.0	31.6
Stomach	8.8	8.8	8.4
Lymph/haematopoietic tissue	8.5	8.3	8.0
Colon	6.5	6.7	6.7
Pancreas	5.2	5.4	5.3
Other	39.8	39.9	39.9

Source: TÜİK, 2013b.

Environmental epidemiological studies range from analysis of social data to individualised on-site data collection (Schenker, 2007; Liu et al., 2012). These can reveal relationships between environmental factors and health outcomes of value to policymakers. Environmental epidemiology also investigates workers' complaints, disease clusters and other unexpected increases in their incidence.

Scientists have ethical and professional responsibilities to research suspected health effects in a timely fashion and to disseminate their findings. Often, however, these actions are limited by vested interests, such as corporations who profit from pollution, as recently noted by Margaret Chan in a WHO meeting (2013).

So-called 'ecological' studies (which, confusingly, have nothing to do with natural ecosystems) are used in environmental epidemiology to analyse group-level spatial and temporal disease distribution. Since these studies rely on aggregated data, it is impossible to correlate exposure with individual health status. The 'ecological fallacy' is the false inference of individual causation from such studies, and is sometimes alleged to discredit all such studies. However, without additional approaches, including individualised data if possible, the ecological fallacy can neither be proven nor disproven. That is, the relationships found in ecological studies may actually be valid (Ojha et al., 2011; Pleil et al., 2012).

The dose–response relationship is central to epidemiological evaluation. Epidemiologists seek to determine the critical level at which effects are detectable and to explore if the effect increases with dose. Many dose–response relationships are based on animal studies. But the measurement of cumulative human exposure is very difficult, and relationship to chronic diseases even more so; such measurements are further complicated by interactions among these exposures. Chronic, low-level environmental exposure can cause chronic damage. However, the determination of such risks is also challenging.

Although epidemiological work reliant on occupational and environmental toxicology is helpful, multidirectional research is necessary to explore hypotheses about factor–consequence relationships.

Some massive sources of industrial pollution cause relatively distinct public health effects. For example a study found the increased incidence of neural tube defects observed in major hospitals in the Black Sea region of Turkey (Mocan et al., 1992). The most plausible hypothesis for this is radiation from the huge 1986 disaster at the Chernobyl nuclear power plant in Turkey's Black Sea neighbour, Ukraine. This was caused by inadequate regulation and a poor safety culture. This affected people from the Republics of Ukraine and Belarus, as well as in Russia and parts of Europe, especially in Scandinavia. By 2005, approximately 5,000–6,000 cases of thyroid cancer had been diagnosed among people who were children or adolescents at the time of the accident, then living in Belarus, the Russian Federation and Ukraine (Bennett et al., 2006;UNSCEAR, 2011). Another notorious industrial accident, with substantial health effects, was the massive methyl isocyanate leakage in Bhopal, India, in 1984. This world's worst industrial disaster raised questions about the implications of the transfer of potentially hazardous technology to developing countries (Varma and Varma, 2005; Eckerman, 2011).

Environmental exposure to asbestos is an important public health issue in Turkey, and the use and trade of asbestos has been forbidden since 31 December 2010. Such exposure is mostly in rural areas, in contrast to the pattern in most developed countries. The number of people estimated to have been exposed to asbestos in rural areas of Turkey in 2012 is approximately one million. The risk of pleural mesothelioma and lung cancer was found to be 799 and 44 times higher, respectively, in women exposed to asbestos in rural areas than in those from the general population (Metintas et al., 2012; Ministry of Health, Republic of Turkey, 2012).

Occupational Determinants

Occupational health, which originated in the Industrial Revolution, is still very important, especially in developing countries. It is multidimensional, encompassing medicine, law, engineering and social sciences. Work has physical, mental, moral, chemical, social and economic aspects (Gül, 2012; Marmot et al., 2012). Occupational health protection requires recognition and, if possible, integrated regulation of these factors. The discipline of occupational health aims to prevent work accidents, injuries and diseases and to advocate long-term health protection. However, especially where employers and unions (if they exist) cooperate, workers can provide a valuable means for epidemiological research and insight, because they constitute a stable social group, some of whose environmental exposures can be quantified.

However, health damage due to industrialisation can be difficult to estimate, due to many interacting factors. For example, in Turkey, Dilovası and the wider, heavily industrialised province of Kocaeli is one of the most polluted provinces in Turkey. In addition, the country's largest highway passes through the city. Fifteen per cent of Turkey's accumulative manufacturing industry is based in Kocaeli. A recent study, though not age adjusted, found that the rate of cancer-related death in Dilovası (33 per cent) was 2.6- and 2.7-fold more than that of the rest of Turkey and the world, respectively (Hamzaoğlu et al., 2011).

Health risks arise at many stages of a production process, from access to the raw material to the finished product. Different forms of business bear specific risks. However, workers are relatively healthy individuals selected from the main population, with an expected probability of death lower than the general population, a phenomenon coined by Tony McMichael as the 'healthy worker effect' (McMichael, 1976).

Many occupational factors are suspected as having a role in disease aetiology, including asbestos, benzene, coal dust, heavy metals, pesticides, aromatic amines, silicon dioxide, chrome, vinyl chloride and radiation. Silicosis had been an important occupational health disease in Turkey because of the sandblasting of denim jeans using silica (Ozturk et al., 2012). Sandblasting work was prohibited in 2009 by the Health Ministry of the Republic of Turkey. But, by then, approximately 600 silicosis cases had been diagnosed in the textile sector, of which 54 had died. But other estimates suggested the real number of cases was nearer 5,000. Another study found an increased incidence of secondary pneumothorax in acute and accelerated forms of silicosis due to denim sandblasting (Kaynar et al., 2012). According to the results of another study, radiological evidence of silicosis (International Labour Organization (ILO) score 1/0 or higher) was present in 53 per cent of 145 sandblasting workers with interpretable chest radiographs (Akgun et al., 2008). Dental prosthetic technicians in Turkey also experience high rates of occupational silicosis, perhaps as high as 10 per cent (Cimrin et al., 2009).

The investigation of environmental exposures will remain challenging. There is significant variation between exposure levels determined by measurements made in the external environment versus exposure levels determined at the point of contact between the environment, the individual and in the human body. This variation can be the result of idiosyncratic variables such as personal lifestyles, physiological characteristics and the time and place of exposure. Another approach is to measure exposure levels from tissue or blood samples taken from humans or animals. In some cases, the impact of industrial pollution cannot be determined by observing acute symptoms, but can be inferred from accumulated effects. However, in such cases, persuading the public and regulators of the causal relationships can be difficult. However, these uncertainties do not mean we dismiss the possibility of risk; epidemiological investigation must continue.

Our understanding and motivation to research these issues has been influenced by Tony McMichael, who taught one of the authors of this chapter (HG) at a course on the epidemiology of cancer, ran by the International Agency for Research on Cancer (IARC) and the World Health Organization, in Lyon, France, in July 2005. HG later encountered Tony at several meetings, including some hosted by the International Society for Environmental Epidemiology (ISEE), of which she became a member in 2007. In fact, it was through ISEE that we first heard of the opportunity to contribute to this book.

Conclusion

A major purpose of this new public health is to control environmental pollution, including occupational exposure, and to protect human health. The socio-economic status of people affects their health and quality of life greatly, so the prevalence and severity of cancer, diabetes, obesity, etc, has increased rapidly in recent years in the developing countries. Climate change, which affects both environmental and socio-economic considerations for all states, plays an increasingly decisive role in sustainable development efforts, both globally and locally. To mitigate climate change and its impacts, states must take the required measures at national as well as international levels, and follow through on their application.

Academics conduct scientific research in order to determine causes of environmental deterioration and exposure. Epidemiological studies analysing the effects of the environment on human health, on an environmental and occupational basis, are a critical aspect of such efforts. Taking into consideration the results of the research carried out for the prevention of risk and the sustainability of measures, the required social and management mechanisms must be created by legislators, and the existing measures must be enforced.

Egalitarian public health policies must be applied with due care for the general public to achieve a fulfilling and healthy life in a clean and safe environment. Environmental and occupational conditions must be investigated from a multidisciplinary perspective, and their impact on public health must be evaluated from all dimensions.

References

Akgun, M., Araz, O., Akkurt, I., Eroglu, A., Alper, F., Saglam, L., et al. 2008. An epidemic of silicosis among former denim sandblasters. *European Respiratory Journal* 32, 1295–303.

Balbus, J.M., Boxall, A.B., Fenske, R.A., McKone, T.E. & Zeise, L. 2013. Implications of global climate change for the assessment and management of human health risks of chemicals in the natural environment. *Environmental Toxicology & Chemistry* 32, 62–78.

Bennett, B., Repacholi, M. & Carr, Z. (eds) 2006. Health Effects of the Chernobyl Accident and Special Health Care Programmes: Report of the UN Chernobyl Forum Health Expert Group. World Health Organization,Geneva, Switzerland. Available at www.who.int/ionizing_radiation/chernobyl/who_chernobyl_report_2006.pdf, accessed 14 February 2015.

Bowen, K., Friel, S., Ebi, K., Butler, C.D., Miller, F. & McMichael, A.J. 2012. Governing for a healthy population: an exploration of how decision-making will determine our global health in a changing climate. *International Journal of Environmental Research and Public Health* 9, 55–72.

Butler, C.D. & McMichael, A.J. 2010. Population health: where demography, environment and equity converge. *Journal of Public Health* 32, 157–8.

Butler, C.D. & Weinstein, P. 2011. Global ecology, global health, ecohealth. *EcoHealth* 8, 253–4.

Capon, A.G. & Rissel, C.E. 2010. Chronic disease and climate change: understanding co-benefits and their policy implications. *NSW Public Health Bulletin* 21, 109–13.

Chan, M. 2013. Opening address at the 66th World Health Assembly. www.who.int/dg/speeches/2013/world_health_assembly_20130520/en/, accessed 14 February 2015.

Cimrin, A., Kömüs, N., Karaman, C. & Tertemiz, K.C. 2009. Pneumoconiosis and work related health complaints in Turkish dental laboratory workers. *Tüberküloz ve Toraks* 57, 282–8.

Dixon, J.K., Hendrickson, K.C., Ercolano, E., Quackenbush, R. & Dixon, J.P. 2009. The environmental health engagement profile: what people think and do about environmental health. *Public Health Nursing* 26, 460–73.

Eckerman, I. 2011. Bhopal gas catastrophe 1984: causes and consequences. In: Nriagu, J.O. (ed.) *Encyclopedia of Environmental Health*. Elsevier, Burlington, Massachusetts, USA, 302–16.

Gül, H. 2011. Sick building syndrome from perspective of occupational and public health. In: Sabah, A. & Al-Sulaiman, A.-W. (eds) *Sick Building Syndrome in Public Buildings and Workplaces*. Springer, USA, 89–104.

Gül, H. 2012. Mobbing at workplaces and the mental health effects on employees. In: Olisah, V. (ed.) *Essential Notes in Psychiatry*. InTech – Open Access Publisher, Croatia.

Hamzaoğlu, O., Etiler, N., Yavuz, C.I. & Cağlayan, C. 2011. The causes of deaths in an industry-dense area: example of Dilovasi (Kocaeli). *Turkish Journal of Medical Sciences* 41, 369–75.

Hanlon, P., Carlisle, S., Hannah, M., Lyon, A. & Reilly, D. 2012. A perspective on the future public health practitioner. *Perspectives in Public Health* 132, 235–39.

Huang, C., Vaneckova, P., Wang, X., FitzGerald, G., Guo, Y. & Tong, S. 2011. Constraints and barriers to public health adaptation to climate change: a review of the literature. *American Journal of Preventive Medicine* 40, 183–90.

IARC. 2012. *Review of Human Carcinogens* (package of 6 volumes A,B,C,D,E,F). IARC Monographs on the Evaluation of Carcinogenic Risks to Humans,Lyon, France.

Karavuş, M., Aker, A., Cebeci, D., Tasdemir, M., Bayram, N. & Çalı, Ş. 2002. Respiratory complaints and spirometric parameters of the villagers living around the Seyitomer coal-fired thermal power plant in Kutahya, Turkey. *Ecotoxicology and Environmental Safety* 52, 214–20.

Kaynar, H., Aydın, Y.A., Akgün, M., Türkyılmaz, A. & Eroğlu, A. 2012. Pneumothorax in the cases with silicosis due to denim sandblasting. *Turkish Journal of Thoracic and Cardiovascular Surgery* 20, 291–4.

Kjellstrom, T. & McMichael, A.J. 2013. Climate change threats to population health and well-being: the imperative of protective solutions that will last. *Global Health Action* 6, 1–9.

Liu, C.-Y., Maity, A., Lin, X., Wright, R. & Christiani, D. 2012. Design and analysis issues in gene and environment studies. *Environmental Health* 11, 93 doi:10.1186/1476-069X-11-93.

McMichael, A.J. 1976. Standardized mortality ratios and the 'healthy worker effect': scratching beneath the surface. *Journal of Occupational Medicine* 18, 165–8.

McMichael, A.J. 2013. Globalization, climate change and health. *New England Journal of Medicine* 368, 1335–43.

McMichael, A.J. & Butler, C.D. 2006. Emerging health issues: the widening challenges for population health promotion. *Health Promotion International* 21, 15–24.

McMichael, A.J. & Lindgren, E. 2011. Climate change: present and future risks to health, and necessary responses. *Journal of Internal Medicine* 270, 401–13.

Marmot, M., Allen, J., Bell, R., Bloomer, E. & Goldblatt, P. 2012. WHO European review of social determinants of health and the health divide. *The Lancet* 380, 1011–29.

Metintas, S., Metintas, M., Ak, G. & Kalyoncu, C. 2012. Environmental asbestos exposure in rural Turkey and risk of lung cancer. *International Journal of Environmental Health Research* 22, 468–79.

Ministry of Health. Republic of Turkey 2012. Strategic Plan for Asbestos Control in Turkey. kanser.gov.tr/Dosya/ar-ge/asbest.pdf, accessed 14 February 2015.

Mocan, H., Aydemir, V., Bozkaya, H., Mocan, M. & Özbay, G. 1992. Incidence of neural tube defects (NTD) in Ankara, Turkey, prior to and after the Chernobyl disaster. *Paediatric and Perinatal Epidemiology* 6, 111–4.

Ojha, R.P., Offutt-Powell, T.N., Evans, E.L. & Singh, K.P. 2011. Correlation coefficients in ecologic studies of environment and cancer. *Archives of Environmental and Occupational Health* 66, 241–4.

Ozturk, A., Cımrın, A.H., Tur, M. & Guven, R. 2012. Prevalence of silicosis among employees in feldspat and quartz mills and associated factors with silicosis. *Tüberküloz ve Toraks* 60, 224–9.

Pleil, J.D., Sobus, J.R., Sheppard, P.R., Ridenour, G. & Witten, M.L. 2012. Strategies for evaluating the environment–public health interaction of long-term latency disease: the quandary of the inconclusive case-control study *Chemico-Biological Interactions* 196, 68–78.

Schenker, M.B. 2007. Appendix: Biostatistics & Epidemiology. In: Ladou, J. (ed.) *Current Occupational & Environmental Medicine* (4th edition). McGraw Hill Medical,New York, USA, 789–813.

TÜİK 2013a. Turkey greenhouse gas inventory 1990–2011 – annual report for submission under the Framework Convention on Climate Change. Ankara: Turkish Statistical Institute, No: 13482. www.turkstat.gov.tr/PreHaberBultenleri.do?id=13482, accessed 14 February 2015.

TÜİK 2013b. Causes of death statistics, 2010, 2011 and 2012. Turkish Statistical Institute, No 15847. Prime Ministry,Ankara, Republic of Turkey. www.turkstat.gov.tr/PreHaberBultenleri.do?id=15847, accessed 14 February 2015.

UNSCEAR 2011. Health effects due to radiation from the Chernobyl accident. *United Nations Scientific Committee on the Effects of Atomic Radiation, Vol 2, Supplement No 46*. United Nations Publication,New York, USA, 47–205.

Varma, R. & Varma, D.Y. 2005. The Bhopal disaster of 1984. *Bulletin of Science, Technology & Society* 25, 37–45.

6

TALES OF OCCUPATIONAL CANCER

(Adapted from *The Secret History of the War on Cancer*)

DEVRA DAVIS AND COLIN D. BUTLER

Abstract

Cancer, once rare, is now the biggest killer of humans. Its rising incidence triggered President Nixon's declaration of war on this still-dreaded diagnosis in 1971. Far less well-known is the coalition of moneyed forces, sometimes corrupting the most eminent of epidemiologists. This coalition has acted effectively to suppress and undermine this war – the secret war on the war on cancer.

The rise in cancer is not due solely to the ageing of the population, but in part to large-scale population exposure to a wide range of carcinogens, many of which are occupational. Once, all carcinogens were naturally occurring, but in the last century, an increasing range of synthetic molecules have been manufactured; some of which are also highly carcinogenic.

This chapter, drawn from *The Secret History of the War on Cancer* (Davis, 2007) gives a taste of many cases in which occupational health has been placed well below the interest of corporations, enabling lower consumer prices.

In some cases, tentative industry sympathy to the worker has given way to active suppression, but in most cases, industry and employers have refused any liability or responsibility. Particular attention is paid in this chapter to the relationship between vinyl chloride and cancer.

From Hippocrates to Percival Pott

Hippocrates depicted, 2,500 years ago, a tumour as a muddled irritable cavity with spindly legs flaring out of control in all directions. Fascinated with its evil, animal-like appearance, he termed it *karkinoma*, the Greek word for *crab*. Like Hippocrates, we are drawn to things of menacing beauty.

In the 1920s, cancer was rare. Nobel Laureate, Andre Cournand, recalled how, during his medical training in Paris, he and his colleagues rushed to see their first case of lung cancer. Today, however, cancer claims one in four persons in most industrial countries. In heavily industrialised areas of China, half of all deaths are due to cancer.

To prevent cancer, the 12th-century Jewish polymath, Moses Maimonides, counselled balanced nutrition, regular exercise and restraint from dust and dirty air. Occupational links with cancer have been recognised for half a millennium. Georgius Agricola noted young miners with chest tumours in the Erz Mountains. His 1556 magnum opus, *De Re Metallica*[1] (with 289 woodcuts) included some of the earliest reports on the ailments of underground work. Those who entered the mines the youngest, fared worst. If they survived trauma, they succumbed to lung diseases and tumours.

Sometimes, it takes centuries to get the message. In 1912, Herbert Hoover[2], then a top mining engineer, and his wife, Lou, a Latin scholar, published the first English translation of Agricola's work in *Mining Magazine* (Nash, 1983). The Hoovers explained that the 16th-century work remained relevant in the 20th century.

By 1714, the Italian physician, Ramazzini, had documented more than three dozen cancerous professions, including mining of coal, lead and iron. Ramazzini recognised many other risky occupations, including smiths, glassmakers, painters, tanners and mirror makers. So, too, were cleaners of privies and cesspits, farmers, fishermen, printers, midwives, wet-nurses and corpse carriers. For each trade, he explained agents or conditions he thought associated with classes of illness. His major work, *De Morbis Artificum Diatriba* (*Diseases of Workers*), showed that the things men and women did in their working lives played major roles in determining their ailments. It laid the foundations of occupational medicine.

1 *See The Secret War on Cancer for full reference details.*

2 Later a U.S. President.

Ramazzini also noted that nuns tended to be free from cervical cancer, then one of the most common fatal tumours of women. Celibate women more often developed breast cancer, and he speculated both were causally related; something now well accepted.

Ramazzini also believed that those who learned of workplace hazards had a moral duty to warn workers of the risks of their employ, and he extended Hippocrates' ancient advice to doctors by advocating an occupational history (Hunter, 1973, p. 35).

In 1775, the English surgeon, Pott, reported that chimney sweeps exposed to soot had an increased risk of scrotal cancer (known by sweeps as 'soot wart'). German sweeps, who wore leather trousers or bathed more often, had a lower incidence. This illustrates four points still relevant. First, workers often know their occupational risks. Second, risk differences can be associated with workplace practices. Third, uncommon events, like cancer of a male reproductive organ, get noticed. Finally, even as clear-cut an association as soot and scrotal cancer reflects multiple causes. Soot is not one chemical but hundreds. Its complex chemistry means that chimney sweeps would have trouble collecting damages in a modern U.S. court. If any were to sue the coal companies for damages, he would be asked to show exactly which of the hundreds of chemicals in coal tar had caused his cancer. The true answer – 'all of them' – is no longer considered acceptable.

New Technologies, New Chemicals, New Risks

Diagnostic radiation, which revolutionised cancer detection and treatment, turned out also to increase disease risk. X-rays damaged erythropoiesis – the capacity of bone marrow to make red blood cells. Girls who hand-painted clock dials with luminescent radioactive paint licked their brushes to craft fine lines. Some lost their jawbones as a result.

That such technological and chemical breakthroughs might harm health was barely imagined by most. Thomas Edison was an exception. After his chief assistant died from radiation, Edison refused to have another X-ray (Montgomery, 1997).

The Curies also died from their own research with radiation. Marie and her husband, Pierre, detailed the phenomenon of radioactivity in pitchblende, the ore that yielded uranium. Years of contact with radioactive material proved harmful. Cataracts fogged their eyes, and constant ringing dulled their ears. In 1906, Pierre was struck by a carriage he could neither see nor hear. Marie died of leukaemia.

The Early 20th Century

In the early 20th century, pioneer American medical researcher, Alice Hamilton, undertook postgraduate studies in Germany, the then acknowledged centre of scientific research. She had direct contact with the manufacturing revolution under way for coal and petroleum-based chemicals including benzene and toluene. Hamilton provided the first comprehensive account of the health effects of benzene, building on European and US case reports of benzene poisoning.

In 1926, the American National Safety Council issued a final report on the hazards of benzol, noting the doses at which it induced narcosis and severe weight loss in animals. It included 125 different references (National Safety Council, 1926). In 1936, Brussels hosted the Second International Congress and Social Campaign against Cancer; recognised carcinogens included hormones, arsenic, sunlight, radiation, benzene and other chlorinated hydrocarbons. By then, tools with which to draw causal inferences regarding cancer included experimental studies of cells and whole animals, and statistical observations of human disease patterns.

The Unusual Candour of the American Petroleum Institute, 1948

In 1948, the American Standards Association, a group of industry experts, maintained that a person could safely be subjected to 100 parts per million of benzene over 8 hours. It is unclear where they got this notion, which made no sense. The American Petroleum Institute (API) offered a contrasting statement: 'Inasmuch as the body develops no tolerance to benzene, and as there is a wide variation in individual susceptibility, it is generally considered that the only absolutely safe concentration for benzene is zero' (Drinker, 1948). The candour in this statement is startling and rare in an industry trade association publication. Today, the API takes a far less precautionary position – actively funding research to try to overturn national benzene standards in many countries.

William Hueper and the National Cancer Institute

In 1949, a report in *Scientific American* (Castleman, 2005, p. 62) expanded on the seminal work of Wilhelm Hueper, who would become the first chief of environmental carcinogenesis at the National Cancer Institute (NCI). Some of its ideas are remarkably contemporary (summarised in Box 6.1).

Box 6.1 Rising rates of cancer cannot be fully explained by ageing and diagnosis (1949 statement)

Scientific and technological progress have exposed humans to new physical and chemical agents. Some are believed associated with the rise of cancer as a cause of death. Customary reasons for increased cancer rates – improved diagnosis and population ageing – fail to explain why approximately 7 per cent of known cancer deaths in 1944 occurred in young people.

An explanation of this increase is thus sought in our environment, so much more complex than in 1900. The cancer increase may be caused by environmental agents hitherto considered comparatively harmless.

Many occupational cancers are unidentified. Physicians are poorly informed of basic symptomatic and sociological factors involved in occupational carcinogenesis and need better education. Occupational histories should reach back as far as 25 years. It is urgent to check medical suspicions of industrial cancer by epidemiological studies of plant workers and paramount to impress plant management with the problem's seriousness.

Control of occupational and environmental carcinogenesis is a public health problem of considerable magnitude. Carcinogens should be:

- eliminated from industrial military and civilian use as far as possible and practical;
- enclosed if used in manufacturing processes;
- separated from communities by reduced discharge in solid waste, effluent and air emissions.

Factories using carcinogens should be licensed and inspected, and their workers provided with protective clothing, equipment and medical supervision, including frequent physical examinations.

Causal Awareness of Cancer Obscured after World War II

In 1936, top scientists understood that much cancer emanated from workplace, hormones, radiation and other external sources, and by 1949 the NCI had begun to train doctors to watch for signs of these health risks and to promote their reduction. What happened to derail programmes to reduce the burden of cancer?

The time of the Belgian cancer congress was an era of mounting hostilities and militarisation. In 1935, the physiologist, Walter Cannon, linked growing nationalism with the lapse of long-term interest in humanitarian science, including the ability of chemicals and radiation to damage human life:

'The worldwide economic depression has greatly reduced the material support for scholarly efforts. What is the social value of the physiologist or biochemist?' (Cannon, 1994).

Cannon coined the term 'fight or flight' to describe the physical response of living beings to life-threatening terrors. Nations may be similar. The prospect of unrestrained global conflict might have changed public priorities, altering the way science was supported and used by its underwriters.

The old knowledge of cancer hazards fell victim to enthusiasm for modern industrial advances and its supporting social and economic forces. Optimism about industrialisation, *bona fide* advances in basic disease biology and darker forces generated a milieu in which the dice were weighted towards industry. The burden of proof for workers, physicians and the community shifted to one that was impossibly heavy. The search for more scientific information morphed into reasons to reject what once was known. The rise of chemotherapy also assisted. If cancer could be cured, then fundamental changes in the nature of modern life could be avoided.

But new chapters have opened due to growing numbers of cancers in young adults, some following therapies allowing them to survive childhood cancer. Other evidence is accruing of the combined effects of low levels of exposures to pesticides, other environmental toxins and persistent materials such as flame retardants and printer inks that put wildlife and humans at risk of cancer and other chronic ailments (Colburn et al., 1996).

Saran Wrap and Stunted Fingers

In 1933, a glass cleaner at Dow Chemical could not get one vial to come clean. It was covered with a tough, transparent film that would become the basis for Saran wrap, formed by linking many molecules of the plastic vinyl chloride. Saran wrap became a common household item.

Vinyl chloride, invented in Germany in the 19th century, was essential to the burgeoning chemical industry. As a slightly sweet-smelling gas under pressure in metal cans, it was once used to propel liquids including whipped cream, vaginal deodorants and hairsprays. More than half of this gas is chlorine, which was used to poison troops in the Great War. But it was presumed, incorrectly, that it lacked the poisonous properties of chlorine. It just turned out to be slower acting.

Commercial production of its solid form – polyvinylchloride (PVC) – skyrocketed. Workers in plastics factories started to notice a strange effect. Stunted fingers had been reported very occasionally in Europe in the 1940s, but not linked to vinyl chloride. Before 1965, only 72 cases of dissolved bone had been recorded globally, mostly in genetically linked families. However, in the 1960s, this rare bone defect was reported in groups of vinyl chloride workers (Lamy and Maroteaux, 1961; Ross, 1970).

A 1964 letter that was sent to a physician at a plant where several cases were found is instructive (see abridged version, Box 6.2) (Trade Secrets, 2014).

Box 6.2 Curious cases of hand disabilities among workers

'We have recently observed several cases of hand disabilities, the causes of which are unknown. We would like to determine as quietly as possible whether similar disabilities might exist in your plant. The disability we have seen is characterized by soreness of finger tips and resorption in the distal phalangeal joints. Several cases exhibit fibrous dermatological changes of the hands.

Please carefully observe the hands of employees if you see them for any reason. If you observe any similarity to this condition, note the individual's job assignment as well as his work history with the company. As yet, we have no firm opinion that these disabilities are occupational in origin.

I appreciate your rapid attention, incidental to other examinations. We do not wish to have this discussed at all, and I request that you maintain this information in confidence.'

In 1967, a report appeared of a man whose fingers had become stunted while working with polyvinyl chloride (Harris and Adams, 1967). His employers considered he must have a genetic defect or a rare disease. But similar reports appeared. In one case, a man's jaw dissolved. The notion that these oddities had common cause became hard to reject.

The vinyl chloride story is a dark moment in occupational medicine. As it looked problematic to humans, companies decided it was logical to see the response in animals. In 1971, Viola reported cancers of the skin, lungs and bones in rats exposed to high levels of vinyl chloride (Viola et al., 1971). Aware of this work and fearful of its implications, a group of companies including Montedison, a major Italian vinyl chloride manufacturer, commissioned a Bologna toxicologist named Maltoni to study it. Maltoni's work proved groundbreaking. For two years, 500 rats were subjected to various levels of the gas. The highest dose group were given 10,000 parts per million (ppm) – a level that nearly anaesthetised them. The lowest dose group were given 250 ppm – an amount that consumers could easily encounter when using aerosolised PVC in hairspray or that workers might inhale in the factory. A third group was unexposed.

One ppm is equivalent to a single minute over two years. Two years, or one million minutes, is the usual time to expose rodents to test compounds. Maltoni's innovation was to allow the rats to live their natural lifetimes, another year that allowed tumours to appear in the last third of life – corresponding to the retirement that human workers look forward to after their factory lives. After the exposures ended and all of the rats – exposed or not – lived out their natural lifetimes, their organs were examined.

The results horrified him. About one in ten of the exposed groups had liver angiosarcoma, an exceptionally rare, untreatable tumour. Not a single unexposed animal did. Maltoni showed a dose–response curve, but some developed this malignancy even at the lowest dose.

By 1972, Maltoni knew vinyl chloride was a serious problem. At first, he honoured his contract and kept quiet. Montedison assured him it would release his findings. Maltoni first expected this would be when the manufacturers met with government officials. But such meetings occurred and his work was not mentioned.

Disgusted, Maltoni violated his agreement in 1974, publishing the results. In Kentucky, a physician noticed that the fingers of a man who worked in B. F. Goodrich's vinyl chloride plant were shortened and stubbed. Within a few weeks, he saw three more in the same plant. His report (Centers for Disease Control and Prevention, 1997; Creech) made Maltoni's work with animals indisputably relevant.

Millions of dollars were at stake. To manufacturers, it made sense to fight any effort to restrain production. From the first reports of harm, the vinyl chloride industry had a simple response: call for more research but release enough information to reassure most people that the problem was trivial. It is cheaper to set up laboratories to evaluate chemicals. It takes time to get things right. Nobody can be opposed to serious scientific investigations. It is also heady for scientists to be told that their work is so important that more is needed. Funding for research on vinyl chloride expanded, as a delaying and distracting tactic.

As with tobacco, asbestos and climate change, attempts to expose the vinyl chloride hazards were met by concerted efforts of obstruction and intimidation. It was argued that case reports were not sufficiently rigorous to justify major changes in vital national production systems on which rested military and industrial foundations. Then, when rodent experiments revealed serious health problems, their relevance to humans was challenged.

Finally, enough time passed for public health studies on large numbers of people with well-documented exposures. But these had to overcome numerous statistical and procedural objections, including court challenges on the grounds that studies of large groups of people were 'mere statistics'. In the meantime, thousands, and sometimes millions, of people continued to be exposed to conditions that had been known decades earlier to be dangerous.

Deceit and Denial

Eventually, the control of vinyl chloride became a regulatory victory. In 1975, the Occupational Safety and Health Administration (OSHA) mandated limit for polyvinyl chloride dropped from 500 ppm to only 1 ppm. Emissions previously released into the community were captured. Contrary to dire warnings that this would mean the end of the plastics industry, business boomed (Ashford, 1984). But deceptions continued.

More than 20 years later, the historians, Markowitz and Rosner, published *Deceit and Denial*, a detailed account of the sordid history of vinyl chloride (Markowitz and Rosner, 2002). This drew the wrath of 20 of the biggest chemical companies in the world, including Dow, Monsanto, B.F. Goodrich and Union Carbide. The chapter that especially rattled these companies was called 'Evidence of an Illegal Conspiracy by Industry'. The title was from a memo by the Manufacturing Chemists Association's lawyers. It warned that concealing evidence of the connection between vinyl chloride and cancer 'could be construed as evidence of an illegal conspiracy by industry if the information were not made public' (Wiener, 2005). The book detailed the machinations of the companies involved in suppressing public awareness of rare and deadly incidents affecting their employees (Markowitz and Rosner, 2002). The authors drew from hundreds of thousands of pages of internal corporate documents.

As a reward, they found themselves at the centre of a major lawsuit. Trying to quash the book's public discussion, chemical firms filed a 'slap suit', a strategic lawsuit against public participation (SLAPP), a widely used tactic to intimidate opponents (Beder, 1998) This charged that they had damaged the reputation of honourable companies, even though they used the industry's own documents to reveal a three-decades-long struggle to keep the public unaware of, or confused about, the dangers of vinyl chloride. Industry subpoenas demanded the records used in writing this book – many from the plaintiffs' own files – and those of the publisher, the book's academic reviewers and the non-profit research organisations that had supported them (Guterman, 2004). To their credit, the authors prevailed and the suit was eventually dropped. The history of vinyl chloride is as sordid as the authors indicated.

Sir Richard Doll

Recognising its danger, the chemical industry employed the best counsel they could afford – Sir Richard Doll, then considered a top epidemiologist. Doll published his own analysis, agreeing that angiosarcoma was associated with vinyl chloride but disputing its links with more common cancers (Doll, 1988). Although he found more cases of brain cancer than expected, he argued this was statistically insignificant (Doll, 1988). However, Doll failed to declare his highly paid consultancy (Doll, 2000) for the Chemical Manufacturer's Association (Sass et al., 2005).

As a result, workers who developed more common tumours after exposures to vinyl chloride were unable to gain compensation. Not until 2000 did it become known that Doll's efforts on vinyl chloride had not been the independent musings of a disinterested expert. A letter found after his death in 2005 indicated that Doll had served as a consultant to Monsanto since at least 1979, at a fee of US$1,500 a day (Roush, 1986).

The Environmental Mutagen Society

Some researchers who received industry funds eventually grew disenchanted. Marvin Legator was one such researcher. He began working in industry in the 1950s, then with the Food and Drug Administration. He was full of ideas but short of funds. In 1969, with three colleagues, he co-founded the Environmental Mutagen Society (EMS). This society sought to investigate environmental factors causing genetic damage. Legator describes being impressed by the Dow Medical Director, who talked of the need to monitor workers continually. He thought, 'we can really find out whether benzene is getting to the bones of these guys!'. But co-EMS founder, Sam Epstein (author of *The Politics of Cancer*, 1978), was unimpressed.

In 1970, Bernard Goldstein was asked by the API to review the benzene literature. He concluded that benzene caused leukaemia. After that, the API withdrew funding. Despite hearing such stories, Legator was unmoved. He did not share Epstein's attitude and believed that solid experimental work would generate reform. He thought Dow Chemical was genuinely interested in basic occupational research. For a while, his was well-funded to perform chromosomal studies in exposed workers. They designed basic methods for detecting structural damage of DNA. Legator remembers this period fondly, until one critical point.

In life, sisters borrow things from one another. But when this happens within chromosomes, it can lead to trouble. 'Sister chromatid exchange' happens when related segments of a chromosome cross over and duplicate unwanted material. Legator's group showed that benzene could induce such genetic damage. The Dow study had collected blood from men when they first began working. Six years later, researchers took additional blood to check on the accrued chromosomal damage. But the results showed that chromosomes had been harmed. Dow pulled the plug on funding.

'Epstein had been perfectly right all along. I was the naïve one.' Legator laughed as he told me (DD) this story. By then, he was riddled with cancer. The disease was no surprise. 'I spent my youth awash in chemicals that can slice right through you. I know what they mean.'

The Weakening of OSHA

There is a widespread belief that OSHA regulates chemical exposures in the workplace – and there was a time, in the late 1970s, when it actively tried to do so. You still hear people complain that OSHA is overzealous. The truth is that it has been a paper tiger for decades.

Nowhere is OSHA's failure clearer than with benzene and vinyl chloride, where even now well-heeled efforts are under way to roll back existing standards. In 1979, OSHA took the radical step of setting a benzene standard of 1 ppm – a level then believed to be as low as feasible. But in 1980, the Supreme Court ruled against the standard, arguing that the agency had failed to prove that this low level would provide measurable health benefits in workers. The court demanded evidence that only time, money and epidemiologists could produce.

Today, OSHA is a shell. For a while, OSHA set standards for an average of one carcinogen a year, but most standards were developed decades ago.

Cancer in China

Since the 1980s, colleagues at the Chinese Academy of Preventive Medicine have been conducting a large epidemiologic study of workers exposed to benzene in Chinese cities. In 1989, they found a statistically significant excess of leukaemia and lung cancer, along with possible increases of liver and stomach cancer, and lymphoma. The NCI is now co-sponsoring further research in China.

Such studies, involving thousands of workers in more than 700 Chinese factories, have finally provided what the Supreme Court asked for two decades ago. Bone marrow disorders, including cancer, are clearly worsened by greater benzene exposures. Recently, these researchers have found that even at exposures of 1 ppm, Chinese shoemakers with certain common genetic traits suffer reduced bone marrow function.

However, these studies could also end up being ignored, because of a brazen act of manufacturing uncertainty that could well lift exposure standards. Unhappy with the efforts under way by the NCI and others in China, five major oil companies have bet millions of dollars that they will be able to 'contradict earlier claims that link low- and mid-levels of benzene to cancers and other diseases from exposure to benzene' (Capiello, 2005).

Personal Notes

The first time one of the authors (Davis) met Tony McMichael was at Cold Spring Harbor,[3] New York, USA in 1980. She explains:

> The first time I met Tony was at Cold Spring Harbor in 1980. I was quite young and naive about the ways that science worked. I had begun working with Marvin Schneiderman of the NCI evaluating the impact of workplace carcinogens and was about to start working on a post-doc with Abe Lilienfeld. We had determined that there appeared to be an increase in cancer not tied with smoking or ageing and had published some of these findings. Tony took the time to look at what we had calculated and admitted that he shared our concerns. Tony and I were among the only people there who raised questions directly to Sir Richard Doll about his proclamation that the only important cause of cancer was tobacco. We were all shocked to learn that at the time that Doll was vociferously arguing against environmental carcinogens being of any major consequence, he had served secretly as a consultant to the chemical

3 www.cshl.edu/About-Us/History.html, accessed 10 April 2015.

> industry, as we describe above. Others pointed out that major funding to Oxford's Green College which Doll led also came from the chemical industry (www.preventcancer.com/losing/other/doll.htm).
>
> When I organized a major international conference on avoidable causes of cancer for the Collegium Ramazzini, Tony was again one of the strong voices urging attention be paid to workplace cancer causes and more general environmental carcinogens. In his refusal to compromise his views and his commitment to impeccable scholarship and integrity, Tony remains a model to us all.

The first time the second author (Butler) met Tony was at Sydney University in 1993, just prior to the 13th International Epidemiology Association conference. His interest in the causes and politics of cancer was piqued by several experiences as a junior family doctor. He recalls that the first patient he ever diagnosed with cancer, in Devonport, Tasmania, in 1989, had asked whether his own exposure to agricultural sprays could have been a factor. His concerns about faint-hearted government enquiries into cancer date to that period, and are described on his blog.[4]

He also recalls reading, later that year, John Goldsmith's keynote talk from the first International Society for Environmental Epidemiology (ISEE) meeting (Goldsmith, 1988). In it, Goldsmith had written:

> We, the environmental epidemiologists of the world, are the canaries, capable of giving warning of impending environmental disaster in time for remedial steps to be taken. Fortunately, our fate is not to have to die as the unfortunate canaries of the coal miners did, but to sing, to call out in clear tones the nature and type of impending health danger that threatens. It is the methods and criteria of scientific detection, analysis, and interpretation that give us our lifesaving potential. (Goldsmith, 1988)

Conclusion

The best wars, to take a line from President McKinley's Secretary of State, are short, splendid little affairs, all pageantry and little fighting. The protracted war on cancer (generally viewed as beginning when US President Richard Nixon signed the National Cancer Act in 1971) has been none of the above. How did we get to this point?

4 globalchangemusings.blogspot.com.au/2013/04/canaries-struggling-to-improve.html, accessed 10 April 2015.

The war on cancer has long been obstructed by vested interests. The ISEE, of which Tony McMichael later became president, has, since its formation, endeavoured to identify and to ameliorate environmental cancer, including among workers. Its ethics committee, in particular, is keenly aware of issues of bias, suppression and repression. Yet, on the whole, proof that the world in which we live and work contributes to cancer has often been systematically overlooked and suppressed.

Prevention has been considerably diluted and diverted to attempts to find, treat and cure the disease. We spend more money than ever to detect and treat cancer (Hanahan, 2014). Today, one subsidiary of Industrial Chemicals Inc. makes cancer-causing pesticides, like atrazine – a compound banned in much of the industrial world –, while another division produces tamoxifen, a widely prescribed anti-cancer drug. Could this paradox be related to the fact that the incidence of cancer not tied to smoking and its treatment options keep increasing, while efforts to restrain environmental causes of the disease limp far behind?

Of course not. Remember that we live in a highly technological, interconnected world. It is safer, and better for your reputation in polite society, to keep reminding yourself that the disease is just so damned complex.

References

Ashford, N.A. 1984. The use of technical information in environmental health and safety regulation: a brief guide to the issues. *Science, Technology, & Human Values* 9, 130–3.

Beder, S. 1998. *Global Spin: The Corporate Assault on Environmentalism*. Scribe Publications, Melbourne, Australia.

Cannon, W.B. 1994. Reflections on the man and his contributions. *International Journal of Stress Management* 1, 145–58.

Capiello, D. 2005. Oil industry funding study to contradict cancer claims: research will analyze effects of benzene on workers in China. *Houston Chronicle*, 29 April 2005.

Castleman, B. 2005. *Asbestos, Medical and Legal Aspects*. Aspen Publishers, New York, USA.

Centers for Disease Control and Prevention 1997. Angiosarcoma of the liver among polyvinyl chloride workers – Kentucky. *Morbidity and Mortality Weekly Report* 46, 97–101.

Colburn, T., Dumanoski, D. & Myers, J.P. 1996. *Our Stolen Future: Are We Threatening Our Fertility, Intelligence and Survival? A Scientific Detective Story*. Dutton, New York, USA.

Creech, J. (deposition) as quoted in Gerald Markowitz and David Rosner, *Deceit and Denial* (University of California Press, Berkeley, California, USA, 2002), 173.

Davis, D. 2007. *The Secret History of the War on Cancer*. Basic Books, New York, USA.

Doll, R.S. 1988. Effects of exposure to vinyl chloride: an assessment of the evidence. *Scandinavian Journal of Work and Environmental Health* 14, 61–78.

Doll, R.S. 2000. Deposition of William Richard Shaboe Doll, Ross V. Conoco, Inc. Case No 90-4837. LA 14th Judicial District Court, London, UK. 27 January, 2000, cited in Sass et al., notes, 811.

Drinker, P. 1948. *API Toxicology Review: Benzene*. American Petroleum Institute. Washington DC, USA.

Epstein, S. 1978. *The Politics of Cancer*. Sierra Club Books, San Francisco, California, USA.

Goldsmith, J. 1988. Improving the prospects for environmental epidemiology. *Archives of Environmental Health* 43, 69–74.

Guterman, L. 2004. Peer reviewers are subpoenaed in cancer lawsuit against chemical companies. *Chronicle of Higher Education*. chronicle.com/article/Peer-Reviewers-Are-Subpoenaed/25295/, accessed 11 February 2015.

Hanahan, D. 2014. Rethinking the war on cancer. *The Lancet* 383, 558–63.

Harris, D.K. & Adams, W.G.F. 1967. Acro-osteolysis occurring in men engaged in the polymerization of vinyl chloride. *British Medical Journal* 3, 712–4.

Hunter, D. 1973. *The Diseases of Occupations, fifth edition*. Hodder and Stoughton, London, 35.

Lamy, M. & Maroteaux, P. 1961. Acro-osteolyse dominante. *Archives Françaises de Pédiatrie* 18, 693–702.

Markowitz, G. & Rosner, D. 2002. *Deceit and Denial*. University of California, Berkeley, California, USA.

Montgomery, J.L. 1997. Diagnostic imaging: finding new ways to see; seeing new ways to cure. *Postgraduate Medicine* 102, 144–8, 155.

Nash, G.H. 1983. *The Life of Herbert Hoover, Volume 1*. W. W. Norton & Co Inc, New York, USA.

National Safety Council 1926. Chemical and Rubber Sections. Final Report of the Committee, Chemical and Rubber Sections, National Safety Council, on Benzol. National Bureau of Casualty and Surety Underwriters, New York, USA, May 1926, 4.

Ross, J.A. 1970. An unusual occupational bone change. In: Jelliffe, A.M. & Strickland, B. (eds) *Symposium Ossium*. Livingstone, London, UK.

Roush, G. 1986. Letter to Richard Doll, dated 29 April 1986, from Doll archives, Oxford University, copy provided by Martin J. Walker.

Sass, J.B., Castleman, B. & Wallinga, D. 2005. Vinyl chloride: a case study of data suppression and misrepresentation. *Environmental Health Perspectives* 113, 809–12.

Trade Secrets. 2014. Available at: www.pbs.org/tradesecrets/program/vinyl.html, accessed 16 February 2014.

Viola, P.L., Bigott, A. & Caputo, A. 1971. Oncogenic response of rat skin, lungs, and bones to vinyl chloride. *Cancer Research* 31, 516–22.

Wiener, J. 2005. Cancer, chemicals and history. *The Nation* 7 February 2005. Available at: www.thenation.com/article/cancer-chemicals-and-history, accessed 20 May 2014.

PART 3

ENVIRONMENTAL AND SOCIAL EPIDEMIOLOGY

Cancer, Chemicals, Radiation and Health Transitions

REPRINT D

Port Pirie Cohort Study: Environmental Exposure to Lead and Children's Abilities at the Age of Four Years

ANTHONY J. MCMICHAEL, P.A. BAGHURST, N. WIGG
G. VIMPANI, E. ROBERTSON AND R. ROBERTS

McMichael, A.J., Baghurst, P.A., Wigg, N., Vimpani, G., Robertson, E. & Roberts, R. 1988. Port Pirie Cohort Study: environmental exposure to lead and children's abilities at the age of four years. New England Journal of Medicine 319, 468–75.

Pages: 125 to 136

PORT PIRIE COHORT STUDY: ENVIRONMENTAL EXPOSURE TO LEAD AND CHILDREN'S ABILITIES AT THE AGE OF FOUR YEARS

ANTHONY J. MCMICHAEL, M.B.B.S., PH.D., PETER A. BAGHURST, M.SC., PH.D., NEIL R. WIGG, M.B.B.S., GRAHAM V. VIMPANI, M.B.B.S., PH.D., EVELYN F. ROBERTSON, M.B.CH.B., AND RUSSELL J. ROBERTS, M.CLIN.PSYCH.

Abstract We studied the effect of environmental exposure to lead on children's abilities at the age of four years in a cohort of 537 children born during 1979 to 1982 to women living in a community situated near a lead smelter. Samples for measuring blood lead levels were obtained from the mothers antenatally, at delivery from the mothers and umbilical cords, and at the ages of 6, 15, and 24 months and then annually from the children. Concurrently, the mothers were interviewed about personal, family, medical, and environmental factors. Maternal intelligence, the home environment, and the children's mental development (as evaluated with use of the McCarthy Scales of Children's Abilities) were formally assessed.

The mean blood lead concentration varied from 0.44 μmol per liter in midpregnancy to a peak of 1.03 μmol per liter at the age of two years. The blood lead concentration at each age, particularly at two and three years, and the integrated postnatal average concentration were inversely related to development at the age of four. Multivariate analysis incorporating many factors in the children's lives indicated that the subjects with an average postnatal blood lead concentration of 1.50 μmol per liter had a general cognitive score 7.2 points lower (95 percent confidence interval, 0.3 to 13.2; mean score, 107.1) than those with an average concentration of 0.50 μmol per liter. Similar deficits occurred in the perceptual-performance and memory scores. Within the range of exposure studied, no threshold dose for an effect of lead was evident.

We conclude that postnatal blood lead concentration is inversely related to cognitive development in children, although one must be circumspect in making causal inferences from studies of this relation, because of the difficulties in defining and controlling confounding effects. (N Engl J Med 1988; 319:468-75.)

ALTHOUGH the health hazards of acute lead toxicity and occupational exposure to lead are well known, uncertainties exist about the adverse effects of environmental exposure to lower levels of lead. Recent epidemiologic studies have indicated that neuropsychological development in children may be impaired by such exposure, but debate persists about methods for ensuring adequate control of the confounding effects of other covariates in such investigations.[1-4]

The early epidemiologic research on the relation between lead and development, which consisted of cross-sectional or case–control studies, was inconclusive. In 1979 Needleman and colleagues, in a community-based study of children in Boston in whom previous exposure to lead was estimated from examinations of deciduous teeth, reported evidence of lead-related neuropsychological deficits.[5] Subsequent research in Germany revealed a similar but statistically insignificant relation.[6] However, in several British studies, adjustment for covariates relating to the social environment greatly attenuated an apparent inverse relation of lead to mental development.[7,8] A recent cross-sectional study of blood lead concentration in relation to cognitive ability and educational attainment in Scottish children six to nine years of age found an inverse relation, with no apparent threshold level of exposure.[9]

From the Department of Community Medicine, University of Adelaide (A.J.M.); the Division of Human Nutrition, Commonwealth Scientific and Industrial Research Organisation (Australia) (P.A.B.); the Child, Adolescent and Family Health Service (N.R.W., R.J.R.); the Department of Paediatrics, Flinders Medical Centre (G.V.V.); and the Department of Chemical Pathology, Adelaide Children's Hospital (E.F.R.). Address reprint requests to Prof. McMichael at the Department of Community Medicine, University of Adelaide, North Terrace, Adelaide, South Australia 5000.

Supported by a series of grants from the National Health and Medical Research Council and additional assistance from the South Australian Health Commission and the University of Adelaide.

These inconsistent results may have arisen because any effect of environmental exposure to lead on children's development is probably small; many coexistent confounding factors also influence children's development; measurement of antecedent exposure to lead is difficult; and there is uncertainty about the selection and measurement of developmental outcomes. The inconsistencies may also reflect interactive effects, in that the deleterious effects of exposure to lead may be greater in socially disadvantaged children.[4]

To overcome some of these methodologic difficulties, cohort studies have been started in several locations. These investigations are seeking more definitive, prospective evidence of the relation between exposure to lead early in life and subsequent neuropsychological development. In a cohort study of 249 children in Boston, the lead concentration in umbilical-cord blood was inversely related, after adjustment for covariates, to cognitive development assessed every six months up to the age of two years.[1] The effect was most evident in the children in the upper and middle tertiles of blood lead concentrations (i.e., predominantly within the range of 0.3 to 1.0 μmol per liter, or 6 to 21 μg per deciliter).

Debate continues over whether there is a threshold, or "safe," level of exposure to lead. At blood lead concentrations as low as 1.0 μmol per liter, various neurophysiologic and enzymatic processes are impaired,[10,11] and disturbances of heme synthesis and altered central nervous system electrophysiologic responses have even been observed at levels below 0.72 μmol per liter (15 μg per deciliter).[12] Within urban and industrial populations, a substantial proportion of young children may have blood lead concentrations above this level; indeed, within the Port Pirie cohort, the mean concentration at the ages of 15 months and 24 months exceeds 1.0 μmol per liter (21 μg per deciliter).[13]

The Port Pirie Cohort Study began in 1979. The industrial town of Port Pirie (population, 16,000) is in South Australia, 200 km northwest of Adelaide. The town is situated immediately downwind of a large and longstanding lead-smelting facility, and there is extensive environmental contamination with lead, particularly in topsoil, yard dust, and house dust.[13]

Earlier results from this study have shown considerable individual variation in blood lead concentration during the first four years of life,[13] with approximately one third of the children having levels above 1.21 μmol per liter (25 μg per deciliter) on one or more occasions. Furthermore, postnatal blood lead concentrations have been found to be inversely associated, albeit weakly, with mental development at the age of two years (assessed by the Bayley Mental Development Index), after adjustment for confounding factors.[14]

This paper presents the results of follow-up to the age of four years, when the children's abilities were evaluated with use of the McCarthy Scales of Children's Abilities (MSCA). The MSCA, which can be used in children three to seven years old, comprises five scales: verbal, perceptual performance, quantitative, memory, and motor.[15] The first three of those scales combined form the general cognitive index (GCI). The GCI provides an age-specific index of cognitive functioning. Formal evaluation has shown that the GCI "assesses the child's reasoning, concept formation, and memory when solving verbal and numerical problems and when manipulating concrete materials."[16] An inverse relation has previously been reported between lead concentrations in the teeth of schoolchildren and perceptual–motor functioning[6]; the perceptual-performance scale of the MSCA measures the equivalent function in preschool children.

Methods

From 1979 to 1982 a total of 723 women were recruited during early pregnancy and followed to the live birth of an apparently healthy child.[17] The children were then entered in a long-term postnatal follow-up study. Recruitment was done through the medical practitioners in and around Port Pirie, who, after a series of meetings with the research team, unanimously agreed to support the study. The recruitment rate, estimated from registrations of births during this period, was 90 percent. Of the 548 children who were followed to the age of four, 397 lived in Port Pirie, and 151 were from the immediate rural area, including several smaller towns. The latter 151 children were included to ensure a range of individual blood lead concentrations, and they were found to have lower mean levels than the children from Port Pirie.[13]

The majority (80 percent) of the children lost to follow-up during the four years of postnatal study were in families that left the Port Pirie district; a few families simply discontinued their participation. Follow-up is continuing, and the final detailed formal neuropsychological assessment is being carried out in children who are seven years old.

Blood samples for measurement of lead concentrations were obtained from the pregnant women at specified times and from each child at delivery (umbilical-cord blood) and at ages 6, 15, and 24 months and annually thereafter. The postnatal samples were obtained from capillaries by finger prick, with use of a rigorous cleansing and collection protocol.[18] A pilot study had demonstrated that blood lead concentrations measured in capillary samples were highly correlated with simultaneously determined venous lead concentrations in 47 children in metropolitan Adelaide who were two to four years of age.[19] The samples were obtained by staff members of the Port Pirie Cohort Study. The capillary–venous blood lead correlation coefficient was 0.97.

Blood lead concentration was estimated with electrothermal atomization atomic absorption spectrometry.[20] Measurements of blood lead levels have been performed by our laboratory (at Adelaide Children's Hospital) for more than 20 years. Throughout this study, both internal and external (interlaboratory) quality-control procedures were used, with consistently satisfactory results. A certified commercially prepared product was employed to monitor intrabatch accuracy and to ensure interbatch standardization. External quality control, entailing assays of regularly supplied samples, was ensured by participation in three major programs: the national quality-control program conducted by the Standards Association of Australia and the international programs run by the health department of Pennsylvania and the Wolfson Research Laboratories (Birmingham, United Kingdom). Estimates were standardized to a packed-cell volume of 35 percent for maternal blood, 50 percent for cord blood, and 35 percent for the children's blood.

Each child's cumulative burden of body lead was estimated by trapezoidal integration of the area under the curve of blood lead concentration, according to age (from birth [cord blood sample] to the age of four years). This method of averaging adjusts for the unequal time periods between successive blood samples. Since blood lead concentrations have approximately log-normal distributions, the reported mean blood concentrations of lead are geometric. To reduce the influence of extreme individual values for blood lead concentration on the statistical analyses, the logarithm (base 10) of the concentration was used in all simple and multiple regression analyses.

At the time the blood samples were obtained, the nurse-interviewer also conducted a structured interview to obtain information on a range of demographic, familial, behavioral, medical, and social environmental factors. All interviews were carried out by one of four trained nurse-interviewers.

The developmental status of each child at the age of four years was assessed with use of the MSCA. This assessment and the blood sampling were carried out on different days. A full-time research psychologist who was blinded to the child's past or current blood lead concentration conducted all testing sessions in a clinic setting. Although the psychologist had also assessed the child's development (using the Bayley Scales of Infant Development) at the age of two years, he was not aware of that earlier result when making the subsequent assessment. The conversion of raw-score data to scale scores was done by computer. The scoring process was thus reliable and accurate. Annual mean MSCA scores during the three years of testing were compared in order to test for temporal observer drift; a variation of only 1 percent was found.

Since there are no Australian standardization data on the MSCA, it was not possible to evaluate the absolute scores obtained in our study population. (A review of the original standardization in the United States, from about 1970, might lead one to expect that the scores would be 100 for the GCI and 50 for the other five scales. However, there is evidence that in developed countries, an upward drift in intelligence scores occurs with successive generations.[21]) Since the MSCA was used in this study solely for the epidemiologic purpose of making intracohort comparisons, our results concern only the relative scores for compared groups of children.

Assessment of the care-giving environment, using the Home Observation for Measurement of the Environment (HOME) inventory, was made during a visit to the children's homes when they were three years of age. This inventory evaluates, by means of observations and interviews, the quality of stimulation of children in their homes.[22] The inventory measures processes that mediate the child's development and has six subscales: emotional and verbal responsiveness of the parents; parental acceptance of the child; maternal involvement with the child; organization of the home environment; appropriateness of play materials; and variety in daily stimulation. These aspects of the home environment correlate well with intellectual and verbal development in early childhood.[22,23] One nurse-interviewer who was trained in the use of the HOME inventory made nearly all the assessments, although the first 30 were done by the psychologist-trainer.

Maternal intelligence was estimated with use of the Wechsler

Adult Intelligence Scale–Revised.[24] This test was administered in full by the research psychologist, who was blinded to the children's blood lead concentrations. The testing was done while the children were in the age range of three to five years.

Results

Blood Lead Concentration at Various Ages

The geometric mean antenatal (maternal) blood lead concentration varied from 0.44 μmol per liter (9.1 μg per deciliter) at 16 weeks of gestation to 0.46 μmol per liter (9.5 μg per deciliter) at delivery. The mean lead concentration in blood from the umbilical cord was 0.40 μmol per liter. The mean values in the children at the ages of 6 months, 15 months, and two, three, and four years were 0.70, 1.01, 1.03, 0.94, and 0.79 μmol per liter, respectively. Maximal uptake of lead appears to occur during the second and third years of life. At the age of two years, when the mean blood lead concentration peaked (at 1.03 μmol per liter, or 21.2 μg per deciliter), individual values ranged from 0.24 to 2.75 μmol per liter. There were no postnatal differences in mean blood lead concentrations between boys and girls. The integrated postnatal average blood lead concentration was 0.92 μmol per liter. The distributions of individual values according to age are indicated in Table 1.

Analysis of autocorrelations of blood lead concentration measured at different ages indicated substantial intraindividual "tracking." The estimated Pearson correlation coefficients for all pairs of measures of blood lead concentrations between the ages of 15 months and seven years (with data still incomplete at six and seven years) were in the range of $r = 0.55$ to 0.80; the value of 0.55 corresponded to the largest possible age difference (69 months). This suggests that for each child, the relative magnitude of the blood lead concentration remained fairly constant with increasing age. This constancy impedes the estimation of the effect of age-specific blood lead concentration on mental development independently of the blood lead concentration at other ages. Correlations between the assessments of lead in the cord blood and postnatal measures were of the order of 0.35 to 0.40.

Results of the MSCA Tests

MSCA testing was completed for 548 children. For 537, it was done within a six-month period around their birthdays, whereas in the other 11, there was an excessive delay before testing. The latter group was excluded from the analysis; among the other 537 children, the time of testing appeared to be unrelated to the blood lead concentration. The mean scores, which were generally higher than the expected values of 100 for the GCI and 50 for other scales, were as follows: verbal, 53.5; perceptual performance, 56.9; quantitative, 50.5; GCI, 107.1; memory, 48.2; and motor, 53.8. The girls scored 2 to 4 percent higher than the boys on all scales. The scores were 2 to 3 percent lower in the children residing in Port Pirie than in those from the surrounding areas.

Comparison of the MSCA test results with the scores on the Bayley Mental Development Index, at the age of two years, showed that the GCI had the highest correlation ($r = 0.58$), whereas the motor scale had the lowest ($r = 0.43$). The MSCA motor scale was only moderately correlated with the Bayley Psychomotor Development Index ($r = 0.28$).

Age-Specific Blood Lead Concentration and MSCA Scores

For each age of the children at which blood sampling was performed, the study population was subdivided into quartiles of blood lead concentration, each of which contained approximately 135 children. Variation in MSCA scores was examined in relation to these quartiles. At each age, there was a consistent inverse relation between blood lead concentration and MSCA scores.

This inverse relation had similar strength for the GCI, the memory

Table 1. Mean MSCA Scores at the Age of Four Years, According to Quartile of Blood Lead Concentration and Time of Blood Sampling.

Blood Lead Level*	Blood Sample								
	Antenatal (Average)	Delivery	Umbilical Cord	6 Mo	15 Mo	2 Yr	3 Yr	4 Yr	Integrated Postnatal Average
Mean blood lead level (μmol per liter)									
1	0.29	0.27	0.21	0.40	0.58	0.64	0.58	0.47	0.60
2	0.42	0.40	0.35	0.61	0.89	0.90	0.84	0.71	0.85
3	0.51	0.53	0.48	0.82	1.18	1.18	1.09	0.92	1.05
4	0.69	0.78	0.72	1.18	1.68	1.63	1.46	1.26	1.36
General cognitive index									
1	108.8	109.5	108.6	111.2	110.1	112.4	112.0	111.1	112.6
2	109.4	108.8	109.3	107.4	109.9	109.4	109.0	109.2	108.3
3	106.7	106.1	104.7	105.9	105.4	104.6	105.7	103.6	104.0
4	104.3	104.2	106.3	104.1	103.6	102.3	102.0	104.7	103.0
Perceptual-performance score									
1	58.4	58.0	57.7	59.2	58.5	59.5	59.0	58.8	59.7
2	57.9	57.9	57.7	57.0	58.5	58.3	58.3	58.7	58.1
3	56.5	56.2	55.2	55.8	56.1	55.7	56.7	54.9	55.6
4	55.2	55.3	57.1	55.6	54.6	54.1	53.6	55.2	54.1
Memory score									
1	48.2	49.1	49.3	49.8	49.2	50.9	51.1	50.7	50.2
2	49.4	49.5	48.6	47.6	49.4	49.0	48.3	48.3	48.1
3	48.0	47.7	47.7	48.0	47.1	47.3	47.3	46.8	46.9
4	47.3	46.9	47.2	47.2	47.1	45.6	45.9	47.0	46.3
Motor score									
1	54.4	54.9	54.5	55.6	55.2	55.6	55.9	55.0	56.0
2	54.4	53.9	54.3	53.6	54.0	55.4	54.2	55.0	54.3
3	53.9	53.9	52.9	53.4	53.5	51.9	53.7	52.0	52.1
4	52.5	52.4	53.2	52.9	52.8	52.2	51.5	52.7	52.8
No. of children	534	479	474	526	527	534	525	530	463

*The first quartile includes those with the lowest blood concentrations of lead and the fourth those with the highest concentrations.

score, and the perceptual-performance score, with the mean values varying by approximately 10 percent between the highest and lowest quartiles of blood lead concentration. Table 1 shows that the range of mean scores was greater for blood lead concentrations measured postnatally than antenatally or at delivery and was greatest at the ages of two and three years. Since the verbal and quantitative scales are subsets of the GCI and the scores obtained on them varied only slightly with the blood lead concentration, they are not listed.

Figure 1 shows the variation in MSCA scores at four years of age in relation to blood lead concentration at three years of age — the age at which there was maximal variation in those scores according to quartile of blood lead concentration (Table 1). For each of the six scores, an inverse gradient extends across the full range of blood lead concentrations. Figure 1 depicts the unadjusted relation between blood lead concentration at the age of three years and MSCA score; the relations at 15 months and two years, as well as with the integrated postnatal blood lead concentration, resembled those shown in Figure 1.

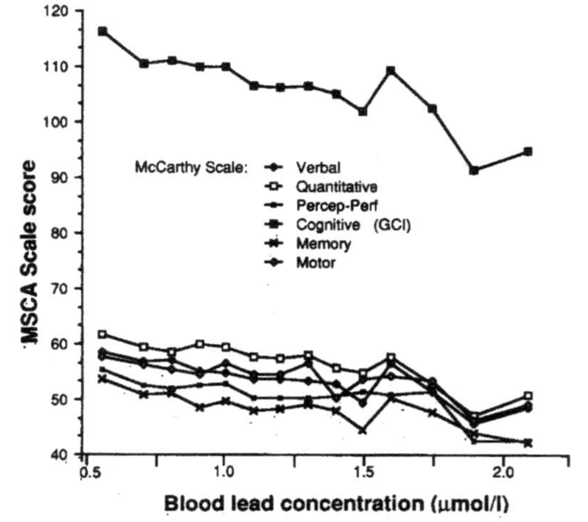

Figure 1. MSCA Scale Scores at the Age of Four Years, According to Blood Lead Concentration at Three Years of Age.

Relation of Other Covariates to MSCA Scores

For the covariates subsequently treated as potential confounders in multivariate analyses, their univariate relations with blood lead concentration and with the GCI and the perceptual-performance and memory scales are shown in Table 2. Many characteristics of the parents (including parental education, the mother's IQ and marital status, and the father's job) were strongly related to the MSCA scores, in the expected direction. Maternal age and the quality of the home environment were positively related to the scores. Obstetrical factors and neonatal characteristics were less strongly related, although the lower values (or the adverse findings) tended to be associated with low MSCA scores.

Regression Analyses of MSCA Scores and Blood Lead Concentration

Table 3 presents the results of simple and multiple linear regression analyses. The multivariate model contained almost all factors identified a priori as potential determinants of developmental abilities — irrespective of the variance in developmental score accounted for by the factor in multiple regression analysis. This approach errs toward overinclusion of covariates, but it does so because of the known difficulty of achieving adequate control of confounding factors in studies of lead and childhood development. The only factors excluded from the original list were two antenatal variables (bleeding during pregnancy and vitamin supplementation), which had no explanatory power in multivariate analysis and for which there were no a priori expectations of the effects on child mental development, and the Apgar score at one minute (which was supplanted by the Apgar score at five minutes). The fit of the linear models was not improved markedly by adding quadratic terms in blood lead concentration and in other continuous covariates (birth weight, maternal age, and HOME score).

The linearity observed with the logarithm of blood lead concentration accords with recent results from studies in schoolchildren in Edinburgh[9] and infants in Cincinnati.[25] Repetition of this analysis, using the untransformed blood lead concentration, did not alter the fit of the model.

The regression coefficients in Table 3 estimate the changes in MSCA score accompanying a 10-fold increase (i.e., one unit on a logarithmic scale) in the corresponding blood lead concentration. Thus, for example, an increase in the integrated postnatal blood lead concentration of from 0.25 to 2.50 μmol per liter would be accompanied by an estimated drop of 28.9 points in the GCI (last entry, first column), ignoring the confounding effects of other covariates. For an increase in the integrated postnatal blood lead concentration of from 0.50 to 1.50 μmol per liter, the expected drop in GCI would be ($\log_{10}3 \times 28.9$) = 13.8 points. After the adjustment for the covariates in the multiple regression analysis, the corresponding drops in GCI (see partial regression coefficients, Table 3) would be 15.0 points (for an increase in blood lead concentration from 0.25 to 2.50 μmol per liter) and 7.2 points (for from 0.50 to 1.50 μmol per liter). The figure of 7.2 points (95 percent confidence interval, 0.3 to 13.2) represents a decrease of approximately 7 percent in GCI score in a child with average values for the other covariates.

In simple regression analyses, blood lead concentration at every age was negatively related to the GCI and the perceptual-performance and memory scales (Table 3). These relations were weakest for the cord blood sample. In multiple regression analyses, the relations between antenatal and perinatal blood lead concentrations and these developmental outcomes

Table 2. Mean MSCA Scores for Covariates That May Confound the Relation between a Child's Ability and His or Her Exposure to Lead.*

COVARIATE	CATEGORY	INTEGRATED MEAN LEAD LEVEL	GENERAL COGNITIVE INDEX		PERCEPTUAL-PERFORMANCE SCALE		MEMORY SCALE	
		µmol/liter	MEAN	P VALUE (% VARIANCE)	MEAN	P VALUE (% VARIANCE)	MEAN	P VALUE (% VARIANCE)
Sex	Male	0.92	105.7	0.058	55.6	0.002	47.5	0.10
	Female	0.92	108.3	(0.5)	58.0	(1.5)	48.8	(0.3)
Residence	Non-Pirie	0.70	109.4	0.06	57.6	0.31	49.6	0.035
	Pirie	1.00	106.4	(0.5)	56.7	(0.0)	47.7	(0.6)
Mother's education (yr)	<10	1.07	102.6	<0.001	54.8	0.003	46.0	0.005
	10	0.96	105.6	(3.2)	55.9	(2.1)	47.4	(1.9)
	11	0.86	107.8		57.7		48.5	
	≥12	0.83	113.2		59.5		50.8	
Mother's work site	Home	0.92	106.4	0.10	56.5	0.10	48.1	0.79
	External	0.92	108.9	(0.3)	57.9	(0.3)	48.4	(0.0)
Mother's marital status	Unmarried	1.13	99.6	<0.001	52.3	<0.001	44.7	0.001
	Married	0.90	107.8	(1.6)	57.3	(1.7)	48.5	(1.0)
Mother's age (yr)	≤21	1.11	102.3	<0.001	54.7	0.02	46.0	0.003
	22–29	0.90	107.3	(2.3)	57.0	(1.1)	48.1	(1.8)
	≥30	0.84	111.3		58.7		50.5	
Antenatal medication use	No	0.91	109.1	0.07	58.2	0.03	49.0	0.18
	Yes	0.93	106.4	(0.4)	56.4	(0.7)	47.9	(0.2)
Mother's IQ	<81	1.11	94.0	<0.001	48.6	<0.001	42.5	<0.001
	81–90	0.98	107.4	(9.1)	57.3	(9.6)	48.7	(6.2)
	91–100	0.88	107.8		57.4		48.3	
	>100	0.80	114.5		61.0		52.0	
	Not measured	0.95	105.5		55.9		47.0	
HOME score	<39	1.08	95.9	<0.001	50.8	<0.001	45.1	<0.001
	39–41	0.99	104.6	(16.0)	55.3	(13.5)	43.7	(9.1)
	42–44	0.92	109.3		58.4		47.0	
	45–47	0.79	110.5		58.9		48.5	
	>47	0.80	116.9		61.7		53.0	
Father's education (yr)	<10	0.96	104.8	<0.001	56.1	<0.001	46.2	0.002
	10	0.91	105.9	(5.9)	56.1	(6.8)	48.0	(2.3)
	11	0.91	108.3		58.0		48.3	
	≥12	0.82	114.6		60.8		51.4	
	Missing	1.09	99.6		51.3		46.6	
Father's work	Unemployed	1.11	97.3	<0.001	52.0	<0.001	43.3	<0.001
	Non-office	0.92	106.5		56.8		47.8	
	Office	0.83	113.8	(6.4)	59.9	(4.7)	51.7	(4.9)
	Unknown	1.13	101.1		52.9		45.6	
Delivery	Occipital	0.92	106.7	0.55	56.8	0.78	47.9	0.52
	Cesarean	0.95	109.1	(0.0)	57.7	(0.0)	48.7	(0.0)
	Other	0.90	107.7		56.9		48.9	
Apgar score at 5 min	9 or 10	0.90	105.5	0.23	56.4	0.55	47.1	0.14
	≤8	1.01	107.5	(0.1)	57.0	(0.0)	48.5	(0.2)
Oxygen use at birth	No	0.90	108.1	0.03	57.4	0.04	48.7	0.04
	Yes	0.99	104.8	(0.7)	55.6	(0.6)	47.0	(0.6)
Neonatal jaundice	No	0.91	107.4	0.59	57.1	0.60	48.4	0.98
	Yes	0.94	106.6	(0.0)	56.6	(0.0)	47.8	(0.0)
Birth weight (g)	<2500	1.06	99.3	0.02	53.0	0.01	44.0	0.17
	2500–2999	0.99	104.5	(1.3)	55.0	(1.6)	48.4	(0.4)
	3000–3499	0.93	107.1		56.6		48.3	
	≥3500	0.88	108.9		58.2		48.4	
Size for dates at birth	Small	1.01	100.7	0.10	53.6	0.01	44.3	0.08
	Appropriate	0.92	107.3	(0.5)	57.0	(1.6)	48.2	(0.6)
	Large	0.90	108.1		56.9		48.5	
Birth rank	First	0.95	106.7	0.62	56.5	0.68	48.4	0.44
	Second	0.91	107.0	(0.0)	57.3	(0.0)	47.6	(0.0)
	Subsequent	0.89	108.5		57.1		48.9	

*The P values indicate the global statistical significance of differences between the categories of each covariate, ignoring all other covariates. HOME denotes home observation for measurement of the environment.

were less strong. However, measures of postnatal blood lead concentration retained clear, negative, and predominantly statistically significant relations with the GCI. For these postnatal measures, including the integrated average value, the regression coefficients were approximately halved relative to their values in the simple regression. Thus, the covariates that were included were, in aggregate, positively confounded with blood lead concentration and accounted (either independently or through their association with exposure to lead) for approximately half the apparent effect of blood lead concentration that was evident in simple regression analysis.

Repeated analysis including stratification according to sex did not significantly improve the fit, although the negative regression coefficient of blood lead concentration in relation to GCI score was slightly higher for girls than for boys. Repeated analysis restricted to children with blood lead concentrations below 1.21 μmol per liter (25 μg per deciliter) showed that the relation at such levels was as strong for this group of children as for the whole cohort (although statistical significance was decreased because of reductions in the range of exposure and the numbers of subjects). For the integrated postnatal average blood lead concentrations, the relation with GCI was actually stronger at values below 1.21 μmol per liter than overall. This could reflect either an actual greater dependence of GCI on blood lead concentration or less confounding by the other covariates, among children with less exposure.

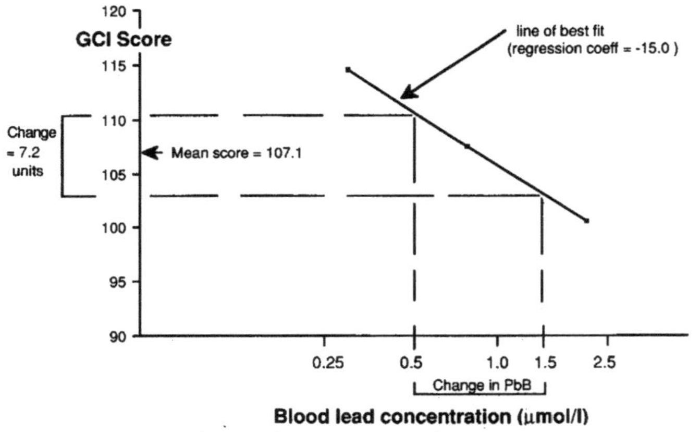

Figure 2. Linear Relation, as Estimated from Multiple Regression Analysis, between the Integrated Postnatal Average Blood Lead Concentration (Shown on a Logarithmic Scale) and the General Cognitive Index (GCI).

The estimated decrease in GCI associated with an increase in blood lead concentration from 0.50 to 1.50 μmol per liter is shown as an example; also see Discussion.

When successive contractions of the age span of the integrated postnatal average blood lead concentration (i.e., spanning the periods from six months to, successively, the fourth, third, and second birthday) were substituted in the regression analyses, small progressive reductions occurred in each of the regression coefficients shown in the bottom row of Table 3. Thus, the integrated measure across the maximal age span (i.e., birth to the age of four years) showed the greatest inverse relation to developmental outcome.

Table 3. Estimated Coefficients of Log Blood Lead Concentration from Simple and Multiple Regression Analyses of MSCA Scores at the Age of Four Years.*

Blood Sample	General Cognitive Index		Perceptual-Performance Scale		Memory Scale	
	simple	partial	simple	partial	simple	partial
	coefficient ±SE (P value)					
Antenatal (average)	−15.1±4.7 (0.001)	−1.8±5.7 (0.75)	−9.5±2.7 (<0.001)	−4.1±3.3 (0.22)	−4.8±2.7 (0.07)	2.0±3.3 (0.54)
Delivery	−10.4±3.9 (0.008)	−0.4±4.5 (0.93)	−5.1±2.3 (0.03)	0.2±2.7 (0.95)	−4.9±2.2 (0.03)	−0.4±2.6 (0.89)
Cord	−6.1±3.4 (0.08)	3.3±4.1 (0.42)	−3.0±2.0 (0.13)	1.6±2.4 (0.50)	−3.0±2.0 (0.12)	2.6±2.4 (0.27)
6 Mo	−15.1±3.8 (<0.001)	−8.5±4.4 (0.05)	−7.8±2.2 (<0.001)	−4.8±2.5 (0.06)	−4.9±2.2 (0.03)	−2.4±2.5 (0.34)
15 Mo	−14.3±3.8 (<0.001)	−3.5±4.8 (0.46)	−8.2±2.2 (<0.001)	−3.2±2.8 (0.26)	−5.3±2.2 (0.01)	−0.5±2.7 (0.87)
24 Mo	−25.8±4.3 (<0.001)	−11.1±5.4 (0.04)	−13.5±2.5 (<0.001)	−6.2±3.2 (0.05)	−13.4±2.4 (<0.001)	−7.3±3.1 (0.02)
36 Mo	−25.1±4.3 (<0.001)	−13.1±5.6 (0.02)	−13.6±2.5 (<0.001)	−7.7±3.3 (0.02)	−12.7±2.4 (<0.001)	−7.2±3.2 (0.27)
48 Mo	−20.1±4.1 (<0.001)	−5.5±5.1 (0.29)	−11.2±2.4 (<0.001)	−4.0±3.0 (0.18)	−10.3±2.3 (<0.001)	−4.1±3.0 (0.17)
Integrated postnatal average	−28.9±5.5 (<0.001)	−15.0±7.3 (0.04)	−15.1±3.2 (<0.001)	−8.3±4.1 (0.05)	−13.3±3.1 (<0.001)	−7.9±4.2 (0.06)

*The partial regression coefficients are from analyses incorporating all the covariates in Table 2. The P values are for assessments of the two-sided hypothesis that the estimates are not zero.

The estimated linear inverse relation between integrated postnatal blood lead concentration and GCI, within the range for which sufficient data were available (0.30 to 2.00 μmol per liter), and with use of the covariate-adjusted coefficient from Table 3, is shown in Figure 2. This fitted line indicates that a child with an average blood lead concentration of 1.50 μmol per liter during the first four years of life will have a GCI score approximately 7.2 points lower (95 percent confidence interval, 0.3 to 13.2) than a child with an average blood lead concentration of 0.50 μmol per liter.

Finally, the change in a child's average blood lead concentration between the first two years and the second two years of life was examined in relation to the change in (rank-ordered) measures of cognitive ability between the ages of two years (according to the Bayley Mental Developmental Index) and four years (according to the GCI). Such an analysis should reveal whether intellectual function at the age of four years is particularly influenced by recent blood lead levels. However, no relation was observed between changes in postnatal blood lead levels and changes in intelligence scores. Futhermore, no such relation existed in the subset of children whose blood lead concentration increased with age, or when we used a regression model designed to control for regression to the mean by including the initial average blood lead concentration (i.e., that during the first two years) along with the difference for the two age periods.

Discussion

Our results corroborate recent findings in several epidemiologic studies,[1,9,25] each of which showed an inverse relation between blood lead concentration and early cognitive development. Among the children in the Port Pirie Cohort Study, there was an inverse relation between the average blood lead concentration in a sequence of samples obtained in early childhood and measures of cognitive functioning. This paper has described that relation at the age of four years; the inverse relation observed at the age of two years has been described elsewhere.[14]

In the Boston cohort study, the inverse relation remained statistically significant after adjustment for 26 covariates consisting of demographic, reproductive, obstetrical, neonatal, and postnatal variables (including maternal IQ and home environment).[1] In our study, 16 covariates that were thought to be potential confounders of the relation of interest were incorporated; thus, we included fewer antenatal and obstetrical variables in the multivariable model than did the Boston study.

In multivariate analyses that incorporate many covariates there is a possibility of "overcontrol."[2] If, for example, the area of residence affects mental development exclusively by determining the child's level of environmental exposure to lead, then it would be inappropriate to control for that covariate. However, while these interrelations remain unknown and controversy persists about whether exposure to lead affects mental development in childhood, inclusion of such covariates is prudent, even though it may cause any true adverse effect of lead to be underestimated.

The fact that the integrated postnatal (birth to the age of four years) average blood lead concentration showed the strongest inverse relation with the GCI score suggests that the adverse effect of exposure to lead on mental development is cumulative during early childhood. The relations of blood lead concentration at the age of four years to concurrent MSCA scores were much weaker in the multiple regression analyses than were those of blood lead concentrations at earlier ages. This finding and the evidence that a change in blood lead concentration between the first two years and the second two years of childhood does not affect development suggest that long-term exposure to lead is the primary determinant of risk of impaired mental development.

The inverse relation is most evident in relation to raised blood lead concentrations during the postnatal period. Within the cohort we studied, any adverse effects of elevations in maternal and fetal blood concentrations of lead are likely to have been overwhelmed by the much higher concentrations in the children because of their direct environmental exposure to high levels of lead during early childhood.

This phase of the Port Pirie Cohort Study indicates that a group of children with an average blood lead concentration of 1.50 μmol per liter will have a decrease in mean GCI score of approximately 7 percent, as compared with children with an average blood lead concentration of 0.50 μmol per liter. The latter blood lead concentration would be typical of a population with little environmental exposure to lead. In public health terms — and assuming that a reduction in mean GCI score reflects a shift in score distribution rather than a change in the shape of that distribution — a downward shift of the distribution of GCI scores of this magnitude represents about half a standard deviation (1 SD equals 15 GCI points[15]). Hence, an additional 15 percent of the children with high exposure to lead could be considered to have developmental delay on the basis of the criterion that a developmental score more than 1 SD below the mean merits clinical attention.

The results of this analysis and those of the earlier analysis of the children at the age of two years[14] suggest that increased exposure to lead results in a developmental deficit, not just developmental delay. The current analysis indicates that cumulative environmental exposure to lead in early childhood is critical in affecting subsequent mental development. Furthermore, the findings of the Port Pirie and Boston cohort studies, which collectively investigated a wide range of blood lead concentrations in very young children, indicate that there may be no clear threshold below which an adverse effect on mental development does not occur.

This cohort study indicates that a raised blood lead concentration in early childhood has an independent deleterious effect on mental development as evaluated at the age of four years. This effect was not accounted for by the known and measurable influences of obstetrical, parental, family, and social environmental factors on mental development. However, because of the intrinsic difficulty of defining and controlling confounding factors when studying the relation between blood lead levels and mental development, causal inferences must be made only with circumspection. The fact that the effect has been observed longitudinally at the ages of two and four years within this cohort and that it is stronger at four years suggests that any adverse effect of lead is cumulative and may result in long-term impairment in development rather than a delay in development.

We are indebted to the families who participated in this study, their doctors, the local hospital staff, the nurse-interviewers (Barbara Hobson, Chris Mavromatis, Mary-Anne Lange, Bronwen Morgan, and Louise Thomson); to the staff of the Department of Chemical Pathology, Adelaide Children's Hospital

(Ms. B. King, Mr. R. Oldfield, and Dr. A.C. Pollard); to Ms. M. Padhye and Ms. A. Bartlett for data management; and to Mr. C. Greeneklee, Commonwealth Health Department Laboratory in Port Pirie.

References

1. Bellinger D, Leviton A, Waternaux C, Needleman H, Rabinowitz M. Longitudinal analyses of prenatal and postnatal lead exposure and early cognitive development. N Engl J Med 1987; 316:1037-43.
2. Yule W. Methodological and statistical issues. In: Lansdown R, Yule W, eds. The lead debate: the environment, toxicology and child health. London: Croom Helm, 1986:193-216.
3. Smith M. Recent work on low level lead exposure and its impact on behavior, intelligence, and learning: a review. J Am Acad Child Psychiatry 1985; 24:24-32.
4. Lansdown R. Lead, intelligence, attainment and behaviour. In: Lansdown R, Yule W, eds. The lead debate: the environment, toxicology and child health. London: Croom Helm, 1986:235-70.
5. Needleman HL, Gunnoe C, Leviton A, et al. Deficits in psychologic and classroom performance of children with elevated dentine lead levels. N Engl J Med 1979; 300:689-95.
6. Winneke G, Krämer U, Brockhaus U, et al. Neuropsychological studies in children with elevated tooth-lead concentrations. II. Extended study. Int Arch Occup Environ Health 1983; 51:231-52.
7. Smith M, Delves T, Lansdown R, Clayton B, Graham P. The effects of lead exposure on urban children: the Institute of Child Health/Southampton Study. Dev Med Child Neurol [Suppl] 1983; 47:1-54.
8. Lansdown R, Yule W, Urbanowicz M-A, Hunter J. The relationship between blood-lead concentrations, intelligence, attainment and behaviour in a school population: the second London study. Int Arch Occup Environ Health 1986; 57:225-35.
9. Fulton M, Raab G, Thomson G, Laxen D, Hunter R, Hepburn W. Influence of blood lead on the ability and attainment of children in Edinburgh. Lancet 1987; 1:1221-6.
10. Hernberg S, Nikkanen J. Enzyme inhibition by lead under normal urban conditions. Lancet 1970; 1:63-4.
11. Otto D, Robinson G, Baumann S, et al. 5-Year follow-up study of children with low-to-moderate lead absorption: electrophysiological evaluation. Environ Res 1985; 38:168-86.
12. Otto D, Benignus V, Muller K, et al. Effects of low to moderate lead exposure on slow cortical potentials in young children: two year follow-up study. Neurobehav Toxicol Teratol 1982; 4:733-7.
13. McMichael AJ, Baghurst PA, Robertson EF, Vimpani GV, Wigg NR. The Port Pirie cohort study: blood lead concentrations in early childhood. Med J Aust 1985; 143:499-503.
14. Wigg NR, Vimpani GV, McMichael AJ, Baghurst PA, Robertson EF, Roberts RJ. Port Pirie Cohort Study: childhood blood lead and neuropsychological development at age two years. J Epidemiol Community Health (in press).
15. McCarthy D. Manual for the McCarthy Scales of Children's Abilities. New York: Psychological Corporation, 1972:1-12.
16. Kaufman AS, Kaufman NL. Clinical evaluation of young children with the McCarthy Scales. New York: Grune & Stratton, 1977:81-106.
17. McMichael AJ, Vimpani GV, Robertson EF, Baghurst PA, Clark PD. The Port Pirie cohort study: maternal blood lead and pregnancy outcome. J Epidemiol Community Health 1986; 40:18-25.
18. Sampling of venous and capillary blood for the determination of lead content. Australian standard 2636 — 1983. North Sydney, Australia: Standards Association of Australia, 1983.
19. Calder IC, Roder DM, Esterman AJ, et al. Blood lead levels in children in the north-west of Adelaide. Med J Aust 1986; 144:509-12.
20. Whole blood — determination of lead — electrothermal atomization atomic absorption spectrometric method. Australian standard 2787 — 1985. North Sydney, Australia: Standards Association of Australia, 1985.
21. Brand C. Bryter still and bryter? Nature 1987; 328:110.
22. Caldwell B, Bradley R. Home observation for measurement of the environment. New York: Dorsey, 1985.
23. Bradley RH, Caldwell BM, Elardo R. Home environment, social status, and mental test performance. J Educ Psychol 1977; 69:697-701.
24. Wechsler D. Wechsler Adult Intelligence Scale — revised. New York: Psychological Corporation, 1981.
25. Dietrich KN, Krafft KM, Bornschein RL, et al. Low-level fetal lead exposure effect on neurobehavioral development in early infancy. Pediatrics 1987; 80:721-30.

END OF REPRINT D

Port Pirie Cohort Study: Environmental Exposure to Lead and Children's Abilities at the Age of Four Years

ANTHONY J. MCMICHAEL, P.A. BAGHURST, N. WIGG,
G. VIMPANI, E. ROBERTSON AND R. ROBERTS

7

ENVIRONMENTAL LEAD EXPOSURE AND CHILDHOOD DEVELOPMENT

The Port Pirie Cohort Study

SHILU TONG

Abstract

'Environmental health' is as broad as it is diverse in scope. As seen from this book, Tony McMichael contributed and advanced many aspects of the discipline, and indeed the field more broadly. In particular, his influence on the direction of the discipline and the policy responses to so many of the key issues that he addressed are recognised throughout this book as being seminal. Lead is one of the topics to which Tony's research contributed. I was fortunate at the time to have been an eager student and the lead project was one in which I participated.

Background

In the late 1970s and early 1980s, another important but unanswered question was whether environmental lead exposure might affect young children's health and development. Lead, from old house paint flakes, car exhaust and some industrial activity was a widespread pollutant. Many cross-sectional studies examined whether exposure to environmental lead at levels previously believed to be innocuous affected neuropsychological development and most of them found an inverse association between exposure measures and neuropsychological performance (Needleman et al., 1979; Smith et al., 1983; Winneke et al., 1983; Harvey et al., 1984; Schroeder et al., 1985; Lansdown et al., 1986; Fulton et al., 1987; Pocock et al., 1987; Hatzakis et al., 1989).

Cross-sectional studies cannot address the temporal relationship between exposure to environmental lead and neuropsychological development because they measure the exposure and outcome(s) at the same time. To test this hypothesis and address the limitations of cross-sectional studies, cohort studies have subsequently been conducted in several countries.

The Port Pirie Lead Smelter Study

Port Pirie, South Australia, has the largest lead smelter in the southern hemisphere. The Port Pirie cohort study (PPCS) commenced in 1979 (McMichael et al., 1988). This was the world's first and largest long-term follow-up study of the influence of early childhood exposure to environmental lead on the neurological and cognitive development of children. The research team had recruited a cohort of 723 children by 1981. These represented an estimated 90 per cent of all pregnancies in and around Port Pirie over a three-year period.

Blood samples were taken from each child at specified ages, and blood lead concentration was measured. Children's 'first teeth' – after they were shed – were collected to provide a further measure of accumulated lead exposure. Lead exposures varied greatly within the community, depending both on the proximity of residence to the smelter and on the levels of lead contamination in house dust and soil. At children's ages 2, 4, 7 and 12, a structured interview was conducted with one of the parents (usually the mother) and neuropsychological tests were administered by a well-trained research psychologist.

I came from China to join Tony and his team in early 1990, to work on the ongoing PPCS. Tony was then Professor of Environmental and Occupational Medicine in the Department of Community Medicine at the University of Adelaide. Shortly after I arrived in Adelaide, Tony wanted me to learn a little about Australian culture and environment and took me to Victor Harbour, which was about 70 km away from the town. Tony and I enjoyed the natural beauty there. By the time I joined the PPCS, the children were around 10 years old. For my PhD research (my supervisors: Tony, Drs Peter Baghurst and Michael Sawyer), I coordinated the follow-up and neuropsychological assessments in the later stage of childhood, at ages 11–13.

Results and Discussion

Of the 723 singleton live births recruited into the study, 601 were assessed at age 2, 548 at age 4, 494 at age 7 and 375 at 11–13 years of age. The geometric mean blood lead concentration of the children in this cohort increased from 8.3

µg/dl (0.40 µmol/l) at birth to 21.2 µg/dl (1.02 µmol/l) at age 2, and decreased to 7.9 µg/dl (0.38 µmol/l) by the age of 11–13. The PPCS collected information on critical features of lead exposure, such as the timing and extent, together with many other socio-environmental factors that might confound the relationship between lead exposure and neuropsychological development. In this study, we found that exposure to lead in this cohort of children was associated inversely with cognitive performance at ages 2, 4, 7 and 11–13, and that this association was still apparent after adjustment for a wide range of confounding factors.

Similar to the PPCS, most other cohort studies (Needleman et al., 1990; Dietrich et al., 1991; Baghurst et al., 1992; Bellinger et al., 1992; Wasserman et al., 1992; Fergusson and Horwood, 1993; McMichael et al., 1994; Lanphear et al., 2005), but not all (Cooney et al., 1989; Ernhart et al., 1989), also found a significant inverse relationship between early exposure to environmental lead and cognitive functioning in childhood after adjustment for confounding factors. However, an important question was raised about whether the apparent deleterious effect of early-life exposure to lead could be reversed when, later in childhood, exposure was reduced. Such exposure reduction could occur either by environmental management or as a consequence of the decreased absorption that appears to accompany growth.

The children's lifetime average blood lead level covered a wide range, from a low level of around 3–5 µg/dl up to around 30 µg/dl (Tong et al., 1996). Figure 7.1 shows that the children are grouped into three exposure categories: low, medium and high, by thirds of lifetime average blood lead concentration up to age 2 (the age when the children's developmental status was assessed for the first time in this cohort study). Their development score, on the vertical axis, changed in a fairly linear way across those three categories, and that was similar at each of the four assessment ages – shown by the four coloured bars. There was an approximately 5 per cent decline in IQ across a whole range of blood lead levels, after potential confounders had been taken into account.

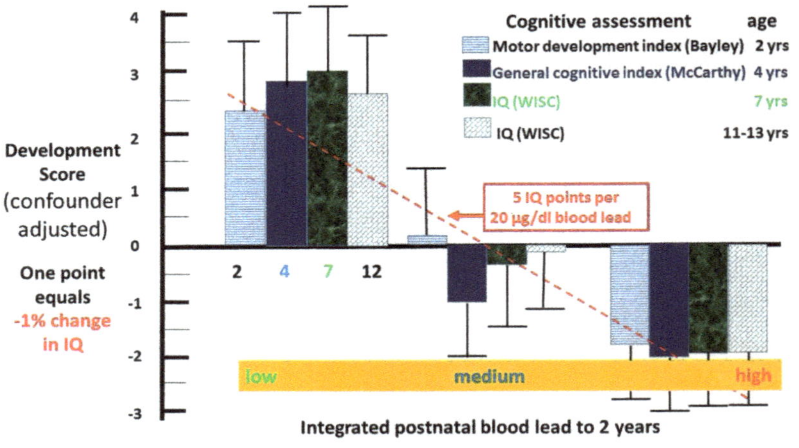

Figure 7.1 Developmental status at different ages by thirds of lifetime average blood lead concentration at age 2.

Source: Author's work.

Additionally, we assessed the reversibility of the apparent effects of lead on cognitive abilities in early childhood by testing whether reductions in blood lead concentrations beyond the age of 2 were associated with improvements in cognition (Tong et al., 1998). The key finding was that the cognitive deficits associated with exposure to environmental lead in early childhood appeared, at most, to be only partially reversed by a subsequent decline in blood lead (Table 7.1). The results from the PPCS indicate that the putative effects of lead on the neuropsychological development of children are genuinely irreversible, and therefore efforts to reduce the exposure of children to environmental lead from a very early age become increasingly important.

Table 7.1 Changes in blood lead concentration and changes in cognitive functioning between 2, 4 and 7 and 11–13 years.

Decline in blood		ΔZ score[a]		
lead (µg/dl)	*N*	Mean (SD)	95% CI	*P*-value[b]
From 2 to 11–13 years				
<10.2	109	0.03 (0.94)	–0.15 to 0.21	
10.2–16.2	108	0.04 (1.01)	–0.15 to 0.23	0.74
>16.2	109	–0.01 (1.02)	–0.20 to 0.18	
From 4 to 11–13 years				
<6.0	109	0.05 (0.90)	–0.12 to 0.23	
6.0–10.3	108	0.01 (0.91)	–0.17 to 0.18	0.42
>10.3	109	0.01 (0.96)	–0.17 to 0.19	

Decline in blood lead (µg/dl)	N	ΔZ score[a] Mean (SD)	95% CI	P-value[b]
From 7 to 11–13 years				
<2.3	109	–5.4 (8.3)	–3.8 to –7.0	
2.3–4.9	108	–5.0 (9.3)	–3.2 to –6.8	0.45
>4.9	109	–3.8 (7.9)	–2.3 to –5.3	

Notes:
[a] ΔZ score = $(Z_{11-13} - Z_2)$ or ΔZ score = $(Z_{11-13} - Z_4)$ or ΔZ score = $(Z_{11-13} - Z_7)$
[b] analysis of variance test.
Source: Tong et al., 1998.

Conclusion

This study provided strong evidence of the detrimental and dose-related impact of lead exposure on early child development, and showed the irreversible nature of lead effects. It demonstrated the importance of prevention and the early treatment of children with lead poisoning. However, lead contamination in a community can last for a long time and is difficult to eliminate. For example, there has not been much reduction in lead smelter emissions, and lead contamination is still widespread in Port Pirie (Taylor et al., 2013).

These results contributed to Australia's move to mandatory lead-free petrol in the 1990s, and were important in the World Health Organization (WHO) and Organisation for Economic Co-operation and Development (OECD) revisions of lead exposure standards soon after. Tony, in conjunction with Drs Peter Baghurst, Graham Vimpani and Neil Wigg, led this seminal study, which made a significant contribution to protecting children from lead effects, both nationally and internationally (Burns et al., 1999; Tong et al., 2000).

Acknowledgements

The author thanks Drs Tony McMichael, Peter Baghurst, Graham Vimpani and Neil Wigg for their constant support and mentoring; Mrs Maureen Wauchope for blood sampling and interviews; Mr Charles Greeneklee for assessing the packed cell volume of blood samples; Ms Elaine Witham for blood lead and iron analyses; Mr Jim Lyster for supervising developmental assessments; and the families who participated in this study.

The PPCS was supported by a series of grants from the National Health and Medical Research Council, the Channel 7 Children's Research Foundation and the University of Adelaide, Australia.

References

Baghurst, P.A., McMichael, A.J., Wigg, N.R., Vimpany, G.V., Robertson, E.F., Roberts, R.J., et al. 1992. Environmental exposure to lead and children's intelligence at the age of seven years: The Port Pirie cohort study. *The New England Journal of Medicine* 327, 1279–84.

Bellinger, D., Stiles, K. & Needleman, H.L. 1992. Low-level lead exposure intelligence and academic achievement: a long-term follow-up study. *Pediatrics* 90, 855–61.

Burns, J.M., Baghurst, P.A., Sawyer, M.G., McMichael, A.J. & Tong, S.L. 1999. Lifetime low-level exposure to environmental lead and children's emotional and behavioral development at ages 11–13 years. The Port Pirie cohort study. *The American Journal of Epidemiology* 149, 740–9.

Cooney, G.H., Bell, A., McBride, W. & Carter, C. 1989. Low-level exposure to lead: the Sydney Lead Study. *Developmental Medicine & Child Neurology* 31, 640–9.

Dietrich, K.N., Succop, P.A., Berger, O.G., Hammond, P.B. & Bornschein, R.L. 1991. Lead exposure and the cognitive development of urban preschool children: the Cincinnati lead study cohort at age 4 years. *Neurotoxicology and Teratology* 13, 203–11.

Ernhart, C.B., Morrow-Tlucak, M., Wolf, A.W., Super, D. & Drotar, D. 1989. Low level lead exposure in the prenatal and early preschool periods: intelligence prior to school entry. *Neurotoxicology and Teratology* 11, 161–70.

Fergusson, D.M. & Horwood, L.J. 1993. The effects of lead levels on the growth of word recognition in middle childhood. *International Journal of Epidemiology* 22, 891–7.

Fulton, M., Raab, G.M., Thomson, G.O.B., Laxen, D.P.H., Hunter, R. & Hepburn, W. 1987. Influence of blood lead on the ability and attainment of children in Edinburgh. *The Lancet* 1, 1221–6.

Harvey, P.G., Hamlin, M.W., Kumar, R. & Delves, H.T. 1984. Blood lead, behaviour and intelligence test performance in preschool children. *Science of the Total Environment* 40, 45–60.

Hatzakis, A., Kokkevi, A., Maravelias, C., Katsouyanni, K., Salaminios, F., Kalandidi, A., et al. 1989. Psychometric intelligence deficits in lead-exposured children. In: Smith, M., Grant, L. & Sors, A. (eds) *Lead Exposure and Child Development: An International Assessment*. Kluwer Academic Publishers, Lancaster, UK, 211–23.

Lanphear, B.P., Hornung, R., Khoury, J., Yolton, K., Baghurst, P., Bellinger, D.C., et al. 2005. Low-level environmental lead exposure and children's intellectual function: an international pooled analysis. *Environmental Health Perspectives* 113, 894–989.

Lansdown, R., Yule, W., Urbanowicz, M.-A. & Hunter, J. 1986. The relationship between blood lead concentrations, intelligence, attainment and behaviour in a school population: the second London study. *International Archives of Occupational Environmental Health* 57, 225–35.

McMichael, A., Baghurst, P., Wigg, N., Vimpani, G., Robertson, E. & Roberts, R. 1988. Port Pirie Cohort Study: childhood blood lead history and neuropsychological development at age four years. *The New England Journal of Medicine* 319, 468–75.

McMichael, A.J., Baghurst, P.A., Vimpany, G.V., Robertson, E.F., Wigg, N.R. & Tong, S.L. 1994. Tooth lead levels and IQ in school age children – The Port Pirie cohort study. *The American Journal of Epidemiology* 140, 489–99.

Needleman, H.L., Gunnoe, C., Leviton, A., Reed, R., Peresie, H., Maher, C., et al. 1979. Deficits in psychologic and classroom performance of children with elevated dentine lead levels. *The New England Journal of Medicine* 200, 689–95.

Needleman, H.L., Schell, A., Bellinger, D., Leviton, A. & Allred, E.N. 1990. The long-term effects of exposure to low doses of lead in childhood: an 11-year follow-up report. *The New England Journal of Medicine* 322, 83–8.

Pocock, S., Ashby, D. & Smith, M. 1987. Lead exposure and children's intellectual performance. *International Journal of Epidemiology* 16, 57–67.

Schroeder, S.R., Hawk, B., Otto, D.A., Mushak, P. & Hicks, R.E. 1985. Separating the effect of lead and social factors on IQ. *Environmental Research* 38, 144–54.

Smith, M., Delves, T., Lansdown, R., Clayton, B. & Graham, P. 1983. The effects of lead exposure on urban children: the Institute of Child Health/Southampton study. *Developmental Medicine & Child Neurology* 47, 1–54.

Taylor, M.P., Camenzuli, D., Kristensen, L.J., Forbes, M. & Zahran, S. 2013. Environmental lead exposure risks associated with children's outdoor playgrounds. *Environmental Pollution* 178, 447–54.

Tong, S.L., Baghurst, P.A., McMichael, A.J., Sawyer, M. & Mudge, J. 1996. Lifetime exposure to environmental lead and children's intelligence at 11–13 years: the Port Pirie cohort study. *BMJ* 312, 1569–75.

Tong, S.L., Baghurst, P.A., Sawyer, M., Burns, J.M. & McMichael, A.J. 1998. Declining blood lead levels and changes in cognitive function during childhood: the Port Pirie Cohort Study. *Journal of the American Medical Association* 280, 1915–9.

Tong, S.L., von Schirnding, Y. & Prapamontol, T. 2000. Environmental lead exposure: a public health problem of global dimensions. *Bulletin of the World Health Organization* 78, 1068–77.

Wasserman, G., Graziano, J.H., Factor-Litvak, P., Popovac, D., Morina, N., Musabegovic, A., et al. 1992. Independent effects of lead exposure and iron deficiency anemia on developmental outcome at age 2 years. *Journal of Pediatrics* 122, 695–703.

Winneke, G., Krämer, U., Brockhaus, U., Ewer, U., Kujanek, G., Lechner, H., et al. 1983. Neuropsychological studies in children with elevated tooth-lead concentrations. II. Extended study. *International Archives of Occupational Environmental Health* 51, 231–52.

8

SHINING LIGHT ON HUMAN IMMUNITY

ROBYN LUCAS, ASHWIN SWAMINATHAN AND KEITH DEAR

Abstract

The immune system is a key interface between environmental exposures and human health. It provides protection against infectious agents and toxins reaching the skin and mucosal surfaces and maintains internal surveillance to destroy abnormal cells. Overactivity of the immune system can result in autoimmune diseases, such as multiple sclerosis, while medicine takes advantage of immune processes to stimulate protection from pathogens, through vaccination. Ultraviolet radiation from the sun can suppress the immune response, potentially decreasing the risk of autoimmune disease development but impairing the immune response to vaccination. This chapter uses these two examples, multiple sclerosis and vaccination, to illustrate a pathway of research that began with observation of variations in disease or vaccination outcomes and proceeded through epidemiological and biomedical studies of increasing depth and sophistication. The end point – yet to be achieved but within sight – will be the translation of the findings into actions to improve public health. Tony McMichael's key contributions to each step of this research pathway are described.

Introduction

In the 1920s, researchers observed that multiple sclerosis, a debilitating degenerative neurological disease, was more common in regions at higher latitude. This finding, replicated in both the northern and southern hemispheres, is an unusual but important feature of the epidemiology of multiple sclerosis. It suggests that environmental factors may play a role in its aetiology. Recent work indicating that the incidence of multiple sclerosis has increased over the past 30 years, after accounting for improved diagnosis, also indicates a role for changing environmental determinants.

A key feature of Tony McMichael's work was to discern and quantify the links between human health and the environment, and the changing ways in which humans interacted with that environment. One facet of that work involved exploring the link between immune function and exposure to ultraviolet (UV) radiation at the population level, particularly in relation to the risk of autoimmune diseases. This chapter begins with a brief sketch of the human immune system, followed by a story of translational public health research: from observation to investigation to testing; and hopefully to prevention.

A Brief Introduction to the Human Immune System

The immune system protects against attack from foreign organisms and maintains internal surveillance to detect and destroy abnormal cells. Humans have both innate and adaptive immune systems, with considerable cross-communication between them. Innate immunity is found in all plants and animals. It provides an immediately maximal but non-specific immune response to injury or pathogen exposure. There is no immunological memory – that is, the innate response is the same each time the system is activated. In contrast, the adaptive immune system is found only in higher animals, specifically, jawed vertebrates. There is a lag of hours or days between pathogen exposure and maximal immune response, but the response is pathogen or antigen specific, and a subsequent exposure to the same pathogen results in a more immediate, targeted physiological attack. This is immunological memory, the basis of vaccination.

The adaptive immune response has two arms that act in concert. Humoral immunity involves the production of antibodies, macromolecules that coat the invading/foreign pathogen and facilitate its destruction. Cell-mediated immunity relies on specialised lymphocytes to recognise and destroy pathogens. Both systems require cells that present antigens (antigen-presenting cells, e.g. dendritic cells) to lymphocytes, including B-lymphocytes and various types of T-lymphocytes (e.g. T-helper cells, T-cytotoxic cells, T-regulatory cells). Different types of cells secrete specific chemicals (cytokines) that permit 'communication' across the immune system during an immunological response.

Multiple Sclerosis and Sun Exposure: From Geography to Prevention

Multiple sclerosis (MS) is an inflammatory disease of the central nervous system, usually leading to progressive deterioration of nerve function. It is the commonest disabling neurological disorder of young adults. MS is thought to be an autoimmune disease, caused by an immune-mediated attack of cells of the adaptive immune system on the myelin-producing cells of the central nervous system, the oligodendrocytes. Myelin is a lipoprotein that coats and insulates nerve fibres, nourishing them and increasing the speed of conduction of nerve impulses. Disruption of myelin results in slowing of conduction and, over time, degeneration of nerve fibres. People with MS generally suffer recurrent bouts of neurological dysfunction, manifesting as weakness, localised altered sensation or visual impairment, eventually followed by cumulative neurological deficits and increasing disability.

Risk Factors for MS

Relatives of a person with MS are also more likely to develop the disease, with the risk increasing according to the closeness of the genetic relationship: for example, the risk in full siblings is approximately 35 times that of the general population, and in monozygotic twins approximately 270 times greater (Ebers, 2008). Despite these high relative risks, with an absolute incidence generally of the order of five to 10 new cases per 100,000 population per year, the absolute risk of MS is low, even in close family members. A growing number of susceptibility genes are recognised, but each of these only slightly increases the risk.

Several lines of evidence indicate the importance of environmental exposures in the pathogenesis of MS, particularly observations of increasing incidence over recent decades and the strong latitudinal gradient seen for incidence, prevalence and mortality. Possible contenders that would account for some of these findings include infections, for example Epstein–Barr virus, canine distemper virus, human herpes virus 6 and others, diet and changing intestinal microbiomes and exposure to the sun or related factors. This story focuses on sun exposure, without discounting the possible importance of other factors that may act independently or interactively.

A positive latitude gradient in MS was first noted by Davenport in 1922, based on data from conscripts to World War I (Davenport, 1922). In 1960, Acheson et al. further explored this finding in an analysis of the place of birth of soldiers in World War II who developed MS. Here, there was a strong correlation between MS prevalence and latitude of birthplace (r = 0.76), and a slightly stronger (inverse) correlation with average daily December solar UV radiation (r = –0.80) (Acheson and Bachrach, 1960; Acheson et al., 1960). A number of other studies over ensuing years have also demonstrated a latitude gradient in several different countries, including Australia, where the prevalence of MS in 1981 was almost seven times higher in Tasmania than in northern Queensland (McLeod et al., 1994).

These ecological studies prompted individual-level observational studies, but the evidence from case-control studies of MS patients and healthy controls was contradictory, variously showing an increase, decrease, or no change in risk in association with self-reported time outdoors.

The Rise of Photoimmunology

The 1970s saw the development of interest in the immune effects of exposure to the sun – photoimmunology. Kripke's work showed that immunosuppression following exposure of the skin to UV radiation contributed to skin cancer development and diminished host resistance to infectious diseases in animals (Kripke, 1994). UV irradiation of the skin was shown to trigger a cascade of immunological events, including decreased antigen-presenting activity, release of the cytokine IL-10 and other immune mediators, and induction of regulatory T-cell activity. The net result was suppression of antigen-specific adaptive immunity, both locally (at the site of immunological challenge) and systemically. In addition, there was a shifting of the balance in T-cell activity towards a suppressive milieu.

Bringing It All Together

Exposure to the UV-B wavelengths of solar radiation (280–315 nm) is the source of over 90 per cent of vitamin D stores in people living in most regions of the world. Accordingly, by 1991, animal studies had tested the effect of administering the active form of vitamin D and shown that high doses completely prevented the development of the animal model of MS, experimental allergic encephalomyelitis (Lemire and Archer, 1991).

By the 1990s, two hypotheses on the causes of MS were in the spotlight: the vitamin D hypothesis that insufficiency leads to an overactive immune system, and an infection hypothesis that a viral infection somehow initiates the autoimmune process. Both hypotheses have been widely tested over the ensuing years. Many case-control and cohort studies have now provided evidence that suggests that lower vitamin D status and a past history of symptomatic infection with Epstein–Barr virus (EBV, glandular fever or infectious mononucleosis) are associated with increased risk of MS.

In 1994, Tony McMichael moved to the London School of Hygiene and Tropical Medicine (LSH&TM), where Sir Donald Acheson was Professor of International Health. Tony was aware of, and intrigued by, Acheson's earlier papers, and the two discussed them. During this period, Tony reviewed the health chapter for the 1994 report of the Environmental Effects Assessment Panel for the Montreal Protocol on Ozone Depletion (Longstreth et al., 1994). This included a review of Kripke's recent work on the immune suppression that occurred following UV irradiation and its importance for skin cancer development. Tony and a colleague at the LSH&TM, Andy Hall, proposed an integrated hypothesis, bringing together this new work with the environmental patterns and the infection hypothesis:

> We therefore propose that UVR-induced suppression of immune function, maximal at low latitudes, attenuates the autoimmune process that underlies MS. This attenuation could occur either by a diminution in the initial sensitization of T-cells to a newly encountered (and myelin basic protein-'mimicking') viral antigen, or by a reduced intensity of cell-mediated immune response to ongoing infection with the virus. (McMichael and Hall, 1997)

This paper was the first to link the apparent protective effect of UV radiation with evidence of risk associated with viral infection. It suggested that UV radiation played a larger role in the MS story than that through vitamin D only, and that viral infection in the presence of impaired environmental immune suppression might be important. It provided a number of testable predictions from the hypothesis, of which some have been supported by empirical evidence, albeit to a limited extent. For example, they hypothesised that 'MS incidence rates (at least in fair-skinned populations) will decline in response to any further increase in population exposure to UVR'. Instead, in many fair-skinned populations, the prevailing public health advice has been to *decrease* exposure to UV radiation to control skin cancer risk. It has been proposed that this may explain the loss of the latitude gradient in MS incidence between successive waves of the Nurses' Health Study in the USA: higher levels of sun protection in the sunnier south may explain greater increases in MS incidence in the south than in the north (Ascherio and Munger, 2007).

In 2003, on his return to Australia, McMichael led the Ausimmune Study that examined sun exposure, vitamin D and infection history in people with a first clinical diagnosis of central nervous system (CNS) demyelination (Lucas et al., 2007), prior to a diagnosis of MS. A weakness of studies of vitamin D levels in people with frank MS is the possibility of reverse causation, whereby people with MS have lower vitamin D status because they have MS, rather than the other way around. This is likely because the disease causes heat intolerance, so that patients tend to avoid the sun, and because the physical disability that develops in later stages makes outdoor exercise difficult. By recruiting people with the first symptoms of an illness that may progress to MS, the Ausimmune Study avoided this possibility. The study was able to examine a wide range of genetic and environmental factors, including infections, and the interactions between them. Key findings of the study were that there was preservation of a latitude gradient of approximately the same magnitude for incidence as had been previously described for prevalence in 1981 data (Taylor et al., 2010); and that lower vitamin D status (Lucas et al., 2011b), past history of infectious mononucleosis and higher levels of EBV antibodies (Lucas et al., 2011a) were all independently associated with increased risk of being a case with a first diagnosis of CNS demyelination. In addition, sun exposure itself, over the life course or the previous three years, was associated with a lower risk of being a case, even after adjustment for other known risk factors.

Based on the weight of accumulating evidence, including that from the Ausimmune Study, a vitamin D prevention trial was initiated in Australia in 2012. The PrevANZ Study will randomly allocate adult participants with a first diagnosis of CNS demyelination to 1,000, 5,000 or 10,000 IU (international units) of vitamin D3 per day, or to placebo (i.e. zero IU), to test whether vitamin D can prevent progression to MS. Importantly, the study will include detailed measurements of sun exposure to distinguish any independent protective effects of sun exposure and vitamin D. Data from questionnaires and blood samples will provide information on past infections, to test integrative hypotheses further, including the one proposed by McMichael and Hall.

Careful observation of disease patterns in ecological studies stimulated the formation of hypotheses about sun exposure, vitamin D and infection, which led to individual-level observational studies to test these hypotheses. Positive findings in relation to vitamin D and sun exposure have further led to clinical trials to test whether observed associations are causal. It has been estimated that if there is a causal association between vitamin D insufficiency and MS incidence, then at least 40 per cent of cases of MS could be prevented (Ascherio and Munger, 2007).

Not Only Benefits

In consideration of human health and the environment, McMichael wrote about the changing nature of the interaction between humans and their environments (McMichael, 2001). Concurrent risks and benefits of environmental exposures for human health, and levels of optimal exposure, are typical of natural selection and survival of the fittest. So, too, for sun exposure. While higher levels of sun exposure may be protective against MS, either independently via vitamin D production or through interaction with viral infection, higher levels also increase the risk of skin cancers and eye diseases. The immunosuppressive effects, potentially beneficial for MS, may impair the immune response to vaccination – a factor that could have considerable importance for those regions at low latitude but with high microbial load. McMichael's research interest in this field continued to explore such risks, through the recently completed Australian Ultraviolet Radiation and Immunity (AusUVI) Study.

Exposure to UV Radiation and Vaccination

Vaccination against common communicable diseases has been one of the most successful public health measures of all time. Any process that might compromise vaccine effectiveness is therefore of profound importance to public health and warrants rigorous scientific investigation. Numerous studies have shown an association between reduced vaccine effectiveness and its administration in high compared with low ambient UV environments (i.e. summer versus winter months and/or low- versus high-latitude regions) (Norval and Woods, 2011). However, these are weak surrogates of an individual's personal sun exposure; that is influenced by a wide range of factors such as how much time they spend outdoors, whether they use sun protection and what types of clothing are worn. Using ecological proxies risks making false inferences about the exposure–outcome relationship (the so-called 'ecological fallacy').

The AusUVI Study, of which Professor McMichael was a key investigator, was conducted to determine the influence of exposure to solar UV radiation, attained through activities of normal daily life, on the primary immune response to subcutaneous vaccination with an experimental vaccine antigen, keyhole limpet haemocyanin (KLH). The advantages of this prospective, two-centre observational study included direct measurement of exposure to UV radiation at an individual level, quantification of potential confounding immune-modulatory factors (e.g. physical fitness, age, psychological well-being) and sophisticated measurement of an array of vaccine-associated immune outcomes.

The results of the AusUVI Study have only recently become available. They show that higher personal exposure to UV radiation in the peri-vaccination period did, indeed, suppress the antigen (KLH)-specific cell-mediated immune response. Exposure to UV radiation in the day prior to vaccination was most influential. Other findings, of a change in the proportion of a circulating subpopulation of T-helper lymphocytes, may have relevance to the pathogenesis of autoimmune diseases (Veldhoen et al., 2008) and the association between sun exposure and autoimmune diseases, such as MS. Interestingly, here, vitamin D status was not associated with immune outcomes, i.e. this was a sun exposure effect rather than a vitamin D effect.

The clinical implications of the findings of the AusUVI Study and related studies are not presently clear. Using immune parameters as a surrogate for increased disease risk (or reduced vaccine effectiveness) is problematic, particularly when those changes are subtle, because the human immune system is endowed with multiple redundancies and functional reserve capacity. However, at a population level (which includes aged, very young and ill individuals), less profound impairment of specific immune processes occurring with high prevalence may manifest as an increased incidence of common infections (e.g. influenza, rhinovirus, otitis media) and/or reduced vaccine effectiveness.

Further well-designed studies using commonly administered vaccines (e.g. measles, pneumococcal) need to be performed where, among other considerations, exposure to UV radiation at an individual level is quantified, confounding variables are accounted for and clinical outcomes (e.g. vaccine effectiveness against disease) measured. Conducting these studies in vulnerable populations may be additionally revealing – e.g. assessing the influence of exposure to solar UV radiation on childhood vaccinations in peri-equatorial regions. If commercial vaccine effectiveness is indeed shown to be compromised by high individual UV radiation exposure, potential public health strategies would include the promotion of sun-protective clothing and sunscreen at around the time of vaccine administration.

Conclusion

McMichael's chief contribution to this story of public health translation was through the bringing together of separate lines of research to generate testable hypotheses, and then exploring predictions from those hypotheses in observational studies. His key insight was that, even in an intensely biomedical field like immunology, untangling disease aetiology could benefit hugely from complementing the laboratory work with epidemiological research undertaken from a global population-level perspective. The work has real potential to decrease the incidence of a disabling, devastating neurological disease, as well as to shed light on new risks related to UV-induced immune suppression that will need to be considered in vaccination delivery.

References

Acheson, E.D. & Bachrach, C.A. 1960. The distribution of multiple sclerosis in U.S. veterans by birthplace. *The American Journal of Hygiene* 72, 88–99.

Acheson, E.D., Bachrach, C.A. & Wright, F.M. 1960. Some comments on the relationship of the distribution of Multiple Sclerosis to latitude, solar radiation and other variables. *Acta Psychiatrica Scandinavica* 35, 132–47.

Ascherio, A. & Munger, K.L. 2007. Environmental risk factors for multiple sclerosis. Part II: Noninfectious factors. *Annals of Neurology* 61, 504–13.

Davenport, C. 1922. Multiple sclerosis from the standpoint of geographic distribution and race. *Archives of Neurology and Psychiatry* 8, 51–8.

Ebers, G.C. 2008. Environmental factors and multiple sclerosis. *Lancet Neurology* 7, 268–77.

Kripke, M.L. 1994. Ultraviolet radiation and immunology: something new under the sun – presidential address. *Cancer Research* 54, 6102–5.

Lemire, J.M. & Archer, D.C. 1991. 1,25-dihydroxyvitamin D3 prevents the *in vivo* induction of murine experimental autoimmune encephalomyelitis. *Journal of Clinical Investigation* 87, 1103–7.

Longstreth, J., de Gruijl, F.R., Kripke, M.L., Takizawa, Y. & van der Leun, J.C. 1994. Effects of increased ultraviolet radiation on human health. In: UNEP (ed.) *Environmental Effects of Ozone Depletion, 1994 Assessment*. UNEP, Nairobi, Kenya, 23–48.

Lucas, R.M., Ponsonby, A.L., McMichael, A.J., van der Mei, I., Chapman, C., Coulthard, A., et al. 2007. Observational analytic studies in multiple sclerosis: controlling bias through study design and conduct. The Australian Multicentre Study of Environment and Immune Function. *Multiple Sclerosis Journal* 13, 827–39.

Lucas, R.M., Ponsonby, A.L., Dear, K., Valery, P.C., Pender, M.P., Taylor, B.V., et al. 2011a. Sun exposure and vitamin D are independent risk factors for CNS demyelination. *Neurology* 76, 540–548.

Lucas, R.M., Ponsonby, A.L., Dear, K., Valery, P.C., Pender, M.P., J.M. Burrows, et al. 2011b. Current and past Epstein–Barr virus infection in risk of initial CNS demyelination. *Neurology* 77, 371–9.

McLeod, J.G., Hammond, S.R. & Hallpike, J.F. 1994. Epidemiology of multiple sclerosis in Australia. With NSW and SA survey results. *Medical Journal of Australia* 160, 117–22.

McMichael, A.J. 2001. *Human Frontiers, Environments and Disease: Past Patterns, Uncertain Futures.* Cambridge University Press, Cambridge, UK.

McMichael, A.J. & Hall, A.J. 1997. Does immunosuppressive ultraviolet radiation explain the latitude gradient for multiple sclerosis? *Epidemiology* 8, 642–5.

Norval, M. & Woods, G.M. 2011. UV-induced immunosuppression and the efficacy of vaccination. *Photochemical & Photobiological Sciences* 10, 1267–74.

Taylor, B.V., Lucas, R.M., Dear, K., Kilpatrick, T.J., Pender, M.P., van der Mei, I.A., et al. 2010. Latitudinal variation in incidence and type of first central nervous system demyelinating events. *Multiple Sclerosis Journal* 16, 398–405.

Veldhoen, M., Hirota, K., Westendorf, A.M., Buer, J., Dumoutier, L., Renauld, J.-C., et al. 2008. The aryl hydrocarbon receptor links TH17-cell-mediated autoimmunity to environmental toxins. *Nature* 453, 106–9.

9

STUDYING THE THAI HEALTH-RISK TRANSITION

ADRIAN SLEIGH AND SAM-ANG SEUBSMAN

Abstract

Since Thailand's first census 100 years ago, its patterns of illness, mortality and fertility have been transformed. Mortality and fertility fell very rapidly in the first 70 years as infectious diseases receded. Healthy childhood and safe motherhood were key benefits. Successive cohorts grew taller, and previously rare chronic diseases became common as families became smaller, incomes rose, people urbanised and the population aged.

Dengue and tuberculosis remain major problems, and in recent decades, HIV/AIDS has become an important cause of mortality among young adults. Traffic injury has become a major threat, and unfamiliar problems such as obesity, anxiety and depression are becoming widespread in Thailand.

These changes have been the focus of a large multidisciplinary study of the Thai health-risk transition funded by the Wellcome Trust and the NH&MRC since 2004, with strong support from senior Thai government officials. The study focuses on the transition of both health risks and outcomes in the Thai population. Guided by conceptual advances in Professor Tony McMichael's approach to population health, it looks beyond the proximate, searching for multilevel drivers of changes under way and the sequences and mediators of transitions. Here, we outline the overall study design – with retrospective and prospective components – including an ongoing cohort study of nearly 90,000 adults already followed for eight years. Progress is summarised and future prospects reviewed.

Introduction

In this chapter, we introduce our longitudinal multidisciplinary international study of the health-risk transition under way in Thailand. The project received critical administrative and intellectual support from Professor Tony McMichael – as Director of the National Centre for Epidemiology and Population Health (NCEPH), as one of the initial Chief Investigators, as advocate for multilevel epidemiology and as a leader of multidisciplinary regional public health research. The legacy of health transition theory established at NCEPH in the 1990s by Professor Jack Caldwell, The Australian National University's (ANU) celebrated demographer, also helped to inspire the work. Another seminal influence arose from the doctoral research experience of the project leaders, as both Adrian Sleigh and Sam-ang Seubsman were engaged in cohort studies at that early stage of their careers. Over the past 10 years, the project has been directed in Australia from ANU (by Sleigh at NCEPH) and in Thailand from the Sukhothai Thammathirat Open University (STOU) (by Seubsman in Bangkok).

The research tackles a significant regional population health issue in middle-income Thailand – transition to modern health risks and the concomitant emergence of chronic disease and injury. The aim is long-term multidisciplinary research that improves understanding of health and its determinants in Thailand while boosting regional health research capacity and collaboration. The questions to be addressed include the progression of the Thai health-risk transition over the past 50 years, its distribution and determinants and potential interventions. Accordingly, we conducted an historical study looking back 50–100 years and also established a large prospective Thai Cohort Study. Regional population health research capacity was also a focus, with a substantial commitment to PhD training in Australia and Master training in Thailand.

We focused on Thailand as an influential country in the region at the geographical head of the Association of Southeast Asian Nations (ASEAN) and bordering more ASEAN neighbours than any other country. It is grappling with unfamiliar health risks and new disease patterns as health-risk transitions unfold. Its responses will be informative to Southeast Asia. To stay relevant, given these changes and mindful of the potential for long-term involvement, we directed capacity-building research to the health-risk transition itself, examining both determinants (risks) and outcomes (health).

We were aware that a demographic transition from high to low fertility and mortality was well advanced in Thailand (Figure 9.1). The country has also experienced an epidemiological transition from infectious to chronic diseases and a health transition from traditional beliefs and practices to science-based health behaviour and services. In addition, Thailand is experiencing a nutrition transition from traditional to 'modern' food, urbanisation and transitions in formal occupation, communication, transport, sexual behaviour, health service access and health service utilisation.

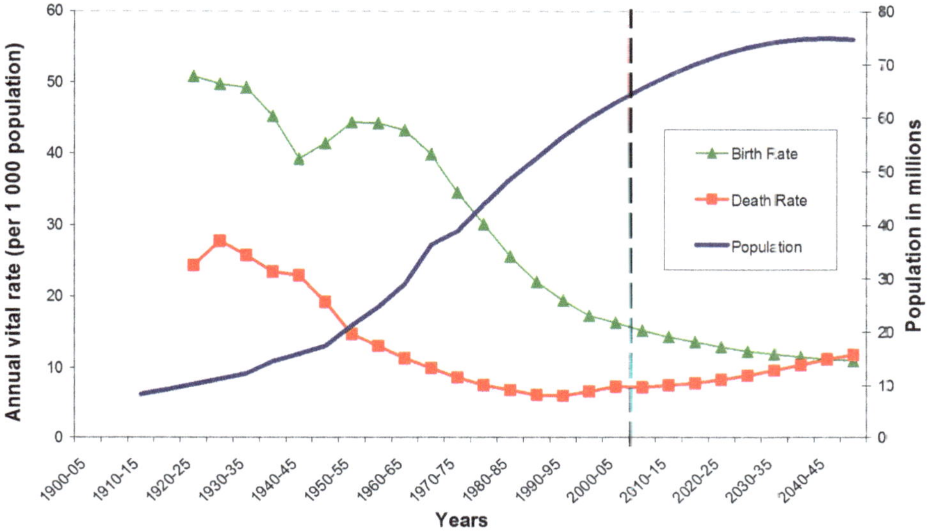

Figure 9.1 The demographic transition in Thailand.

Multiple sources, from Sleigh et al., 2008 (with permission). Population before 1940: Hirshman (1994); birth and death rates before 1950 adapted from estimates of crude birth rate and crude death rate for each year (1920–50) from the Economic and Social Commission for Asia and the Pacific (1976); from 1960: Population Division of the Department of Economic and Social Affairs of the United Nations Secretariat (2003).

The study began in 2004 and was funded competitively for the first five years under the International Collaborative Research Grants Scheme, a once-only opportunity created by the combined efforts of the Wellcome Trust (UK) and the Australian National Health and Medical Research Council (NH&MRC). These funders created an unusual opportunity to form an international research team to investigate a regional public health problem that neither threatened Australia directly nor promised bioscience patents of direct benefit to the Australian economy. In 2009, the NH&MRC launched its new competitive global health project grant funding, enabling our project to win support for five more years.

The research involves a Thai–Australian partnership including STOU, the Thai National Economic and Social Development Board reporting to the Thai Prime Minister and Cabinet, the Thai Ministry of Public Health, Chiang Mai University and several Australian partners (see acknowledgements).

Health-Risk Transitions

In recent years, understanding of the dynamics and determinants of population health transitions has been enhanced by diverse international syntheses on social, demographic and health trends (Caldwell, 1993; Harper et al., 1994; World Health Report, 2002). This has involved insights from sociologists, historians, demographers, nutritionists and ecologists. Newly characterised upstream health determinants have been identified as drivers of population health transitions, either under way or completed in many regions – for survival and longevity (Caldwell and Caldwell, 1993), for diet and nutrition (Drewnowski and Popkin, 1997) and for epidemiologic patterns, environmental risks and human ecology (McMichael, 2001).

This knowledge is complemented by the growing insights of social epidemiology, showing how sociocultural and economic factors also act as upstream drivers of many health outcomes (Berkman and Kawachi, 2000). Also important was the realisation that the distribution of risk factors within populations was the best target for many interventions (Rose, 1992; Laaser et al., 2001). Every population should understand the local dynamics of the distributions and upstream determinants of its own health risks before devising national intervention strategies.

The economic causes and consequences of the interrelated demographic, epidemiological and nutritional transitions have become a central concern for health and development planners and financiers (Jamison et al., 1993; World Bank, 1993). Economic debate on whether health is an 'input' or 'output' of 'development' has culminated in the recognition that health is both, and the international health economics agenda for the new millennium opened with the World Health Organization's *Report of the Commission on Macroeconomics and Health* (Commission on Macroeconomics and Health, 2001). This comprehensive and persuasive dossier shows that health has been a key determinant of the economic development and wealth of nations over the past 200 years. For example, it showed that in low-income countries, an additional investment of US$34 per head in health would prevent about eight million deaths per year, around one-fifth of the annual toll worldwide. This would boost life expectancy at birth (LEB), and for every 10 per cent improvement of LEB, after controlling for other factors, the economy of a country would grow 0.3–0.4 percentage points. The report lays out compelling economic arguments for investing in population health and has exerted considerable influence over the past decade. Notwithstanding these considerations, there are also growing concerns about the long-term consequences of continuous economic growth, with implications for public health, as considered below.

Preventive thinking has moved beyond old debates over the relative contributions of material advances, social modernisation or deliberate public health interventions. Well-governed societies distribute health knowledge and technology via responsive and fair health systems within supportive civil institutions and cultural norms (Warren, 1997), and invest in health to boost wealth creation and development. Experiences in Japan, Korea and Singapore show that population health patterns can change over just two to four decades, from high to low mortality and fertility, with increased longevity, control of infectious diseases and large reduction of maternal–child mortality. Transitions that took Western countries 150 years can be telescoped into shorter periods, if all goes well. But, economic progress may consume ecological (i.e. natural) capital, leaving overly large 'environmental footprints', or induce health-impairing consumer behaviours, thus jeopardising population health (McMichael, 2001c).

The foregoing considerations are highly relevant to Thailand, now undergoing its own rapid risk and health transition, with years of high economic growth but limited societal capacity to detect and contain health-endangering environmental, economic and social changes. Some countries recently achieved risk and health transitions with lower per capita gross domestic product (GDP) than previously (Wilson, 2001). Over the decades, 1976–96, Thais experienced a remarkable 11-year rise in LEB (from 59 to 70 years for males and from 64 to 75 years for females) and equally dramatic falls in infant mortality and fertility. The Thai population is now nearly 65 million, and its growth rate has slowed. Mean per capita income has passed US$3,000 per year, and 36 per cent of the export-oriented economy's GDP now derives from manufacturing, while only 12 per cent is from agricultural production (National Statistical Office of Thailand, 2003; World Bank, 2013).

Other transitions are visible in Thailand. Chronic disease and injury are emerging as unfamiliar sources of most of the years of healthy life now being lost. The twin epidemics of obesity and (Type 2) diabetes loom. By 2000, diabetes incidence was rising 10 per cent per year, reaching 13.2 new cases reported per 100,000 (Bureau of Health Policy and Planning, 2002), and obesity now affects around one-third of the adult population (Aekplakorn et al., 2007). Fatal injury has also appeared as a major problem over the past two decades, with rates among males about four times those for females, mostly associated with motorcycles (Wilbulpolprasert, 2008).

The transitions in Thai health and risk were not automatic; they co-evolved with and reflected social attitudes and other aspects that were conducive. National identity remains strong, religious freedom is entrenched, there is no male child preference and female autonomy is evident. So, Thai men and women are free to embrace changes in family dynamics, lifestyle and even in core values. To some extent, this freedom has affected national governance and integration into the world economy. For example, over the past two decades parliamentary democracy initially strengthened, Thailand joined the World Trade Organization in 1995 and the country adopted its first popular democratic constitution in 1997. Governments changed peacefully several times, but consensus broke down in the last decade and was replaced by civil disturbances and conflict between political factions, yet to be resolved.

Economic changes have also been important influences on health and risks. Forty years of rapid national economic growth ceased in 1997, completing the low-wage phase of industrialisation. Now, the Thai economy is growing again, but with increasing need for a skilled workforce and an economic strategy to take the country forward towards a higher-wage future. Population health status will be both an input and an output of future skill development and the expanding Thai economy.

Bearing in mind the complex forces, as discussed above, that determine population health status in Thailand, we adopted a multilevel eco-social model to guide our ongoing study of the health-risk transition under way (Figure 9.2).

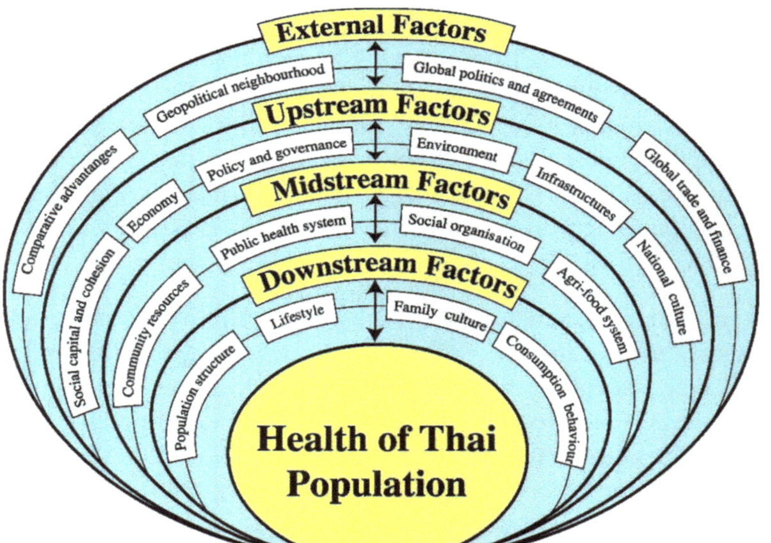

Figure 9.2 Multilevel eco-social health model.

Source: Sleigh et al., 2008 (open access).

Rationale for a National Cohort Study in Thailand

Our research is generating novel Thai data on population risk and health transitions. The country is moving on from its 'old agenda' of high maternal and infant mortality and poverty-related environmental and microbial risks, but needs new knowledge to reduce its emerging health problems – chronic disease and injury. As Thailand modernises, its population is adapting to Western medical services. In addition, dietary habits are changing, urbanisation and associated environmental pollution proceed, oncoming population segments are reaching higher education and scientific capacity is growing. To design appropriate prevention programmes, Thais need comprehensive information on the trends and determinants of current risk and health transitions.

Prospective cohort studies follow individuals into the future, periodically monitoring their health and other potential risk factors over time. This research design enables the investigation of multiple risk factors as well as the multiple health effects of given risks, such as smoking, specific diets, exercise levels, residential conditions and occupational exposures, including climate change and heat stress. All-cause mortality and major morbidity are estimable and can be characterised further for specific health outcomes. Distributions of risk exposures are measurable, and their upstream socioecological determinants can also be investigated within the cohort study – with implications for national interventions. For common morbid outcomes (such as transport or occupational injury, or effects of air pollution), detection of incident cases enables case-control analysis and socioecological research on upstream causal webs.

Some general population cohort studies, in other parts of the world, have lasted many decades and have provided much valuable information for public health policy. Taking peer-reviewed research publications as one indication of overall scientific productivity, we note that the Nurses' Health Study in the USA (n = 121,900) has produced nearly 1,000 original articles since 1976 (Figure 9.3). It has also trained many national and international leaders in public health (www.channing.harvard.edu/nhs/).

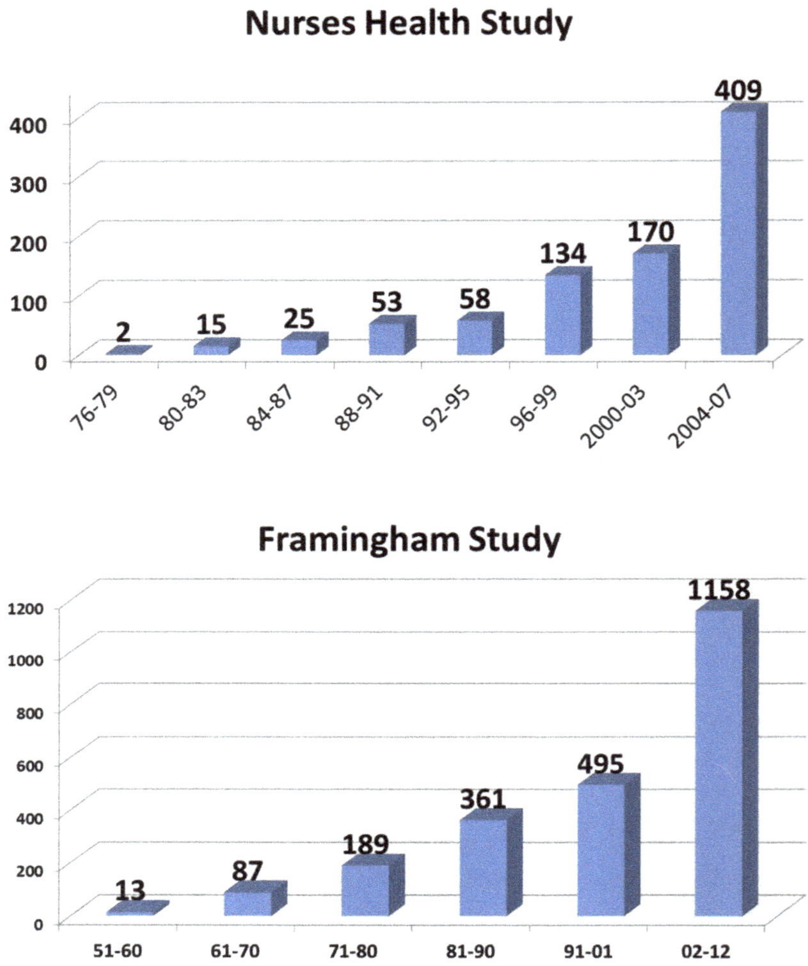

Figure 9.3 Publications over time for two seminal cohort studies. Data not cumulative.

Source: Nurses and Framingham cohort project websites.[1] Not previously published.

Another famous community cohort study continues in Framingham, Massachusetts, USA. It began in 1948 with 5,200 men and women and has lasted for 53 years. Problems arising from the small size of the original cohort were tackled by creating second- and third-generation cohorts, children and grandchildren of the original group. This study is a powerhouse of new health knowledge, with publications now appearing at the rate of 100 per year, totalling over 2,000 since inception (Figure 9.3). Framingham's cohorts now enable studies

1 www.channing.harvard.edu/nhs, accessed 10 April 2015; www.framinghamheartstudy.org, accessed 10 April 2015.

of many outcomes, beyond the initial focus on heart disease, including stroke, dementia, osteoporosis, arthritis, nutrition, diabetes, eye diseases, hearing disorders, lung diseases and genetic disorders.

There have been many other useful cohort studies, large and small, over the past 40 years. But no such general cohort studies have been conducted in the developing world, owing to the unequal distribution of global resources for such research. Our project, developing a large national cohort study in Thailand, helps to fill that significant research gap. Our Thai Cohort Study is of special value because that country is undergoing a rapid health and risk transition and is a public health leader for the ASEAN region, especially Indochina.

This is the first prospective cohort study addressing the health-risk transition, a set of emerging health problems centred around chronic disease and injury and arising with socio-economic development. It is the first nationwide cohort study to be conducted in Thailand and therefore is a landmark in the development of epidemiology in the region. These data reveal trends in population health in Thailand bearing on an emerging public health issue in the Asia-Pacific – transition from traditional patterns of risk, infection and maternal–child health problems, to the dominance of chronic disease and injury with concomitant implications for prevention and health services.

Overview of Thai Cohort Study Design

We developed our Thai Cohort Study by recruiting cohort members nationally, collaborating with STOU, Thailand's largest established distance learning open university (Sleigh et al., 2008). Its 200,000 students are an accessible group of emerging educated Thais, who aspire to an educated world view and are those most likely to be affected by the health-risk transitions under way. The open university status of STOU means there are no course fees; hence, students need not be socially or economically advantaged, and may live all over Thailand. This student population thus represents Thai adults well for age, sex, occupation, geographic residence and socio-economic status (Seubsman et al., 2012). Furthermore, these adult students are uniquely accessible by mail and are adept at filling in optically scanned sheets, because such forms are in use for multiple-choice examinations in the STOU system.

We recruited 87,134 students at baseline in 2005, with ages ranging from 15 to 87 years (median 29 years) and with 54 per cent females. Among them, we could determine distributions and rates of change for multiple proximal and upstream risk factors, many of which were generalisable to the wider Thai population (Ponsonby et al., 1996). The first follow-up in 2009 reached over 60,000 (more than 70 per cent) of the baseline cohort. These data are yielding valuable information on relative risk trends, transitions and upstream drivers, and comparative data on the effect of risk exposures – knowledge needed to plan multilevel population interventions (Table 9.1).

Table 9.1 Risk hierarchy – three levels of analysis for five risk factors.

	Levels of analysis		
Risk factors	**Proximal (downstream) Level 1**	**Structural (upstream) Level 2**	**Systemic (distal) Level 3**
Diet – cardiovascular disease	Intake of fat, sugar, protein, fruit, carbohydrate, vegetables, alcohol	Social class, income, food costs, household management, transport	Culinary culture, risk perceptions, market–regulation, socioecology
Energy expenditure – obesity and diabetes	Housework, shopping, work, recreation, travel to work	Social class, income, transport cost–availability, ease of exercise	Knowledge–perceptions, marketing, built environment, ecology
Motor cycle use – traffic injury	Motorcycle–alcohol, size–quality, helmet, driver–pillion	Social class, income, transport cost, peers, time–weather, work	Laws, marketing, risk perceptions, roads–vehicles–alcohol
Social integration – mental illness, violence and suicide	Social network, friends, family, positive community, upbringing	Marital status, education, income, employment, health services	Temperament, culture, social capital, urban–rural location
Tobacco – cardiopulmonary disease	Smoking duration and frequency, addiction, environmental smoke	Social class, income, family size, social cluster effects, work stress	Anti-smoking laws, taxes, marketing, perceptions, knowledge

Source: Thai cohort study team (2004-15).

Topics covered for the cohort study include social demography, socio-economic status, health service use and finance, contraceptive use, vision, hearing and dental health and occupation and associated hazards. Further, using questions based on standards indicated in parentheses (with the sources given when they are used), we measured overall health (SF8),[2] psychological distress (Kessler),[3] personal well-being (Cummins),[4] happiness (Yiengprugsawan et al., 2012a) and social capital (Putnam)[5]. We also collected self-reported data on the lifetime record of injury and of 25 important medical conditions including depression, diabetes, hypertension, stroke and common varieties of cancer. In addition, participants provided information on smoking and alcohol consumption, transport and related safety behaviour, family health history, body size at birth, current height and weight and food purchasing and consumption habits.

2 www.sf-36.org/tools/sf8.shtml, accessed 10 April 2015.

3 www.beyondblue.org.au/the-facts/depression/signs-and-symptoms/anxiety-and-depression-checklist-k10.

4 tinyurl.com/potge6s, accessed 10 April 2015.

5 bowlingalone.com/, accessed 10 April 2015.

Information generated from the cohort baseline in 2005 (including embedded retrospective components) has been substantial. The cohort productivity in terms of new knowledge about population health trends in middle-income transitional Thailand will continue to increase as person-time accumulates. Our current analyses (in 2013) are concentrated on the first four years of longitudinal data (2005–09). The first eight years (2005–2009–2013) will be available in 2015, a rich source of new longitudinal information.

In the following sections, we summarise Phase I (2004–09) of our Thai health-risk transition research, as well as the first part of Phase II (2010–15), in regard to both the research findings and capacity building.

Key Research Findings

Analyses of 2005 baseline data from the large national (STOU) cohort led to a number of key findings. For example, injury was more frequent than expected. Its risk factors included being male, having poor vision, having low income and being young (for traffic injury) or old (for falls) (Stephan et al., 2010). Social capital influenced self-assessed health, psychological health and personal well-being (Yiengprugsawan et al., 2011a). In transitional Thailand, we found that mental health and well-being were affected adversely by psychosocially or physically hazardous jobs, a pattern similar to that found in affluent countries (Yiengprugsawan et al., 2013). Self-reported health also mirrors patterns found in developed countries, with females reporting more frequent 'poor' or 'very poor' health (odds ratio (OR) = 1.35) (Seubsman et al., 2011). Also, emulating patterns in affluent settings are some unfortunate consequences of improved nutrition and smaller families. Taller women had an increased risk of breast cancer (OR = 2.3), as did women with non-insulin-dependent diabetes mellitus (OR = 8.4). Women with older siblings had a reduced risk of breast cancer compared to those firstborn (OR = 0.3) (Jordan et al., 2009).

By Asian standards of self-reported height and weight, 16 per cent of the cohort was obese (body mass index (BMI) >25) and 15 per cent overweight (BMI >23–24.9). Obesity was associated with urban residence, inactivity and with spending more than four hours a day watching television or using computers. We found a 33 per cent reduction in obesity risk for cohort members reporting daily housework/gardening (Banwell et al., 2009). Further longitudinal analyses have also revealed the strong relationship between short sleep hours and weight gain in the cohort (Yiengprugsawan et al., 2012b). A most interesting finding was the association of obesity with sex and socio-economic status in our cohort. The relationship was direct for males (i.e. higher status linked to more obesity) but strongly inverse for females, suggesting that educated Thai women had already developed a rich-country pattern of an inverse relationship between social class and obesity. The OR for obesity associated with higher income was 1.54 for males and 0.68 for females (Seubsman et al., 2010).

Another transition-related finding was the strong relationship between life-course urbanisation status and health outcomes. The rural–urban group (those who moved to cities after age 12 years) constituted almost one-third of the cohort members and were significantly different from other groups in many ways (e.g. more one-person or couple-with-no-children households). Health and other social outcomes of urbanisers were closer to those in the urban–urban group and were worse than the rural–rural group, with lower self-assessed health and a higher prevalence of hypertension, depression and obesity (Lim et al., 2009; Seubsman et al., 2010, 2011; Thawornchaisit et al., 2013).

Another important finding to date relates to the progressive increase in the attained height of young adult Thais over the past 50 years. We studied this in 34,000 20-year-old military recruits measured in Bangkok from 1972 to 2006, finding a five-centimetre increase to 169 centimetres over that period. The best explanation was that poor children around Bangkok became progressively better nourished and healthier from 1952 to 1986 (Seubsman and Sleigh, 2009). Biological nationwide evidence of such an historical health-risk transition was also obtained among age cohorts born from the 1940s to the 1990s. Such data for both sexes were available from STOU students who were members of the Thai Cohort Study (Jordan et al., 2012) (Figure 9.4). This analysis supported the military recruit data and showed that urban Thais became taller than rural counterparts, reflecting healthier childhoods on average, with the gap growing wider over this 50-year period. However, rural Thais also grew taller, but at a slower rate, suggesting increased inequality. Both males and females had similar trends (female data not shown). This growing divergence reflects, and possibly underpins, much of the rural-urban tension still evident in Thailand.

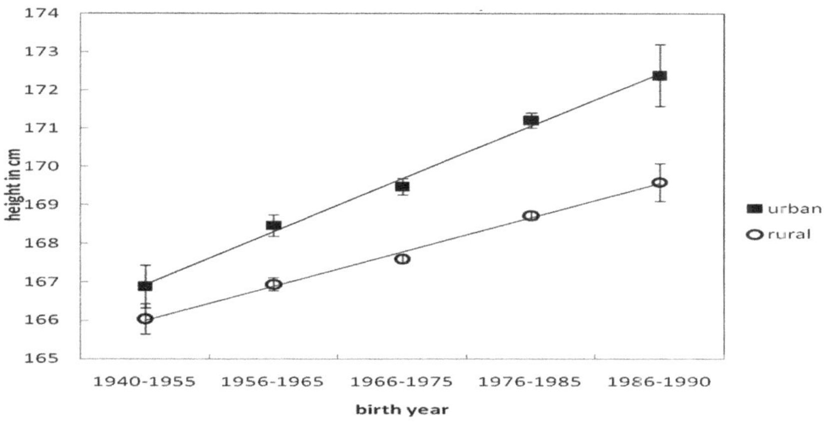

Figure 9.4 Mean heights (95 per cent CIs) among Thai men classified by their location (whether rural or urban) at age 10–12.

Source: Thai Cohort Study analysis, with permission (Jordan et al., 2012).

An important issue for future population health in Thailand concerns the effects of heat stress, particularly in the workplace (Kjellstrom et al., 2009). At baseline in 2005, around 20 per cent of working cohort members reported experiencing uncomfortably high temperatures at work, and in 2009, around 30 per cent reported being bothered by high temperatures when either sleeping, doing housework, working, exercising or daily travelling. Our study has revealed such heat stress in Thailand is associated with kidney disease (Tawatsupa et al., 2012a), poorer overall well-being (Tawatsupa et al., 2012b) and increased risk of occupational injury (Tawatsupa et al., 2013). These associations will be of particular concern if global temperatures increase under climate change. Mortality in Thailand may be expected to increase 5–13 per cent if predicted temperature increases of 4°C by 2100 are realised (Tawatsupa et al., 2012c).

As the Thai population ages and chronic disease and disability become more prevalent, the need for caring support will also increase. In the absence of sufficient state-supported social security measures, this caring burden falls largely to family members, as it would traditionally. However, in the past, aged people were less prevalent and larger families were normal. Around one-third of our Thai cohort reported currently being a carer for a sick or disabled individual. Caring had significant impacts on cohort members, with carers reporting more prevalent lower back pain, psychological distress and, among females, worse self-rated overall health than their non-carer counterparts (Yiengprugsawan et al., 2012c). However, caregiving was also associated with higher levels of self-esteem and contentment with life, particularly where caregivers retained social contacts with those outside the household, indicating the importance of social support for those in caregiving roles (Yiengprugsawan et al., 2012d).

The effects of increased longevity, as well as changes in lifestyles, are being revealed in other aspects of our study. Oral health is one example where age is important, with older cohort members having a much higher prevalence of poor oral health, which is then associated with poor quality of life (Yiengprugsawan et al., 2011b, 2011c). Around 8.5 per cent of cohort members had trouble with their hearing (Yiengprugsawan et al., 2012e), and one-third of the cohort had vision impairment (Yiengprugsawan et al., 2012f). Both of these problems were strongly associated with poor self-rated health and psychological distress.

Building Regional Population Health Capacity

We have developed a productive international research partnership involving senior policymakers and academics in Thailand and specialists in epidemiology, international health, demography, sociology, economics and development in Australia. Further, we have boosted public health research capacity through doctoral and Masters training. By May 2014, directly associated with the project, there were eight completed or current Master's graduates in Thailand; in addition, six Thais and two Australians had completed PhDs in Australia and three more were under way. Among these 19 young public health scholars, 16 are Thai and three are Australasian.

By May 2014, the research has generated a substantial output on risk trends, transitions and health outcomes, with 80 published or in press papers, seven books or book chapters, and eight submitted papers. Of the 21 first authors for these 80 published papers, eight were Thai and 12 authors were PhD students or project postdoctoral researchers.

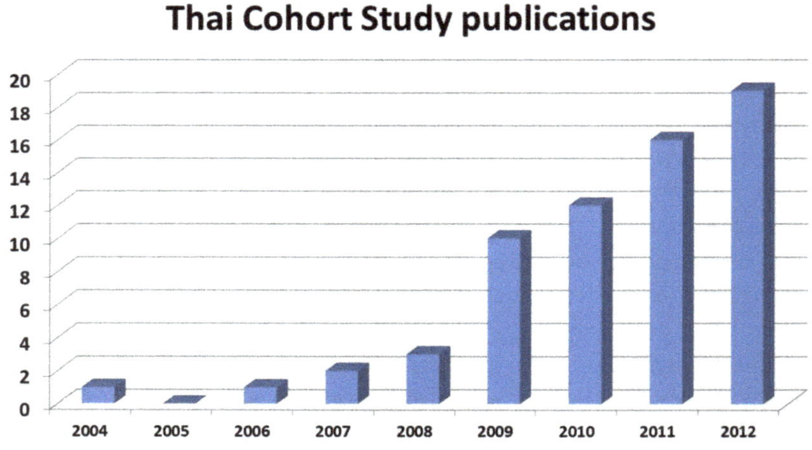

Figure 9.5. Publications arising from the Thai Cohort Study each year.

Source: Authors' work.

Conclusions

The mean height trends suggest that Thai modernisation is about half completed, but that rural disadvantage is growing. Public health campaigns are urgently needed to reduce traffic injury. We also recognise a new public health focus is needed on urban health, social capital and healthy cities. There are serious emerging problems of stress and psychological distress at work and at home, and an urgent need exists for dietary education and regulation of the food environment, decreasing exposure to calorie-dense processed foods. As well, there is a need to encourage physical activity and a permissive built environment, especially for Thai children. There also appears to be an emerging problem of underweight young Thai females, particularly noticeable in the cohort.

Other project data (not discussed above) also indicate the great importance of maintaining the successful anti-smoking campaigns, especially for females, whose non-smoking behaviour is set culturally and is enormously beneficial (Pachanee et al., 2011). It is also important to monitor the Universal Coverage Scheme of health insurance, especially for the poor (Yiengprugsawan et al., 2009), and to provide new sexual health services for Thai adolescents (Tangmunkongvorakul et al., 2010). Continued improvement in occupational health and safety is needed as the Thai workforce formalises (Yiengprugsawan et al., 2009; Kelly et al., 2010; Tangmunkongvorakul et al., 2010; Berecki-Gisolf et al., 2013).

Our results are available to assist health policy development in Thailand, and we already have two senior policymakers as Chief Investigators. We have also succeeded in linking our cohort data (which includes Citizen ID numbers) with the existing national databases for deaths (Ministry of Interior, Ministry of Public Health). We continue to seek links to Thai cancer registries and health-service databases (civil servant and universal health insurance) to improve our analytic capacity.

The Thai–Australian partnership has worked productively in terms of capacity building, regional collaboration and research. Professor McMichael was both inspirational and supportive, especially at the start, as we were finding our way. He was also an excellent host on many social occasions, and this helped to motivate the team.

Acknowledgements

Phase I of the project (2004–10) was supported by the International Collaborative Research Grants Scheme, with joint grants from the Wellcome Trust UK (GR071587MA) and the Australian NH&MRC (268055). Phase II (2010–14) was supported by the Australian NH&MRC (585426). We thank the staff at Sukhothai Thammathirat Open University who assisted with student contact, and STOU students who are participating in the cohort study. We thank our research collaborators at Monash University, The University of Queensland and the Queensland Institute of Medical Research in Australia.

Finally, we thank the members of the Thai cohort study team, who worked together over many years to make this project happen. The team members are listed here. Thailand: Jaruwan Chokhanapitak, Chaiyun Churewong, Suttanit Hounthasarn, Suwanee Khamman, Daoruang Pandee, Suttinan Pangsap, Tippawan Prapamontol, Janya Puengson, Yodyiam Sangrattanakul, Boonchai Somboonsook, Nintita Sripaiboonkij, Sam-ang Seubsman, Pathumvadee Somsamai, Benjawan Tawatsupa, Arunrat Tangmunkongvorakul, Duangkae Vilainerun, Wanee Wimonwattanaphan. Australia: Chris Bain, Emily Banks, Cathy Banwell, Janneke Berecki-Gisolf, Bruce Caldwell, Gordon Carmichael, Tarie Dellora, Jane Dixon, Sharon Friel, David Harley, Susan Jordan, Matthew Kelly, Tord Kjellstrom, Lynette Lim, Roderick McClure, Anthony McMichael, Tanya Mark, Adrian Sleigh, Lyndall Strazdins, Tam Tran, Vasoontara Yiengprugsawan, Jiaying Zhao.

References

Aekplakorn, W., Hogan, M.C., Chongsuvivatwong, V., Tatsanavivat, P., Chariyalertsak, S., Boonthum, A., et al. 2007. Trends in obesity and associations with education and urban or rural residence in Thailand. *Obesity* 15, 3113–21.

Banwell, C., Lim, L.L.Y., Seubsman, S., Bain, C., Dixon, J. & Sleigh, A.C. 2009. Body mass index and health-related behaviours in a national cohort of 87 134 Thai open university students. *Journal of Epidemiology and Community Health* 63, 366–72.

Berecki-Gisolf, J., Tawatsupa, B., McClure, R., Seubsman, S, Sleigh, A. & the Thai Cohort Study Team 2013. Determinants of workplace injury among Thai Cohort Study participants. *BMJ Open*, pii:e003079, doi:10.1136/bmjopen-2013-003079.

Berkman, L.F. & Kawachi, I. (eds) 2000. *Social Epidemiology*. Oxford University Press, Oxford, UK, and New York, USA.

Bureau of Health Policy and Planning 2002. *Annual Morbidity Statistics*. Ministry of Public Health, Thailand.

Caldwell, J.C. 1993. Health transition: the cultural, social and behavioural determinants of health in the Third World. *Social Science & Medicine* 36, 125–35.

Caldwell, J.C. & Caldwell, P. 1993. The South African fertility decline. *Population and Development Review* 19, 225–62.

Commission on Macroeconomics and Health 2001. *Macroeconomics and Health: Investing in Health for Economic Development*. Report of the Commission on Macroeconomics and Health. World Health Organization, Geneva, Switzerland.

Drewnowski, A. & Popkin, B.M. 1997. The nutrition transition: new trends in the global diet. *Nutrition Reviews* 55, 31–4.

Harper, A.C., Holman, C.D.J. & Dawes, V.P. 1994. *The Health of Populations*. Churchill Livingston, South Melbourne, Victoria, Australia.

Hirshman, C. 1994. Population and society in twentieth-century Southeast Asia. *Journal of Southeast Asian Studies* 25, 381–416.

Jamison, D.T., Mosley, W.H., Measham, A.R. & Bobadilla, J.L. (eds) 1993. *Disease Control Priorities of the Developing World*. Oxford University Press, New York, USA.

Jordan, S., Lim, L.L.Y., Vilainerun, D., Banks, E., Sripaiboonkij, N., Seubsman, S., et al. 2009. Breast cancer in the Thai Cohort Study: an exploratory case-control analysis. *The Breast* 18, 299–303.

Jordan, S., Lim, L.L.Y., Seubsman, S., Bain, C., Sleigh, A.C. & the Thai Cohort Study Team 2012. Secular changes and predictors of adult height for 86105 male and female members of the Thai Cohort Study born between 1940 and 1990. *Journal of Epidemiology and Community Health* 66, 75–80.

Kelly, M., Strazdins, L., Dellora, T., Khamman, S., Seubsman, S. & Sleigh, A.C. 2010. Thailand's work and health transition. *International Labour Review* 149, 373–86.

Kjellstrom, T., Homer, I. & Lemke, B. 2009. Workplace heat stress, health and productivity – an increasing challenge for low- and middle-income countries during climate change. *Global Health Action* 2, 10.3402/gha.v2i0.2047.

Laaser, U., Breckenkamp, J., Ullrich, A. & Hoffmann, B. 2001. Can a decline in the population means of cardiovascular risk factors reduce the number of people at risk. *Journal of Epidemiology and Community Health* 55, 179–84.

Lim, L.L.Y., Kjellstrom, T., Sleigh, A.C., Khamman, S., Seubsman, S., Dixon, J., et al. 2009. Associations between urbanisation and components of the health-risk transition in Thailand. A descriptive study of 87,000 Thai adults. *Global Health Action* 2, doi:10.3402/gha.v52i0.1914.

McMichael, A.J. 2001. *Human Frontiers, Environments and Disease: Past Patterns, Uncertain Futures*. Cambridge University Press, Cambridge, UK.

National Statistical Office of Thailand 2003. Core Economic Indicators of Thailand, and Key Statistics of Thailand, 2001. Available at: www.nso.go.th/, accessed 20 October 2010.

Pachanee, C., Lim, L.L.Y., Bain, C., Wibulpolprasert, S., Seubsman, S. & Sleigh, A.C. 2011. Smoking behavior among 84 315 open-university students in Thailand. *Asia Pacific Journal of Public Health* 23, 544–54.

Ponsonby, A.-L., Dwyer, T. & Couper, D. 1996. Is this finding relevant? Generalisation and epidemiology. *Australian and New Zealand Journal of Public Health* 20, 54–6.

Population Division of the Department of Economic and Social Affairs of the United Nations Secretariat 2003. World Population Prospects: The 2004 Revision and World Urbanization Prospects: The 2003 Revision. Now available at: www.un.org/en/development/desa/population/publications/pdf/trends/population-projections.pdf, accessed March 2015.

Rose, G. 1992. *The Strategy of Preventive Medicine*. Oxford University Press, Oxford, UK, and New York, USA.

Seubsman, S. & Sleigh, A.C. 2009. Change in mean height of Thai military recruits from 1972 through 2006. *Journal of Epidemiology* 19, 196–201.

Seubsman, S., Lim, L.L.Y., Banwell, C., Sripaiboonkit, N., Kelly, M., Bain, C., et al. 2010. Socioeconomic status, sex and obesity in a large national cohort of 15–87 year old open university students in Thailand. *Journal of Epidemiology* 20, 13–20.

Seubsman, S., Kelly, M.J., Yiengprugsawan, V. & Sleigh, A.C. 2011. Thai Cohort Study Team. Gender, socioeconomic status, and self-rated health in a transitional middle-income setting: evidence from Thailand. *Asia Pacific Journal of Public Health* 23, 754–65.

Seubsman, S., Yiengprugsawan, V., Sleigh, A.C. & the Thai Cohort Study Team 2012. A large national Thai cohort study of the health-risk transition based on Sukhothai Thammathirat Open University students. *ASEAN Journal of Open Distance Learning* 4, 58–69.

Sleigh, A.C., Seubsman, S., Bain, C. & the Thai Cohort Study Team 2008. Cohort profile: the Thai cohort of 87,134 open university students. *International Journal of Epidemiology* 37, 266–72.

Stephan, K., McClure, R., Seubsman, S., Kelly, M., Yiengprugsawan, V., Bain, C., et al. 2010. Review of injuries over a one year period among 87,134 adults studying at an open university in Thailand. *Southeast Asian Journal of Tropical Medicine and Public Health* 41, 1220–30.

Tangmunkongvorakul, A., Carmichael, G., Banwell, C., Seubsman, S. & Sleigh, A.C. 2010. Intimate relationships amongst adolescents in different social groups in Northern Thailand. *Southeast Asian Journal of Tropical Medicine and Public Health* 41, 1475–93.

Tawatsupa, B., Lim, L.L.Y., Kjellstrom, T., Seubsman, S., Sleigh, A.C. & the Thai Cohort Study Team 2012a. The association between occupational heat stress and kidney disease among 17 402 males and 20 414 females in the Thai Cohort Study (TCS). *Journal of Epidemiology* 22, 251–60.

Tawatsupa, B., Yiengprugsawan, V., Kjellstrom, T., Seubsman, S., Sleigh, A.C. & the Thai Cohort Study Team 2012b. Heat stress, health, and wellbeing: findings from a large national cohort of Thai adults. *BMJ Open* 2, e001396, doi:10.1136/bmjopen-2012-001396.

Tawatsupa, B., Dear, K., Kjellstrom, T. & Sleigh, A.C. 2012c. The association between temperature and mortality in middle income Thailand from 1999 to 2008. *International Journal of Biometerology*, doi:10.1007/s00484-012-0597-8.

Tawatsupa, B., Yiengprugsawan, V., Kjellstrom, T., Berecki-Gisolf, J., Seusbman, S. & Sleigh, A.C. 2013. Association between heat stress and occupational injury among Thai workers: findings of the Thai Cohort Study. *Industrial Health* 51, 34–46.

Thawornchaisit, P., de Looze, F., Reid, C.M., Seubsman, S. & Sleigh, A.C. 2013. Thai Cohort Study Team. Health risk factors and the incidence of hypertension: 4-year prospective findings from a national cohort of 60569 Thai Open University students. *BMJ Open* 3, doi:10.1136/bmjopen-2013-002826.

Warren, K.S. 1997. Rationalising health care in a changing world: the need to know. *Health Transition Review* 7, 61–71.

Wilbulpolprasert, S. (ed.) 2008. *Thailand Health Profile 2005–2007*. Ministry of Public Health, Bangkok, Thailand.

Wilson, C. 2001. On the scale of global demographic convergence 1950–2000. *Population and Development Review* 27, 155–71.

World Bank 1993. *Investing in Health. World Development Report 1993*. Oxford University Press, Oxford, UK.

World Bank 2013. World Data Bank: World Development Indicators. Online database. Available at: databank.worldbank.org/ddp/home.do?Step=3&id=4, accessed 8 March 2013.

World Health Report 2002. *Reducing Risks, Promoting Healthy Life*. World Health Organization, Geneva, Switzerland.

Yiengprugsawan, V., Lim, L.L.Y., Carmichael, G. & Sleigh, A.C. 2009. Tracking and decomposing health and disease inequality in Thailand. *Annals of Epidemiology* 19, 800–7.

Yiengprugsawan, V., Khamman, S., Seubsman, S., Lim, L.L.Y. & Sleigh, A.C. 2011a. Social capital and health in a national cohort of 82,482 Open University adults in Thailand. *Journal of Health Psychology* 16, 632–42.

Yiengprugsawan, V., Somkotra, T., Seubsman, S., Kelly, M., Sleigh, A.C. & the Thai Cohort Study Team 2011b. Factors associated with self-reported number of teeth in a large national cohort of Thai adults. *BMC Oral Health* 11, 31, doi:10.1186/1472-6831-11-31.

Yiengprugsawan, V., Somkotra, T., Seubsman, S., Sleigh, A.C. & the Thai Cohort Study Team 2011c. Oral health-related quality of life among a large national cohort of 87,134 Thai adults. *Health and Quality of Life Outcomes* 9, 42, doi:10.1186/1477-7525-9-42.

Yiengprugsawan, V., Somboonsook, B., Seubsman, S. & Sleigh, A.C., 2012a. Happiness, mental health, and socio-demographic associations among a national cohort of Thai adults. *Journal of Happiness Studies* 13, 1019–29.

Yiengprugsawan, V., Banwell, C., Seubsman, S. & Sleigh, A.C. 2012b. Short sleep and obesity in a large national cohort of Thai adults. *BMJ Open*, doi:10.1136/bmjopen-2011-000561.

Yiengprugsawan, V., Harley, D., Seubsman, S., Sleigh, A.C. & the Thai Cohort Study Team 2012c. Physical and mental health among caregivers: findings from a cross-sectional study of Open University students in Thailand. *BMC Public Health* 12, 1111, doi:10.1186/1471-2458-12-1111.

Yiengprugsawan, V., Seubsman, S. & Sleigh, A.C. 2012d. Psychological distress and mental health of Thai caregivers. *Psychology of Well-Being: Theory, Research and Practice* 2, doi:10.1186/2211-1522-2-4.

Yiengprugsawan, V., Hogan, A., Harley, D., Seubsman, S., Sleigh, A.C. & the Thai Cohort Study Team 2012e. Epidemiological associations of hearing impairment and health among a national cohort of 87 134 Adults in Thailand. *Asia Pacific Journal of Public Health* 24, 1013–22.

Yiengprugsawan, V., Seubsman, S. & Sleigh, A.C. 2012f. Associations of vision impairment and health among a national cohort of 87,134 Thai Adults. *Asia Pacific Journal of Public Health*, doi:10.1177/1010539511433049.

Yiengprugsawan, V., Strazdins, L., Lim, L.L.Y., Kelly, M., Seubsman, S., Sleigh, A.C., et al. 2013. Physically and psychologically hazardous jobs and mental health in Thailand. *Health Promotion International*, doi:10.1093/heapro/dat080.

10

CLIMATE CHANGE AND ENVIRONMENTAL INFLUENCES ON AUSTRALIA'S POPULATION DISTRIBUTION

GRAEME HUGO AND JANET WALL

Abstract

Australia has a distinctive population distribution characterised by a concentration in major metropolitan centres and coastal areas, with much of the continent being sparsely settled. This has been strongly shaped by historical, environmental and economic processes, but it is likely that climate change may have some influence in the future. The current generation of climate change models have limited spatial resolution, so it is difficult to be precise about the areas that will be most impacted by climate change. This paper investigates six major non-metropolitan regions that have been identified as areas likely to be most affected by climate change. While effects on coastal cities will be substantial, they are not considered in detail here. The six non-metropolitan 'hotspots', however, are each considered in turn and the potential health and population distribution effects discussed. It is argued that Australian discourse on climate change has not focused sufficiently on intranational variations in the potential effects of that change.

Introduction

Tony McMichael's contribution extended beyond epidemiology and public health disciplinary boundaries to influence the social sciences more broadly. His work linking the dynamics of change in people, place and health and the impacts of climate change was influential in geography and demography. He drew attention to the health implications of climate change and their potential effects on population distribution and redistribution, and provided insights into how particular types of climate change would have both direct and indirect impacts on health (McMichael, 2001; McMichael et al., 2006, 2010). In this context, the spatial dimensions of climate change, the location of 'hotspots' of significant changes in temperature, rainfall and extreme weather events are important. Yet this aspect of climate change remains neglected. Accordingly, this chapter seeks to identify these potential hotspots of severe climate change impact in Australia and relate them to present and potential future patterns of population distribution.

The current distribution of population in Australia is a function of the location of resources, environmental amenity, transport routes, historical forces, liveability, past and present government policy and global and national markets. Environment and climate have interacted to be influential in shaping this distribution. Accordingly, climate change can influence that distribution, such as by affecting the extent to which the inhabitants of an area can earn a local livelihood or by changing a location's liveability. Health dimensions are an important factor in the latter (McMichael et al., 2010).

This chapter begins by discussing briefly the current patterns of Australian population growth and distribution, and the forces that have shaped it. It then examines what is currently known about possible spatial differences in the impact of climate change across Australia. It is shown that there is at present a concentration of population in areas anticipated to experience significant detrimental climate change effects, especially rainfall decline. Moreover, many Australian hotspots of population growth are also hotspots of substantial anticipated impact by climate change.

Australia's Contemporary Population Distribution

Although the Aborigines' hunting and gathering economy meant larger numbers inhabited the well-watered eastern and south-western margins where food was more abundant, Table 10.1 shows that, compared with the contemporary population, the Aboriginal population had a more dispersed distribution. Contemporary Australia is one of the most spatially concentrated populations of all nations, with 89 per cent living in urban areas, 65 per cent in capital cities and 82 per cent living within 50 km of the coast. Few countries have a more uneven distribution of the population, with 0.34 per cent of the population living in 84.2 per cent of the land area of the continent, with a population density of less than 0.1 persons per km^2, and 90.5 per cent of the people living in the 0.22 per cent of the land area, with 100 persons or more per km^2. Moreover, there is a strong clustering on the east coast and south-east and south-west regions.

Table 10.1 Australia: Estimated distribution of Aboriginal population at the time of initial European settlement and total Australian population in 2011.

State	1776 Aboriginal population		2011 Total Australian population		Per cent of area
	Number	Per cent	Number	Per cent	
New South Wales (incl. ACT)	48,000	15.3	7,274,877	33.8	10.5
Victoria	15,000	4.8	5,354,040	24.9	3.0
Queensland	120,000	38.2	4,332,737	20.1	22.5
South Australia	15,000	4.8	1,596,570	7.4	12.8
Western Australia	62,000	19.7	2,239,170	10.4	32.9
Tasmania	41,500	1.5	495,350	2.3	0.9
Northern Territory	50,000	15.9	211,944	1.0	17.5
Total	314,500	100.0	21,504,688	100.0	100.0

Source: Smith, 1980, p. 69; Australian Bureau of Statistics (ABS), 2011 Census of Population and Housing.

What forces explain this stark contrast in population distribution? Clearly, the changing nature of the economy involving a contracting proportion of the population required to produce food and an increase in urban-based secondary, tertiary and quaternary activities is a major factor. Historical elements, such as the fact that each state was formerly a separate colony with its capital being an entrepot linkage point with Britain, have also played a role. In the contemporary context location of key resources, differences in the amenity of areas for retirees and tourists, strategic location in relation to transport and accessibility are important. A crucial element, however, is environment, as it was to Aboriginal Australia. The extent to which the environment affects the potential to earn a living is of basic importance. Moreover, 'prevailing climatic conditions, and in weather variability affect human well-being, safety, health and survival' (McMichael et al., 2010, p. 195).

The role of the environment and climate in shaping population settlement in Australia after European colonisation was recognised by geographers a century ago (Price, 1939). Arguably, however, the environmental role has been neglected with the decline in the proportion of the population working in primary industry, massive developments in transport and communication, medical advances and technological development such as air conditioning. Almost a century ago, Griffith Taylor argued that:

> the contemporary margins of settlement in Australia already closely approximated the limits which had been set by the very nature of the physical environment: whether people, plants or animals were considered, the appropriate environmental controls could be ignored only at a cost. (quoted in Powell, 1984, p. 87)

There is much to support Taylor's argument that the fundamental structure of Australian settlement was already established by the second half of the 19th century (Rowland, 1982).

A further aspect relates to spatial patterns of population growth. Not only is the Australian population distribution highly concentrated but also there is considerable spatial variation in the pattern of *population change* – growth and decline. This is evident in Table 10.2, which shows the pattern of recent population change by remoteness categories. In both numerical and relative terms, recent population growth is concentrated in the major cities (those with 100,000 or more inhabitants) that are, apart from Canberra, located in the south-east and south-west coastal areas. The impact of the mining boom on very remote areas since 2006 is also evident.

Table 10.2 Australia: Population change by remoteness area, 1996–2012.

	Population change (thousands)		Growth rate (%) p.a.			
Remoteness area category	**1996–2006**	**2006–12**	**1996–2001**	**2001–06**	**2006–11**	**2011–12**
Major cities of Australia	2069.2	1790.4	1.8	1.4	1.7	1.8
Inner regional Australia	330.2	66.1	0.3	1.4	1.2	1.2
Outer regional Australia	9.3	80.7	–0.7	0.8	0.6	1.0
Remote Australia	–12.2	5.0	–0.7	0.0	0.7	1.3
Very remote Australia	–5.7	39.8	–0.5	–0.2	2.6	1.3
Total	2390.8	1982.1	1.2	1.3	1.5	1.6

Source: Authors' work, calculated from ABS censuses.

In summary, in Australia there is strong spatial differentiation of population distribution, population density and population growth, which have been shaped by economic and historical forces along with environmental and climate elements.

Spatial Differences in the Impact of Climate Change in Australia

In this section, we consider how the spatial patterns described above interact with the predicted effects of climate change. Before that, however, it is instructive to consider some of these relationships over recent decades.

One major effect of climate change is anticipated to be a change in rainfall and water run-off. The recent 13-year drought in south-eastern Australia, together with the continuing droughts in south-western Australia, is consistent with long-term rainfall declines associated with climate change (State of the Environment, 2011). Figure 10.1 presents analysis by the Commonwealth Scientific and Industrial Research Organisation (CSIRO) and the Bureau of Meteorology (BOM) (2010) relating to national rainfall trends between 1960 and 2009. The long-term rainfall increase in north-western Australia is balanced by a significant decline in the closely settled south-eastern and south-western parts of the nation. Of interest is that, in 2011, the majority of Australians lived in areas experiencing a long-term decline in rainfall, although the population was growing faster in this area experiencing an increase in rainfall.

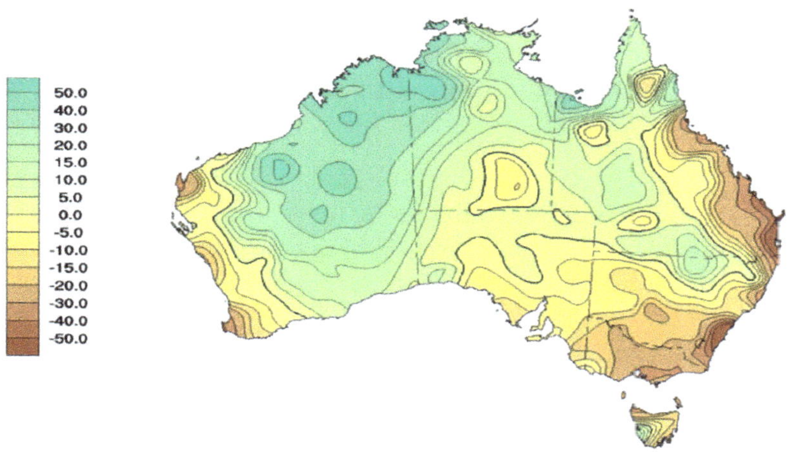

Figure 10.1 Trends in annual total rainfall, 1960–2009 (millimetres per decade).

Source: CSIRO and BOM, 2010, with permission from the Bureau of Meteorology.

Table 10.3 Australia: Population growth in long-term rainfall trend areas, 2006–11.

Long-term rainfall trend (mm)	2006 population	2011 population	Change 2006–11	Change 2006–11 (%)	Growth rate per annum (%)
Increase (+10 or greater)	462,629	545,947	83,318	18.01	3.37
Stable (between +10 and –10)	2,285,712	2,459,589	173,877	7.61	1.48
Decline (–10 or less)	16,923,224	18,439,950	1,516,726	8.96	1.73
No data	26,234	13,245	–12,989	–49.51	–12.78
Total	**19,697,799**	**21,458,731**	**1,760,932**	**8.94**	**1.73**

Source: Authors' work, from BOM, Trend in Annual Total Rainfall 1960–2009 (2011) and ABS Censuses (2006, 2011). Population data based on ABS Census 2006 CD centroid and 2011 SA1 centroid population counts (usual resident). Annual average growth rate has been calculated over a five-year period (2006–11).

It is difficult to identify precisely locations in Australia that will be impacted most severely by climate change. This section summarises current understanding of likely spatial variation in climate change in Australia over the next few decades. The climate change models used here are the widely used CSIRO–BOM regional climate change projections for 2030, 2050 and 2070, and the assumptions underlying them are detailed in CSIRO and BOM (2007). These models have a spatial resolution of around 250 km between grid squares, and provide only an average over those grid squares so that 'within square' heterogeneity is not captured.

With respect to rainfall, it is projected that by 2030 there will be little change in precipitation in the north and decreases of 2–5 per cent elsewhere. The decreases are highest in winter and spring, especially in the south-west, where they reach 10 per cent. In summer and autumn, decreases are smaller, with slight increases in the east. Daily precipitation intensity increases in the north and decreases in the south. The models show that droughts will increase in frequency over most of Australia, but especially in the south-west. It is also shown that there is a substantial increase in fire-weather risk, especially in south-eastern Australia. Regarding temperature, it is projected that by 2030 there will be an increase of around 1°C in average temperature – 0.7–0.9°C in coastal areas and 1–1.2°C inland. There is little variation in the results over the full range of climate change scenarios in the 2030 projections. However, there is greater variation in the projections to 2050 and 2070. The major regional variations are of less warming in the southern and north-east and more inland areas.

Turning to sea level rise, the CSIRO and BOM (2007, p. 92) point out that the Intergovernmental Panel on Climate Change (IPCC) projects an 18–59 cm rise in sea level by 2100, with the east coast of Australia anticipated to record a rise above the global mean (Climate Commission, 2011, p. 12).[1] The impact of sea level rise, however, can be exacerbated by storm surges that enable inundation and damaging waves to penetrate further inland (CSIRO and BOM, 2007, p. 94). On average, sea levels have risen globally by 3.2 mm/year since the early 1990s.

Projection of future climate change is improving, but the inherent uncertainty is exacerbated when it is spatially disaggregated. It is not yet possible to anticipate precisely the climate change impacts at local and community levels in Australia, but some generalisations can be made:

- Rainfall is likely to be reduced in the southern areas of Australia, especially in winter, and in southern and eastern areas in spring, due to a southerly contraction in the rainfall belt. Intense rainfall events in most areas will become more extreme and frequent, although future changes in summer tropical rainfall in northern Australia remain uncertain.
- As temperatures and dryness increase, so too does the frequency of extremely hot days, especially in inland Australia, with consequent increased bushfire risk.

The Climate Action Network (2006) has identified six major hotspots of potential high impact of climate change in Australia, shown in Figure 10.2. This classification focuses predominantly on non-metropolitan areas and hence misses the effects of climate change on large metropolitan centres, such as:

1. Potential inundation and storm surge impacts along coasts.
2. Constraints on urban water supplies created by the reduced rainfall and run-off in the watersheds of large mainland metropolitan centres and in the Murray–Darling Basin, which supplies a significant part of the water supply of Adelaide and Melbourne. Decreased run-off, especially in inland catchments, will be exacerbated by increased evaporation due to higher temperatures. For example, for Sydney, it is projected that there will be a 22 per cent increase in pan evaporation in inland catchments and a 9 per cent increase in coastal catchments by 2070 (Department of Climate Change and Energy Efficiency (DCCEE), 2011a, p. 1).
3. There will be increased risk of extreme bushfires near several capitals. For Sydney, for example, fire seasons will start earlier and end later and the number of extreme fire danger days will rise from 9 at present to 15 by 2020 (DCCEE, 2011a).

1 It should be noted that the IPCC put substantial qualifications on these numbers – for example, they do not include the full ice melt factors.

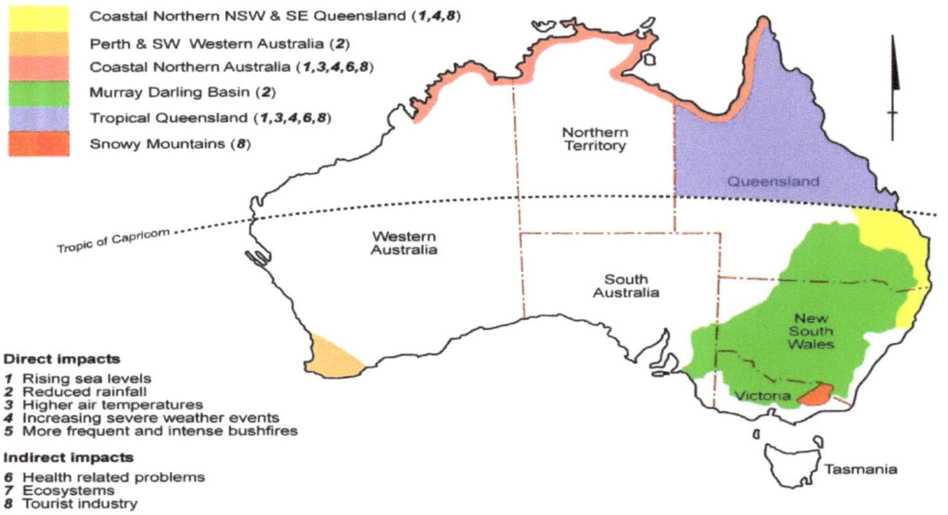

Figure 10.2 Broadly defined non-metropolitan climate change impact hotspots in Australia.

Source: Chris Crothers, Faculty of Arts, University of Adelaide, using information from Climate Action Network, 2006.

In this context, it is important to note that several potential negative health outcomes from climate change are especially important in large cities. Gamble et al. (2008) have identified climate-sensitive health outcomes in US cities that provide insights into the likely health effects of climate change in Australian metropolitan areas. These include thermal extremes involving both heatwaves and coldwaves. In Sydney, for example, extreme heat days are projected to increase from 3.5 per annum currently to 12 by 2070 (DCCEE, 2011a).

Climate Change Hotspots, Population and Health

We will now turn to each of the six hotspot areas, examining the potential health and population impacts of climate change more closely, using a framework developed by McMichael et al. (2010, p. 196). Table 10.4 summarises these impacts.

Table 10.4 Potential health risks in Australian climate change hotspot areas.

Categories of health risk (after McMichael et al., 2010, p. 196)	Coastal NSW S.E. Qld	Perth and S.W. WA	Coastal northern Australia	Murray–Darling Basin	Tropical Qld	Snowy Mountains
Direct acting risks						
Injury and death from extreme events – floods, storms, fires	X	X	X	X	X	X
Illness and death from more frequent and intense heatwaves	X	X	X	X	X	
Increased risk of respiratory illnesses from high air pollution		X	X	X	X	X
Exacerbation of respiratory allergic condition from pollen		X	X	X	X	X
Indirect acting risks						
Impoverishment by impaired/failed agriculture or other livelihood	X	X	X	X	X	X
Increased risk of gastroenteritis			X		X	
Change in seasonal outbreak of mosquito-borne infection			X		X	
Health risk associated with displacement	X	X	X	X	X	
Increased mental health risks	X	X	X	X	X	X

Source: Authors' work.

Coastal northern New South Wales and south-east Queensland

This region has one of the most rapidly growing populations of any region in Australia in recent decades, with metropolitan peri-urban and coastal development associated with the Brisbane–Gold Coast and Sunshine Coast complex. Two major elements of climate change – increased sea levels and increased severe weather events – are likely to affect the area. The rapid recent growth of population in this region has been associated with increased tourism and lifestyle-related in-migration including young families and retirees (Burnley and Murphy, 2004). The imminent retirement of baby boomers is likely to see a substantial future influx of people in their 60s, and of a working-age population to service them. The pattern of coastal areas with rapid population growth and in-migration being at substantial risk of significant impact of climate change is one that is replicated in many parts of the world (McGranahan et al., 2007).

It has been estimated that between 43,900 and 65,300 residential buildings with a current value of between A$14 and 20 billion are at risk of inundation in coastal New South Wales if sea levels were to rise by 1.1 m. While this rise is substantially higher than current IPCC projections for 2100, it is potentially possible if there are no mitigation interventions. Such a rise would put at risk up to 4800 km of roads, 320 km of railways and up to 1200 commercial buildings (DCCEE, 2011b). Queensland shows similar patterns for a similar sea level rise. From a health perspective, Table 10.4 indicates that this devastation would result in increased injury and death. Moreover, the region will also be influenced by greater frequency and intensity of heatwaves, with likely pronounced health effects, especially for the large numbers of older people in the area. Indirect effects include the loss of livelihood in agriculture and tourism, increased exposure to mental health problems and displacement from coastal areas. In the face of such trends, it would be difficult in the longer term to sustain the current rapid rates of population growth.

Perth and south-west Western Australia

One of the most consistent findings in climate change modelling in Australia (CSIRO and BOM, 2007) is a reduced rainfall in the south-western corner of the Australian continent. This has clear implications for the wheat–sheep as well as viticulture and other intensive agriculture in that region. In addition, Perth is currently Australia's most rapidly growing capital city, but the reduction in rainfall anticipated in its hinterland has dire implications for the water supply of the capital and has already seen the increasing use of desalination technology.

Rainfall has already fallen by around 15 per cent in south-western Western Australia since the 1970s. The annual average stream flow into Perth dams has fallen from 338 gigalitres over 1911–74 to 177 in 1975–2000 to 75 in 2000–10. Modelling suggests that there could be a 7 per cent decrease in rainfall and a 14 per cent decrease in run-off over the 2021–50 period, and that the region could experience 80 per cent more drought months by 2070 (DCCEE, 2011c). Furthermore, the number of very hot days per year in Perth over 35°C will increase from 28 currently to 67 in 2070.

The potential health impacts shown in Table 10.4, with the impacts from loss of livelihood, heatwaves and displacement of significant coastal populations, are likely to be significant. Again, this is a very rapidly growing population in this region and it will be difficult to sustain these high population growth rates in the longer term without reduced per capita water consumption. Moreover, the sustainability of primary industry will depend on the development of new methods and new mixes of agricultural activation.

Coastal northern Australia

The entire north coast of the continent is designated a climate change hotspot in Figure 10.2. All climate change models suggest that this region is likely to experience little change in precipitation, or even a small increase. This has led to some calls for encouraging population growth in the region, based partly on transferring some primary industry into these areas. There is a long history of such calls, and mostly ill-fated attempts, to establish intensive agriculture in the north (Davidson, 1965). However, the region is at risk to a number of other negative climate change impacts – rising sea levels, higher temperatures and increased severe weather events. These will impinge on the liveability of these areas, as well as the potential to expand their primary production, especially food production. The outlook for increasing demand for the types of foods produced in Australia among the rapidly growing middle classes of Asia is positive, but climate change will present challenges for the expansion of extensive and intensive agriculture and animal production in the region. The location of the region in close proximity to Asian markets is clearly a potential advantage to economic development in the area. Implications of these changes for health include a possible extension of the area receptive to *Ae. aegypti* mosquitoes, and hence the risk of more dengue fever and perhaps other vector-borne diseases (McMichael et al., 2006). This view is supported by others, including Newth and Gunasekara (2010). There have been calls to capitalise on the anticipated increase in the rainfall in northern Australia to increase the region's population significantly and alter Australia's population distribution significantly. Any such planning needs to consider fully, however, the liveability impacts of that climate change.

Murray–Darling Basin

The release of the Murray–Darling Basin report in November 2011 has underscored its significance to the national economy and the threats to the integrity of the system posed by excessive withdrawal of water from it for agricultural and urban uses (Murray–Darling Basin Authority, 2011). The 13-year drought that broke in 2010 showed the necessity to reduce water withdrawal from the basin significantly if it was to survive as a healthy system. Projected climate change exacerbates this situation. All models suggest that there is likely to be a reduction in rainfall in the watershed. Moreover, run-off reductions will exceed that of rainfall decrease, with important implications for irrigated agriculture along the system and for the cities that draw water from it. One study by Cullen and Eckard (2011) has suggested that these changes may see a significant relocation in Australia's dairying industry over the next few decades, perhaps to Tasmania.

As mentioned, these changes in rainfall and run-off in this region will affect the water supply to major cities in the south-east of Australia. Cities affected include Canberra (DCCEE, 2011d). In addition, the increased temperatures could increase bushfire risk in the ACT.

The Garnaut Climate Change Review (Garnaut, 2008) summarised the effects of climate change on Australian states in the absence of any mitigation. It found that climate change would potentially have a major effect on primary industry activity in each state. For example, it is suggested that, by mid-century, irrigated agriculture output in the Murray–Darling Basin could be reduced by half. It would seem, therefore, that the population supported by agricultural activity in the Murray–Darling Basin will be reduced, and in the absence of alternative economic activity, there will be population declines.

Tropical Queensland

Tropical Queensland contains some of the fastest growing communities in the country. In coastal areas, tourism, at least until recently, has been expanding exponentially, while mining activity has also been growing apace. Again, several significant impacts of climate change are anticipated in the region. These include rising sea levels, increased temperatures and increased incidence and severity of extreme weather events. The effects will vary between the coast and inland, but will be severe in both cases. Table 10.4 indicates that the area as a whole will be susceptible to both direct and indirect risk factors, including a southward extension of the area at risk of dengue fever (McMichael et al., 2006). As in northern coastal areas, liveability impacts of climate change need to be considered when assessing future regional development, but population growth in the region is likely to continue.

Snowy Mountains

Climate change is likely to have a disproportionate effect on temperatures in mountain areas compared with sea level (CSIRO and BOM, 2007). Rising mountain temperatures will reduce snow in Australia's alpine areas, with consequences for run-off to irrigation and water reserves, as well as for tourism. Under an extreme emissions scenario with increased temperatures and decreased rainfall, the duration of the snow season in the Australian Alps could fall by 96 per cent by 2050, with disastrous consequences for vulnerable alpine flora and fauna (DCCEE, 2011a).

While those six areas are quite large and heterogeneous, it is useful to examine some of their population characteristics, including their vulnerability, which is relevant to health (Few, 2007). The Intergovernmental Panel on Climate Change (2008, p. 883) defines vulnerability to climate change as 'the degree to which a system is susceptible to, or unable to cope with, adverse effects of climate change, including climate variability and extremes'.

There is strong evidence that vulnerability and constraints on adaptation increase as the economic situation of individuals and communities declines (Brooks et al., 2005; Sevoyan and Hugo, 2014), though non-socio-economic factors also play a role. This is relevant to negative health risks. It is thus valid to consider the socio-economic situation of populations in hotspot areas, although analysis here is limited to averages across the entire hotspot area. In fact, within each area, there is considerable variation. The measures used are the Socio-economic Indexes for Areas (SEIFA) (Australian Bureau of Statistics (ABS), 2008), derived from 2006 census data. The averaged measure was obtained as a mean from all Census Collection Districts included in each of the hotspot areas. Only two hotspot areas have a SEIFA score average above that of the non-hotspot areas (see Table 10.5). These are coastal New South Wales and south-east Queensland, and the very large Murray–Darling Basin. In most areas, however, there is below average socio-economic status. This raises questions of the capacity of the communities in those areas to adapt to the impacts of climate change, including those related to health. There are especially low SEIFA scores in coastal Northern Australia.

Table 10.5 Australia: Climate change hotspot areas by SEIFA index,[a] 2006.

Climate change hotspot regions	Mean SEIFA score 2006
Non-hotspot areas	972.59
Coastal northern Australia	690.81
Coastal northern NSW and S.E. Qld	981.55
Murray–Darling Basin	978.96
Perth and S.W. Western Australia	938.51
Snowy Mountains	795.72
Tropical Queensland	932.55

[a] There are four different SEIFA indexes developed by the ABS. The one used here is the Index of Relative Socio-Economic Disadvantage.

Source: ABS, 2008.

Ethnicity is also of relevance to vulnerability. Cultural and language factors can limit social inclusion, increasing vulnerability to the risk of harm from deteriorating economic, social or environmental situation. Table 10.6 shows the proportion of the population in the hotspot areas born overseas at the 2006 census. This is below the national average in all but one, and due to the exclusion of metropolitan areas other than Perth. Most migrants to Australia, especially from mainly non-English speaking (NES) countries, concentrate in major metropolitan areas (Hugo, 2011). The one hotspot area with a high proportion of the population overseas-born is Perth and south-western Australia. Although the NES origin population are under-represented in hotspot areas, they are highly vulnerable to the effects of climate change, because of social exclusion and cultural isolation. Recent patterns of settlement of refugee-humanitarian migrants in non-metropolitan areas in Australia are relevant (Hugo, 2014). Recent displacement of Sudanese men living in caravans by floods in Queensland in 2012–13 points to the potential of being 'twice displaced' – ousted by war in their homeland and by the environment in their destination. One-fifth of new refugee (rather than total migrant) arrivals in Australia settle in non-metropolitan areas. Many carry a high risk of physical and mental health problems. This can be exacerbated by their isolated location and may be worsened by climate change.

Table 10.6 Australia: Birthplace composition of hotspot areas of climate change impact, 2006.

Climate change hotspot regions	Per cent Australia-born	Per cent mainly English-speaking countries	Per cent mainly non-English-speaking countries	Per cent of Aboriginal/ Torres Strait Islander descendant
Coastal northern Australia	77.1	5.6	8.4	23.0
Coastal northern NSW and S.E. Qld	74.4	10.7	8.1	2.1
Murray–Darling Basin	82.7	4.8	6.6	2.9
Perth and S.W. Western Australia	64.0	15.3	13.3	1.6
Snowy Mountains	77.1	5.6	4.7	0.5
Tropical Queensland	79.7	6.4	5.3	7.3
Non-hotspot areas	67.4	7.7	17.7	1.8
Total	70.9	8.4	13.7	2.3

Source: ABS (2011) Census of Population and Housing.

Another very important dimension of ethnicity is the representation of Indigenous Australians in the hotspot areas. Table 10.6 shows that there is a striking pattern in evidence. In the coastal northern Australian hotspot area, almost one-quarter of the resident population are Aboriginal and Torres Strait

Islanders. This has significant implications for any adaptation strategies to be culturally sensitive and has important interactions with health impacts. It is also noticeable that the Indigenous population is also over-represented in the small population in the Snowy Mountains and in the Murray–Darling Basin.

In addition, demographic age structures can affect community capacity to adjust to climate change and have health implications. Some older populations experience impacts of particular climate change more intensely than other groups. For example, the heatwave in Adelaide and Melbourne in 2010 resulted in amplified death rates among older residents.

Table 10.7 shows that there is significant variation between hotspot areas in the proportion of the resident population aged 65 years and over. Older populations are under-represented in coastal northern Australia. Elsewhere, there is little variation in the proportion of the population in the older age groups, but they are a substantial fraction in each hotspot area.

Table 10.7 Australia: Climate change hotspot areas – percentage of the population 65 years and over, 2006.

Climate change hotspot regions	Number	Per cent
Coastal northern Australia	7,103	4.81
Coastal northern NSW and S.E. QLD	454,372	13.45
Murray–Darling Basin	352,672	13.21
Perth and S.W. Western Australia	204,733	12.82
Snowy Mountains	1,645	16.05
Tropical Queensland	71,833	10.64
Non-hotspot areas	1,548,199	13.66
Total	2,640,557	13.33

Source: ABS (2011) Census of Population and Housing.

In addition to looking at the characteristics of the population in each of the hotspot areas, the effects of climate change on families and households and the housing they occupy is important. Table 10.8 shows that average household sizes are bigger in coastal northern Australia and tropical Queensland than in non-hotspot areas. While the proportion of residents in single person households is only above the national average in Perth–south-west Australia and the Murray–Darling Basin, it is more than one-fifth of the population living in hotspot areas. Such households are more vulnerable on average (Sevoyan and Hugo, 2014), many are older and frail people, especially women. The proportion of the population renting their housing is also higher in hotspot areas than elsewhere; this is another factor associated with vulnerability.

Table 10.8 Australia: Climate change hotspot areas – household characteristics, 2006.

Climate change hotspot regions	Average household size	Per cent lone person households	Per cent who own or are purchasing their own home
Coastal northern Australia		19.5	51.9
Coastal northern NSW and S.E. Queensland		22.0	67.6
Murray–Darling Basin		23.5	73.5
Perth and S.W. Western Australia		24.6	71.5
Snowy Mountains		23.2	65.0
Tropical Queensland		20.9	63.8
Non-hotspot areas		23.7	70.0
Total		23.3	69.8

Source: ABS 2006 Census and Climate Action Network 2006 (manually digitised for GIS analysis).

Conclusion

Tony McMichael's work alerted many to the health implications of climate change and that these impacts required consideration not only of the nature of that change but its complex interactions with place, society and economy. The complexity is deepened by spatial variation, not only in the effects of climate change but also in the nature of environments and affected populations. Our understanding of this complexity is extremely limited, and this is a major barrier to developing effective policy responses. This chapter has sought to assemble current knowledge of domestic climate change effects in Australia and how these relate to population distribution dynamics and characteristics. It is imperative that our empirical understanding of climate change is expanded so that there can be greater certainty in locating the hotspots of greatest impact and thus taking steps to alleviate their impacts. Without this, impacts will fall disproportionately on the most vulnerable; social exclusion will worsen. It is important that Tony McMichael's work in linking health, place and people in the context of climate change in Australia be built on, not only by epidemiologists but also by population scientists and geographers.

References

Australian Bureau of Statistics (ABS) 2008. *Information Paper – An Introduction to Socio-Economic Indexes for Areas (SEIFA) 2006*. Catalogue No. 2039.0. ABS, Canberra, Australia.

Brooks, N., Adger, N.W. & Kelly, P.M. 2005. The determinants of vulnerability and adaptive capacity at the national level and the implications for adaptation. *Global Environmental Change* 15, 151–63.

Burnley, I. & Murphy, P. 2004. Why sea changers move: income support recipients. In: Burnley, I. & Murphy, P. (eds) *Sea Change: Movement from Metropolitan to Arcadian Australia*. UNSW Press, Sydney, Australia, 161–74.

Climate Action Network 2006. Social Impacts of Climate Change, Australia, Population. Available at: www.cana.net.au/socialimpacts/australia/population.html, accessed 28 November 2006.

Climate Commission 2011. *The Critical Decade: Climate Science, Risks and Responses*. Department of Climate Change and Energy Efficiency, Canberra, Australia.

CSIRO & Bureau of Meteorology 2007. *Climate Change in Australia: Technical Report 2007*. CSIRO, Melbourne, Australia.

CSIRO & Bureau of Meteorology 2010. *State of the Climate, Australian Government*. CSIRO, Melbourne, Australia.

Cullen, B.R. & Eckard, R.J. 2011. Impacts of future climate scenarios on the balance between productivity and total greenhouse gas emissions from pasture based airy systems in south-eastern Australia. *Animal Feed Science and Technology* 166–167, 721–35.

Davidson, B.R. 1965. *The Northern Myth: A Study of the Physical and Economic Limits to Agricultural and Pastoral Development in Tropical Australia*. Melbourne University Press, Melbourne, Australia.

Department of Climate Change and Energy Efficiency 2011a. Climate Change – Potential Impacts and Costs: Queensland – Factsheet. Australian Government, Canberra, Australia.

DCCEE 2011b. Climate Change – Potential Impacts and Costs: New South Wales – Factsheet. Australian Government, Canberra, Australia.

DCCEE 2011c. Climate Change – Potential Impacts and Costs: Western Australia – Factsheet. Australian Government, Canberra, Australia.

DCCEE 2011d. Climate Change – Potential Impacts and Costs: Australian Capital Territory – Factsheet. Australian Government, Canberra, Australia.

Few, R. 2007. Health and climatic hazards: framing social research on vulnerability, response and adaptation. *Global Environmental Change* 17, 281–95.

Gamble, J.L., Ebi, K.L., Sussman, F.G. & Wilbanks, T.J. 2008. Analyses of the effects of global change on human health and welfare. Human Systems, Synthesis and Assessment Product 4.6. Climate Change Science Program, Washington, DC, USA.

Garnaut, R. 2008. *The Garnaut Climate Change Review – Final Report*. Cambridge University Press, Cambridge, UK.

Hugo, G.J. 2011. Changing spatial patterns of immigrant settlement. In: Clyne, M. & Jupp, J. (eds) *Multiculturalism and Integration – A Harmonious Combination*. ANU E Press, Canberra, Australia, 1–40.

Hugo, G.J. 2014. Immigrant settlement in non-metropolitan Australia: patterns and processes. In: Dufty-Jones, R. & Connell, J. (eds) *Rural Change in Australia: Population, Economy, Environment*. Ashgate, Farnham, UK, 52–87.

Intergovernmental Panel on Climate Change 2008. *Climate Change 2007: Climate Change Impacts, Adaptation and Vulnerability. Contribution of Working Group II to the Fourth Assessment Report of the Intergovernmental Panel on Climate Change*. Cambridge University Press, Cambridge, UK.

McGranahan, G., Balk, D. & Anderson, B. 2007. The rising tide: assessing the risks of climate change and human settlements in low elevation coastal zones. *Environment and Urbanization* 19, 17–37.

McMichael, A.J. 2001. *Human Frontiers, Environments and Disease: Past Patterns, Uncertain Futures*. Cambridge University Press, Cambridge, UK.

McMichael, A.J., Woodruff, R.E. & Hales, S. 2006. Climate change and human health: present and future risks. *The Lancet* 367, 859–69.

McMichael, A.J., McMichael, C.E., Berry, H.L. & Bowen, K. 2010. Climate-related displacement: health risks and responses. In: McAdam, J. (ed.) *Climate Change and Displacement: Multidisciplinary Perspectives*. Hart Publishing, Oxford, UK, and Portland, Oregon, USA, 191–220.

Murray–Darling Basin Authority 2011. Proposed Basin Plan. Murray–Darling Basin Authority, Canberra, www.mdba.gov.au/sites/default/files/archived/proposed/proposed_basin_plan.pdf, accessed 18 March 2015.

Newth, D. & Gunasekera, D. 2010. Climate change and the effects of dengue upon Australia: an analysis of health impacts and costs. *IOP Conference Series: Earth and Environmental Science* 11, 012020.

Powell, J. 1984. Home truths and larrikin prophets 'Australian Unlimited': the interwar years. In: Birrell, R., Hill, D. & Nevill, J. (eds) *Populate and Perish: The Stresses of Population Growth in Australia*. Fontana, Sydney, Australia, 47–79.

Price, A.G. 1939. *White Settlers in the Tropics*. American Geographical Society, New York, USA.

Rowland, D.T. 1982. Population growth and distribution. *Population of Australia, Volume 1, ESCAP Country Monograph Series No. 9*. United Nations, New York, USA, 10–33.

Sevoyan, A. & Hugo, G.J. 2014. Vulnerability to climate change among disadvantaged groups: the role of social exclusion. In: Palutikof, J., Boulter, S., Barnett, J. & Rissik, D. (eds) *Applied Studies in Climate Adaptation*. Wiley-Blackwell, Hoboken, NJ, USA, 258–65.

Smith, L.R. 1980. *The Aboriginal Population of Australia*. Australian National University Press, Canberra, Australia.

State of the Environment 2011. State of the Environment Report 2011. Independent Report to the Australian Government Minister for Sustainability, Environment, Water, Population and Communities, Canberra, Australia.

11

GLOBALISATION AND THE EPIGENETIC LANDSCAPE

PAOLO VINEIS

Abstract

One of the most inspirational books by Tony McMichael has been *Human Frontiers, Environments and Disease*. In the present chapter, I expand on some of the thoughts that book put forward. There are a few good examples of how environmental changes have modified the genetic make-up of some populations. It is likely, however, that much more important changes have taken place and will take place in humankind's epigenetic landscape, i.e. acquired and transgenerationally transmissible changes in DNA expression. A mounting body of evidence on the importance of epigenetic changes related, for instance, to *in utero* dietary exposures or deficiencies is now available. The past 30–40 years have seen unprecedented modifications in markets, industrial food availability and other aspects of lifestyle. Is it plausible that these changes could have an enduring effect on humankind's epigenetic landscape? In this chapter, I review some of the existing evidence.

In *Human Frontiers, Environments and Disease* (McMichael, 2001), McMichael describes in a wonderful way the interplay between human evolution and environmental changes. This chapter is a tribute to that book, with reference to some recent developments in epigenetics that I believe are consistent with Tony's original ideas.

Introduction

The evolution of living organisms is the expression of different and sometimes opposing forces. The main tension is between the need for stability and the need for change. The first is expressed, for example, by the great structural stability of DNA and of its coding system, conserved almost intact across all species. However, without the ability to change, organisms would not be able to adapt to changing environments and their continuous threats. Transposons (transposable elements), crossing over at meiosis and epigenetic changes, are some of the mechanisms that ensure the variety of genetic configurations that allow variation, adaptation and evolution.

It was Barbara McClintock's (awarded the Nobel Prize in 1983: see Figures 11.1 and 11.2) great merit to first understand the relevance of transposable elements and to promote the field of epigenetics after its foundation by Conrad Waddington. The latter defined epigenetics in 1942 as 'the branch of biology which studies the causal interactions between genes and their products, which bring the phenotype into being'. McClintock, on the one hand, hypothesised the existence of 'jumping genes' (transposable elements) through her studies of maize; on the other hand, she first speculated in 1951 that DNA expression was permitted by what today we identify as DNA methylation, or the acetylation of histones:

> The progeny of two (such) sister cells are not alike with respect to the types of gene alteration that will occur ... This inactivity or suppression is considered to occur because the genes are 'covered' by other non-genic chromatin materials ... Gene activity may be possible only when a physical change in this covering material allows the reactive components of the gene to be 'exposed' and thus capable of functioning. (McClintock, 1951)

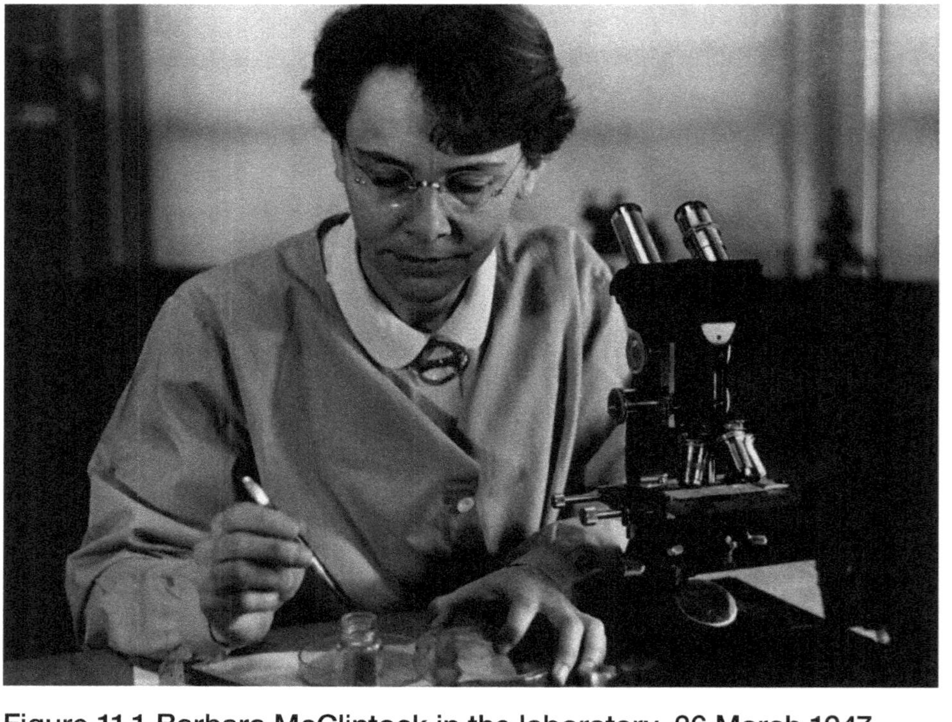

Figure 11.1 Barbara McClintock in the laboratory, 26 March 1947.

Source: profiles.nlm.nih.gov/ps/access/LLBBPP_.jpg, accessed 20 March 2015, courtesy National Library of Medicine, USA.

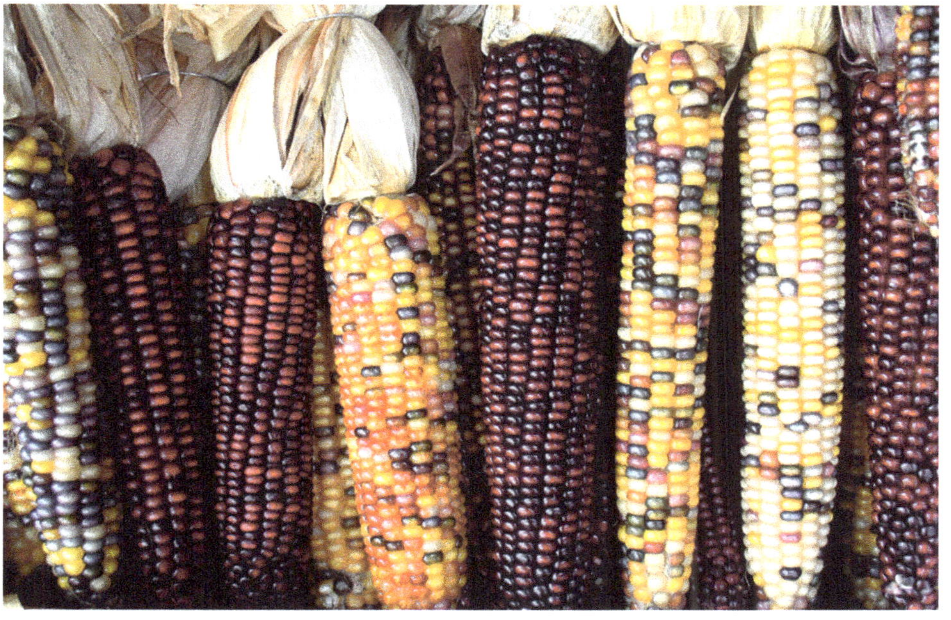

Figure 11.2 Varieties of maize.

Source: Wikimedia commons, en.wikipedia.org/wiki/Blue_corn#mediaviewer/File:Corncobs.jpg, accessed 14 February 2015.

As a very general rule, environmental stresses tend to increase (epi)genomic instability (via DNA demethylation, for example, or increasing activity of transposable elements), and this is both a mechanism to enhance diversity and respond to threats and a potentially harmful mechanism leading to disease. Over the past two decades, much research has gone into the role of epigenetic changes in the development of diseases like cancer (Feinberg and Tycko, 2004; Salnikow and Zhitkovich, 2008). The most broadly researched and studied epigenetic mechanism is DNA methylation (Christensen and Marsit, 2011). First observed in the early 1980s in studies of carcinogenesis (Feinberg and Tycko, 2004), DNA methylation occurs mainly at CpG dinucleotides, which are found grouped together in promoter regions of around 50 per cent of all human genes (so-called CpG islands). DNA methylation involves the addition of a methyl group to a CpG dinucleotide (Christensen and Marsit, 2011). Methylation of CpG islands can cause gene silencing. If this affects tumour suppressor genes, there may be the induction of cancer. Cancer cells have been seen, in fact, to have unusual patterns of methylation, including both hypermethylation of tumour suppressor genes and hypomethylation of proto-oncogenes or transposable elements (Tabish et al., 2012).

Another epigenetic mechanism is dysregulation through histone modifications due to the phosphorylation, methylation or acetylation of histone tails (Feinberg and Tycko, 2004), which are predominantly responsible for maintaining nucleosome structures (Luger et al., 1997; Ren et al., 2011). Disruption of normal histone modification mechanisms can cause changes in gene expression and has been observed in the development of some cancers (Luger et al., 1997; Jo et al., 2009). For example, *in vitro* studies conducted on human cells by Jensen et al. in 2008 described alterations of histone H3 acetylation and changes in gene expression of genes linked to histones, due to the exposure to arsenicals (Jensen et al., 2008). Likewise, in 2009, Zhou et al. (2009) found that arsenite exposure in human lung carcinoma cells led to increased methylation of H3K4 and caused repression of cellular transcription (Luger et al., 1997) (we refer to arsenic because this is one of the environmental exposures best studied from the epigenetic perspective).

A third main mechanism by which epigenetic changes occur is through micro-RNA (miRNA) expression. miRNAs are described as small, non-coding RNA molecules of approximately 22 nucleotides. miRNAs are involved in genomic and cellular regulation and are thought generally to suppress gene expression. There are many hundreds of miRNAs in humans, and it is believed that up to 30 per cent of genes in mammals are influenced by miRNAs (Luger et al., 1997). Dysregulation of miRNA expression has been suggested to play a role in various diseases (Abdellatif, 2012) such as arsenic-related kidney and bladder cancers (Hoffman and Cairns, 2011).

Exposure to environmental carcinogens and the associated epigenetic changes such as the ones described above can also occur *in utero*; epigenetic programming may play a major role in embryonic development and the health of an individual in the long term (Christensen and Marsit, 2011). A study conducted on rats by Martínez et al. in 2011 showed that arsenic exposure during gestation resulted in altered patterns of DNA methylation of brain cells affecting memory, thus suggesting that arsenic exposure *in utero* could have long-standing effects on growth and development (Martínez et al., 2011).

Diabetes, Migrants and Epigenetics

Birth cohort studies show that maternal undernutrition, low birth weight and rapid post-natal child growth are all associated with an increased risk of diabetes in the offspring. These risks appear to be mediated through epigenetic modification and may be transgenerational.

The vast majority of low birth weight (<2500 g) cases occur in the developing world, with the highest incidence in South Asians (31 per cent of live births). The results of The Pune Maternal Nutrition Study, a prospective population-based observational study of rural South Asian women and their offspring, showed that Asian mothers were shorter and thinner than their European counterparts and that full-term South Asian neonates were ~700 g lighter than the average European. These neonatal differences are accompanied by changes in body composition, with greater reduction in lean muscle tissue than truncal fat.

Birth cohort studies in India confirm the association of maternal undernutrition, low birth weight and thinness in infancy with the subsequent development of impaired glucose tolerance (IGT) and type 2 diabetes (T2D) (Yajnik et al., 2003). Risk of IGT and T2D was highest among South Asians who had shorter mothers or parents with lower body mass index (BMI), or were themselves of low birth weight, thin during infancy but with greater weight gain during childhood and adolescence, independent of their adult BMI. The risk of IGT/T2D was increased six times among South Asians who were in the lowest third of BMI as children but progressed to be in the highest third of BMI as adults, compared with adults who had high BMI as children but became thin adults (Raghupathy et al., 2010). These observations of adverse intrauterine and post-natal exposures in South Asians raise the possibility that epigenetic modification of gene expression may contribute to age-dependent changes in key metabolic genes, and increased susceptibility to T2D.

Diet and Epigenetics

Diet influences the methylation status of cells in several ways. A major focus of interest has been the 1-carbon metabolism pathway, because this is the main conduit for methyl group donation at a cellular level.

Folate deficiency has been associated with an increased risk of cancer at different sites. The two most commonly hypothesised mechanisms by which folate inadequacy may contribute to carcinogenesis are DNA hypomethylation and uracil misincorporation during DNA synthesis, leading to genomic instability (Crider et al., 2012). While 1-carbon metabolism and folate availability have, to date, been a major focus of attention, it is increasingly apparent that altered DNA methylation is not simply an issue of the bioavailability of methyl groups. For example, the isoflavone, genistein, has profound effects on DNA methylation but has no involvement in 1-carbon metabolism (King-Batoon et al., 2008).

A striking example of the impact of diet on epigenetic changes is evident in bees. The behaviourally and reproductively distinct queen and worker female castes (same genome) are a result of differential intake of royal jelly (diet-controlled phenotypes) implemented in concert with DNA methylation (brain methylomes). Thus, nutritional control of the reproductive status in honeybees seems to occur via DNA methylation. Australian researchers have recently imitated the effects of royal jelly by turning off the enzyme that labels DNA with methyl groups in bee larvae. These larvae all turned into queens – without any royal jelly (Lyko et al., 2010).

Evidence of the effects of maternal malnutrition on offspring comes from a historical cohort of Dutch individuals whose mothers were exposed during the wartime famine of 1944–45. The offspring of women exposed to malnutrition during early pregnancy were more likely to develop the metabolic syndrome in adulthood compared to the offspring of women pregnant before or after the famine. The effects were dependent on the trimester of gestation in which famine was experienced. Epigenetic analyses of these individuals nearly 60 years later show differential methylation in several genes involved in growth and metabolic control, which are dependent on gender and time of exposure during gestation (de Rooij et al., 2007). Hypomethylation of the promoter of *IGF2*, a maternally imprinted gene implicated in growth and development, has also been observed in those exposed during the peri-conceptional period relative to unexposed siblings, although the effect is small (Heijmans et al., 2008).

In other more recently established cohorts, individuals exposed *in utero* and during infancy to the Nigerian civil war famine of 1968–70 were at increased risk of hypertension, IGT and being overweight about 40 years later (Barouki et al., 2012). Similarly, women exposed during gestation or early childhood to the 1959–61 famine in China are reported to have a greater risk of metabolic syndrome (Barouki et al., 2012).

Can a 'Healthy' Diet Stabilise the Epigenome?

We have conducted a randomised dietary intervention study that consisted of enrichment with flavonoids, derived mainly from cruciferous vegetables. We then investigated the methylation status of the promoter regions of cyclin-dependent kinase inhibitor 2A, methylenetetrahydrofolate reductase, Ras-association domain family 1 isoform A, mutL homologue 1 genes and of the LINE-1 repetitive sequence (Scoccianti et al., 2011). LINE-1 transposable elements are a surrogate marker for global DNA methylation levels, and loss of methylation in LINE-1 has been associated with risk of cancer and neurological and cardiovascular diseases (Scoccianti et al., 2011).

In this study, we observed increased global methylation in peripheral blood cells among the participants, consistent with a role of DNA methylation in controlling retrotransposon mobility by lowering their activities and consequently stabilising the genome. We also observed a decrease of inter-individual methylation levels for three of the panel of five genes after dietary intervention. Together, the increase in global methylation and the decrease of dispersion in the distribution of individual methylation levels may reflect a form of increased epigenetic stability. Epigenetic stability could be the counterpart of genetic stability and may play a role in cancer prevention, since it has been shown that loss of genetic stability promotes tumour progression.

Globalisation and the Epigenetic Landscape

There are different definitions of globalisation, but a common theme is 'the process of extending social relations across world space'. Such extensions arise from the movements of people, things and ideas (en.wikipedia.org/wiki/Globalization).

If we consider some of the evidence available on both genetic and (possibly) epigenetic changes in populations, we find that these often come from migrations: lactose tolerance, skin colour and (possibly) diabetes in Asian migrants are examples. One of the features of globalisation is certainly mass migration, but there is much more to it. In fact, it seems that existing populations – as we have known over the last centuries – are the product of long-term adaptation to local circumstances, like the characteristic phenotypes of pygmies, Watusi or Eskimos, probably resulting from a combination of genetic selection and epigenetic features. Local circumstances are now changing very rapidly, and it is difficult to imagine that this will not impact, if not on the genetic make-up, almost certainly on the epigenetic landscape of many population groups.

An example of a rather dramatic secular change is the constantly decreasing age at menarche in girls, which parallels increasing height. These changes are likely to be mediated by epigenetic mechanisms (Demetriou et al., 2013) In addition, as explained by Gluckman and Hanson in their book, *Mismatch* (Gluckman and Hanson, 2006), the earlier and earlier sexual maturation of girls is mismatched with psychosocial maturation, which is more and more delayed in both girls and boys. The global market exploits both the 'infantilisation' of society and earlier sexual maturation to increase consumerism and target the marketing of commodities for pre-teens.

Conclusion

The epigenetic landscape of many population groups is likely to be affected by globalisation. Changes are related to global economic and environmental phenomena, mass migration and the extension to the whole world of features characteristic of Western societies, such as physical inactivity, tobacco smoking, regular alcohol consumption, energy-dense foods and chemical contamination (e.g. endocrine disruptors). The likely consequences of these changes include the spreading epidemic of obesity and diabetes, the spread of cancer to African countries and the decreasing age at menarche in girls.

New insights from epigenetic research might influence policy and practice – for example, by demonstrating mechanisms by which environmental factors influence disease, thus providing stronger evidence for policymakers and for civil society. Indeed, showing how epigenetic changes are linked to specific exposures could be more powerful than statistical associations between risk factors and disease, and might lead to innovative legislation. The study of the life-course, transgenerational epigenetic consequences of globalisation should be a top priority for a 21st-century research agenda on environmental diseases.

References

Abdellatif, M. 2012. Differential expression of microRNAs in different disease states. *Circulation Research* 110, 638–50.

Barouki, R., Gluckman, P.D., Grandjean, P., Hanson, M. & Heindel, J.J. 2012. Developmental origins of non-communicable disease: implications for research and public health. *Environmental Health* 11, 42 doi: 10.1186/1476-069X-11-42.

Christensen, B.C. & Marsit, C.J. 2011. Epigenomics in environmental health. *Frontiers in Genetics* 2, 28–44.

Crider, K.S., Yang, T.P., Berry, R.J. & Bailey, L.B. 2012. Folate and DNA methylation: a review of molecular mechanisms and the evidence for folate's role. *Advances in Nutrition* 3, 21–38.

de Rooij, S.R., Painter, R.C., Holleman, F., Bossuyt, P.M. & Roseboom, T.J. 2007. The metabolic syndrome in adults prenatally exposed to the Dutch famine. *American Journal of Clinical Nutrition* 86, 1219–24.

Demetriou, C.A., Chen, J., Polidoro, S., van Veldhoven, K., Cuenin, C., Campanella, G., et al. 2013. Methylome analysis and epigenetic changes associated with menarcheal age. *PLoS One* 8, e79391.

Feinberg, A.P. & Tycko, B. 2004. The history of cancer epigenetics. *Nature Reviews Cancer* 4, 143–53.

Gluckman, P. & Hanson, M. 2006. *Mismatch – The Lifestyle Diseases Timebomb*. Oxford University Press, Oxford, UK.

Heijmans, B.T., Tobi, E.W., Stein, A.D., Putter, H., Blauw, G.J., Susser, E.S., et al. 2008. Persistent epigenetic differences associated with prenatal exposure to famine in humans. *Proceedings of the National Academy of Sciences (USA)* 105, 17046–9.

Hoffman, A.M. & Cairns, P. 2011. Epigenetics of kidney cancer and bladder cancer. *Epigenomics* 3, 19–34.

Jensen T.J., Novak P., Eblin K.E., Gandolfi A.J., Futscher B.W. 2008. Epigenetic remodeling during arsenical-induced malignant transformation. *Carcinogenesis*. 29(8):1500–8.

Jo, W., Ren, X., Chu, F. Aleshin M., Wintz H., Burlingame A., Smith M.T., Vulpe C.D., Zhang L. 2009. Acetylated H4K16 by MYST1 protects UROtsa cells from arsenic toxicity and is decreased following chronic arsenic exposure. *Toxicology and Applied Pharmacology* 241, 294–302.

King-Batoon, A., Leszczynska, J.M. & Klein, C.B. 2008. Modulation of gene methylation by genistein or lycopene in breast cancer cells. *Environmental and Molecular Mutagenesis* 49, 36–45.

Luger, K., Mader, A.W., Richmond, R.K., Sargent, D.F. & Richmond, T.J. 1997. Crystal structure of the nucleosome core particle at 2.8 A resolution. *Nature* 389, 251–60.

Lyko, F., Foret, S., Kucharski, R., Wolf, S., Falckenhayn, C. & Maleszka, R. 2010. The honey bee epigenomes: differential methylation of brain DNA in queens and workers. *PLoS Biology* 8, e1000506.

McClintock B. 1951. Chromosome Organization and Genic Expression. Cold Spring Harbor Symposia on Quantitative Biology 16,: 13-47.

McMichael, A.J. 2001. *Human Frontiers, Environments and Disease: Past Patterns, Uncertain Futures*. Cambridge University Press, Cambridge, UK.

Martínez, L., Jiménez, V., García-Sepúlved, C., Ceballos, F., Delgado, J.M., Niño-Moreno, P., et al. 2011. Impact of early developmental arsenic exposure on promotor CpG-island methylation of genes involved in neuronal plasticity. *Neurochemistry International* 58, 574–81.

Raghupathy, P., Raghupathy, P., Antonisamy, B., Geethanjali, F.S., Saperia, J., Leary, S.D., Priya, G., et al. 2010. Glucose tolerance, insulin resistance and insulin secretion in young South Indian adults: relationships to parental size, neonatal size and childhood body mass index. *Diabetes Research and Clinical Practice* 87, 283–92.

Ren, X., McHale, C.M., Skibola, C.F., Smith, A.H., Smith, M.T. & Zhang, L. 2011. An emerging role for epigenetic dysregulation in arsenic toxicity and carcinogenesis. *Environmental Health Perspectives* 119, 11–9.

Salnikow, K. & Zhitkovich, A. 2008. Genetic and epigenetic mechanisms in metal carcinogenesis and cocarcinogenesis: nickel, arsenic, and chromium. *Chemical Research in Toxicology* 21, 28–44.

Scoccianti, C., Ricceri, F., Ferrari, P., Cuenin, C., Sacerdote, C., Polidoro, S., et al. 2011. Methylation patterns in sentinel genes in peripheral blood cells of heavy smokers: influence of cruciferous vegetables in an intervention study. *Epigenetics* 6, 1114–9.

Tabish, A.M., Poels, K., Hoet, P. & Godderis, L. 2012. Epigenetic factors in cancer risk: effect of chemical carcinogens on global DNA methylation pattern in human TK6 cells. *PLoS One* 7, e34674.

Zhou, X., Li, Q., Arita, A., Sun, H., Costa, M. 2009. Effects of nickel, chromate, and arsenite on histone 3 lysine methylation. *Toxicology and Applied Pharmacology*. 236(1):78–84.

Yajnik, C.S., Fall, C.H.D., Coyaji, K.J., Hirve, S.S., Rao, S., Barker, D.J.P., et al. 2003. Neonatal anthropometry: the thin-fat Indian baby. The Pune Maternal Nutrition Study. *International Journal of Obesity and Related Metabolic Disorders* 27, 173–80.

12

USES AND MISUSES OF EPIDEMIOLOGY

ALISTAIR WOODWARD

Abstract

Tony McMichael was at the centre of an important debate in the 1990s about the scope and range of epidemiology. His own research included both influential traditional risk factor-oriented studies and paradigm-shifting investigations of large-scale environmental and social issues. One of the best examples of effective 'micro-epidemiology' is work done on the health effects of passive smoking. Tony contributed as a researcher, a commentator and an expert witness. Among all the legal challenges to the tobacco industry, notable is the case of the Australian Federation of Consumer Organisations (AFCO) versus the Tobacco Institute of Australia (1988–90). This action in the Australian Federal Court tested the Tobacco Institute claim that 'there is little evidence, and nothing which proves scientifically that cigarette smoke causes diseases in non-smokers'. What was at stake was the status of epidemiological research; what were debated before the presiding judge, Justice Morling, were the uses and misuses of epidemiology. Tony McMichael was the principal witness for the AFCO. His testimony on the current knowledge and appropriate interpretation of epidemiological studies of passive smoking was critical to the outcome of the case, and in turn, Morling's judgement set the direction for tobacco control in Australia in succeeding decades.

Introduction

This chapter is concerned with Tony McMichael's contribution to epidemiology, the study of diseases and their causes in populations. I do not attempt to tell the full story – there is not space, and I know that others will have more to say elsewhere in the book. I will focus on epidemiology close up, research into environmental and behavioural factors that are proximal to the disease of interest. This is 'micro' epidemiology, as distinct from the study of the big picture phenomena that are high up in the causal chain.

I will tell of one court case, of great importance to public health, that hinged on the interpretation of micro-epidemiology, and in which Tony McMichael was at the centre.

Background – The Development of Modern Epidemiology

Origins are personal constructs. For me, modern epidemiology begins in 1957, the year in which Jerry Morris's book, *The Uses of Epidemiology*, was published. It was the first text to consider seriously the application of epidemiology to health problems other than infectious diseases (Smith, 2001). The book was very popular and the third edition (Morris, 1975) was my entry to public health studies in the late 1970s. The style was informal, the examples surprising, and the text fizzed and darted in unexpected and telling directions. *The Uses of Epidemiology*, like its author, aged extraordinarily slowly. (I met Jerry Morris only once, at Tony and Judith's house in North London, in the early 2000s. I remember him as a small man, full of good humour and bounce, even though he was into his 90s. Recently, he had been forced to give up his daily swim, Jerry told me, because every time he started on his ten laps of the local pool, the lifeguards would dive in and save him.)

I was captured immediately. Here was a book that laid out all the wonderful things that could be done with epidemiology. Not only could the epidemiologist turn her or his hand to an almost limitless number of health issues but also the ways of working were multivalent – there was potential here to connect with sociologists, economists, clinicians, biomedical scientists. Morris applied this catholic approach in his own work, which stretched from malaria control in India in World War II to the effects on the heart of regular physical activity (Morris et al., 1953; Blair and Morris, 2009), to the question of a minimum healthy wage (Morris et al., 2000).

But for some, the Morris free-range conception of epidemiology was too easy and breezy. It was not just a matter of where we wanted to go, people argued, but how to get there. What exactly was there under the epidemiological bonnet? If you listened carefully, the action seemed to run a little rough. Was it time for some fine-tuning, perhaps even a major overhaul?

It was not the case that Morris ignored methods – he argued frequently that epidemiology's contribution depended on a critical and methodical approach to population health. But Morris foregrounded the applications of the discipline, and he drew on a wide range of techniques. As Nancy Krieger commented, 'the challenge was to think big and small at the same time; to see the details of disease mechanisms while not losing sight of the social production of disease' (Krieger, 2007).

In the last quarter of the 20th century, attention was paid, increasingly, to methods, and in particular to the methods of micro-epidemiology. This was illustrated among the textbooks by classics such as *Modern Epidemiology* (Rothman, 1986), and subsequently, a multiplication of subspecialty volumes, including *Molecular Epidemiology* (Schulte and Perera, 1998). Tony McMichael made important contributions to the technical literature. There was, for example, his early work in North Carolina on aspects of occupational epidemiology, including an elegant dissection of standardised mortality ratios that launched the 'healthy worker effect' (McMichael, 1976).

The epidemiological engine certainly did operate more strongly and more reliably as a result of these methodological improvements. But did a sharper focus in epidemiology entail limiting the field of vision?

Ken Rothman and colleagues put the case for a restricted version of epidemiology (Rothman and Poole, 1998; Rothman et al., 1998). They argued the most rapid gains came from the study of disease mechanisms in individuals. In their account, better knowledge of the fine detail of exposures and disease outcomes is the best way to reduce error, increase precision and identify health interventions.

Rothman et al. were arguing for microscope epidemiology. In their world-view, poverty and other upstream factors were not unimportant, it was just that they were out of range. Instead, they believed the discipline was most profitably employed close to disease occurrence, identifying proximal causes such as specific nutrient deficiencies, or particular carcinogens in the workplace, or pathogens that might provide the basis for effective vaccines.

Proponents of a broader view of the scope of epidemiology included Neil Pearce (Pearce, 1996), Steve Wing (Wing, 1998) and Tony McMichael. They argued that an exclusive 'close to disease occurrence' focus missed an important part of the public health picture. After all, there are epidemiological equivalents of 'failing to see the wood for the trees'. There are qualities of populations, such as levels of immunity to infectious disease, that affect the risk of ill health and may be overlooked if epidemiological studies concentrate downstream. It is not true that a finer scale of resolution necessarily takes us closer to the truth (Susser, 1998) and preoccupation with narrowly defined error reduction, risked in Tony's terms, making the epidemiologist a 'prisoner of the proximate' (McMichael, 1999).

An alternative approach is to work on the scale of analysis that makes most sense for the particular problem at hand. In place of microscopes, the appropriate metaphor might be spectacles with a variable focal length. It would be daft if prevailing methods determined what epidemiology did and did not pay attention to – surely, there should be some flex in the discipline's methods, to accommodate the most pressing issues of the time. Within limits, of course, epidemiologists will never have a great deal to offer particle physics, the fine detail of macroeconomics, or the important question of how to grow a broccoli that is both cancer preventing and tastes good. But, assuming a relatively broad field of operation, and depending on need, Tony McMichael and colleagues were arguing, the focus of our craft might range from chromosome to continent, from molecule to meta-analysis, from healthy worker to healthy planet.

At a micro level, there is a host of local, direct-acting toxic exposures that affect individuals. At the whole community level, there are problems such as air pollution from motor vehicles and power generation. Moving upscale, there are issues such as acid rain and brown haze. When planetary systems are affected, the problem takes on a global dimension – climate change is one example.

In other chapters, colleagues will populate the far reaches of the epidemiological matrix, reflecting on the meso and macro topics that Tony had been most concerned with recently. But here, I will concentrate on a near-field topic, environmental tobacco smoke, or passive smoking. This is partly for completeness – Tony's career spanned all the levels that have been mentioned here, and it would be a serious omission if the Festschrift neglected his important contributions to the traditional heartland of environmental epidemiology. I have chosen passive smoking because this is a success story, in which public health advances depended to a large extent on the knowledge provided by epidemiological research.

And this is also the topic that I first worked on with Tony, as a PhD student, when he and Bob Douglas were my supervisors.

The Case Against Passive Smoking

Progress towards the control of passive smoking was not straightforward. The road blocks and obstructions, the challenges, both personal and professional, are illustrated by one important case in law. This is AFCO versus the Tobacco Institute of Australia.

On 1 July 1986, the Tobacco Institute of Australia, the public relations arm of the tobacco industry, published an advertisement in 14 Australian newspapers, entitled 'A message from those who do ... to those who don't'. The institute assumed to speak on behalf of all those who smoked cigarettes, and aimed to reassure non-smokers that their concerns about the effects on health of second-hand smoke were unfounded. 'Often our [sic] own concerns about health can take an unproven claim and magnify it out of all proportion; so that what begins as a misconception turns into a frightening myth.' The solution proposed was common courtesy: smokers should be more considerate of the annoyance that may be caused, and non-smokers should be more tolerant, taking into account 'each other's rights and feelings'.

The advertisement anticipated two significant events: the public launch of the first report from the Australian National Health and Medical Research Council (NH&MRC) on the health effects of passive smoking (National Health and Medical Research Council, 1987), and the biennial conference of the Australian Labor Party, at which it was known a resolution would be tabled to ban smoking on all public transport, including airlines. The Labor Party was in government at the time, and if the resolution was passed, it would likely be translated into legislation (Chapman and Woodward, 1991).

The sticking point in the advertisement was the claim: 'there is little evidence, and nothing which proves scientifically that cigarette smoke causes diseases in non-smokers'. This conclusion was based, allegedly, on work from the World Health Organization, the American Cancer Society and the UK Institute of Cancer Research.

Advocacy groups responded angrily, through letters and press releases, pointing out that the relevant science was seriously misrepresented. The Australian Council on Smoking and Health took a case to the Advertising Standards Council, and gained a partial retraction from the tobacco industry.

But the most substantial challenge came, unexpectedly, from AFCO, which took its concerns to the Federal Trade Practices Commission. The Trade Practices Commission was the body responsible, among other duties, for discouraging deceptive and misleading advertising, and it ruled that this particular advertisement was not acceptable, in its original form. But AFCO was not satisfied. It sought an undertaking that the Tobacco Industry of Australia (TIA) would not repeat its claim 'that there is little evidence and nothing which proves scientifically...'. The TIA did not agree, so AFCO took action in the Federal Court.

The case was a long-running and expensive saga – it has been estimated the TIA spent about A$5 million on legal fees and expenses for witnesses. It was heard by Justice Morling, who was well known at the time for his role in the royal enquiry into the death of Azaria Chamberlain. (This enquiry was based on a re-evaluation of the scientific evidence, and led to the acquittal of Lindy Chamberlain.)

Before Morling, on behalf of AFCO, appeared toxicologists (Bernard Stewart), clinicians and a royal cast of epidemiologists. Tony McMichael was central to the case, as he had chaired the NH&MRC report. He was quizzed closely by Morling on the contents of the report, and the judge was evidently impressed by the answers he received. ('I formed the opinion' he wrote in his judgement 'that Professor McMichael is highly skilled and that his opinions are entitled to great respect' (Everingham and Woodward, 1991).)

The QC for the tobacco industry was predictably hostile and pressed for any opportunity to undermine and discredit the expert witnesses on the other side. For instance, he attempted to show that Tony had a close relationship with the advocacy group, Action on Smoking and Health (ASH), and therefore could not be regarded as an unbiased witness. As part of this inquisition, Tony was ordered to supply lecture notes and teaching materials so the legal team for the TIA could comb through them in search of incriminating references. This was the day of the overhead transparency – kilograms of paper and plastic sheets were retrieved from filing cabinets and delivered to the court. (Nothing came to light that could be used against the AFCO case.)

The witnesses who appeared for the TIA were mostly imported from the USA and, on the whole, did not impress Justice Morling. For instance, the judge said of Layard, a consulting statistician, 'plainly he has a close association with the tobacco industry and depends on it for most of his income… I do not think that Dr Layard expressed opinions that he does not hold, but I do think his hyper-critical approach to the epidemiological studies may not be disassociated with his close connection with the tobacco industry'. The industry witnesses were statisticians, or toxicologists; they did not include a single epidemiologist.

The court sat for 90 days; the judgement, when it was handed down almost five years after the offending advertisement, ran to over 200 pages (Everingham and Woodward, 1991). It covered a host of contentious scientific issues that were relevant to AFCO's case. I will pick out just a couple.

Relevant evidence – when we call on the authority of science, what data are admissible? Do peer-reviewed studies have precedence? What weight (if any) should be given to the grey literature? These questions, familiar to all of us who have been involved in contentious assessments, were explored in court.

The industry argued that meta-analyses and other forms of review should be discounted – that the relevant research included only the primary, empirical studies, and that these had to be treated one by one. The AFCO case was built on what Morling called a 'mosaic' approach to science, with constituents building up a picture that was greater than the sum of its parts. This approach, the AFCO version, was the one the judge preferred.

The starting point for the industry was that observational studies, of any kind, were not persuasive, on the basis that 'if science is the sun, statistics are Pluto'. This expression is not found in the judgement, but I think it represents fairly the arguments that were tabled before Morling.

The full quote runs:

> We really don't know whether the statistical associations identified through epidemiology are real or not. After all, we've only identified them through statistics, and statistics are not science. If science is the sun, statistics are Pluto. In fact, all sorts of wacky associations can be identified through statistics.

And the source is Steve Milloy, at the website junkscience.org. Milloy was not involved with the AFCO case, as far as I know, but his name is familiar to those who have studied the 'merchants of doubt', and the argument that association is not the same as cause has been launched against epidemiology on many occasions (Oreskes and Conway, 2010). It gained no purchase here. Nor did a subsequent foray from industry trenches, brandishing statistics in the form of significance testing and arguing that *p* values were pass/fail arbiters of causal validity.

In hindsight, the TIA would have been in a much stronger position if the advertisement had said no more than 'nothing that proves scientifically'. To claim 'there was little evidence' put the industry in a very exposed position, and Morling's finding was unambiguous. 'There is compelling scientific evidence' he concluded 'that cigarette smoke causes lung cancer in non-smokers', and 'the evidence establishing a causal relationship between passive smoking and respiratory disease in very young children is overwhelming. The evidence is of such strength that it constitutes scientific proof' (Everingham and Woodward, 1991). To rub salt into the wound, he ordered the TIA to pay the costs of the other side.

What were the consequences of the Morling judgement? It carried political weight, for a start. The tobacco industry's expert witnesses had performed woefully in court, and the credibility of the industry took a dive. Remember this was the 1980s and '90s, when tobacco companies had not yet fallen to pariah status – respectable universities still accepted industry money for what it, the university, believed was honest medical research with no strings attached.

The judgement affirmed the value of epidemiology in sorting out difficult, contested environmental problems, and it contained a very useful summary of the science that was being debated at the time. But perhaps what was most important was that Morling was a springboard for regulation, policy and a large-scale shift in public attitudes to tobacco. Other factors played a part, of course, but the Morling judgement skewered the argument that 'common courtesy' would suffice, and provided the foundation for intervention. There were questions still about how much ill health could be attributed to this cause, but not about whether second-hand smoke was harmful.

It is easy to forget how much has changed. In the late 1980s, smoke-free policy in Australia (and other countries) was partial, ineffective and apologetic. Twenty years post-Morling, in Australia and many other parts of the world, policies are comprehensive, widely accepted and assertive (International Agency for Research on Cancer, 2009).

There have been important advances also in the epidemiology of passive smoking. For a start, the quantity of evidence has increased manyfold. When the TIA advertisement appeared, claiming 'little evidence that cigarette smoke causes disease in non-smokers', there were fewer than a dozen studies of lung cancer and passive smoking. A review published in 2001 counted 43 epidemiological studies of this kind (Taylor et al., 2001). More important than the mushrooming number of studies is the consistency of the findings: the odds of lung cancer among non-smoking women married to men who smoked did not change materially between 1987 and 2001, although the statistical uncertainty around the pooled estimate has reduced considerably.

At the heart of the objections raised before Morling by the TIA was the issue of biological plausibility. How could it be, witnesses for the industry asked, that such small exposures, compared with the amount of smoke inhaled by an 'active' smoker, caused such large effects? The disjunction between dose and outcome seemed particularly large with cardiovascular diseases. A woman who smoked 10–15 cigarettes a day increased her risk of a heart attack by about 100 per cent; for the non-smoking wife of a man who smoked, the excess risk was roughly 30 per cent, although she breathed in much less than one-third of the dose of toxic agents in tobacco smoke. Research carried out in the last 20 years has solved this puzzle. Clinical studies have demonstrated clearly the ways in which second-hand smoke affects the heart and blood vessels, and epidemiology has filled in the gaps in the dose–response curve. The findings of the early studies on second-hand smoke are not inconsistent with the research on active smoking, because the nature of the dose–response is non-linear. What were thought to be 'small' exposures to tobacco smoke were clearly sufficient to bring about potentially dangerous changes such as vascular inflammation and increased platelet activity. However, these biological responses are saturated or buffered in some way at higher doses, and if graphed on a linear scale, the dose–response curve flattens out in the active smoking range (Pope et al., 2009).

The arguments before Morling focused very much on lung cancer – much less attention was paid to other diseases that might be related to second-hand smoke. But subsequent work on the burden of ill health attributable to passive smoking has shown that cases of lung cancer are a small proportion of the total. It has been estimated that in 2004, worldwide, 40 per cent of children, 33 per cent of male non-smokers and 35 per cent of female non-smokers had been exposed to second-hand smoke (Öberg et al., 2010). This exposure was estimated to have caused, each year, about 21,400 deaths from lung cancer (about 3.5 per cent of all mortality attributable to second-hand smoke). Much more numerous were 379,000 attributable deaths from ischaemic heart disease, 165,000 from lower respiratory infections and approximately 36,900 from asthma.

Although the burden of disease due to passive smoking remains considerable, worldwide, there have been significant advances. One of the most important has been the introduction in many countries of comprehensive smoke-free policies in the workplace. These policies have been shown to reduce the prevalence of smoking at work, and to cut exposures to second-hand smoke dramatically. (In New Zealand, it was estimated that smoke-free laws reduced exposures in bars and hotels by 90 per cent (Fernando et al., 2007).) What has also become apparent is that laws of this kind have substantial beneficial and rapid effects on public health. Up to 2009, there were nine studies published on the effect of smoke-free legislation on hospital visits for acute coronary disease. What was seen was a reduction of 15–20 per cent in the first 12 months after legislation, consistent with falling exposures to second-hand smoke in the workforce and in the population at large, and it was unlikely that this effect could be explained by other changes that took place at the same time as smoke-free laws were introduced (International Agency for Research on Cancer, 2009).

Conclusion

For his 1999 paper, Tony drew a figure to illustrate the dimensions in which epidemiology might operate (Figure 12.1). He argued that we should think adventurously, beyond common presumptions, which tend to huddle in the bottom left-hand corner of the picture. (And for good reason – look at the far right-hand corner – doing epidemiology in the future? Goodness, that is a big ask.)

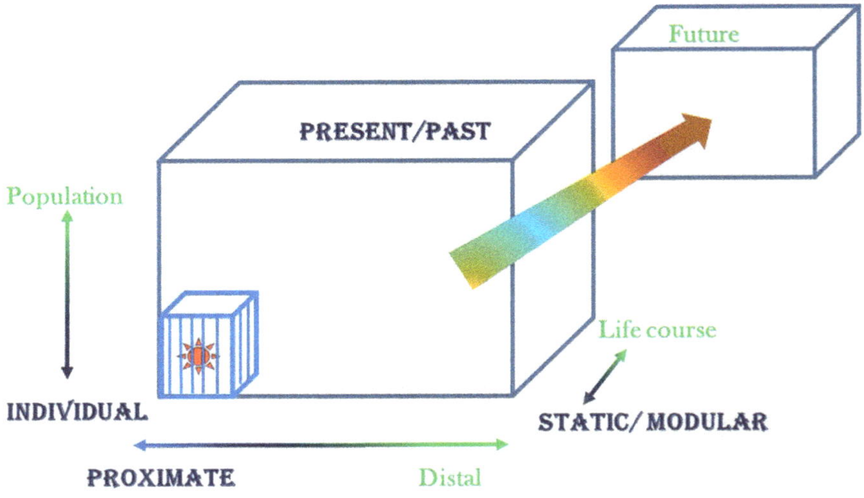

Figure 12.1 The dimensions of epidemiological research.
Source: McMichael, 1999 (redrawn with permission from Oxford University Press).

The zone of comfort is marked by what could be a jail cell containing a crystal ball, or a child's playpen with a beach ball. Tony was at pains to defend the use of proximal epidemiology, where it was appropriate, and passive smoking was one case in which the bottom left-hand corner was the right place to be. But he urged us: if the need arises, leave the playpen, because purpose trumps technique.

To my mind, Tony McMichael and Jerry Morris were very much on the same page. 'One of the urgent needs of highly developed and rapidly changing societies', Jerry Morris wrote in his textbook, 'is to determine ways of healthy living, the wisdom of body and mind and the principles of social organization that can inform the quality of life and lighten the burden of disease. The quest for this knowledge is the main use of epidemiology.'

References

Blair, S.N. & Morris, J.N. 2009. Healthy hearts – and the universal benefits of being physically active. *Annals of Epidemiology* 19, 253–6.

Chapman, S. & Woodward, S. 1991. Australian court rules that passive smoking causes lung cancer, asthma attacks, and respiratory disease. *BMJ* 302, 943–5.

Everingham, R. & Woodward, S. 1991. *Tobacco Litigation. The Case Against Passive Smoking AFCO v TIA*. Legal Books, Sydney, New South Wales, Australia.

Fernando, D., Fowles, J., Woodward, A., Christophersen, A., Dickson, S., Hosking, M., et al. 2007. Legislation reduces exposure to second-hand tobacco smoke in New Zealand bars by about 90%. *Tobacco Control* 16, 235–8.

International Agency for Research on Cancer 2009. *IARC Handbooks of Cancer Prevention, Tobacco Control, Vol. 13: Evaluating the Effectiveness of Smoke-free Policies*. IARC, Lyon, France.

Krieger, N. 2007. Commentary: Ways of asking and ways of living: reflections on the 50th anniversary of Morris' ever-useful *Uses of Epidemiology*. *International Journal of Epidemiology* 36, 1173–80.

McMichael, A.J. 1976. Standardized mortality ratios and the 'healthy worker effect': scratching beneath the surface. *Journal of Occupational Medicine* 18, 165–8.

McMichael, A.J. 1999. Prisoners of the proximate: loosening the constraints on epidemiology in an age of change. *American Journal of Epidemiology* 149, 887–97.

Morris, J.N. 1975. *The Uses of Epidemiology. Third Edition*. Churchill Livingstone, London, UK.

Morris, J.N., Heady, J.A., Raffle, P.A., Roberts, C.G. & Parks, J.W. 1953. Coronary heart disease and physical activity of work. *The Lancet* 265, 1053–7.

Morris, J.N., Donkin, A.J.M., Wonderling, D., Wilkinson, P. & Dowler, E.A. 2000. A minimum income for healthy living. *Journal of Epidemiology & Community Health* 54, 885–9.

National Health and Medical Research Council 1987. *The Heath Effects of Passive Smoking. A Scientific Information Paper*. NH&MRC, Canberra, ACT, Australia.

Öberg, M., Jaakkola, M.S., Woodward, A., Peruga, A. & Prüss-Ustün, A. 2010. Worldwide burden of disease from exposure to second-hand smoke: a retrospective analysis of data from 192 countries. *The Lancet* 377, 139–46.

Oreskes, N. & Conway, E.M. 2010. *Merchants of Doubt. How a Handful of Scientists Obscured the Truth on Issues from Tobacco Smoke to Global Warming*. Bloomsbury Press, New York, USA.

Pearce, N.E. 1996. Traditional epidemiology, modern epidemiology and public health. *American Journal of Public Health* 86, 678–83.

Pope, C.A. 3rd, Burnett, R.T., Krewski, D., Jerrett, M., Shi, Y., Calle, E.E., et al. 2009. Cardiovascular mortality and exposure to airborne fine particulate matter and cigarette smoke. Shape of the exposure–response relationship. *Circulation* 120, 941–8.

Rothman, K.J. 1986. *Modern Epidemiology*. First Edition. Little, Brown and Company, Boston, Massachusetts, USA.

Rothman, K.J. & Poole, C. 1998. Our conscientious objection to the epidemiology wars. *Journal of Epidemiology & Community Health* 52, 1–2.

Rothman, K.J., Adami, H.-O. & Trichopoulos, D. 1998. Should the mission of epidemiology include the eradication of poverty? *The Lancet* 352, 810–2.

Schulte, P.A. & Perera, F.P. (eds) 1998. *Molecular Epidemiology. Principles and Practices*. Academic Press, Boston, Massachusetts, USA.

Smith, G.D. 2001. The uses of '*Uses of Epidemiology*'. *International Journal of Epidemiology* 30, 1146–55.

Susser, M. 1998. Does risk factor epidemiology put epidemiology at risk? Peering into the future. *Journal of Epidemiology & Community Health* 52, 608–11.

Taylor, R., Cumming, R., Woodward, A. & Black, M. 2001. Passive smoking and lung cancer: a cumulative meta-analysis. *Australian & New Zealand Journal of Public Health* 25, 203–11.

Wing, S. 1998. Whose epidemiology, whose health? *International Journal of Health Services* 28, 241–52.

PART 4

NUTRITION AND FOOD SYSTEMS

REPRINT E

Diet and Cancer of the Colon and Rectum: A Case-Control Study

JOHN D. POTTER AND ANTHONY J. MCMICHAEL

Potter, J.D. & McMichael, A.J. 1986. Diet and cancer of the colon and rectum: a case-control study. *Journal of the National Cancer Institute* 76, 557–69.

Pages: 221 to 236

Diet and Cancer of the Colon and Rectum: A Case-Control Study [1]

John D. Potter [2] *and* **Anthony J. McMichael** [2,3]

ABSTRACT—In 1979-81, 419 patients with incident cases of colon and rectal cancer and 732 controls were questioned regarding diet and alcohol. Cancer cases were a population-based series reported to the South Australian Central Cancer Registry, were 30-74 years of age, and were residing in Metropolitan Adelaide. Controls were selected from the electoral roll and individually age- and sex-matched to cancer cases. The most consistent risk factor for colorectal cancer was dietary protein, which was associated with a twofold-to-threefold relative risk for colon cancer and for rectal cancer in women for all levels of consumption above the base line (i.e., the lowest consumption quintile). For male colon cancer the corresponding relative risk was similar; but for male rectal cancer, risk was elevated only at old ages. Total energy intake and, less clearly, meal frequency were also positively associated with increased risk. Total alcohol intake (but not specifically beer) was associated with increased risk of both colon and rectal cancer in women; in both sexes, there was an increased risk of colon and rectal cancer associated with spirits consumption. A reduced risk of rectal cancer was associated with vitamin C but not with vitamin A. The increased risk associated with high protein and total energy was confined to those consuming a low fiber diet, particularly among women; but some other aspects of the relationship between fiber consumption and risk of colorectal cancer were more complex. Some modifications and extensions of the current fat-to-bile acid-to-fiber theory of bowel carcinogenesis were suggested.—JNCI 1986; 76:557-569.

Previous studies of large bowel cancer [international correlation studies (*1*), case-control studies (*2-5*), and metabolic epidemiology (*6, 7*)], despite their inconsistent findings, have suggested a role for dietary factors in some stage of the cancer process. The currently prevailing model of colorectal carcinogenesis includes fat (*8, 9*) (associated with increased risk) and fiber (*8, 9*) (reduced risk) as well as a role for alcohol (*10-12*) (increased risk) and hormonal factors (*13-17*) each, partly or wholly, exerting influence via effects on hepatic and intestinal BA metabolism.

In previous studies, little attention has been paid to the possibility that relationships between risk and these dietary and hormonal factors may vary by site (colon vs. rectum) and within the colon by subsite, sex, and age. The arguments for considering these effects separately have been detailed elsewhere (*18*) but rest on the evidence for systematic variation in the age-sex-subsite distribution of bowel cancer and on the evidence for differences in etiology and perhaps histopathology of tumors from different subsites.

The present study investigated the relationship between nutrient intake and bowel cancer risk, including examination of postulated variations in diet-related risk by age, sex, and subsite (*13, 15*).

SUBJECTS AND METHODS

Subjects.—All those with newly incident cases of cancer of the colon and rectum who were reported to the South Australian Cancer Registry during 1979 and 1980, with additional inclusion of those with rectal cancer during early 1981, who resided in Metropolitan Adelaide, who were between the ages of 30 and 74 years, and who are alive at the time of reporting, made up the eligible case series. Of these 576 cases, 70 died before being contacted. Of the remaining 506, permission to interview was refused by the attending surgeon for 55 (10.9%), usually because the patient was terminally ill. Twenty-two (4.3%) refused to be interviewed and 10 (2.0%) were not found. To establish comparability with controls, the electoral roll status (*see further*) of the first 100 cases was determined. Of these, 99 were on the electoral roll.

Among controls there were 216 (20.4%) refusals, and 112 (10.6%) were not located out of a total of 1,060 eligible living individuals. Controls were selected from the Metropolitan Adelaide community via the electoral roll [voter registration is compulsory and more than 98% of those over 30 years of age are enrolled (*19*)]. Two controls were individually matched to each case by sex and age. The inclusion of the rectal cancer cases reported in early 1981 (37 males, 19 females) was undertaken to increase the number of rectal cancer cases to enable them to be studied as a separate cancer site. As no combined matched analyses were contemplated, these additional cases were each matched to 2 randomly selected controls for colon cases. Therefore, in the analyses that follow, the control populations for colon and rectum study contained 112 persons in common.

Data collection.—In all, 419 cases and 732 controls (*see* table 1) completed a self-administered dietary questionnaire and were interviewed regarding demographic variables, medical and family history, and dietary changes. Two trained interviewers—one male, one female—collected all information; each case-control triplet was interviewed by the same individual.

ABBREVIATIONS USED: BA = bile acid; CI = confidence interval; OR = odds ratio; RR = relative risk(s); VFA = volatile fatty acid(s).

---

[1] Received December 18, 1984; revised October 16, 1985; accepted December 2, 1985.

[2] Division of Human Nutrition, Commonwealth Scientific and Industrial Research Organization, Kintore Ave., Adelaide, SA 5000, Australia.

[3] We thank Ms. Sally Record for technical assistance with the computing; Ms. Maria Juras for interviewing; Dr. Anton Bonett, Central Cancer Registry of the South Australian Health Commission; and the many surgeons in Adelaide who facilitated the conduct of the study.

TABLE 1.—*Study population: Age, sex, and site distribution of cases and controls*

Age, yr	Colon				Rectum			
	Males, No.		Females, No.		Males, No.		Females, No.	
	Cases	Matched controls	Cases	Matched controls	Cases	Matched controls	Cases	Matched controls
30-54	20	35	21	40	15	33	19	43
55-59	17	39	13	30	27	55	16	26
60-64	29	49	15	28	27	60	12	33
65-69	28	59	18	32	26	43	16	25
70-74	27	59	32	67	29	57	12	21
Total[a]	121	241	99	197	124	248	75	148

[a] As described in the text, there is some overlap between colon and rectum control groups.

The dietary questionnaire, a quantitative food-frequency questionnaire developed by our research group, has been used extensively in a variety of settings and has been tested for repeatability and against biochemical measures (*20-22*). Recent evidence suggests that, in general, food frequency questionnaires provide reliable and repeatable data (*22-24*). The version used recorded frequency of consumption of 141 food items, as well as alcohol consumption and a variety of qualitative questions regarding cooking methods, fat use, bread type, etc., which were used in deriving nutrient indices.

Where changes had occurred recently, respondents (both cases and controls) were asked to describe their diets as they had been 12 months prior to interview. This procedure was to preclude, in unbiased fashion, those who had changed after diagnosis and treatment. Usual diet was asked for to preclude changes in diets that had resulted from symptoms. It was decided that interviews were to be conducted in the home rather than in the hospital to allow resumption of usual dietary (and other) habits and to ensure that there was comparability in the interview setting between cases and controls. Cases were contacted after they had been reported to the cancer registry. Mean time from operation to interview was 9.1±0.1 months.

Food frequency data were converted to nutrient consumption via FREQUAN (*21*) by using food table data [based on the McCance and Widdowson data base (*25*) modified where appropriate and possible with local nutrient analyses] and standard serve sizes (*26*). No direct comparisons between the sexes were planned or undertaken, so the use of a single serve size created no additional problems.

During the latter part of the study, 106 cases and 222 controls were specifically questioned regarding recent changes in diet. Twenty-seven cases (25.5%) and 28 controls (12.6%) indicated that their present diets had changed in the previous 12 months. These 2 groups were compared with all cases and all controls, respectively. The difference between the females in this "changed" group and the study as a whole were minimal and tended to make the results reported somewhat conservative. The reverse was true for the male "changed" group where the differences were also greater.

Cancers were all histologically confirmed and only adenocarcinomas were included. They were categorized by subsite according to the International Classification of Diseases (Ninth Revision) and aggregated for some analyses into proximal colon (cecum, ascending colon, hepatic flexure), distal colon (transverse colon to sigmoid), and rectum (including rectosigmoid).

Demographic data, including usual occupation as a measure of social class, were collected at interview.

Presentation of analyses.—Analyses were presented initially as comparisons of means and as matched OR (approximating RR) and 95% confidence intervals. For the dietary variables, exposure was categorized into quintiles based on the total study population; a conditional logistic regression model was used to determine the OR associated with each quintile (*27*). To control for the simultaneous effects of several variables, the data were analyzed either stratified on potential confounders or by the use of conditional logistic regression models (*27*).

RESULTS

Means.—The mean consumption levels of major nutrients thought to be relevant to the genesis of large bowel cancer are shown in table 2. For colon cancer in women, mean consumption of most nutrients, including fiber, was statistically significantly higher in cases than in controls. For male colon cancer, the differences between cases and controls in consumption of saturated fat, total energy, and alcohol approached statistical significance. These observations were also generally consistent with those for rectal cancer, although there appeared to be even less of a difference in consumption between male cases and controls. Expressed as a percentage of total energy intake, there were no differences in intakes of nutrients between cases and controls in either sex, with the exception of alcohol consumption, which was higher in female colon cancer cases than in controls.

Major nutrients; colon.—The combined population of cases and controls formed the basis for stratification into exposure quintiles separately for males and females. The quintiles were approximately one step apart for males and females for most nutrients: i.e., in absolute consumption terms, the "base-line" quintile in males

TABLE 2.—*Colorectal cancer: Mean ± SEM daily consumption of nutrients*

Nutrient	Colon						Rectum					
	Males			Females			Males			Females		
	Cases, n=121	Controls, n=241	P	Cases, n=99	Controls, n=197	P	Cases, n=124	Controls, n=248	P	Cases, n=75	Controls, n=148	P
Protein, g	95.5±2.4	93.8±2.0	.306	84.8±2.1	78.9±1.5	.012	91.4±2.5	90.5±1.7	.384	85.1±3.2	77.2±2.2	.020
Fat, g	113.5±3.7	108.0±2.7	.116	89.2±3.0	83.8±1.8	.062	110.7±4.3	104.5±2.4	.106	91.6±3.9	82.5±2.8	.028
Saturated fat, g	46.8±1.7	44.1±1.1	.091	37.3±1.4	35.2±0.9	.097	46.4±1.9	43.0±1.0	.058	38.2±1.8	34.4±1.3	.044
Cholesterol, mg	418.9±14.9	413.0±14.7	.390	326.3±12.3	300.9±8.7	.047	405.5±16.4	384.8±10.6	.138	319.7±16.2	300.4±11.9	.172
Energy, MJ[a]	10.5±0.3	10.0±0.2	.084	8.4±0.2	7.8±0.1	.010	10.2±0.3	9.8±0.2	.155	8.5±0.3	7.6±0.2	.003
Fiber, g	20.2±0.7	20.3±0.6	.952	22.4±0.8	19.7±0.6	.009	19.7±0.7	20.0±0.5	.381	21.7±1.0	19.4±0.6	.044
Alcohol, g	22.4±2.6	17.7±1.5	.063	6.8±1.1	4.3±0.6	.020	18.5±2.1	19.2±1.5	.387	6.7±1.4	5.4±0.8	.200

[a] MJ=1 kilocalorie×0.004184.

approximated the second quintile in females. The only major exception to this was fiber, where male and female absolute intakes were similar (*see* table 3).

Table 3 shows the relationship between exposure quintiles of major nutrients and risk of colon cancer. For males, there was a consistent elevation of RR associated with protein consumption above the base line. For females, protein and total energy consumption showed a stepwise increase in RR for the first quintile of exposure above the base line but no further increase. Fat, saturated fat, and cholesterol showed a similar pattern. For alcohol in women, there may be a similar, but less marked, increase at the fourth exposure quintile. Fiber consumption was associated with an increasing estimate of RR for each quintile of exposure. Analyses with nutrients expressed as a percentage of total energy intake were less clear and showed few differences between cases and controls.

TABLE 3.—*Colon cancer and diet—univariate matched RR (95% CI) by exposure quintiles*

Nutrient	RR (95% CI) for quintile:[a]				
	1	2	3	4	5
Males					
Protein	1.0	2.2 (1.0–4.8)	2.3 (1.1–4.8)	1.9 (0.9–4.0)	2.1 (1.0–4.5)
Fat	1.0	1.0 (0.5–2.1)	1.0 (0.5–2.2)	1.2 (0.6–2.4)	1.4 (0.7–2.9)
Saturated fat	1.0	0.6 (0.3–1.3)	1.3 (0.7–2.6)	1.3 (0.7–2.6)	1.1 (0.6–2.3)
Cholesterol	1.0	1.5 (0.7–3.2)	1.0 (0.5–2.0)	1.6 (0.8–3.2)	1.5 (0.7–3.0)
Energy	1.0	1.1 (0.5–2.3)	1.6 (0.8–3.2)	1.3 (0.7–2.6)	1.8 (0.9–3.7)
Alcohol	1.0	0.6 (0.3–1.3)	0.4 (0.2–1.0)	0.8 (0.4–1.7)	1.0 (0.5–2.1)
Fiber	1.0	1.2 (0.6–2.4)	2.1 (1.0–4.3)	1.0 (0.5–2.1)	1.3 (0.6–2.6)
Females					
Protein	1.0	2.6 (1.1–6.1)	2.1 (0.9–5.0)	2.2 (1.0–4.9)	2.8 (1.5–5.2)
Fat	1.0	1.9 (0.8–4.3)	1.9 (0.8–4.5)	1.8 (0.6–5.2)	1.7 (0.8–3.6)
Saturated fat	1.0	1.6 (0.7–3.7)	2.4 (1.0–5.5)	1.0 (0.4–2.4)	2.1 (0.9–4.8)
Cholesterol	1.0	2.0 (0.8–4.7)	2.2 (1.0–5.3)	1.3 (0.6–2.8)	2.7 (1.2–6.1)
Energy	1.0	6.2 (2.1–18.0)	3.4 (1.1–9.8)	5.3 (1.8–15.7)	4.8 (1.7–13.9)
Alcohol	1.0	1.4 (0.7–2.7)	1.2 (0.5–2.6)	2.0 (0.9–4.4)	2.0 (0.9–4.5)
Fiber	1.0	1.8 (0.7–4.3)	2.2 (0.9–5.4)	2.9 (1.3–6.8)	4.1 (1.7–10.0)

[a] Quintile cut points—for males: protein (g/day): 68.4, 81.4, 94.8, 113.8; fat (g/day): 76.9, 91.4, 110.6, 136.8; saturated fat (g/day): 29.7, 37.8, 46.2, 57.5; cholesterol (mg/day): 247.0, 327.0, 426.0, 533.0; energy (MJ/day): 7.6, 9.0, 10.5, 12.2; alcohol (g/day): 0.1, 4.0, 12.8, 31.8; fiber (g/day); 13.2, 17.1, 21.2, 26.8. Quintile cut points—for females: protein (g/day): 60.5, 71.2, 84.5, 97.5; fat (g/day): 59.5, 75.1, 89.0, 108.6; saturated fat (g/day): 24.1, 30.9, 37.6, 47.0; cholesterol (mg/day): 204.0, 257.0, 311.0, 395.0; energy (MJ/day): 6.0, 7.2, 8.3, 9.6; alcohol (g/day): 0.01, 0.95, 3.9, 12.9 (the 38% nondrinkers comprise the lowest quintile; the remaining cut points are at 55, 70, and 85% of the distribution); fiber (g/day): 14.0, 17.9, 21.0, 25.7.

As modifying effects of age had been postulated and, specifically, as the possibility that dietary factors may differ in their relative influence before and after menopause in women (*13, 15*), patterns of differences in dietary intakes were investigated between cases and controls at various ages. It was found that the youngest cases of colon cancer in women had low intakes of fiber compared with intakes of controls but that older cases showed both higher mean intakes and greater variability than did respective controls. This pattern was confined to women with distal (transverse to sigmoid) colon cancer (data not shown separately), the sex-subsite group that largely accounted for the association between increased RR and higher fiber consumption overall.

On the basis of these observations the question arose as to what, among other measured variables, distinguished females who were low fiber consumers from females who were high fiber consumers. It was striking that, although other nutrients increased approximately linearly as fiber intake increased among controls, the same was not true for cases. In cases, low fiber consumption was associated with consumption of other major nutrients at a level approaching that of those in the highest fiber intake group; the lowest intake of other nutrients was found among the "middle fiber" intake group of cases. Thus the case-control differences in consumption of major nutrients and energy were largely confined to those women who had low intakes of fiber. Nondietary variables did not distinguish between low and high fiber-consuming groups of women. Table 4 shows the estimates of RR associated with tertiles of consumption of major nutrients after stratifying on tertiles of fiber per megajoule of energy (to control for the association between amounts of fiber and total energy in the diet).

For females, there was a gradient of increased RR with increasing consumption of total fat, saturated fat, and protein at low consumption levels of fiber. This finding also indicated, however, that there was the same unexpected increase in RR associated with increasing consumption of fiber as seen in table 3, even after controlling for total energy intake.

For males, the first of these two observations holds—namely, that a higher estimate of RR was associated with higher consumption of nutrients at lower levels of fiber intake; but there was also evidence that a reducing risk was associated with increasing fiber at high levels of nutrient intake.

The overall pattern associated with age suggested that dietary-related RR were more marked at young ages in women and at older ages in men [for details, *see* (*18*)].

Major nutrients; rectum.—Table 5 shows the corresponding findings for rectal cancer cases and controls. For males, there was no significant variation from 1.0 associated with any major nutrient. Alcohol consumption was unexpectedly associated with a nonsignificant reduction in RR for all categories of drinker. For females, protein, total fat, saturated fat, and total dietary energy were associated with increases in RR with increasing levels of consumption. The top 20% of the

TABLE 4.—*Colon cancer and diet: RR (95% CI) associated with tertiles of major nutrients after stratification on fiber intake controlled for total energy intake*

Nutrient	Level	Fiber per MJ of energy		
		Low	Mid	High
Females				
Protein	Low	1.0	0.5 (0.1-2.7)	1.3 (0.3-5.0)
	Mid	0.6 (0.1-3.0)	3.3 (0.9-11.8)	3.8 (1.1-12.9)
	High	2.3 (0.7-7.4)	1.7 (0.5-6.3)	2.3 (0.6-8.4)
Total fat	Low	1.0	1.6 (0.3-7.3)	2.7 (0.7-10.6)
	Mid	1.7 (0.4-7.8)	2.8 (0.7-11.1)	3.2 (0.8-12.6)
	High	2.4 (0.6-9.0)	2.1 (0.5-8.9)	3.1 (0.7-14.0)
Saturated fat	Low	1.0	2.1 (0.4-12.1)	3.2 (0.7-15.2)
	Mid	2.1 (0.4-11.1)	3.8 (0.8-18.3)	6.0 (1.3-27.4)
	High	3.2 (0.7-14.8)	2.3 (0.4-12.3)	2.3 (0.4-13.8)
Males				
Protein	Low	1.0	0.8 (0.2-2.7)	1.3 (0.4-3.8)
	Med	1.3 (0.4-4.2)	1.7 (0.6-5.1)	1.5 (0.5-4.7)
	High	1.6 (0.5-4.6)	1.6 (0.5-4.9)	1.1 (0.3-3.7)
Total fat	Low	1.0	1.2 (0.4-3.6)	1.5 (0.5-4.3)
	Med	1.5 (0.5-4.6)	1.9 (0.7-5.3)	1.9 (0.7-5.6)
	High	2.1 (0.8-5.7)	1.8 (0.6-5.1)	1.0 (0.3-3.5)
Saturated fat	Low	1.0	1.4 (0.4-5.5)	2.6 (0.8-8.5)
	Med	3.5 (1.0-12.3)	2.8 (0.9-9.1)	2.5 (0.7-8.9)
	High	3.3 (1.0-10.3)	4.0 (1.2-13.4)	2.3 (0.6-8.9)

consumption distributions of almost all of these variables was associated with a doubling or greater RR of rectal cancer.

Stratification on age suggested little variation of RR of rectal cancer for women but showed a marked interaction of most nutrient consumption levels with age for men. Text-figure 1 shows relative risks at various ages derived from fitting the total energy consumption levels

TABLE 5.—*Rectal cancer and diet: Univariate matched RR (95% CI) by exposure quintiles*

Nutrient	RR (95% CI) for quintile:				
	1	2	3	4	5
Males					
Protein	1.0	0.9 (0.4-1.9)	1.3 (0.7-2.6)	1.1 (0.6-2.2)	1.0 (0.5-1.9)
Fat	1.0	0.7 (0.4-1.6)	1.8 (0.9-3.6)	1.1 (0.6-2.2)	1.3 (0.7-2.6)
Saturated fat	1.0	1.3 (0.6-2.6)	1.6 (0.8-3.2)	1.2 (0.6-2.5)	1.7 (0.9-3.4)
Cholesterol	1.0	1.3 (0.7-2.7)	1.2 (0.6-2.3)	1.1 (0.6-2.0)	1.2 (0.6-2.4)
Energy	1.0	0.8 (0.4-1.7)	1.2 (0.6-2.4)	1.0 (0.5-2.0)	1.2 (0.6-2.4)
Fiber	1.0	1.2 (0.6-2.5)	0.7 (0.3-1.3)	0.5 (0.3-1.1)	1.3 (0.6-2.7)
Alcohol	1.0	0.7 (0.3-1.3)	0.8 (0.4-1.5)	0.6 (0.3-1.2)	0.7 (0.4-1.5)
Females					
Protein	1.0	2.5 (1.0-6.7)	2.3 (0.9-6.1)	2.1 (0.7-6.1)	3.0 (1.2-7.6)
Fat	1.0	3.2 (1.2-8.4)	3.1 (1.1-8.4)	3.6 (0.9-13.8)	2.5 (1.1-6.0)
Saturated fat	1.0	2.7 (1.0-7.1)	2.1 (0.9-5.2)	1.8 (0.7-4.6)	2.3 (1.0-5.4)
Cholesterol	1.0	1.5 (0.6-3.5)	0.7 (0.3-1.9)	1.6 (0.7-4.0)	1.4 (0.6-3.2)
Energy	1.0	2.4 (0.9-6.7)	1.2 (0.5-3.4)	2.6 (0.9-7.1)	4.6 (1.7-12.5)
Fiber	1.0	1.4 (0.6-3.5)	0.9 (0.3-2.3)	1.2 (0.5-3.2)	2.4 (1.0-5.7)
Alcohol	1.0	0.6 (0.2-1.3)	1.7 (0.7-3.9)	1.1 (0.5-2.5)	1.5 (0.6-3.7)

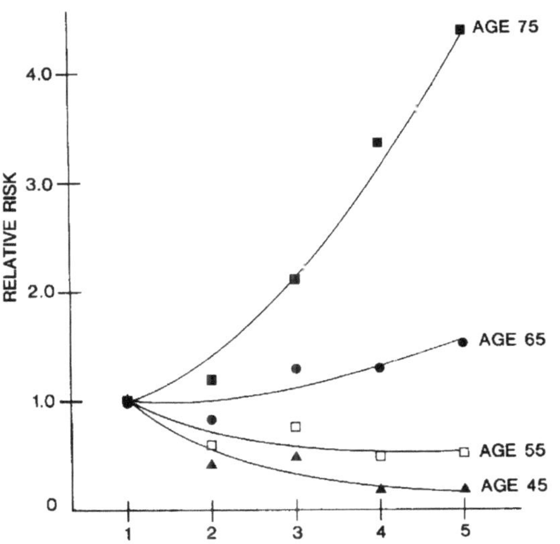

TEXT-FIGURE 1.—Estimates of matched RR for male rectal cancer associated with quintiles of total energy consumption at various ages (yr). Estimates are derived from a conditional logistic regression model that incorporated the primary variables (energy consumption quintiles) and age-interaction terms. Smoothed curves are for clarification of relationships only.

TABLE 6.—*Colon and rectal cancer and micronutrients: Univariate matched RR (95% CI) by exposure quintiles by sex*

Nutrient	RR (95% CI) for quintile:[a]				
	1	2	3	4	5
Male colon					
β-carotene	1.0	0.6 (0.3–1.5)	0.2 (0.4–1.5)	0.8 (0.4–1.6)	0.8 (0.4–1.6)
Vitamin C	1.0	1.2 (0.6–1.3)	1.5 (0.8–3.1)	1.8 (0.9–3.8)	1.0 (0.5–2.1)
Retinol	1.0	1.1 (0.6–2.3)	1.5 (0.7–2.9)	1.1 (0.5–2.1)	1.4 (0.8–2.4)
Female colon					
β-carotene	1.0	0.8 (0.4–1.6)	1.4 (0.5–3.5)	0.9 (0.4–2.0)	2.2 (1.0–4.7)
Vitamin C	1.0	1.4 (0.6–3.2)	1.2 (0.6–2.6)	1.3 (0.6–2.9)	2.2 (1.0–4.8)
Retinol	1.0	1.0 (0.4–2.1)	1.1 (0.5–2.4)	1.0 (0.5–2.2)	1.6 (0.7–3.5)
Male rectum					
β-carotene	1.0	0.9 (0.4–1.7)	1.1 (0.6–2.2)	0.5 (0.2–1.1)	0.9 (0.4–1.7)
Vitamin C	1.0	0.7 (0.4–1.4)	0.7 (0.4–1.4)	0.6 (0.3–1.2)	0.6 (0.3–1.1)
Retinol	1.0	0.8 (0.4–1.4)	0.7 (0.3–1.3)	0.8 (0.4–1.6)	0.7 (0.4–1.4)
Female rectum					
β-carotene	1.0	0.9 (0.4–2.2)	0.9 (0.3–3.2)	1.2 (0.5–3.0)	1.5 (0.6–3.6)
Vitamin C	1.0	0.4 (0.1–1.0)	0.8 (0.3–1.7)	0.9 (0.4–2.4)	0.3 (0.1–0.8)
Retinol	1.0	1.0 (0.4–2.3)	1.5 (0.7–3.4)	1.2 (0.5–2.7)	1.3 (0.6–3.0)

[a] Quintile cut points—for males: β-carotene (μg/day): 2,360, 3,560, 4,770, 7,000; vitamin C (mg/day): 59.6, 104.5, 158.5, 223.0; retinol (μg/day): 300, 446, 816, 1,436. Quintile cut points—for females: β-carotene (μg/day): 2,970, 4,290, 5,750, 8,180; vitamin C (mg/day): 72.8, 127.0, 178.0, 255.0; retinol (μg/day): 252, 379, 585, 1,410.

and age interaction terms in a logistic model. The pattern was consistent for each nutrient, including fiber and alcohol, with higher consumption of each associated with reduced RR at younger ages but with markedly increased RR at older ages. The net effect across all ages combined was no apparent relationship between nutrient consumption levels and risk of rectal cancer as seen in table 5. However, the observed pattern was consistent in both age-stratified analyses (not shown) and fitted models and was therefore not simply artifactually produced by the constraints of the fitted model. The confidence limits were wide and tended to include 1.0, except for higher consumption at older ages.

Micronutrients.—Consumption of some specific micronutrients (vitamin C, β-carotene, retinol) showed little relationship to risk of colon cancer in either sex; for rectal cancer there was a reduction in RR associated with vitamin C in both sexes but more marked in women (*see* table 6). In male rectal cancer, stratification by age showed that vitamin C consumption was particularly associated with reduced RR at younger ages, this effect disappearing only by 70 years of age. This pattern was consistent, however, with that for major nutrients noted above (*see* text-fig. 1) and may reflect only that young male rectal cancer cases appeared to eat much less than did either older cases or controls. However, no marked increased was observed in RR associated with high consumption of vitamin C at older ages.

Fiber source.—Table 7 shows that the increased RR associated with higher levels of consumption of dietary fiber in women was confined primarily to consumption of cereal fiber. Furthermore, the increased risk was confined to the distal colon (data not shown separately) and rectum.

Alcohol source.—Table 8 shows the RR associated

TABLE 7.—*Colon and rectal cancer and fiber consumption: Univariate matched RR (95% CI) by exposure quintiles*

Fiber source	RR (95% CI) for quintile:				
	1	2	3	4	5
Male colon					
Vegetable fiber	1.0	1.2 (0.6–2.5)	2.0 (0.9–4.1)	1.2 (0.6–2.5)	1.3 (0.6–2.6)
Cereal fiber	1.0	1.5 (0.8–2.9)	1.3 (0.6–2.6)	1.2 (0.6–2.4)	1.4 (0.7–2.8)
Female colon					
Vegetable fiber	1.0	1.1 (0.5–2.5)	1.4 (0.7–3.0)	0.8 (0.3–1.8)	1.7 (0.8–3.6)
Cereal fiber	1.0	3.1 (1.3–7.9)	2.0 (0.8–5.3)	4.6 (1.9–11.3)	5.1 (2.1–12.7)
Male rectum					
Vegetable fiber	1.0	1.1 (0.6–2.1)	0.8 (0.4–1.6)	0.6 (0.3–1.2)	0.9 (0.4–1.8)
Cereal fiber	1.0	1.3 (0.6–2.6)	1.8 (0.9–3.7)	1.6 (0.8–3.3)	1.2 (0.6–2.3)
Female rectum					
Vegetable fiber	1.0	0.5 (0.2–1.1)	0.5 (0.2–1.3)	0.6 (0.3–1.4)	0.7 (0.3–1.5)
Cereal fiber	1.0	2.7 (1.0–7.3)	1.3 (0.5–3.8)	2.3 (0.9–6.0)	4.4 (1.7–12.0)

TABLE 8.—*Colon and rectal cancer and alcohol: Matched univariate RR and 95% CI by alcohol type*

Source	β	χ^2	RR[a]	95% CI
Male colon[b]				
Beer	−0.00	0.00	1.00	0.99–1.01
Wine	0.02	0.93	1.02	0.98–1.06
Spirit	0.08	9.33	1.08	1.03–1.13
Female colon[b]				
Beer	0.01	0.06	1.01	0.95–1.06
Wine	0.04	2.06	1.04	0.98–1.11
Spirit	0.13	4.51	1.13	1.01–1.27
Male rectum[c]				
Beer	−0.00	0.30	1.00	0.98–1.01
Wine	−0.02	1.42	0.98	0.95–1.01
Spirit	0.04	3.67	1.04	1.00–1.09
Female rectum[b]				
Beer	−0.03	1.06	0.97	0.92–1.03
Wine	0.11	5.22	1.11	1.02–1.22
Spirit	0.05	0.67	1.05	0.94–1.17

[a] RR expressed/glass/wk.
[b] These results are essentially unaltered when all three exposures are included in a single model.
[c] Inclusion of all three alcohol variables for male rectum in a single model raises RR (95% CI) for spirit consumption to 1.05 (1.01–1.10).

with alcohol consumption expressed per glass per week for both colon and rectum. Only spirits consumption was associated with increased RR at each site, significantly so in three of four sex-site categories. For colon cancer, these figures indicated approximately a doubling of risk for a glass per day of spirits in women and for two glasses per day in men. There was no association, in these data, between beer consumption and risk at either site. Separate analyses by subsite within the colon showed that the RR of distal colon cancer, the numerically predominant subsite, accounted for most of the above-mentioned risk variation and that risk of proximal (cecum and ascending) colon cancer was unrelated to alcohol consumption.

Eating frequency.—Table 9 shows the relationship between eating frequency (number of times per day, irrespective of size of meal) and RR of colon and rectal cancer, after controlling for total energy intake. There may be an increase of risk of colon, but not rectal, cancer associated with higher frequency of eating.

TABLE 9.—*Colon and rectal cancer and diet: Conditional logistic regression models; meal frequency (controlling for total energy intake) by sex*

Daily meal frequency	RR	95% CI
Male colon		
≤3	1.0	
4	1.3	0.7–2.4
≥5	1.6	0.9–2.7
Female colon		
≤3	1.0	
4	0.8	0.4–1.6
≥5	1.7	0.9–3.1
Male rectum		
≤3	1.0	
4	1.1	0.6–1.8
≥5	1.3	0.8–2.1
Female rectum		
≤3	1.0	
4	1.0	0.5–2.0
≥5	1.0	0.6–1.9

TABLE 10.—*Male colon cancer: Conditional logistic regression model*[a]

Variable	β	χ^2	RR	95% CI
Protein quintiles				
1			1.0	
2	0.78	3.39	2.2	1.0–5.0
3	1.04	6.73	2.8	1.3–6.2
4	0.76	3.40	2.2	1.0–4.8
5	0.91	4.40	2.5	1.1–5.8
Fiber per MJ of energy quintiles				
1			1.0	
2	−0.07	0.03	0.9	0.4–2.0
3	0.01	0.00	1.0	0.5–2.1
4	−0.28	0.44	0.8	0.3–1.7
5	0.10	0.06	1.1	0.5–2.4
Spirits consumption[b]	0.08	7.42	1.08	1.02–1.15
Occupation				
Professional and/or managerial			1.0	
Other	−1.17	16.06	0.3	0.2–0.6

[a] Overall risk function: Likelihood ratio, $\chi^2_{10}=36.01$; $P<.0001$.
[b] RR expressed/glass/wk.

Combined models.—Tables 10 and 11 show logistic regression models detailing the association between nutrients and RR of colon cancer controlling in women for reproductive variables (*16*) and in men for socioeconomic status, which proved to be a significant explanatory variable. All variables in these models are shown.

Colon cancer.—In summary, this study found that, for colon cancer, protein was the major nutrient associated

TABLE 11.—*Female colon cancer: Conditional logistic regression model*[a]

Variable	β	χ^2	RR	95% CI
Protein quintiles				
1			1.0	
2	0.97	4.34	2.6	1.1–6.6
3	0.77	2.57	2.2	0.8–5.5
4	1.16	6.19	3.2	1.3–8.0
5	1.35	7.08	3.9	1.4–10.4
Fiber per MJ of energy quintiles				
1			1.0	
2	−0.25	0.27	0.8	0.3–2.0
3	0.93	3.10	2.5	0.9–7.2
4	0.57	1.56	1.8	0.7–4.3
5	0.68	2.06	2.0	0.8–5.0
Spirits consumption[b]	0.12	2.96	1.12	0.98–1.28
OC use (mo)				
0			1.0	
1–24	−0.77	1.75	0.5	0.2–1.5
≥25	−1.42	2.93	0.2	0.1–1.2
Parity				
0			1.0	
1–2	−0.16	0.16	0.9	0.4–1.9
≥3	−1.07	6.42	0.3	0.2–0.8

[a] Overall risk function: Likelihood ratio $\chi^2_{13}=36.97$; $P=.0004$.
[b] RR expressed/glass/wk.

with increased RR in both sexes, showing about a doubling of risk in males and about a twofold-to-fourfold increase in females for the four upper quintiles relative to the lowest.

Age interacted with nutrient consumption so that the effect for males tended to be greater at older ages (the greatest RR was associated with total energy), whereas, for females, for left colon cancer and for the colon as a whole, RR estimates were higher at younger ages [*see* (*18*)].

Increased intakes of total fat, saturated fat, cholesterol, and total energy were more clearly associated with increased RR in females.

The increase in RR estimates for fiber exposure, particularly in women, was due partly to the complex relationship that fiber and energy bore to each other. The increased RR estimates for energy and protein, etc., are only evident at low fiber intake, but there was also an association between increasing fiber consumption and increasing estimates of RR.

Micronutrients did not appear to be related to the risk of colon cancer.

Overall, alcohol was associated with increases in RR of colon cancer in women but not in men. However, when analyzed by alcohol type, consumption of spirits was associated with about a 10% increase in RR per glass per week for both sexes.

Rectal cancer.—Protein, fat, saturated fat, and total energy were each associated with increased RR of rectal cancer in females consistently across all age groups and in males at older ages. Vitamin C was associated with a reduced RR of rectal cancer in women at all ages and in men until around 60 years of age. Spirits consumption in males and wine in females were associated with an increase of 5-10% in RR per glass per week.

At young ages, there was an increased RR of rectal cancer in males associated with a generalized low dietary intake. One possible interpretation of this was that protective factors such as vitamin C (and possibly fiber) were critically reduced by low total intakes at young ages. The crossover from reduced RR to increased RR at high consumption occurred a decade later for vitamin C than for the major nutrients; vitamin C was not associated with significantly increased RR, even at 75 years of age.

DISCUSSION

There are a series of issues that this study raises, the first items of which are methodologic.

This is the first community-based case-control study of large bowel cancer to be reported. Previous studies have relied on hospital cases (exclusively) and hospital controls (all studies except one). The use of a population-based cancer registry for cases and a population register for controls eliminates several of the biases inherent in hospital-based studies, particularly studies of dietary etiology; diets postulated to be related to colon cancer are also thought to bear on the risk of many other chronic diseases. Even traffic crashes (alcohol) and conditions such as osteoarthritis (obesity) are not free of this potential.

The dietary method chosen for this study is one that is well established for etiologic studies of cancer—a food frequency method (20-24). The use of standard serve (rather than self-described) sizes results in some misclassification and thus biasing of the RR toward 1.0. The method, in addition to satisfactory repeatability characteristics, is consistent with "common-sense" checks such as women reporting lower total consumptions than men and older persons reporting less total consumption than younger. Repeatability data suggest that even reports of past dietary patterns though "contaminated" by current practice allow ready differentiation into groups (*22*). Note was taken of the extent to which the presence of disease altered the current dietary practice. The inclusion of those whose diet had changed recently (both cases and controls) tended to bias the RR estimates toward 1.0 in women, arguing that the above estimates for women are somewhat conservative. The reverse, however, was true for the males.

Fat, protein, total energy, and meal frequency.—A central finding of this study is that total energy or protein or some other nutrient for which these are good markers in this study population (e.g., fat and saturated fat) are associated with increased risk of large bowel cancer—a finding consistent with the prior hypothesis and previous work. The judgment as to which nutrient is the relevant one, however, is very much determined by the biologic model invoked to explain the development of the disease; fat or saturated fat have usually been considered the most likely, since they stimulate increased BA excretion with subsequent initiation or promotion of a mucosal cancer (*8, 9*).

The absence of a monotonic dose-response effect both of protein (but *see* table 11) and of energy in relation to colon cancer indicates the possibility of a risk saturation point with at least 80% of the population exceeding it (*18, 28*). Factors other than diet, particularly genetic susceptibility, and, in women, reproductive behavior will therefore determine the additional individual variation in likelihood of developing colon cancer. We have discussed more extensively elsewhere the possible relevance of dose-response relationships and the problem of categorization of universal exposures (*18*). A linear dose-response relationship is only one of various possible and plausible models. The major argument for its applicability to cancer biology appears to rest only on crude analogy with pharmacologic and toxicologic models.

The only previous study in which the role of specific nutrients, as opposed to food groups, was able to be considered concluded that, on the strength of the relationships between RR estimates and dietary constituents, saturated fat was the most likely major dietary constituent to be part of the causal chain (*5*). That study expressed the results in terms of tertiles of exposure and presented them separately for males and females and for colon and rectum. The major methodologic difference between that study and this present one was the use of 2 control groups in the former study—one hospital group and one neighborhood group. They found RR for the highest tertile of saturated fat consumption compared with the lowest of approximately 2.5 for men and women.

Two earlier studies (*3, 4*)[4] had described a relationship between frequency of consumption of foods high in saturated fat and increased risk of large bowel cancer. Haenszel et al. (*29*) (studying the Hawaiian Japanese), Bjelke in Norway (*2*), and Phillips (*3*) each describe an association between meat consumption and risk. Several studies, however, have failed to find such a relationship.

Both nutrients and individual foods, while perhaps important in their own right, are also acting as markers for dietary intake in general. In the international correlation studies, no study has examined the relationship between mean energy intake and colon cancer; the commonest finding is a relationship between increased risk and consumption of animal protein, fat, and meat (*1*), these variables being closely correlated with each other and with total energy intake.

In examining smaller agglomerations of populations, e.g., States of the United States (*30*), United Kingdom, United States, Australia, and New Zealand over time (*31*), the relationship with these variables has not emerged as strongly. Liu et al. (*32*) have suggested cholesterol as the candidate exposure. Less direct evidence from earlier case-control studies concerns the relationship of nonmeat protein consumption—nutmeat, milk, fish—to *reduced* risk (*3*).

Most of the animal experiments and the human metabolic epidemiology have focused on the fat-BA model, with little attention paid to the possible role of protein or overall food intake. Reddy et al. (*33*), however, noted that high protein in the diet of rats, irrespective of source, is associated with elevated levels of bacterial β-glucuronidase activity in the large intestine, one of the enzymes postulated as relevant to the bile acid theory. Reddy et al. (*34*) have shown similar effects in humans on high meat vs. low meat diet. More recently, Wise et al. (*35*) have shown that dietary protein levels influence several bacterial enzymes, postulated to be relevant to bowel carcinogenesis, in the rat cecum.

Reddy et al. (*36*) have further shown that carcinogenesis is more likely to occur on a high fat, high protein diet than a low fat, low protein diet, irrespective of the fat and protein source. Topping and Visek (*37*) have shown that of rats fed 7.5% (low) dietary protein fewer than half developed tumors compared with those fed higher protein diets (15 or 22% protein) and that tumor numbers per rat were only 50% of that in the other 2 groups. (There was no evidence of a dose-response effect in relation to protein exposure in this animal experiment.) However, a high protein, low fat experiment has not been conducted.

[4] Phillips' criteria (*3*) for "high-saturated fat foods" are not defined; Dales et al. (*4*) used the criteria of foods containing ≥5% saturated fat.

Fiber.—There are several possibilities in relation to the apparent implausibility of an increased intake of dietary fiber itself being part of a causal chain leading (directly or indirectly) to increased risk of large bowel cancer.

One possibility is that the dietary instrument used varies in its capacity to provide an accurate picture of nutrient consumption. The data on repeatability (*22, 28*) do indeed suggest that dietary fiber is not as consistently reported as, e.g., alcohol or fat. However, this kind of essentially random inaccuracy ought to produce a conservative, but not reversed, estimate of the RR associated with that variable; there is no a priori reason to believe that this dietary misclassification might differ between cases and controls.

Another possibility is that cases may well have (in some instances, are known to have) increased their fiber intake postoperatively on the advice of their surgeon. This would indeed produce exactly the pattern noted, inasmuch as cases would be more likely to have an increased intake of fiber. However, *both* cases and controls were asked to describe their intake as it had been 12 months earlier if they had changed it either as a result of recent illness or for some other reason. As noted in "Subjects and Methods," only marginal differences were seen between those (both cases and controls) who had changed their diets recently and the rest of the population. Further, it was reasoned that the only increase in dietary fiber likely to be recommended would be the addition of bran to the daily intake. A variable—"fiber minus bran"—behaved in almost identical fashion to "all fiber"; bran accounted for very little of total dietary fiber intake (0.5–1.0% in males, 1.0–3.6% in females).

Lyon et al. (*38*) have recently argued that as numerous major nutrients, especially fat, protein, and fiber, are highly correlated with total energy intake, then, if cases consume more food than controls, each of these nutrients will be associated with increased RR. Thus, while only guilty by association, a putative protective factor may appear to increase the risk.

It was considered, reasoning as had Lyon (*38*), that the most likely explanation for increased risk associated with fiber was that total dietary fiber intake is closely associated with total food intake. Several other studies of free-living Australian populations (*20*) have shown intake of dietary fiber to be correlated with total energy intake. If, as in this study, total energy intake is associated with increased risk of bowel cancer, the increased risk associated with fiber is likely a problem of multicollinearity, the fiber merely acting as a marker for total energy or other major nutrient intakes.

Fiber from vegetable and cereal sources were considered in separate analyses. There appears to be little relationship between fiber consumption of both kinds and risk of colon cancer in males (and little difference between subsites). For females, cereal fiber is associated with increased risk and in dose-response fashion. This result is largely explained by its strong positive association with risk of distal colon cancer.

Despite our result appearing to be paradoxic for dietary fiber, it may cast some light on previously puzzling findings, which have been ignored in other studies.

The two studies of Haenszel et al. (*29, 39*) found an increased RR for colon cancer associated with high rice consumption in Japanese both in Japan and Hawaii. They comment on this finding on *both* occasions, only to say that it runs counter to the known low colon cancer risk of rice-eating populations. Despite their low risk, Japanese consume levels of fiber almost identical with this Australian population (*40*). Wynder et al. (*41*) found fruit intake to be associated with an increased RR of colorectal cancer, and Haenszel et al. (*29*) found legumes (particularly string beans) to be a risk factor. Martinez et al. (*42*) found an increasing RR of large bowel cancer associated with increasing fiber consumption and considered recall bias as a possible explanation.

Hill et al. (*43*) noted that dietary fiber and total dietary intake, as well as fat intake, increase with income in the Hong Kong population and that this in turn is positively associated with increasing risk of colorectal cancer. Although several correlation studies have found negative relationships between risk and cereal or fiber consumption (*44, 45*), the consistent "protective" factor in analytic studies has been vegetables rather than cereals. Thus Stocks (*46*), Bjelke (*2*), Phillips (*3*), Graham et al. (*47*), and Haenszel et al. (*39*) describe reduced risks associated with some variety of vegetable foods. Modan et al. (*48*) and Dales et al. (*4*) constructed high-fiber indices that showed a protective effect against large bowel cancer, but the overwhelming majority of the dietary constituents in these indices were vegetable rather than cereal. Further, of Modan's 73 high fiber items (≥0.5% of fiber), four were consumed *more* often by cases than by both sets of controls. Two of these were bourghul (cracked wheat) and oats (*48*). Jain et al. (*5*) found no relationship between *crude* fiber intake and risk of colorectal cancer.

Thus the finding in this present study, that cereal fiber is associated with increased risk of colon cancer in women, is not inconsistent with previous analytic studies, though it differs from popular belief and current hypotheses. In summary, the important observations on fiber are these: 1) High fiber consumption is associated with increased estimates of RR for colon cancer, particularly in women; and, within this group, it is particularly associated with risk of distal colon cancer and possibly only at older ages. 2) The relationship between fiber intake and consumption of other nutrients is complex among female cases but not among controls (and not among male cases and controls); female cases who consume low fiber also consume high intakes of other nutrients and food in general. Thus the increased estimates of RR for large bowel cancer observed for the female population as a whole were shown to be largely explained by the increased RR in those with a low fiber intake. 3) If there is *any* real increase in RR associated with high fiber consumption in women (independent of this complex relationship with other nutrients or total energy), then it is confined to an association with cereal fiber.

The differences between men and women with regard to fiber-related risk may partly reflect more accurate responses from women. The complex relationship between total energy and fiber noted above for women argues against its being a sole explanation; findings from several human and animal studies are relevant: Bowel transit time, fecal weight, and aspects of fecal biochemistry (e.g., pH) are each related to dietary fiber intake and have each been shown to vary between the sexes even when diets were controlled (*15*); cereal fiber has been shown to provoke cell proliferation differentially within the rat colon (*49*) and to enhance carcinogenesis (*50*); cellulose is associated with a distal shift and older age at appearance of tumors (*51, 52*).

Differences by age.—This study provides information on the way in which age interacts with dietary exposures. The interaction is with age at presentation (not age at, e.g., initial exposure) and therefore may reflect a relationship between dietary exposures and a critical exposure time *or* between such exposures and the biologic behavior of a cancer (perhaps, e.g., accelerating or retarding the rate of growth between transformation and clinical presentation).

The most striking feature related to the age interaction is the fact that, in fitted models (and in age-stratified analyses), the strength of the relationships between dietary exposures and risk of colon cancer is greater in women that are younger but in men that are older [for details *see* (*18*)].

Colon cancer has an overall sex ratio of around 1.0 but a female colon cancer excess for those between 25 and 55 years of age (*13, 15*). A higher risk at younger ages in relation to dietary exposures for women and the reverse for men is consistent with this overall pattern of colon cancer incidence.

One study (*53*), which has investigated both age and sex in the 1,2-dimethylhydrazine-induced rat model of large bowel carcinogenesis, found that males were approximately equally susceptible to developing bowel cancer at several ages while females had both lower incidence overall and declining susceptibility with age. Castration of males produced a susceptibility pattern similar to that of the females, while castration of females had no effect on age-related susceptibility (*53*). These age-sex patterns are also consistent with those noted in the present study for colon cancer.

For rectal cancer, age-associated risk for dietary variables is maximal at older ages in males and unaffected in females. This finding too is consistent with the descriptive epidemiology for rectal cancer, where the sex ratio is around 1.0 at younger ages but increases steadily with age, suggesting perhaps that older males are more susceptible to cumulative insults whether due to dietary or other exposures.

Micronutrients.—Vitamin C (*2*) and vitamin A (*54*) indices (constructed with reference to foods high in these micronutrients) have been postulated to be related to reduced risk of epithelial cancers as well as specifically cancer of colon and rectum. In the present study, vitamin C is associated with reduced estimates of RR for rectal cancer but no association is noted between either micronutrient and risk of colon cancer.

Jain et al. (*5*) failed to find a consistent relationship between vitamin C exposure and risk of colorectal cancer. DeCosse et al. (*55*) have described a decreased incidence of rectal polyps following vitamin C administration to patients with familial polyposis. Bruce et al. (*56*) noted a reduction of fecal mutagens as a consequence of vitamin C administration. Possible mechanisms are not established, but vitamin C is an antioxidant and is also known to reduce the absorption of nitrosamines (*56*).

Alcohol and beer.—In view of the extensive literature on the possible relationship between beer and, particularly, rectal cancer (*10-12*), the failure to find a relationship in this population is puzzling. Seven previous case-control studies have collected data on alcohol consumption; three of these found a relationship. A study in alcoholics (*57*) and a follow-up study in Norway (*58*) have also showed an excess rectal cancer risk for beer drinkers, but possibly no more marked than that for spirits drinkers. Of the two follow-up studies of brewery workers, one showed a relationship to rectal cancer (*11*) while the other did not (*59*).

No study has found a negative relationship between beer consumption and risk of colorectal cancer. Thus it may be that differences in the beer itself (brewing practices, other constituents) may be significant in determining risk; it may also be, however, that characteristics of the study design itself (e.g., the quality of the instrument) determine whether a relationship is detected.

In this study, a consistent colorectal cancer relationship was noted not specifically with beer but with spirits.

Tuyns et al. (*60*) have reported a slightly, but not significantly, elevated RR of rectal cancer in association with alcohol consumption; Wynder and Shigematsu (*61*) noted a higher percentage of heavy drinkers among male rectal cancer cases than among one of their control groups, but much of this appears to be due to differences in beer consumption. Modan et al. (*48*) described colon cancer cases as consuming a significantly different amount of alcohol from controls but specified neither the direction of this difference nor the beverage types involved.

The relationship between RR and alcohol consumption appears, as with most other dietary variables, to be stronger for colon cancer in females than in males. In regard to the reasons, similar considerations to those already examined for diet may be canvassed for the differences for alcohol.

However, females report consumption at lower levels than males; thus, even if males are misreporting their consumption overall, it still may be that women are more sensitive to the effects of alcohol on risk of large bowel cancer. This approach would be consistent with other observations about male-female responses to alcohol (*62*).

Nutrients, alcohol, and large bowel cancer; conclusions.—In the light of the findings discussed above, it is proposed that the fat-BA theory is incomplete and that this present study provides some evidence for a more extensive multifactorial hypothesis.

In addition to the role of fat (and possibly protein) stimulating BA production and in addition to fiber as a BA-sequestering agent and bacterial substrate (thus producing VFA and altering gut pH), a role is proposed for total dietary intake (including feeding frequency), for alcohol, and for sex hormone differences. Vitamin C is proposed as a protective agent against rectal cancer.

The level of total dietary intake is suggested to influence the rate of colon cell renewal and therefore to influence the rate at which cell transformation or at which malignant progression is likely to occur. Further, the frequency of feeding influences the profile of circulating BA—increased feeding frequency will increase the recirculation of the BA pool and thus the proportion of secondary BA.

Against this background, BA production will be influenced particularly by fat (and possibly protein), alcohol, female sex hormones, and possibly other endogenous influences producing a BA profile that has both long-term features and short-term fluctuations. Menopause will alter hormone levels—one long-term influence. BA profile will have a greater influence on proximal colon, but this effect will be reduced more distally where the general background stimulation associated with total dietary intake will be more important (*63*).

Low protein intake may improve the capacity of the liver to deal with exogenous carcinogens (*64*).

Fiber intake will exert several influences. In the presence of high energy (and fat) intake, low fiber will be associated with an increased risk, both as a consequence of increased BA exposure for the colon mucosa and the reduced VFA production; the VFA would normally act as differentiating agents for the colon cells, lower gut pH, and therefore reduce the effectiveness of BA-degrading bacterial enzymes (*65*).

High fiber intake may influence colon cell turnover rates proximally but not distally, in the same way that it does in rats.

In a susceptible population (and this may be tested by a longitudinal study), high fiber intakes will delay the appearance of cancer, thus being associated with paradoxic increase in (particularly distal) tumors among the old.

Female sex hormones influence not only BA production but other aspects of gut physiology, so that the female colon is more susceptible to dietary-associated carcinogenesis at a younger age. In addition to the established effects on transit time, fecal bulk, and pH, one should consider that bacterial populations may be directly influenced by female hormones, as may colon mucosal cells.

Rectal carcinoma will be influenced in part by the biologic and chemical activity of the fecal mass, therefore by some of the above factors (but probably not by VFA and pH), and also by the integrity of the mucosal cells that may be influenced by micronutrients, particularly by vitamin C.

REFERENCES

(1) ARMSTRONG B, DOLL R. Environmental factors and cancer incidence and mortality in different countries, with special reference to dietary practices. Int J Cancer 1975; 15:617-631.

(2) BJELKE E. Case-control study of cancer of the stomach, colon, and rectum. Oncology 1970; proceedings of the 10th International Cancer Congress. Chicago: Yearbook Medical Publ., 1971.

(3) PHILLIPS R. Role of life-style and dietary habits in risk of cancer among Seventh-Day Adventists. Cancer Res 1975; 35:3513-3522.

(4) DALES LG, FRIEDMAN GD, URY HK, et al. A case-control study of relationships of diet and other traits to colorectal cancer in American Blacks. Am J Epidemiol 1979; 109:132-144.

(5) JAIN M, COOK GM, DAVIS FG, et al. A case-control study of diet and colo-rectal cancer. Int J Cancer 1980; 26:757-768.

(6) REDDY BS, HEDGES AR, LAAKSO K, et al. Metabolic epidemiology of large bowel cancer, fecal bulk and constituents of high-risk North American and low-risk Finnish populations. Cancer 1978; 42:2832-2838.

(7) JENSEN OM, MACLENNAN R, WAHRENDORF J. Diet, bowel function, faecal characteristics and large bowel cancer in Denmark and Finland. Nutr Cancer 1982; 4:5-19.

(8) HILL MJ. Metabolic epidemiology of dietary factors in large bowel cancer. Cancer Res 1975; 35:3398-3402.

(9) IARC Intestinal Microecology Group. Dietary fibre, transit time, faecal bacteria, steroids, and colon cancer in two Scandinavian populations. Lancet 1977; 2:207-211.

(10) ENSTROM JE. Colorectal cancer and beer drinking. Br J Cancer 1977; 35:674-683.

(11) DEAN G, MACLENNAN R, MACLOUGHLIN H, et al. Causes of death in blue collar workers at a Dublin brewery 1954-73. Br J Cancer 1979; 40:581-589.

(12) POTTER JD, MCMICHAEL AJ, HARTSHORNE JM. Alcohol and beer consumption in relation to cancers of bowel and lung; an extended correlation analysis. J Chronic Dis 1982; 35:833-842.

(13) MCMICHAEL AJ, POTTER JD. Reproduction, endogenous and exogenous sex hormones, and colon cancer: A review and hypothesis. JNCI 1980; 65:1201-1207.

(14) WEISS NS, DALING JR, CHOW WH. Incidence of cancer of the large bowel in women in relation to reproductive and hormonal factors. JNCI 1981; 67:57-60.

(15) MCMICHAEL AJ, POTTER JD. Do intrinsic sex differences in lower alimentary tract physiology influence the sex-specific risks of bowel cancer and other biliary and intestinal diseases? Am J Epidemiol 1983; 118:620-627.

(16) POTTER JD, MCMICHAEL AJ. Large bowel cancer in women in relation to reproductive and hormonal factors: A case-control study. JNCI 1983; 71:703-709.

(17) MCMICHAEL AJ, POTTER JD. Parity and death from colon cancer in women: A case-control study. Community Health Stud 1984; 8:19-25.

(18) ———. Diet and colon cancer: Integration of the descriptive, analytic, and metabolic epidemiology. NCI Monogr 1985; 69:223-228.

(19) Australian Electoral Office. A quantitative assessment of electoral enrollment in Australia. Research Report, Australian Electoral Office. Canberra: AEO, 1983.

(20) BAGHURST KI, BAGHURST PA. The measurement of usual dietary intake in individuals and groups. Trans Menzies Found 1981; 3:139-160.

(21) BAGHURST KI, RECORD SJ. A computerised dietary analysis system for use with diet diaries or food frequency questionnaires. Community Health Stud 1984; 8:11-18.

(22) ROHAN TE, POTTER JD. Retrospective assessment of dietary intake. Am J Epidemiol 1984; 120:876-887.

(23) JAIN M, HOWE GR, JOHNSON KC, et al. Evaluation of a diet history questionnaire for epidemiologic studies. Am J Epidemiol 1980; 111:212-219.

(24) WILLETT WC, SAMPSON L, STAMPFER MJ, et al. Reproducibility and validity of a semiquantitative food frequency questionnaire. Am J Epidemiol 1985; 122:51-65.

(25) PAUL AA, SOUTHGATE DA. McCance and Widdowson's The Composition of Foods, 4th ed. London: Her Majesty's Stat Off, 1978.

(26) THOMAS S, CORDEN M. Tables of composition of Australian foods. Canberra: Australian Govt Printing Service, 1970.

(27) THOMAS DC. General relative-risk models for survival time and matched case-control analysis. Biometrics 1981; 37:673-686.

(28) POTTER JD. The aetiology of colorectal cancer with particular reference to diet, alcohol and reproductive status: A case-control study. PhD thesis. Brisbane: University of Queensland, 1984.

(29) HAENSZEL W, BERG JW, SEGI M, et al. Large bowel cancer in Hawaiian Japanese. J Natl Cancer Inst 1973; 51:1765-1779.

(30) ENSTROM JE. Colorectal cancer and consumption of beef and fat. Br J Cancer 1975; 32:432-439.

(31) MCMICHAEL AJ, POTTER JD, HETZEL BS. Time trends in colorectal cancer mortality in relation to food and alcohol consumption: US, UK, Australia and New Zealand. Int J Epidemiol 1979; 8:295-303.

(32) LIU K, STAMLER J, MOSS D, et al. Dietary cholesterol, fat and fibre, and colon cancer mortality. Lancet 1979; 2:782-785.

(33) REDDY BS, MANGAT S, WEISBURGER JH, et al. Effect of high-risk diets for colon carcinogenesis on intestinal mucosal and bacterial β-glucuronidase activity in F344 rats. Cancer Res 1977; 37:3533-3536.

(34) REDDY BS, WEISBURGER JH, WYNDER EL. Fecal bacterial β-glucuronidase: Control by diet. Science 1974; 183:416-417.

(35) WISE A, MALLETT AK, ROWLAND IR. Dietary protein and cecal microbial metabolism in the rat. Nutr Cancer 1983; 4:267-272.

(36) REDDY BS, NARISAWA T, WEISBURGER JH. Effect of a diet with high levels of protein and fat on colon carcinogenesis in F344 rats treated with 1,2-dimethylhydrazine. J Natl Cancer Inst 1976; 57:567-569.

(37) TOPPING DC, VISEK WJ. Nitrogen intake and tumorigenesis in rats injected with 1,2-dimethylhydrazine. J Nutr 1976; 106:1583-1587.

(38) LYON JL, GARDNER JW, WEST DW, et al. Methodological issues in epidemiologic studies of diet and cancer. Cancer Res 1983; 43:2392s-2396s.

(39) HAENSZEL W, LOCKE FB, SEGI M. A case-control study of large bowel cancer in Japan. JNCI 1980; 64:17-22.

(40) MINOWA M, BINGHAM S, CUMMINGS JH. Dietary fibre intake in Japan. Hum Nutr Appl Nutr 1983; 37A:113-119.

(41) WYNDER EL, KAJITANI T, ISHIKAWA S, et al. Environmental factors of cancer of the colon and rectum. II. Japanese epidemiological data. Cancer 1969; 23:1210-1220.

(42) MARTINEZ I, TORRES R, FRIAS Z, et al. Factors associated with adenocarcinomas of the large bowel in Puerto Rico. Adv Med Onc Res Educ 1975; 3:45-52.

(43) HILL M, MACLENNAN R, NEWCOMBE K. Diet and large-bowel cancer in three socioeconomic groups in Hong Kong (letter). Lancet 1979; 1:436.

(44) SCHRAUZER GN. Cancer mortality correlation studies. II. Regional associations of mortalities with the consumption of foods and other commodities. Med Hypotheses 1976; 2:39-49.

(45) BINGHAM S, WILLIAMS DR, COLE TJ, et al. Dietary fibre and regional large bowel cancer mortality in Britain. Br J Cancer 1979; 40:456-463.

(46) STOCKS P. Cancer incidence in North Wales and Liverpool region in relation to habits and environment. In: British Empire Cancer Campaign. 35th annual report. Suppl to part 2. 1957:1-127.

(47) GRAHAM S, DAYAL H, SWANSON M, et al. Diet in the epidemiology of cancer of the colon and rectum. JNCI 1978; 61:709-714.

(48) MODAN B, BARELL V, LUBIN F, et al. Low-fiber intake as an etiologic factor in cancer of the colon. J Natl Cancer Inst 1975; 55:15-18.

(49) JACOBS LR, WHITE FA. Modulation of mucosal cell proliferation in the intestine of rats fed a wheat bran diet. Am J Clin Nutr 1983; 37:945-953.

(50) JACOBS LR. Enhancement of rat colon carcinogenesis by wheat bran consumption during the stage of 1,2-dimethylhydrazine administration. Cancer Res 1983; 43:4057-4061.

(51) FREEMAN HJ, SPILLER GA, KIM YS. A double-blind study on the effects of differing purified cellulose and pectin fiber diets on

1,2-dimethylhydrazine-induced rat colonic neoplasia. Cancer Res 1980; 40:2661-2665.

(52) ———. A double-blind study on the effect of purified cellulose dietary fiber on 1,2-dimethylhydrazine-induced rat colonic neoplasia. Cancer Res 1978; 38:2912-2917.

(53) MOON RC, FRICKS CM. Influence of gonadal hormones and age on 1,2-DMH-induced colon carcinogenesis. Cancer 1977; 40:2502-2508.

(54) PETO R, DOLL R, BUCKLEY JD, et al. Can dietary betacarotene materially reduce human cancer rates? Nature 1981; 290:201-208.

(55) DECOSSE JJ, ADAMS MB, KUZMA JF, et al. Effect of ascorbic acid on rectal polyps of patients with familial polyposis. Surgery 1975; 78:608-612.

(56) BRUCE WR, VARGHESE AJ, WANG S, et al. The endogenous production of nitroso compounds in the colon and cancer at that site. In: Miller JA, Miller EC, Sugimura T, et al., eds. Naturally occurring carcinogens, mutagens and modulators of carcinogenesis. Baltimore: University Park Press, 1979.

(57) SUNDBY P. Alcoholism and mortality. New Brunswick: Rutgers Centre on Alcohol Studies, 1967.

(58) BJELKE E. Frequency of use of alcoholic beverages and incidence of cancer of the large bowel and other sites: Prospective study of 12,000 Norwegian men. Meeting on alcohol and cancer. Lyon: IARC, 1974.

(59) JENSEN OM. Cancer morbidity and causes of death among Danish brewery workers. Int J Cancer 1979; 23:454-463.

(60) TUYNS AJ, PEQUIGNOT G, GIGNOUX M, et al. Cancers of the digestive tract, alcohol and tobacco. Int J Cancer 1982; 30:9-11.

(61) WYNDER EL, SHIGEMATSU T. Environmental factors of cancer of the colon and rectum. Cancer 1967; 20:1520-1561.

(62) Editorial. The female alcoholic. Lancet 1977; 2:1015-1016.

(63) MCMICHAEL AJ, POTTER JD. Guest editorial: Host factors in carcinogenesis: Certain bile-acid metabolic profiles that selectively increase the risk of proximal colon cancer. JNCI 1985; 75:185-191.

(64) KARI FW, JOHNSTON JB, TRUEX CR, et al. Effect of dietary protein concentration on yield of mutagenic metabolites from 1,2-dimethylhydrazine in mice. Cancer Res 1983; 43:3674-3679.

(65) THORNTON JR. High colonic pH promotes colorectal cancer. Lancet 1981; 1:1081-1083.

END OF REPRINT E

Diet and Cancer of the Colon and Rectum: A Case-Control Study

JOHN D. POTTER AND ANTHONY J. MCMICHAEL

13

MONOCULTURES

A Blight on Human and Planetary Health

JOHN D. POTTER

Abstract

Naturally occurring ecosystems are highly complex almost everywhere. Human impact on the environment has, over tens of thousands of years, resulted in their transformation and simplification. The rate at which this has occurred has been accelerating with increases in population size and the development of industrial economies. Much of the impact is the result of food-raising practices, but other human choices regarding land and water use, including mining, forestry and the growth of cities, have also contributed.

The hallmark of the human footprint is monoculture, a result of deliberate choices in agriculture, the raising of animals for meat and dairy, and forestry, but now appearing, as an unintended by-product of human activity, in the oceans and soil. By definition, monoculture represents a decline of species over some particular area. As monoculture has become the widespread norm in food raising, species decline is occurring almost everywhere. There are other quantifiable, mostly detrimental, changes that extend out from monocultures and their impact on the simplification of ecosystems as chains and nets of causes and consequences. These span an array of intentional human behaviours designed to maintain monocultures and unforeseen outcomes for the planet and its inhabitants. Such inputs and outcomes include:

- kidnapping and slavery
- distortions of production systems
- fold changes over time of consumption of foods and nutrients, with impacts on human behaviour and health
- widespread and increasing antibiotic and hormone use
- similar increases in pesticide and herbicide use

- combinations of genetic modification of plants and pesticide use
- thus, selection against beneficial species and for unwanted species: microbial, animal and plant
- soil loss
- soil degradation
- pollution of soil, freshwater, oceans
- habitat destruction
- climate disruption.

It is not yet clear how we can reverse many of these trends, but monoculture is one of the central problems we need to solve in order to slow the decline of planetary and human health.

Introduction

Humans began as gatherer-hunters.[1] At varying times in the past 10–15,000 years and in various parts of the world, we began to domesticate animals and cultivate specific crops (Ponting, 1992). For much of our subsequent history, cultivated grains (sometimes as mixed-crop agriculture, sometimes more extensively planted as a single crop) have provided the majority of human energy intake, often supplemented by hunting, fishing and gathering, as well as by raising domesticated sources of animal protein in the form of eggs and dairy products and, relatively less importantly until quite recently, meat.

The following nutrients are rare in nature: sugar, salt, fat, meat, alcohol. The following sources of mood-altering drugs are similarly rare: tobacco, poppies, coca, marijuana, coffee, tea, cocoa. We have a taste for them all and, because they are rare and thus consumed at a high level infrequently, there have been no deleterious evolutionary consequences. Hence, we have not evolved any natural curbs on their frequent overconsumption. Based on our experience of crop raising, humans increasingly focused on raising these specific crops in more organised fashion. Today, this approach has led us to a high intake of energy-dense food and various combinations of drugs (alcohol has the dubious distinction of being an energy-dense drug). Thus, our response to the rarity of specific nutrients and drugs – once we had established that we did not have

1 The usual designation of hunter gatherers appeals to the Tarzanist fantasies of some commentators, but gathering has almost always been a much more secure source of dietary energy than hunting, across the world and throughout history.

just to gather and hunt – was to cultivate them to keep ourselves in calories and comfort. Our commitment to this approach has led us to more and more intensity in the way we raise our food (and drugs). This is the problem of monoculture.

From Gatherer-Hunters to Industrial Agriculture

The agriculture of settled communities is one of several human strategies aimed at ensuring a regular food supply. It has benefits as well as drawbacks when contrasted with the gatherer-hunter economy. It may be, as Ponting (1992) has suggested, that a population of around four million was all that could be supported by a gatherer-hunter lifestyle. However, there is good evidence that humans contributed to the reduced carrying capacity of the environment by hunting out megafauna over a relatively short period almost everywhere (Rule et al., 2012) – although climate change has also been important, whenever humans appeared in numbers, food animals became scarce, both locally and continent wide (Flannery, 1997, 2001; Lorenzen et al., 2011). This pattern has persisted to the present day. Settling down and raising crops overcomes the problem of the human-induced scarcity of hunted animals. Further, settlements can be established near a secure water supply and defended against animals, nomads, gatherer-hunters, other settled groups and refugees. Such settlements allow food storage, which evens out variations in supply, both seasonal and weather related. Settlement facilitates cooperation and builds communities, although these processes clearly began much earlier with gatherer-hunters. It allows specialisation and leisure for increased development of art and science (although, again, surely among the greatest human art is the work of gatherer-hunters at Chauvet and Lascaux, France, and other palaeolithic art galleries (Valladas et al., 2001; Balter, 2008)). Essentially, of course, settlement provides food security – dependent, always, on climate and weather.

The drawbacks of the peasant agricultural economy include a decline in the variety of food consumed; deficiency diseases, both because of this decline and because of the potential for crop failure; increased crowding compared to the gatherer-hunter lifestyle, with increasing risk of epidemic and endemic infectious diseases. There is always the possibility of multi-year crop failure and consequent starvation; a settled community finds it harder to move again and recapture the nomadic gatherer-hunter lifestyle. The Greenland cattle-raising community refused to acknowledge that the climate was worsening and that the growing season was shortening; this had disastrous consequences for the settlers (Gribbin and Gribbin, 1990). Nonetheless, some humans have been able to show appropriate flexibility: the north American (Iowa) Indians of Mill

Creek adapted to worsening climatic conditions by reverting to hunting and gathering as primary strategies after being successful grain farmers (Gribbin and Gribbin, 1990).

Much of subsequent human history has involved: small decentralised local populations; animal-assisted agriculture; a relatively 'inefficient' human labour-intensive production system, often with storage and loss problems, a low crop yield compared with what is now achieved with industrial farming and less intensive land use. Many of these aspects of inefficiency, however, are much closer to the behaviours needed to maintain long-term ecologic balance. The food production system, moreover, was efficient enough to ensure the growth of cities, especially in Europe, even if some of the impetus was provided by a decades-long recovery following huge human die-off as a result of epidemic disease (Tuchman, 1979). The food production system was highly dependent on weather, rainfall and temperature. Food distribution was via small-scale local markets, or even family/village self-contained production. Distances over which food was traded were small (though trade in more durable goods was over much longer distances). Finally, this economy also involved a distribution of wealth and power (e.g. peasant farmers and warrior/landowners in Europe) that ensured food security for the few and more tenuous survival for the many.

Initially, humans made transitions to something approaching monocultures with crops like sugarcane (see below). However, as the power of the ruling classes ensured a better transition from feudal states to a capitalist economy for the aristocrats and landowners than peasant farmers, much of the shared land, common land, 'wasteland' and woodland was seized and enclosed (nowhere more obviously than in England (Hoskins, 1970)). This allowed grain crops to be grown over larger areas, with some benefits from the resulting production efficiency but substantial loss of livelihood for the landless workers and smallholders, who, to survive, migrated to the cities, providing cheap labour for the Industrial Revolution.

Thus, we moved from a gatherer-hunter economy to peasant agriculture, with its mixed-cropping subsistence and focus on immediate needs for energy (mostly grain) supplemented by small quantities of animal protein. We became increasingly urban with an industrialised agriculture. By the 20th century, all was different: there had been a massive decrease in human labour and a corresponding increase in fossil fuel use to supply energy – the success of the Industrial Revolution in creating wealth in cities was increasingly used as a blueprint for agriculture. This energy use, along with the Haber–Bosch process of fixing atmospheric nitrogen to make inorganic fertilisers, allowed a vast increase in production capacity and was an essential driver of the 20th-century population rise (Smil, 1999). These changes were further augmented by the development of pesticides and herbicides, and from the middle of the

20th century, the intensive development (and restriction) of crop species; this 'Green Revolution' further increased food production capacity. The resulting industrialised agriculture is conducted over large areas, with reduced human labour input and no animals to provide either energy or fertilisers. It supplies large centralised populations and, with major changes in transport, allows extensive trade over large distances. The power and centralisation of control of production have increased (albeit with corporations having taken the place of warrior landowners), with many workers in the system (needed for harvest, particularly) living marginal lives on low wages and no job security. Much of this system, however, does not function according to neoliberal market models, but is highly subsidised by governments, further distorting the distribution of power and wealth.

It has been estimated that 30–50 per cent (1.2–2 billion tonnes (Bt)) of all human food produced is never consumed (Institution of Mechanical Engineers, 2013). Another estimate suggests that total production is around 19 megajoules (MJ) per person per day, but what is available for human consumption is around 8 MJ per person per day (McIntyre et al., 2008b). Yet today, we are trapped by the manufactured, but widespread, belief that we need to increase food production to supply a massive and still increasing human population. What is actually needed is an integrated food distribution and security system that is not driven by profit and protection but by human need and human-scale solutions (Nierenberg et al., 2011). Indeed, as Tudge (2013) has noted, industrial monocultures – the farming practices supposed to be feeding the world – in reality provide less than one-third of the world's food. Twenty per cent comes from fishing, hunting and back gardens, and half comes from small, mixed traditional farms (McIntyre et al., 2008a).

Our capacity for food production stretches the boundaries of what is possible for the planet. Industrialised agriculture, incarnated as extensive monoculture, is regarded as the norm for supplying the world's food. That, itself, is a false claim, but its deleterious consequences – to the planet and human health – abound. Three examples, sugar, meat and cereals, follow.

Sugar

Sugarcane, a grass initially from South Asia, provided a local luxury for much of human history. It began to be cultivated intensively in the 19th century, as a crop that has remained labour-intensive in many parts of the world to this day. In order to supply that labour, cane plantation owners turned to the African slave trade from the 18th century (Richardson, 1987), and to its marginally more benign South Pacific descendant in the 19th (Price and Baker, 1976). Almost zero-cost labour to produce a lucrative crop meant huge profits as a result of growing sales to an increasingly addicted population (Rönnbäck, 2007).

Sugar consumption in the UK around 1700 was less than 2 kg per year from multiple sources (Mintz, 1985); by 1990, in Australia, it was more than 40 kg per year (Espinel and Innes-Hughes, 2010) – a more than 20-fold increase, with comparable rises throughout the industrialised world. In the USA, sugar in soft drinks alone now accounts for about 13 per cent of daily dietary energy intake among teenagers (Jacobson, 2005).

The industry began (like tobacco) with kidnapping, slavery and casual murder to acquire the relevant workforce (Solow, 1987). As with agricultural workers in many parts of the world, sugarcane cutters often remain members of an informal, 'casual' labour force on low wages, with few rights or benefits. Even in high-income countries, cane cutting was a brutally hard seasonal job in hot conditions until largely replaced by mechanisation.

The deliberate human inputs into sugarcane production over the past 150 years have included 'clearing' of land for plantations; an early (1935) attempt at biologic control of pests (Phillips et al., 2006); use of conventional pesticides and herbicides; fertiliser use; and mechanisation and fossil fuel use.

Some of the unplanned outcomes for human health (see Table 13.1) include high consumption of sugar itself (Monteiro et al., 2011), leading to obesity, diabetes, caries, etc (Jacobson, 2005; Lustig et al., 2012); high alcohol consumption leading to alcoholism, trauma, violence and chronic disease, including cancer (Pelucchi et al., 2011); loss of jobs requiring physical labour, resulting in declining employment and declining physical activity in the population, but also reduction of workplace accidents and increased longevity.

Table 13.1 Sugar monoculture: Deliberate human inputs and unplanned outcomes.

Planned products	Planned inputs	Unplanned outcomes (human health)	Unplanned outcomes (planetary health)
Sugar		Obesity, diabetes, caries	
Alcohol		Alcoholism, trauma, violence, chronic disease, including cancer;	
	Sugar plantations		Habitat loss, decline in diversity
	Kidnapping and slavery (18th and 19th century)	Reduced longevity	Shifts in human populations
	Biologic pest control		Unchecked cane toads (*Bufo marinus*)
	Mechanization and fossil fuel use	Declining physical activity Declining employment Reduction of workplace accidents and increased longevity	Climate disruption
	Pesticides		Disruption of chemical cues, including those involved in reproduction
	Herbicides		Mangrove dieback Deleterious consequences for coral ecosystems
	Fertilizers		Decline in coral reef health particularly the rise in Crown of Thorns starfish (*Acanthaster planci*)

Source: Author's work.

Some of the unplanned outcomes for planetary health (Table 13.1) include habitat loss and decline in diversity (Gomiero et al., 2011); unchecked, rapidly evolving cane toads (*Bufo marinus*), which now have a range of more than 1 million square kilometres (Phillips et al., 2006); contributions to climate disruption as a result of industrialisation and mechanisation of agriculture (Rockström et al., 2009); decline in coral reef ecosystem health, particularly the rise in crown-of-thorns starfish (*Acanthaster planci*) as a result of fertiliser use and nutrient run-off (Brodie et al., 2005); mangrove dieback (Duke et al., 2005) and consequences for coral ecosystems (Lewis et al., 2009) as a result of herbicide exposure; disruption of chemical cues, including those involved in reproduction (Luccio-Camelo and Prins, 2011) in a variety of organisms by pesticides, which are widespread in coral ecosystems (Johnson and Ebert, 2000).

Meat

Humans have a long history of meat consumption, although our closest primate relatives are vegetarian (*Gorilla gorilla*) or low, but clearly not zero, meat consumers (*Pan troglodytes* and *Pan paniscus*) (Nishida and Uehara, 1983; Stanford, 1996; Hofreiter et al., 2010). Further, there is good evidence that some of our hominin cousins (*Australopithecus bahrelghazali*, *Paranthropus robustus* and *Australopithecus sediba*) were largely plant eaters (Balter et al., 2012; Henry et al., 2012a; Lee-Thorp et al., 2012). Evidence from contemporary gatherer-hunters suggests that the majority of their dietary energy is derived from plants. Nonetheless, by the end of the last ice age, some 10–12,000 years ago, humans demonstrated both extensive hunting skills and a taste for meat (Smil, 2002), devastating the megafauna on all continents except Africa, including Australia, as well as on islands (Flannery, 1997, 1999, 2001; Rule et al., 2012).

With the transition to a pastoral lifestyle, humans began to raise animals for meat and milk, in settlements or as seasonal nomads (these usually also raised crops) or fully nomadic (Ponting, 1992). In this economy, animals were raised on land not used for crops. As with the gatherer-hunter economy, the majority of dietary energy is derived from plant foods.[2] This land use ensured that the best soil was used for raising plant foods. It also allowed other land to be cleared of scrubby plants and improved by fertilisation with animal manure. Further, crop stubble could be used as animal food and, again, the fields fertilised and then allowed to lie fallow. The practices of crop rotation, mixed cropping and raising animals on more marginal land were central features of human agriculture across the world, although the crops and animals varied widely. Indeed, these practices still persist in many parts of the world. However, in those areas where agriculture has been replaced by industrial farming, much has changed: crops are not rotated; land does not lie fallow; animals have become a dominant 'crop'; and land of any quality, including land hacked out of pristine rainforest, is used. Livestock now occupy 30 per cent of the Earth's entire land surface, mostly permanent pasture but including 33 per cent of the global arable land, which is dedicated to producing feed. In Latin America, about 70 per cent of former Amazon forest has been turned over to grazing (Steinfeld et al., 2006); animals are irrelevant to soil fertility (indeed CAFOs[3] ensure that the soil and groundwater are damaged by excretions); artificial fertilisers and consequent soil degradation are common; animals have often ceased to feed on grass and consume far more energy-dense food in the form of grains and legumes.

2 There were and are clearly some exceptions to this, particularly among nomadic pastoralists and among humans who live at northern extremes but, even there, plant foods are important, including those harvested from the stomach contents of herbivores.

3 Concentrated animal feeding operations, now used extensively for cattle in the USA and for pigs and chickens in many parts of the world.

This approach to animal raising increases greatly the availability of meat (refrigeration and freezing have also been important). This, in turn, has increased demand for meat, such that the current level of consumption in rich countries is unprecedented in human history. Meat consumption in traditional agricultural societies was rarely higher than 5–10 kg a year; in most subsistence peasant societies of the Old World, meat was eaten once a week or less, with relatively larger amounts consumed only during festive occasions. (Smil, 2002). Meat consumption in Australia, the USA and New Zealand is now around 110–120 kg per year (a 12- to 24-fold increase). India, in contrast, has a per capita consumption around 4 kg a year (Espinel and Innes-Hughes, 2010) (see also FAOSTAT: faostat3.fao.org/home/index.html#COMPARE).

There are unplanned consequences (see Table 13.2) of this shift from raising animal protein as a modest supplement to a plant-based diet to providing as much as 15–20 per cent of total energy (in India, the proportion is less than 1 per cent). For human health, those consequences include elevated disease – obesity, cardiovascular disease, diabetes and cancer – as a result of high consumption of meat and fat (Linos et al., 2008); accelerated human sexual development either as a result of meat and fat consumption itself (Rogers et al., 2010) or possibly arising from low-dose, naturally occurring or exogenous growth-promoting hormones in meat (Courant et al., 2008); extensive antibiotic resistance among organisms that affect humans, e.g. *Salmonella*, *Escherichia coli*, following antibiotic use to promote animal growth (Health Council of the Netherlands, 2011) – about 80 per cent of all antibiotics sold in the USA are used in animals (Food and Drug Administration, 2013). There has been a reduction of available human food (and consequent hunger for those reliant on grain and subsistence agriculture) as cattle are fed energy-dense grains and legumes: more than 97 per cent of the soymeal produced globally is fed to livestock (Steinfeld et al., 2006). There are higher risks of bacterially infected meat from animals raised in the highly crowded settings of feedlots and CAFOs (Price et al., 2007; also www.cdc.gov/salmonella/typhimurium-groundbeef/010512/index.html); this leads to recommendations to consume heavily cooked meat, a source of colorectal carcinogens (Potter, 1999); crowding also increases the risk of *Salmonella*-infected eggs. Pig CAFOs act as a point source and 'mixing vessel' for recombination of epidemic influenza strains (Gray and Kayali, 2009; Forgie et al., 2011) and mixing animal vaccines has been shown, on at least one occasion, to lead to the emergence of a virulent field strain as a result of the recombination of two attenuated strains in the setting of a factory farm (Lee et al., 2012). Current feeding practices have also ensured the ill health of the animals themselves. Some of the resultant diseases are zoonoses: bovine spongiform encephalopathy was a direct result of recycling infected animal parts as food to obligate herbivores (Matthews, 1990).

Table 13.2 Meat monoculture: Deliberate human inputs and unplanned outcomes.

Planned products	Planned inputs	Unplanned outcomes (human health)	Unplanned outcomes (planetary health)
Meat and eggs **Animal fat** **Overcooked meat**		Chronic disease, including cardiovascular disease, obesity, diabetes, cancer, etc.	
	Clearing of prairie, woodland, etc, for cattle		Habitat loss, decline in biodiversity
	Hard-footed animals on fragile topsoil		Topsoil loss
	Rainforest destruction		Habitat loss, decline in biodiversity, climate disruption
	Water use		Aquifer depletion
	Total biomass of cattle four times that of humans		Methane production leading to climate disruption
	Hormone use to stimulate growth, e.g. cattle, fowl	Effects on human sexual development	Environmental/ reproductive effects, e.g. on fish
	Antibiotic use to stimulate growth, e.g. pigs	Antibiotic resistance among organisms that affect humans, e.g. *Salmonella, Escherichia coli*	
	Switch to grain feeding	Reduction of human food supply	
	Concentrated animal feeding operations (CAFOs)	*E. coli*-infected meat supply *Salmonella*-infected eggs Influenza point source Vaccine recombination leading to virulent field strain from two attenuated strains	Groundwater pollution
	Culls to protect cattle against tuberculosis, e.g. of bison, badgers		Decline in biodiversity

Source: Author's work.

Some of the unplanned outcomes for environmental and planetary health (Table 13.2) include habitat loss and decline in diversity (some decline in biodiversity is quite deliberate, with the intensive culling of badgers (Steinfeld et al., 2006) and bison from specific regions, with the dubious goal of protecting cattle from tuberculosis); rainforest destruction (Steinfeld et al., 2006);

topsoil loss, particularly in Australia (Fanning, 1999); disruption of reproduction in fish and amphibians following exposure to environmentally relevant concentrations of steroid hormones (Vandenberg et al., 2012); the depletion of aquifers (Steinfeld et al., 2006) – it takes more than 110,000 litres of water to produce 1 kg of meat protein (Mekonnen and Hoekstra, 2010). The production of methane is now estimated to be 65 million tonnes (Mt) per year from beef and dairy cattle enteric rumination, another 20 Mt from other ruminants and a further 18 Mt from animal manure, accounting for 37 per cent of anthropogenic methane (with 23 times the global warming potential of CO_2) and for 65 per cent of anthropogenic nitrous oxide (almost 300 times the potential of CO_2), the great majority from manure. Livestock are also responsible for groundwater pollution, as well as 64 per cent of anthropogenic ammonia emissions, which contribute significantly to acid rain and acidification of ecosystems (Steinfeld et al., 2006). There are major contributions to global climate disruption from the combination of rainforest destruction and the production of greenhouse gases: at 18 per cent of all greenhouse gases, the livestock sector generates more than transport (Steinfeld et al., 2006).

In a world of stalling cereal production, grain is now being used to make biofuels and to feed cattle. Meat and dairy animals now account for about 20 per cent of the total terrestrial animal biomass – about four times that of humans (Steinfeld et al., 2006). Accordingly, world meat production and consumption is continuing to increase, but with marked inequalities and new attitudes to food; whereas, once, plant foods were staples and meat was the garnish, now, increasingly, meat is seen as essential and plants much less so. Nonetheless, of course, grain remains the major source of human dietary energy that it became with the establishment of settled farming communities. What has changed is that cereals, too, are a central part of how we raise food as monocultures.

Cereals

The features of medieval European (and probably continuously from much earlier) village farming included shared fields and shared labour; mixed crops; rotation to allow fallowing and grazing; and (obviously) the use of animals for ploughing. This pattern has been particularly well characterised by Hoskins for England (Hoskins, 1970), who also chronicled the changes to the mid-20th century.

Enclosures meant more private property and much clearer title to land; loss of woodland; loss of shared labour; loss of common land. It also meant marginalising smallholders, and often deprivation of their livelihood. John Clare (1793-1864), the working class romantic poet, put it like this in *The Fallen Elm*:

> It grows the cant term of enslaving tools
> To wrong another by the name of right;
> Thus came enclosure – ruin was its guide,
> But freedom's cottage soon was thrust aside
> And workhouse prisons raised upon the site.
> E'en nature's dwellings far away from men,
> The common heath, became the spoiler's prey
> The rabbit had not where to make his den
> And labour's only cow was drove away.
> No matter – wrong was right and right was wrong,
> And freedom's bawl was sanction to the song...
>
> In freedom's name the little that is mine.
> And there are knaves that brawl for better laws
> And cant of tyranny in stronger power
> Who glut their vile unsatiated maws
> And freedom's birthright from the weak devour.

The loss of woodland meant loss of biodiversity. Hedgerows, which from then increasingly marked field boundaries, still provided some cover for birds and beneficial insects.

Since then, this pattern (which we think of as quintessentially defining the English countryside (Hoskins, 1970)) has given way to increasing 'prairie-isation'; this pattern is not like the boundary-free fields that had existed earlier, particularly because a great deal of the woodland and wild land disappeared with enclosures. Over the past 50 years or so, the hedgerows have been eliminated and mechanised farming has been facilitated – both ploughing and harvesting; short-term efficiency has thereby been improved and immediate financial costs reduced. However, much else has deteriorated, much has been lost.

Other farming systems, for example in Australia and North America, already used very large areas and were extensively mechanised relatively quickly. However, much was lost in the USA as the real biodiversity of the prairie succumbed to the plough – elegiacally chronicled by Aldo Leopold (1949).

Rice, the predominant staple in 17 countries in Asia and the Pacific, as well as in countries in the Americas and Africa, provides 20 per cent of the world's dietary energy supply, about the same proportion as wheat and about four times that of maize (FAO, 2012). Grown largely in necessarily flat, flooded fields and extensively on smaller holdings, rice is less amenable both to very large single areas under cultivation and to mechanisation (Van den Berg et al., 2007). However, there are increasing approaches to mechanisation, both for planting (Dixit et al., 2007) and harvesting (Horio, 2009).

The major benefit of widespread cereal cultivation, rather than mixed crops, crop rotation and small-scale animal/plant raising, is the ability to secure a more predictable supply of dietary energy. Indeed, the cereal monocultures of Australia and North America, particularly, allow an extensive export trade; other former importers have become exporters following the 'Green Revolution'. The major planned inputs in cereal monocultures include not only the extensive 'clearing' of land – woodland, prairie and rainforest – but also considerable increases in mechanisation and the use of fertilisers, herbicides and pesticides.

Unplanned consequences for human health (see Table 13.3) include the fact that maize and other cereals are now used to provide not only whole food but also increasing numbers of food fractions unrecognisable by our ancestors. These include high-fructose corn syrup (HFCS), which is widely used as an energy-dense sweetener in many manufactured foods. Many of the metabolic consequences of high exposure to fructose are like those of alcohol (Lustig, 2010). HFCS also provides empty calories, increasing the incidence of chronic disease, including obesity and diabetes (see above). Grain is also used to produce alcohol, high consumption of which also elevates chronic diseases, including cancer and alcoholism, as well as contributing extensively to trauma and violence. The use of human food to make biofuel, alcohol and high-value food fractions also means reduced food availability in marginal economies (Mitchell, 2008). Although the 'Green Revolution' produced multiple problems (Shiva, 1991; Hazell, 2009), it did increase crop yield substantially. In contrast, the use of genetically modified (GM) varieties shows little or no improvement in yield, and indeed, often a lower yield than conventional strains (Gurian-Sherman, 2009). Declining physical activity, as well as declining employment, follow from widespread mechanisation of farming, although the reduction in the number of workers who spend their lives in very hard physical labour has contributed to increased longevity in some settings. Use of specific pesticides and herbicides has increased risk of lymphoma among the highly exposed (Kogevinas et al., 1997); there may be a less detectable burden across the population.

Table 13.3 Cereal monoculture: Deliberate human inputs and unplanned outcomes.

Planned products	Planned inputs	Unplanned outcomes (human health)	Unplanned outcomes (planetary health)
Cereals **Derived food fractions (including white flour, corn syrup)**		Obesity, diabetes, caries, etc.	
Alcohol		Alcoholism, trauma, violence, chronic disease, including cancer	
Biofuels		Reduced food availability in marginal economies	
	Cereal fields, cleared from prairie, forest, etc, or concentrated by enclosures and later by elimination of hedgerows (UK)		Habitat loss, decline in diversity
	Mechanisation and fossil fuel use	Declining physical activity Declining employment Increased longevity	Climate disruption
	Pesticides, particularly neonicotinoids		Colony collapse disorder among honeybees (*Apis mellifera*, etc.) Loss of other beneficial insects and bird-eating insects Development of pesticide resistance in unwanted species, which leads, in turn, to increased use of pesticides (vicious circle)
	Herbicides	Lymphoma	Herbicide resistance among unwanted plants, leading to greater herbicide use (vicious circle) leading to 'need' for development of genetically modified (GM) strains
Genetically modified (GM) strains		No improvement in yield; often a lower yield than conventional strains	Loss of beneficial insects, e.g. from insertion of *Bacillus thuringiensis* genes Increased herbicide use on GM herbicide-resistant maize further increased as herbicide resistance develops among unwanted plants
	Fertilisers		Soil degradation

Source: Author's work.

Some of the unplanned outcomes for environmental and planetary health (Table 13.3) include increasing habitat loss and decline in diversity as a consequence of land clearing (Chamberlain et al., 2000); fresh water loss and aquifer depletion – in 2000, agriculture accounted for 70 per cent of the world's fresh water consumption (Steinfeld et al., 2006); greenhouse gases and climate disruption that follows from mechanisation of farming and fossil fuel (Potsdam Institute for Climate Impact Research and Climate Analytics, 2012). Pesticides (particularly neonicotinoids) have a major influence on marked declines in honeybees (*Apis mellifera*) and other pollinators (Gill et al., 2012; Henry et al., 2012b; Whitehorn et al., 2012). Use of pesticides ensures both loss of other beneficial insects and bird-eating insects and the development of pesticide resistance in unwanted species (Heckel, 2012), which leads, in turn, to increased use of pesticides (vicious circle). Herbicide resistance among unwanted plants leads to greater herbicide use (another vicious circle) and, together with insecticide resistance among unwanted species, has led to justifications for the development of GM strains that are resistant to herbicides or that carry genes for pesticides (e.g. insertion of *Bacillus thuringiensis* genes). However, this has increased biocide use, which, in turn, has accelerated herbicide resistance among unwanted species in an ever-tightening vicious circle (Benbrook, 2012). There are now more than 200 herbicide-resistant species across the world (www.weedscience.org/summary/home.aspx). GM insecticide-producing crops also contribute to the loss of beneficial insects (Hilbeck et al., 2012). There are more contested data that suggest that use of GM cereals and the associated high use of glyphosate may have consequences for mammalian health as well (European Food Safety Authority, 2012; Séralini et al., 2012).

Other Monocultures

Other monocultures include those consequent upon wide-scale use of forests of pine, eucalyptus and other trees. Clearing for such forests means soil loss, acidification and salinisation; reduced biodiversity; species and habitat loss; and reduced water availability for nearby communities (Cannell, 1999; Jackson et al., 2005; Karumbidza and Menne, 2011). Large-scale fishing operations look a lot like strip-mining of the oceans (Puig et al., 2012) and have produced the emergence of untoward unplanned monocultures (Acuña et al., 2011; Condon et al., 2011). Increasing reliance on small numbers of plant species means loss of varieties and loss of genetic variation. This is particularly concerning for important human crops like bananas (D'Hont et al., 2012) and tomatoes (The Tomato Genome Consortium, 2012).

A Counterfactual World

It is possible to ask what the world might be like if we had not developed industrialised food production. Certainly, the fixing of nitrogen was a key step in improving productivity (Smil, 2000), which contributed, in turn, to rapid changes in human population size. Now, of course, we could not feed the world's population without inorganic fertilisers (Smil, 1999), but it is equally true that we would not have had the growth of population without the food the fertilisers made possible. Could we have lowered infant mortality rates and improved longevity without markedly increasing the size of the human population (itself now the greatest burden on planetary health and a cause of the Anthropocene mass extinctions)? Could we have somehow made a transition to a world where life was not nasty, brutish and short for most? It seems as though, if industrialised agriculture supplied only one-third of all food, we might have been able to do it – but not within the structure of current-day oligopoly capitalism and massive protectionism for large food-producing corporations. Now, it has become hard to picture a way back – or forward.

Events and Trends

Humans have become good at rapid disaster management. However, we are very poor at slow disaster management, including increasingly hostile environmental conditions and climate disruption. Although the short-term advantages of monocultures are definable and include the provision of adequate food for a large proportion of the seven billion humans now alive (benefits for the many), as well as power and control of much of that food supply by a small number of individuals and corporations (benefits for the few), there are obvious and growing problems that we need to solve quickly if we are not to live in a world dominated by catastrophic collapse across the environment. We are now facing, not necessarily in order of importance or imminence: the accelerating disappearance of birds, which are key insectivores, and thus, the increasing appearance of insects in plague proportions (consequences include declining crop yields and increasing insect-borne diseases); the accelerating disappearance of bees, which are not relevant for cereals and legumes but, of about 100 crops that provide 90 per cent of the world's food, 71 are pollinated by bees (United Nations Environment Programme (UNEP), 2010); out-of-control herbicide-resistant weeds, competing for food-producing land; accelerating loss of rainforest; increasing climate disruption with effects on coastal lands, temperatures, water supplies, rainfall and weather patterns; growing loss of biodiversity; increasing use of human food for cattle; more frequent crop failure as a result of degraded soil, lack of new arable land and falling water supplies;

perhaps GM crop failure as a result of unforeseen weaknesses in the newly cobbled genomes – and, as a result of these, increasing food deprivation for the poor but increasing obesity, diabetes, coronary heart disease and cancer for the rich.

Although much of this could flow just from increasing human numbers and our neglect and abuse of the only planet we have (Jenkins, 2003), energy-profligate, herbicide- and pesticide-addicted monoculture is making these problems that much more severe, that much closer at hand and that much more urgently in need of attention.

One of the reviewers of this chapter properly noted that I needed to acknowledge that all was not dismal and that there were alternatives (both goals and practices) to the road we were on, involving, for instance improved distribution (Nierenberg et al., 2011); scrutiny and labelling of GM food (European Commission Directorate General for Health and Consumers, 2010) (although evidence of effective field control is scant (Bauer-Panskus et al., 2013) and expenditure on misinformation is extensive – see the Proposition 522 fight in Washington, USA (www.organicconsumers.org/essays/did-anti-gmo-movement-really-lose-washington); alternative pest-control systems (Lewis et al., 1997; Chandler et al., 2011); ecologic agricultural management (Buck and Scherr, 2011; La Via Campesina, 2013); and the food sovereignty movement (Claeys, 2012; La Via Campesina, 2013). I acknowledge, applaud and support these activities (among other things, I grow organic food and keep bees), but I remain sceptical of long-term beneficial outcomes when these trends are arrayed against the power of sociopathic international capitalism.

Charles Darwin begins the final paragraph of *Origin of Species* with the following:

> It is interesting to contemplate a tangled bank, clothed with many plants of many kinds, with birds singing on the bushes, with various insects flitting about, and with worms crawling through the damp earth, and to reflect that these elaborately constructed forms, so different from each other, and dependent upon each other in so complex a manner, have all been produced by laws acting around us. (Darwin, 1883)

He then enumerates those laws, which include growth and reproduction, inheritance, variability, 'a ratio of Increase so high as to lead to a Struggle for Life', natural selection, divergence of character and extinction. We seem, increasingly, to find ways to disrupt, mock or intensify the impact of these laws. We do so at growing peril to ourselves and to the planet.

References

Acuña, J.L., López-Urrutia, Á. & Colin, S. 2011. Faking giants: the evolution of high prey clearance rates in jellyfishes. *Science* 333, 1627–9.

Balter, M. 2008. Going deeper into the Grotte Chauvet. *Science* 321, 904–5.

Balter, V., Braga, J., Telouk, P. & Thackeray, J.F. 2012. Evidence for dietary change but not landscape use in South African early hominins. *Nature* 489, 558–60.

Bauer-Panskus, A., Hamberger, S. & Then, C. 2013. *Transgene Escape: Global Atlas of Uncontrolled Spread of Genetically Engineered Plants*. Testbiotech, Munich, Germany.

Benbrook, C. 2012. Impacts of genetically engineered crops on pesticide use in the U.S. – the first sixteen years. *Environmental Sciences Europe* 24, 24. doi:10.1186/2190-4715-24-24.

Brodie, J., Fabricius, K., De'ath, G. & Okaji, K. 2005. Are increased nutrient inputs responsible for more outbreaks of crown-of-thorns starfish? An appraisal of the evidence. *Marine Pollution Bulletin* 51, 266–78.

Buck, L.E. & Scherr, S.J. 2011. Moving ecoagriculture into the mainstream. In: Nierenberg, D., Halweil, B.A., Androa, R.G., Benbrook, C., Binagwaho, M-A., Buck, L.E., et al. (eds) *State of the World 2011. Innovations that Nourish the Planet*. Worldwatch Institute, New York, USA, 15–26.

Cannell, M.R. 1999. Environmental impacts of forest monocultures: water use, acidification, wildlife conservation, and carbon storage. *New Forests* 17, 239–62.

Chamberlain, D.E., Fuller, R.J., Bunce, R.G.H., Duckworth, J.C. & Shrubb, M. 2000. Changes in the abundance of farmland birds in relation to the timing of agricultural intensification in England and Wales. *Journal of Applied Ecology* 37, 771–88.

Chandler, D., Bailey, A.S., Tatchell, G.M., Davidson, G., Greaves, J. & Grant, W.P. 2011. The development, regulation and use of biopesticides for integrated pest management. *Philosophical Transactions of the Royal Society B: Biological Sciences* 366, 1987–98.

Claeys, P. 2012. The creation of new rights by the food sovereignty movement: the challenge of institutionalizing subversion. *Sociology* 46, 844–60.

Condon, R.H., Steinberg, D.K., del Giorgio, P.A., Bouvier, T.C., Bronk, D.A., Graham, W.M., et al. 2011. Jellyfish blooms result in a major microbial respiratory sink of carbon in marine systems. *Proceedings of the National Academy of Sciences (USA)*. 108, 10225–30.

Courant, F., Antignac, J.-P., Laille, J., Monteau, F., Andre, F. & Le Bizec, B. 2008. Exposure assessment of prepubertal children to steroid endocrine disruptors. 2. Determination of steroid hormones in milk, egg, and meat samples. *Journal of Agricultural and Food Chemistry* 56, 3176–84.

D'Hont, A., Denoeud, F., Aury, J.-M., Baurens, F.-C., Carreel, F., Garsmeur, O., et al. 2012. The banana (*Musa acuminata*) genome and the evolution of monocotyledonous plants. *Nature* 488, 213–7.

Darwin, C. 1883. *The Origin of Species by Means of Natural Selection or the Preservation of Favoured Races in the Struggle for Life*. John Murray, London, UK.

Dixit, A., Khurana, R., Singh, J. & Singh, G. 2007. Comparative performance of different paddy transplanters developed in India – a review. *Agricultural Review* 28, 262–9.

Duke, N.C., Bell, A.M., Pederson, D.K., Roelfsema, C.M. & Bengtson Nash, S. 2005. Herbicides implicated as the cause of severe mangrove dieback in the Mackay region, NE Australia: consequences for marine plant habitats of the GBR World Heritage Area. *Marine Pollution Bulletin* 51, 308–24.

Espinel, P. & Innes-Hughes, C. 2010. Apparent consumption of selected foods and household food expenditure. Monitoring Update. PANORG, University of Sydney, Sydney, NSW, Australia.

European Commission Directorate General for Health and Consumers 2010. Evaluation of the EU legislative framework in the field of GM food and feed: Framework Contract for evaluation and evaluation related services – Lot 3: Food Chain. Final Report. European Commission, Brussels, Belgium.

European Food Safety Authority 2012. Final review of the Séralini et al. (2012a) publication on a 2-year rodent feeding study with glyphosate formulations and GM maize NK603 as published online on 19 September 2012 in Food and Chemical Toxicology. *EFSA Journal* 10, 2986.

Fanning, P.C. 1999. Recent landscape history in arid western New South Wales, Australia: a model for regional change. *Geomorphology* 29, 191–209.

FAO 2012. *FAO Statistical Year Book 2012*. FAO, Rome, Italy.

Flannery, T.F. 1997. *The Future Eaters. An Ecological History of the Australasian Lands and People*. Reed New Holland, Sydney, NSW, Australia.

Flannery, T.F. 1999. Debating extinction. *Science* 283, 182–3.

Flannery, T.F. 2001. *The Eternal Frontier. An Ecological History of North America and its Peoples*. Grove Press, New York, USA.

Food and Drug Administration 2013. 2011 Summary Report on Antimicrobials Sold or Distributed for Use in Food-Producing Animals. Food and Drug Administration, Department of Health and Human Services, Washington, DC, USA.

Forgie, S.E., Keenliside, J., Wilkinson, C., Webby, R., Lu, P., Sorensen, O., et al. 2011. Swine outbreak of pandemic Influenza A virus on a Canadian research farm supports human-to-swine transmission. *Clinical Infectious Diseases* 52, 10–8.

Gill, R.J., Ramos-Rodriguez, O. & Raine, N.E. 2012. Combined pesticide exposure severely affects individual- and colony-level traits in bees. *Nature* 491, 105–8.

Gomiero, T., Pimentel, D. & Paoletti, M.G. 2011. Environmental impact of different agricultural management practices: conventional vs. organic agriculture. *Critical Reviews in Plant Sciences* 30, 95–124.

Gray, G.C. & Kayali, G. 2009. Facing pandemic influenza threats: the importance of including poultry and swine workers in preparedness plans. *Poultry Science* 88, 880–4.

Gribbin, J. & Gribbin, M. 1990. *Children of the Ice*. Basil Blackwell Ltd, Oxford, UK.

Gurian-Sherman, D. 2009. *Failure to Yield. Evaluating the Performance of Genetically Engineered Crops*. UCS Publications, Cambridge, Massachusetts, USA.

Hazell, P.B.R. 2009. The Asian Green Revolution. IFPRI Discussion Paper. International Food Policy Research Institute (IFPRI), Washington, DC, USA.

Health Council of the Netherlands 2011. *Antibiotics in Food Animal Production and Resistant Bacteria in Humans*. Health Council of the Netherlands, The Hague, the Netherlands.

Heckel, D.G. 2012. Insecticide resistance after *Silent Spring*. *Science* 337, 1612–4.

Henry, A.G., Ungar, P.S., Passey, B.H., Sponheimer, M., Rossouw, L., Bamford, M., et al. 2012a. The diet of *Australopithecus sediba*. *Nature* 487, 90–3.

Henry, M., Beguin, M., Requier, F., Rollin, O., Odoux, J.-F., Aupinel, P., et al. 2012b. A common pesticide decreases foraging success and survival in honey bees. *Science* 336, 348–50.

Hilbeck, A., Meier, M. & Trtikova, M. 2012. Underlying reasons of the controversy over adverse effects of Bt toxins on lady beetle and lacewing larvae. *Environmental Sciences Europe* 24, 9.

Hofreiter, M., Kreuz, E., Eriksson, J., Schubert, G. & Hohmann, G. 2010. Vertebrate DNA in fecal samples from bonobos and gorillas: evidence for meat consumption or artefact? *PLoS One* 5, e9419.

Horio, H. 2009. Stripping process for removing grains: history and consequence. *Engineering in Agriculture, Environment and Food* 2, 120–3.

Hoskins, W. 1970. *The Making of the English Landscape*. Penguin Books, London, UK.

Institution of Mechanical Engineers 2013. *Global Food: Waste Not, Want Not*. Institution of Mechanical Engineers, London, UK.

Jackson, R.B., Jobbágy, E.G., Avissar, R., Roy, S.B., Barrett, D.J., Cook, C.W., et al. 2005. Trading water for carbon with biological carbon sequestration. *Science* 310, 1944–7.

Jacobson, M.F. 2005. *Liquid Candy: How Soft Drinks are Harming Americans' Health*. Center for Science in the Public Interest, Washington, DC, USA.

Jenkins, M. 2003. Prospects for biodiversity. *Science* 302, 1175–7.

Johnson, A.K.L. & Ebert, S.P. 2000. Quantifying inputs of pesticides to the Great Barrier Reef Marine Park – a case study in the Herbert River catchment of North-East Queensland. *Marine Pollution Bulletin* 41, 302–9.

Karumbidza, B. & Menne, W. 2011. *CDM Carbon Sink Tree Plantations in Africa: A Case Study in Tanzania*. The Timberwatch Coalition, Mayville, South Africa.

Kogevinas, M., Becher, H., Benn, T., Bertazzi, P.A., Boffetta, P., Bueno-de-Mesqurta, H.B., et al. 1997. Cancer mortality in workers exposed to phenoxy herbicides, chlorophenols, and dioxins an expanded and updated international cohort study. *American Journal of Epidemiology* 145, 1061–75.

La Via Campesina 2013. La Via Campesina's Open Book: Celebrating 20 Years of Struggle and Hope. Published on Wednesday, 15 May 2013 17:42 ed. La Via Campesina. viacampesina.org/en/index.php/publications-mainmenu-30/1409-la-via-campesina-s-open-book-celebrating-20-years-of-struggle-and-hope, accessed 19 February 2015.

Lee, S.-W., Markham, P.F., Coppo, M.J.C., Legione, A.R., Markham, J.F., Noormohammadi, A.H., et al. 2012. Attenuated vaccines can recombine to form virulent field viruses. *Science* 337, 188.

Lee-Thorp, J., Likius, A., Mackaye, H.T., Vignaud, P., Sponheimer, M. & Brunet, M. 2012. Isotopic evidence for an early shift to C4 resources by Pliocene hominins in Chad. *Proceedings of the National Academy of Sciences (USA)* 109, 20369–72.

Leopold, A. 1949. *A Sand County Almanac and Sketches Here and There*. Oxford University Press, Oxford, UK.

Lewis, S.E., Brodie, J.E., Bainbridge, Z.T., Rohde, K.W., Davis, A.M., Masters, B.L., et al. 2009. Herbicides: a new threat to the Great Barrier Reef. *Environmental Pollution* 157, 2470–84.

Lewis, W.J., van Lenteren, J.C., Phatak, S.C. & Tumlinson, J.H. 1997. A total system approach to sustainable pest management. *Proceedings of the National Academy of Sciences (USA)* 94, 12243–8.

Linos, E., Willett, W.C., Cho, E., Colditz, G. & Frazier, L.A. 2008. Red meat consumption during adolescence among premenopausal women and risk of breast cancer. *Cancer Epidemiology Biomarkers & Prevention* 17, 2146–51.

Lorenzen, E.D., Nogues-Bravo, D., Orlando, L., Weinstock, J., Binladen, J., Marske, K.A., et al. 2011. Species-specific responses of late Quaternary megafauna to climate and humans. *Nature* 479, 359–64.

Luccio-Camelo, D.C. & Prins, G.S. 2011. Disruption of androgen receptor signaling in males by environmental chemicals. *The Journal of Steroid Biochemistry and Molecular Biology* 127, 74–82.

Lustig, R.H. 2010. Fructose: metabolic, hedonic, and societal parallels with ethanol. *Journal of the American Dietetic Association* 110, 1307–21.

Lustig, R.H., Schmidt, L.A. & Brindis, C.D. 2012. Public health: the toxic truth about sugar. *Nature* 482, 27–9.

McIntyre, B.D., Herren, H.R., Wakhungu, J. & Watson, R.T. 2008a. International Assessment of Agricultural Knowledge, Science and Technology for Development (IAASTD) Global Report. IAASTD, Island Press, Washington, DC, USA.

McIntyre, B.D., Herren, H.R., Wakhungu, J. & Watson, R.T. 2008b. International Assessment of Agricultural Knowledge, Science and Technology for Development (IAASTD). Synthesis Report. A Synthesis of the Global and Sub-Global IAASTD Reports, Island Press, Washington, DC, USA.

Matthews, W.B. 1990. Bovine spongiform encephalopathy. *BMJ* 300, 412–3.

Mekonnen, M.M. & Hoekstra, A.Y. 2010. The green, blue and grey water footprint of farm animals and animal products. *Value of Water Research Report Series*. UNESCO-IHE, Delft, the Netherlands.

Mintz, S.W. 1985. *Sweetness and Power: The Place of Sugar in Modern History*. Penguin Books, London, UK.

Mitchell, D. 2008. A note on rising food prices. *World Bank Policy Research Working Paper*. World Bank, Washington DC, USA.

Monteiro, C.A., Levy, R.B., Claro, R.M., de Castro, I.R.R. & Cannon, G. 2011. Increasing consumption of ultra-processed foods and likely impact on human health: evidence from Brazil. *Public Health Nutrition* 14, 5–13.

Nierenberg, D., Halweil, B., Androa, R.G., Benbrook, C., Binagwaho, M.-A., Buck, L.E., et al. (eds) 2011. *State of the World 2011. Innovations That Nourish the Planet*. Worldwatch Institute, New York, USA.

Nishida, T. & Uehara, S. 1983. Natural diet of chimpanzees (*Pan troglodytes schweinfurthii*): long-term record from the Mahale mountains, Tanzania. *African Study Monographs* 3, 109–30.

Pelucchi, C., Tramacere, I., Boffetta, P., Negri, E. & Vecchia, C.L. 2011. Alcohol consumption and cancer risk. *Nutrition and Cancer* 63, 983–90.

Phillips, B.L., Brown, G.P., Webb, J.K. & Shine, R. 2006. Invasion and the evolution of speed in toads. *Nature* 439, 803.

Ponting, C. 1992. *A Green History of the World*. Penguin Books, London, UK.

Potsdam Institute for Climate Impact Research and Climate Analytics 2012. *Turn Down the Heat: Why a 4°C Warmer World Must Be Avoided*. International Bank for Reconstruction and Development/The World Bank, Washington, DC, USA.

Potter, J.D. 1999. Colorectal cancer: molecules and populations. *Journal of the National Cancer Institute* 91, 916–32.

Price, C.A. & Baker, E. 1976. Origins of Pacific island labourers in Queensland, 1863–1904: a research note. *The Journal of Pacific History* 11, 106–21.

Price, L.B., Graham, J.P., Lackey, L.G., Roess, A., Vailes, R. & Silbergeld, E. 2007. Elevated risk of carrying gentamicin-resistant *Escherichia coli* among U.S. poultry workers. *Environmental Health Perspectives* 115, 1738–42.

Puig, P., Canals, M., Company, J.B., Martin, J., Amblas, D., Lastras, G., et al. 2012. Ploughing the deep sea floor. *Nature* 489, 286–9.

Richardson, D. 1987. The slave trade, sugar, and British economic growth, 1748–1776. *The Journal of Interdisciplinary History* 17, 739–69.

Rockström, J., Steffen, W., Noone, K., Persson, A., Chapin, F.S., Lambin, E.F., et al. 2009. A safe operating space for humanity. *Nature* 461, 472–5.

Rogers, I.S., Northstone, K., Dunger, D.B., Cooper, A.R., Ness, A.R. & Emmett, P.M. 2010. Diet throughout childhood and age at menarche in a contemporary cohort of British girls. *Public Health Nutrition* 13, 2052–63.

Rönnbäck, K. 2007. From extreme luxury to everyday commodity. Sugar in Sweden, 17th to 20th centuries. *Göteborg Papers in Economic History*. Göteborg University School of Economics and Commercial Law, Göteborg, Sweden.

Rule, S., Brook, B.W., Haberle, S.G., Turney, C.S.M., Kershaw, A.P. & Johnson, C.N. 2012. The aftermath of megafaunal extinction: ecosystem transformation in Pleistocene Australia. *Science* 335, 1483–6.

Séralini, G.-E., Clair, E., Mesnage, R., Gress, S., Defarge, N., Malatesta, M., et al. 2012. Long term toxicity of a Roundup herbicide and a Roundup-tolerant genetically modified maize. *Food and Chemical Toxicology* 50, 4221–31.

Shiva, V. 1991. *The Violence of the Green Revolution. Third World Agriculture, Ecology and Politics*. Zed Books Ltd, London, UK.

Smil, V. 1999. Detonator of the population explosion. *Nature* 400, 415.

Smil, V. 2000. *Enriching the Earth: Fritz Haber, Carl Bosch, and the Transformation of World Food Production*. MIT Press, Cambridge, Massachusetts, USA.

Smil, V. 2002. Eating meat: evolution, patterns, and consequences. *Population and Development Review* 28, 599–639.

Solow, B.L. 1987. Capitalism and slavery in the exceedingly long run. *The Journal of Interdisciplinary History* 17, 711–37.

Stanford, C.B. 1996. The hunting ecology of wild chimpanzees: implications for the evolutionary ecology of Pliocene hominids. *American Anthropologist* 98, 96–113.

Steinfeld, H., Gerber, P., Wassenaar, T., Castel, V., Rosales, M. & de Haan, C. 2006. *Livestock's Long Shadow*. Food and Agricutural Organization, Rome, Italy.

Tomato Genome Consortium, The 2012. The tomato genome sequence provides insights into fleshy fruit evolution. *Nature* 485, 635–41.

Tuchman, B.W. 1979. *A Distant Mirror: The Calamitous 14th Century*. Ballantine Books, New York, USA.

Tudge, C. 2013. The Founding Fables of Industrialised Agriculture. Available at: www.independentsciencenews.org/un-sustainable-farming/the-founding-fables-of-industrialised-agriculture, accesssed 20 January 2015.

United Nations Environment Programme (UNEP) 2010. *UNEP Emerging Issues: Global Honey Bee Colony Disorder and Other Threats to Insect Pollinators*. UNEP., Nairobi, Kenya.

Valladas, H., Clottes, J., Geneste, J.-M., Garcia, M.A., Arnold, M., Cachier, H., et al. 2001. Evolution of prehistoric cave art. *Nature* 413, 479.

Van den Berg, M.M., Hengsdijk, H., Wolf, J., Van Ittersum, M.K., Guanghuo, W. & Roetter, R.P. 2007. The impact of increasing farm size and mechanization on rural income and rice production in Zhejiang province, China. *Agricultural Systems* 94, 841–50.

Vandenberg, L.N., Colborn, T., Hayes, T.B., Heindel, J.J., Jacobs, D.R., Lee, D.-H., et al. 2012. Hormones and endocrine-disrupting chemicals: low-dose effects and nonmonotonic dose responses. *Endocrine Reviews* 33, 378–455.

Whitehorn, P.R., O'Connor, S., Wackers, F.L. & Goulson, D. 2012. Neonicotinoid pesticide reduces bumble bee colony growth and queen production. *Science* 336, 351–3.

14

GLOBAL FOOD SECURITY, POPULATION AND LIMITS TO GROWTH

COLIN D. BUTLER

Abstract

Egalitarians have long called for a fairer global distribution of the determinants of health and nutrition. But the progress made towards global health for all, especially between 1960 and 1990 is now faltering, though some emerging technologies and social movements may still have the potential to reverse this trend. This chapter will argue that the struggle for global development is placed at risk by insufficient high-level recognition of the nexus between emerging 'limits to growth' manifested by high energy prices, climate change and the diversion of food crops to fuel. These, with other issues, such as inequality, neoliberalism, and the general refusal of the West to accept its role in the genesis for the 'War on Terror' have profound implications for human well-being that are immensely troubling over the next few decades and beyond.

The most important academic response that is needed to cope with these interlinked crises, including for food security, is not to call for more agricultural investment or for better technology (until recently the main mantras), but for genuine, multidisciplinary appreciation of the interlinked, systemic, nature of these problems. Together with increased food production, humanity has also to slow population growth by improving human rights-based determinants of lower fertility, especially better education for girls.

In fact, it can be argued that the moral compass of the global elite, largely based in the West, supported and corrupted by lobbyists, has, in recent decades, been set to excessive consumerism during the neoliberalism-fuelled 'cornucopian enchantment'. Some might suggest that it has always been thus, but the reduction in inequality between the end of World War II and the ascent of neoliberalism was for several decades complemented by aspirational language of health and food for all. This recent decay in morality and global responsibility has influenced government and academia in ways that disguise awareness of these larger risks. Its continuation will lead to the managed retreat of civilisation, or disorderly rout. Urgent reform is thus needed.

Introduction: Nutrition, Hunger, Famine and Their 'Eco-social' Determinants

> This latest *Lancet* Series concludes, not surprisingly perhaps, that the international nutrition system is broken. (Horton, 2008)

This chapter has a very broad scope. Lack of space prevents in-depth discussion of many issues it raises; I can thus only give impressions. From the argument that causation is rarely purely ecological or social, the chapter ranges to the Green Revolution, hunger targets and measures, and how impinging limits to growth threaten the attainment of hunger targets. It also touches on neoliberalism and the follies of conventional economists.

Good nutrition is essential for health, both at the individual and population levels. Many health determinants are social, such as inequality and companionship, but many products of social factors manifest physically. Too often, the public health literature in recent decades has been biased towards social causal factors (Butler and Friel, 2006, McMichael et al., 2015). Even more deficient, however, is the failure of academics and politicians (though not the military) to sufficiently consider the interaction of social with physical (including environmental) determinants, such as has very plausibly contributed to the current Syrian conflict (Kelly et al., 2015). This leads to oversimplification and to inadequate remedies.

One such example of 'either/or' thinking is to consider the causes of food distribution and famine. Nutritional causation is *not* binary; that is, it is neither purely social (as extreme interpretations of Amartya Sen's work might suggest) nor is it purely environmental (as an extreme interpretation of Lester Brown or Paul Ehrlich's work might suggest) (e.g. Ehrlich, 1968; Brown, 2011).

Even overnutrition (another form of *mal*nutrition) has ecological as well as social causes; for example, cheap, nutrient-poor calorie –rich food (such as corn syrup) is grown and stored more easily and, consequently, is more abundant than many more nutritious alternatives (e.g. raspberries). All food is derived from the environment, whether gathered or hunted from the wild, cultivated from the soil, raised via animal (including fish) farming, or even through hydroponics.

Food is not produced from ideas alone, though of course ingenuity can increase food production. Laboratory produced meat remains a research project, though insect farming, which of course also depends on the environment, is increasing.

Food availability and consumption, together with its ingestion and absorption, are shaped by a myriad of social elements, but environmental factors (including the cost of energy, the supply of phosphorus and a sufficiently favourable climate) are *always* involved. If food supplies were to fail due to drought or some other catastrophe (e.g. war or volcanic activity, as happened globally after the explosion of Mount Tambora, leading to the Year Without a Summer in 1816 (Wood, 2014)), and if the failure is sufficiently widespread or prolonged so that trade or aid cannot fully compensate, then population nutrition must suffer.

Beyond a threshold of scarcity, redistribution fails, by definition. That is, redistribution can successfully prevent crises, but extremes exist beyond which redistribution is not enough. Redistribution can also be more difficult to implement if at times of approaching crisis, elites capture dwindling supplies, restricting sharing (Motesharrei et al., 2014). A recent historical example is the Rwandan genocide of 1994. While there was little frank starvation preceding the genocide, there was great scarcity (especially of arable land), marked inequality and the apprehension that scarcity would deepen (André and Platteau, 1998; Butler, 2000a). Other examples are of the Russian and French revolutions, each of which was driven – but not exclusively, by extreme social inequality.[1]

Macronutrient insufficiency and the 'Green' Revolution

In developed countries, most nutritional attention is focused on the search for elixirs to maximise healthy life (such as a putative optimal balance of micronutrients) and the avoidance of overnutrition and obesity. Undernutrition also occurs (and is increasing), but is generally restricted to micronutrient deficiencies among the extremely poor; some of whom are homeless, some of whom suffer chronic alcoholism and many of whom have untreated mental illness.

In contrast, in developing countries, undernutrition of 'macronutrients' (carbohydrates, fat and protein, vital for energy and amino acids, the building blocks of protein) are important problems, no more so in absolute terms than in the world's second most populous nation, India. In 2012, the Food and Agricultural Organization (FAO) of the UN estimated that 48 per cent of

1 A strong El Niño may have contributed to poor harvests leading to the French revolution (Grove, 1998).

Indian children were stunted (FAO, 2012). This represents an enormous loss of human potential. More people (287 million) were reported as undernourished between 2010 and 2012 in South Asia than in sub-Saharan Africa (234 million) (FAO, 2012).

The 'Green Revolution' expanded total food production greatly, including on the Indian sub-continent. However, in India, extreme inequality is ancient, illustrated by its still-entrenched caste system, described in 2006 by then Indian Prime Minister Singh as a human rights scourge worse than apartheid was in South Africa (Rahman, 2006). Indian-born Nobel Laureate economist, Amartya Sen, is renowned for his work on 'effective' food 'entitlement', which he defines as the capacity to acquire food by cultivation or purchase.[2] His most famous book on this topic, published in 1981, arose, in part, from his childhood experience in Calcutta (now Kolkata), during World War II (Sen, 1981). Put simply, the year of maximum famine (1943) was not the year of minimum food production (1941). Social factors clearly played a role.

A lesser-known famine in North Vietnam, also in World War II, killed a similar number of people to that in Bengal (Gunn, 2011). Unlike in India, and ignoring deep underlying factors of resource competition that contributed to Japanese aggression in World War II, this famine can be considered *entirely* of social origin, due to the forced acquisition of locally grown food by the occupying Japanese. The horrific famine in China, from 1958 to 1962, was predominantly caused socially, as was the Ukrainian famine in the 1920s. But the social dimension to these famines (and revolutions) does not mean there is no environmental component; this implies that we should not exclusively rely on social factors to prevent all future famine and revolution. We need to also consider environmental resources.

The Measurement of Global Hunger: A Black Art?

In 1996, at the World Food Summit, an ambitious target was announced to halve macronutrient hunger by 2015, from 850 to 425 million. Only four years later this target was amended, making it easier, as part of the first Millennium

2 'Starvation is ... some people not having enough food to eat. It is not the characteristic of there being not enough food to eat. While the latter can be a cause of the former, it is but one of many possible causes' (Sen, 1981, p. 1). His insight is not unique. Mallory (1926) wrote, 'There are some famines that are due almost certainly to "natural" causes (i.e. drought, locusts, plant disease), and there are scarcely any to which natural phenomena do not contribute.' This implies that Mallory recognised that the cause of famines was not *exclusively* environmental.

Development Goal (MDG) (Pogge, 2004). The revised target (about 570 million depending on assumptions of global population in 2015) permitted almost 150 million people more to remain hungry (see Figure 14.1).

Since 1999, the FAO has produced an annual report called *The State of Food Insecurity in the World* (SOFI), which is widely regarded as the most authoritative source of global hunger data. In response to growing criticism, SOFI 2012 (FAO, 2012) reported new global hunger data for the period from 1990 (see Figure 14.1). Without comment, explanation or criticism, the FAO in this report also redefined a target of the Millennium Development Goal for hunger (see Box 14.1). This error was subsequently corrected in later reports, with no acknowledgement of the 2012 mistake.

However, the main reason for the revision in data is that, since 2012, the FAO has also used a new measurement and definition of hunger. This has been criticised for using, in part, a caloric intake threshold, lasting for more than a year, at a level below that required for a sedentary lifestyle (Lappé et al., 2013). However, in defence of the FAO, this is only one component of a new, complex assessment of hunger that also reflects population nutrition using median height as a composite indicator of the interaction between calorie ingestion, absorption, energy output and metabolism. I think it is too early to judge the success of this measure, but it is nevertheless puzzling how hunger could be found to have fallen in recent years at the same time as food prices, adjusted for inflation, have risen so much (Butler, 2015). Until the 2012 FAO revision, this hunger target looked hopelessly beyond reach; but it can only be considered a modest failure. The second revised target of 700 million is only 152 million fewer than the revised number of hungry in 2010. In other words, it is not badly out of reach (if the new numbers are accepted).

Repositioning the Hunger Targets

Even less well recognised, but consistent with the perhaps excessive optimism that surrounds the topic of global hunger, is that limits to growth (see Box 14.2) are combining with inequality to reawaken the curse of famine. Old and 'sleeping' infectious disease scourges (e.g. plague, tuberculosis) could return in future if population-level immunity is weakened by worse nutrition due to rising food prices and increased social disorganisation (Butler, 2012). In combination with this is the risk of harm from human groups behaving essentially as predators, attacking those who are weaker and vulnerable (Motesharrei et al., 2014).

Adequate responses by government and public health authorities are also being eroded, as is now evident in parts of sub-Saharan Africa and South Asia. For example, the recent famine in a large part of Somalia was worsened by the extreme Islamist group, Al Shabaab, who targeted relief workers (Maxwell et al., 2012).

Box 14.1 The FAO's inadvertent and brief redefinition of the MDG hunger target.

Part of the first Millennium Development Goal (MDG) target is 'to halve the proportion of people who suffer from hunger between 1990 and 2015'. But in 2012, the FAO reported this as to 'halve the prevalence of under-nourishment in the *developing world* by 2015'. Partly because of this revision, the FAO also concluded that the MDG target was 'within reach' (FAO, 2012). However, a far more important reason for this conclusion was that the estimate of hunger in 1990 was revised upwards from 850 million to over one billion, and that for years after 2000 it was lowered (Butler, 2015). Consequently, using these revised data, the MDG target requires a fall between 2013 and the end of 2015 of less than 120 million; prior to the revisions, the required decline was 340 million (see Figure 14.1).

Estimates of hunger assembled by the FAO, based on surveys, have long been criticised, but, at the moment, remain dominant. Barrett (2013) and others have argued that there are inadequate resources (financial and/or political) to conduct sufficient high-quality surveys to measure hunger in developing countries accurately. It seems clear that these hunger data are only approximately correct, and even trends are uncertain. But this does not justify data nihilism; for example, there is strong evidence, from multiple sources, that undernourishment is excessive in India (Sainath, 1996; Black et al., 2008) and in parts of sub-Saharan Africa.

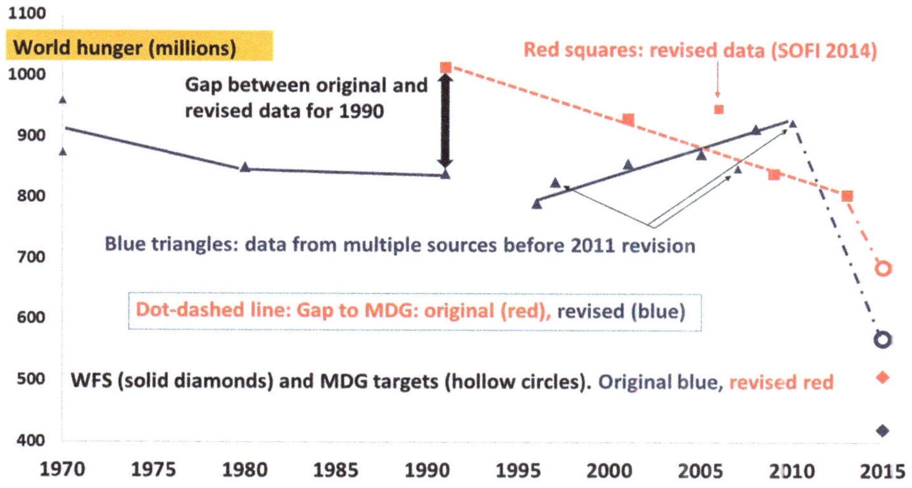

Figure 14.1. World hunger (millions) and 2015 hunger targets, 1990–2015.

The blue triangles show global hunger points using data reported by the FAO until 2010. The red squares refer to FAO data reported in 2014. The data points reported in SOFI 2012 and 2013 are similar to these, but not shown for simplicity. Focussing on the blue points a decline in hunger between 1970 and 1996 is evident, followed by an obvious increase until 2010, the last year for which data using the pre-2011 method are available. The spike in hunger to over a billion in 2009 (reported in SOFI 2009 and 2010) is not shown, for simplicity. In contrast, the red squares show a generally declining trend between 1990 and 2013, including the period of rising global food prices.

In addition, four hunger targets are shown for 2015. The hollow blue circle (568 m) shows the original MDG target (converted from a percentage). Its revision (687 m) is shown as a solid red circle. The revised trend looks far more encouraging, but its credibility is uncertain. The solid blue diamond (420 m) shows the original WFS target. Its revision (507 m) is shown as a solid red diamond. The revised trend looks far more encouraging, but its credibility is uncertain Note, too, that the revised estimate of hunger in 1990 (1.01 billion) is substantially higher than previously reported for 1970 (920 million). This implies (implausibly) either that hunger increased between 1970 and 1990, the heyday of the Green Revolution (see figure 14.2), or that the percentage of the world's population who were hungry in 1970 was closer to 30 per cent than the 25 per cent it was then thought to be. A third variant is that the revised hunger estimates are wrong. World population data were taken from FAOSTAT.

Source: Author's work, from raw FAO data (not previously published).

Persistent Hunger: Rising Concerns, Possible Solutions

One hundred million hungry people is immense; it should be an unacceptably large number in today's world. Yet, the actual number of people deprived of sufficient macronutrients for health or economic productivity is at least seven times as large, even using the more optimistic FAO measure. This is an abysmal state of affairs for the world's ultra-poor, though it seems unlikely that few of them fully realise this, in part from a lack of the necessary pedagogical components of the oppressed (Freire, 1970). In addition, up to two billion *additional* people suffer micronutrient deficiencies, especially iron and zinc. Iron, especially, is vital for stamina, learning and earning capacity. Chronic undernutrition of both macro- and micronutrients also increases the risk of chronic illnesses, occurring at relatively young ages, should undernourished infants survive into mid- or later life (Victora et al., 2008).

Now, after several decades of widespread complacency about global food security, academic interest is returning, not only in hunger but also in the issue of limits to growth more broadly (Turner, 2008; Ehrlich and Ehrlich, 2013; Motesharrei et al., 2014). Not only climate change but also other forms of 'planetary overload' (as Tony McMichael (1993) called it) deepen the challenge of sufficient and sustainable food production (see Box 14.2). Agricultural intensification, particularly of livestock, is only a partial solution. While it can help preserve biodiversity-rich ecosystems, such as forests (Garnett et al., 2013), intensive animal farming still requires *extensive* inputs, particularly of feed and shipping. Intensive animal farming can also generate novel and virulent strains of infectious diseases, affecting humans and animals alike (Liverani et al., 2013). Intensive crop production (monoculture) has its own problems, and in any case is already used widely. Rice intensification has been promoted for more than a decade, by some, as a miracle method of raising more food on a given area, but with little compelling evidence (Sheehy et al., 2004).[3] Similarly, genetically modified crops promise far more for food security than has been delivered to date.

In addition, but discussed inadequately in recent decades by most agricultural scholars, including the FAO, high rates of human population growth continue in many regions that are poor and already famine struck, such as Niger (Royal Society, 2012).

3 However, persistent reports from India continue to intrigue (e.g. www.agriculturesnetwork.org/resources/extra/bihar-sri, accessed 12 February 2015).

Box 14.2 Limits to growth

Energy

The steep rise in the price of energy from about 2005 to late 2014 is due mainly to falling supplies of the most accessible, high-quality forms of fossil fuel (Murray and King, 2012). The sustained high price of energy early in that period made many forms of unconventional fossil fuel economically feasible, at least for a period. But such energy is no bargain, and its combustion will use up the remaining 'carbon budget', risking critical climate change (Hansen et al., 2013). In late 2014, in a little-foreseen development, Saudi Arabia flooded the market with oil at a price at which it appears only it can sustain for long. Seen by some as a tactic to hurt Iran and Russia (Cooper, 2014), and by others as a means to cripple its high-cost competitors such as oil from fracking or tar sands (Moran, 2014), few if any commentators argue that such low prices can be sustained for many years (Heinberg, 2014). Optimists hope that by the time oil prices again rise substantially, the price of renewables will be so low as to also drive energy from 'tight' oil from the market.

Other metals

Similar to oil, the most accessible forms have been preferentially accessed. What remains, whether of copper, gold, lead and nickel is in a similar position (Michaux, 2014).

Phosphorus

This element must be mined or recycled. Reserves are now concentrated in only three countries, and its price is rising. Peak phosphorus may occur before 2050 (Cordell et al., 2009).

Climate change

Though not conventionally considered a form of limit to growth, climate change is, for two reasons: (i) the capacity of the Earth system to absorb waste gases is limited; consequently, waste gas concentration is rising; (ii) climate change will limit real economic growth, such as is the case with Typhoon Haiyan, which devastated the Filipino city of Tacloban in 2013 (Vidal, 2013).

Food fuels

The rising cost of energy has stimulated alternative liquid fuels made from crops, which could be used to supply food; especially maize, sugarcane and palm oil. The potential of numerous other crops for ethanol and other biofuels is being explored (de Vries et al., 2010). Already, about 40 per cent of US maize is used for fuel, not food.

Crop yield limits

All animal and plant species have limits to height and weight. The annual rate of increase of many crop yields, in many countries, is now flattening, including in China, India, the USA and Europe (Grassini et al., 2011; Ray et al., 2013).

Fertile land and water

Diminishing tracts of potentially fertile land exist, though many forest areas are inhabited by Indigenous peoples. Such areas provide vital regulating and cultural ecosystem services and have inherent existence value. We surely destroy them at our peril. Water scarcity is increasing, including from aquifer depletion.

Diminishing returns to additional complexity

The Collapse of Complex Societies (Tainter, 1988) suggests that human societies, like other organisms, have an optimal size for optimal function. Some megacities have exceeded this optimum.

Increased Vegetarianism to Ameliorate Global Hunger?

In 1971, *Diet for a Small Planet* (Lappé and Collins, 1971) pointed out that a substantial fraction of grain that could be fed to humans was instead used to feed animals to supply meat. Because animals convert plants to flesh inefficiently, advocates for vegetarianism argue that if this edible food were ingested by people, ample food would exist, even as the population rises. Since 1971, the 'feed conversion' rates of animals grown for meat have greatly improved (Godfray et al., 2010), due in part to more crowding, reduced exercise and the selection of rapidly growing breeds of animal. However, the nutritional properties of such animals has probably declined, due, in part, to their decreased exercise and, perhaps, a less favourable composition of fatty acids in their diet. Undoubtedly, though, the grain and soy animals eat would feed more people if ingested directly by humans.

There are two main reasons why advocates of complete, or even predominant, vegetarianism meet limited success, globally. First, complete vegetarianism is often neither culturally preferred nor ecologically possible, particularly in cultures traditionally based on pastoralism, hunting or fishing. In such regions, where crop growing is often difficult, animals convert indigestible grass and scraps, to humans, adding to the total human food supply.

The second reason why complete vegetarianism is impossible, from an anthropocentric perspective, is nutritional. Complete vegetarianism (even with synthetic vitamin B12 supplementation) is physiologically inadequate for many people due to low absorption of iron and probably zinc. Low iron levels are especially likely in vegetarians who lack the gene for haemochromatosis, a condition that enhances iron absorption (Naugler, 2008). Other genes and cultural habits (such as certain spices) that have a similar function may also exist.

However, perhaps one to two billion people eat more animal products, especially meat and dairy products, than is needed for good nutrition. Lowering the ingestion by this population, especially of red meat from digastric mammals that emit methane, will improve their health and slow the rate of greenhouse gas accumulation (McMichael et al., 2007). Increased vegetarianism by so many people would also reduce pressure on global food supplies.

The argument that the cause of global hunger cannot be solved simply by more food production (Carolan, 2012, Garnett et al., 2013), including agricultural intensification, is correct. Improved social determinants of food security are also needed. Such 'productionist' views appear to finally be becoming less influential. For example, while the main FAO (2013) report for *The State of Food and Agriculture* stresses investment in farmers and in agriculture as the main solution to hunger, and is silent on increased vegetarianism and even on food redistribution, it does discuss the need for a 'food systems' approach to under- and overnutrition. Also, though the report does not mention that treating parasites and other chronic illnesses that rob or cost nutrients will improve nutrition, it does mention improved sanitation, hand washing and other ways to improve public health.

Reduced Food Waste, Including of Offal

Recent FAO reports also give increasing attention to food waste, whether pre-harvest, post-harvest or pre- or post-purchase (Institution of Mechanical Engineers, 2013). The custom of eating offal has all but vanished among most affluent populations, though not in China; less waste of offal would also extend food supplies (and possibly benefit health).

Critics of the Green Revolution

Arguments in favour of greater global sharing of food resources are made by prominent critics of the Green Revolution, such as the physicist Vandana Shiva (1991). However, Shiva's conceptualisation of this agricultural technology seems inseparable from that of the unfair social structures of many of the societies that have employed it. It is true that industrialised agriculture associated with the Green Revolution favoured large over small farmers, and in many cases helped to perpetuate or enhance inequality. But, it is overly simplistic to blame an agricultural technology, operated and controlled by humans, for the inequality.

There are many interlocking reasons for inequality and poverty, and it is simplistic to blame only the new crop varieties or pesticides. The criticism of Shiva and others would be more accurate if directed towards the *societies* that implement *unfair* versions of the Green Revolution.

Food Redistribution

The appeals for a fairer distribution of food have, to date, not been very successful. While *excessive* inequality cannot be sustained indefinitely in either human society or many animal groups, all human and many animal groups are, in fact, characterised by numerous forms of inequality, whether of status, power, experience, strength or ability. The reduction of human inequality on a scale sufficient to abolish hunger completely is certainly desirable, at least to egalitarians who subscribe to the principle of social justice, but it is currently utopian.

Despite the uncertainty concerning hunger data, there was, until 2012, consensus that the proportion of global hunger (and the absolute number) fell substantially between about 1970 and 1990, the heyday of the Green Revolution, when supplies of grain and soy per person were rising sharply (see Figure 14.2). This reduction in hunger probably had more to do with rising food production (thus endorsing support for 'productionism') and falling food prices than with deliberate redistribution policies, although the ideological competition of the Cold War probably did encourage more international cooperation than the subsequent period of neoliberalism (Butler, 2000b). A virtuous feedback may have also developed (a component needed to improve the pedagogy of the oppressed) (Freire, 1970), in which better-nourished people organised to demand other factors that contributed to increased prosperity, including education, lower fertility and greater human rights. That success in hunger reduction appears to form the basis for today's dominant strategies to reduce hunger, but this approach is influenced by denial, selective data interpretation and think tanks funded by and loyal to fossil fuel industries and other vested interests.

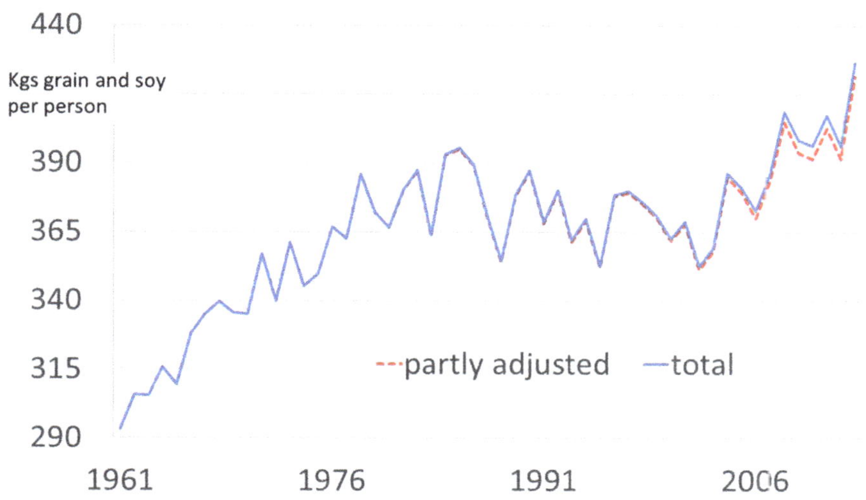

Figure 14.2. Global per capita production of grain and soy, 1961–2013, total and partly adjusted for ethanol from US maize.

Grain and soy are both durable and transportable. Rice is fed mostly to humans, but other grains, especially maize, are used both for animal feed and biofuels. Almost all soy (reported as much as 97 per cent) is fed to animals (Steinfield et al., p. 46). In 2013 the production of grain and soy reached a new record. Claims that food production per person has recently been at all-time highs do not tell the whole story, due to the lack of easily accessible data adjusted for (animal) feed and for 'fuel' foods. However, the production reported in 2013 is striking, and it may be a record, even after accounting for feed and fuel. Importantly, however, the diversion of so much food away from human mouths does not mean that hunger for the poorest 700 million is overcome.

Source: Author's work, from raw FAO data (not previously published).

Climate Change, Food, Security and More Wishful Thinking

There is increasing scientific doubt that an average global temperature increase due to anthropogenic climate change can be limited to 2°C (Peters et al., 2013). The current warming already appears to be harming crop production (Butler, 2014a, 2014b), and the World Bank (2012) recently added its weight to warnings that a rise of 4°C would have profound and adverse consequences for agricultural production and undernutrition.

Despite these warnings, the rapidly increasing scientific literature about agriculture, nutrition and climate change remains conservative (Butler, 2010, 2014b). For example, the fourth report of the Intergovernmental Panel on Climate Change (IPCC) concluded that climate change would generate a modest *increase* in global food production, provided that the global average temperature increase did not exceed 3°C (Easterling et al., 2007). This conclusion was based partly on an optimistic assessment of the benefits to crops from the carbon fertilisation effect (CFE),[4] and partly on a failure to account properly for extreme weather events and excessive optimism concerning adaptation to climate change. There is also a long tradition of unrealistic optimism by the FAO concerning climate change and food security (Goldsmith and Hildyard, 1991).

The 2007 IPCC report also has estimates for hunger in 2080 (in the absence of climate change) that appear wildly optimistic. Scenarios are characterised by general economic development, with seeming dismissal or incomprehension about the feedbacks discussed in this chapter and by many others. Even the *worst* scenario shows a marked improvement compared to 2010, while the three best scenarios predicted that macronutrient hunger would almost vanish (Easterling et al., 2007). The agricultural chapter of the Fifth IPCC Assessment, published as this chapter was being completed, is less optimistic, especially if the average level of warming reaches beyond 3 degrees (Porter et al., 2014).

There is also insufficient recognition, including among health workers, of the potential for climate change to trigger systemic, interacting, socially propagated 'tertiary' adverse effects, on a sufficient scale to endanger civilisation (Butler, 2014c). Such consequences include conflict, large-scale migration and impaired global governance. However, on the other hand, there is a long history of recognition, dating at least to the birth of the United Nations, including the FAO and its founding Director General, Boyd Orr, of the relationship between food insecurity and conflict (Staples, 2003). Any significant deterioration in regional or global food security has consequences for conflict and governance.

Excessive hope also affects the recent estimates of food production For example, Josette Sheeran, head of the World Food Programme in 2011, claimed that food production per person was at a record high (Sheeran, 2011). However, the data she (and many others) use to support such claims fails to account for food-crop diversion to biofuels, such as 40 per cent of US maize and 98 per cent of Brazilian sugarcane. A substantial number of other crops are also used for biofuels, and these 'food fuels' should *not* be counted as crops for human consumption. From 2011 until very recently, the rise in food prices also suggests that food production (excluding biofuels) per person has further declined (Butler, 2014b). If food per person is really so abundant, why have global food prices been so persistently near record highs? Note, however, that at the time of revising this chapter (March 2015), food prices had fallen (though are still well above

4 The 2007 IPCC food chapter included a detailed discussion of the CFE literature, without a conclusion. In my view, and that of other critics (Long et al., 2006) sufficient evidence then existed then to conclude that the CFE was weaker than earlier believed, especially for C4 crops such as maize. However, I have not identified any authors who have specifically commented on this with regard to the IPCC.

levels earlier this century), and, as figure 14.2 shows, grain and soy may have reached a record high in 2013, even accounting for biofuels. Time will tell if this production can be sustained and if food prices continue to fall.

The Distracting Debate between Advocates for Consumption and Population

In 1970, Norman Borlaug, 'father' of the Green Revolution, was awarded the Nobel Prize. His acceptance speech warned in part:

> There can be no permanent progress in the battle against hunger until the agencies that fight for increased food production and those that fight for population control unite in a common effort. (Borlaug, 1970)

In 1966, a famine was emerging in the chronically impoverished, caste-ridden northern Indian state of Bihar. Its ecological causes included drought and, in some parts, floods. At that time, there was little extraction of groundwater (contaminated by naturally occurring arsenic) using tube wells. In response, US State officials recommended large shipments of American grain as relief aid. President Johnson agreed, on condition that India's family planning programme be strengthened (Califano, 1981). This was the time of maximum concern about global population growth, which peaked in 1968 at 2.1 per cent per annum. Paul Ehrlich's book, *The Population Bomb*, was a major bestseller, globally.

Yet, exactly at this time (but then underappreciated), global food supplies per person were rising steeply, due to the Green Revolution (see Figure 14.2), achieved entirely without genetic modification, by selective plant breeding, economies of scale and the extensive use of fossil fuel (including to manufacture pesticides). This allowed far more food to be grown in a given area, provided there was adequate fertiliser and water. It thus helped to preserve biodiversity. I am unaware of any scholar, including Shiva, who proposes how the widespread famines perceived by many as plausible in the 1970s could have been averted without some form of the Green Revolution.

In the following two decades, food supplies rose spectacularly on a per person basis (see Figure 14.2). World hunger also declined, both proportionally and in absolute terms. While a few famines occurred from 1970 to 2000, their scale was modest compared to what had been feared.

Until Reagan became US president, his predecessors, from Eisenhower to Carter, had recognised, to varying degrees, like Borlaug, that high population growth posed a risk to global food and other forms of human security (Butler, 2004). These presidents supported not only the Green Revolution but also policies (direct and indirect) that slowed global population growth. In 1984, Reagan broke this consensus, declaring that the importance of human population size had been 'vastly exaggerated' (Finkle and Crane, 1985). Since then, on the Right, neoliberal supporters and their policies have downplayed the importance of population, while critics on the Left have, unhelpfully, generally argued that consumption is far more important (Monbiot, 2008).

In reality, both matter. Population matters: principally in rich countries, where too many of us consume too much; our collective footprint is the main cause of planetary overload (McMichael and Butler, 2011). High population size and growth in poor countries also matters. This is not because of the contribution of the global poor to the global 'footprint', but because it helps trap such populations in poverty (Campbell et al., 2007). Finally, population in poor countries matters because their elevation from poverty (if it ever occurs) will increase their environmental footprint greatly, unless they rely almost exclusively on solar and other environmentally preserving technologies, including the recycling of phosphate.

Conclusion

This chapter has a very broad scope. Lack of space prevents in-depth discussion of many issues it raises, for which I apologise. Collectively, limits to growth, including climate change, are generating a slow-moving, global, intergenerational crisis. I believe that our collective political leadership is in denial, demonstrated, for example, by the embarrassing failure of the Rio +20 summit in 2012, which was attended by few leaders of wealthy countries.

For decades, agricultural companies and their neoliberal, techno-optimistic supporters have claimed that genetic manipulation is the best means to trigger a new agricultural revolution. But, little progress has been made, at least relative to the required challenge, and long-predicted (Steinbrecker, 1996) adverse effects increasingly are documented, including pesticide-resistant weeds (Bonny, 2011) and harm to health (Séralini et al., 2011). A Green Revolution could enhance food production in Africa (Ejeta, 2010), but this is made much more challenging by the high price of energy. As important as are arguments for more food, ways to alter the determinants of fertility so as to increase child survival and the demand for education and lower population growth are at least as urgent.

The moral compass of the global elite, cheered on by lobbyists and advertisers, has, in recent decades, been set to indulgence and selfishness, manifest not only by declining foreign aid by most rich countries but also by excessive consumerism during the 'cornucopian enchantment' (Butler, 2007). This decay has also affected government and academia, in ways that have inhibited public awareness of these larger risks. Continuation of this behaviour will lead either to the managed retreat of civilisation or to its disorderly rout (Ehrlich and Ehrlich, 2013).

The most important academic response to the gathering crisis of food and governance is not to call for more agricultural investment. While necessary, this is insufficient. Instead, multidisciplinary recognition of these fundamental, interlinked crises is required, along with planetary mobilisation on the scale of a global war, to transform the entire industrial system (Ehrlich and Ehrlich, 2013). This task is seemingly impossible, but its scale is less forbidding if this task is considered incrementally. To start, policymakers and politicians need to show courageous leadership, including challenging what could be called the 'other Rome Consensus'; that is, the belief that all is well and that hunger will gradually decline if we follow business as usual.

One step is to change the focus from the effort to increase supply in order to meet wants and needs, to instead develop ways in which humanity can slow resource consumption in both the near and long-term future, including by slowing population growth by providing determinants of lower fertility using human rights-based approaches, especially better education for girls and women (Campbell et al., 2007). Non-government organisations and civil society, such as Climate Justice, the foundation established by Mary Robinson, are also vital.

References

André, C. & Platteau, J.-P., 1998. Land relations under unbearable stress: Rwanda caught in the Malthusian trap. *Journal of Economic Behavior and Organization* 34, 1–47.

Barrett, C.B. 2010. Measuring food insecurity. *Science* 327, 325–8.

Black, R.E., Allen, L.H., Bhutta, Z.A., Caulfield, L.E., de Onis, M., Ezzati, M., et al. 2008. Maternal and child undernutrition: global and regional exposures and health consequences. *The Lancet* 371, 243–60.

Bonny, S. 2011. Herbicide-tolerant transgenic soybean over 15 years of cultivation: pesticide use, weed resistance, and some economic issues. The case of the USA. *Sustainability* 3, 1302–22.

Borlaug, N. 1970. Nobel Prize Acceptance Speech. Available at: www.nobelprize.org/nobel_prizes/peace/laureates/1970/borlaug-acceptance.html, accessed 20 April 2014.

Brown, L.R., 2012. World in serious trouble on food front Earth Policy Institute, www.earth-policy.org/plan_b_updates/2012/update104, accessed 22 March 2015.

Butler CD. 2000a. Entrapment: global ecological and/or local demographic? Reflections upon reading the BMJ's 'six billion day' special issue. *Ecosystem Health* 2000;6(3):171–80.

Butler, C.D. 2000b. Inequality, global change and the sustainability of civilisation. *Global Change and Human Health* 1, 156–72.

Butler, C.D. 2004. Human carrying capacity and human health. *Public Library of Science Medicine* 1, 192–4.

Butler, C.D. & Friel, S. 2006. Time to regenerate: ecosystems and health promotion. Public Library of Science Medicine 3, e394.

Butler, C.D. 2007. Globalisation, population, ecology and conflict. *Health Promotion Journal of Australia* 18, 87–91.

Butler, C.D. 2010. Climate change, crop yields, and the future. *SCN News* 38, 18–25.

Butler, C.D. 2012. Infectious disease emergence and global change: thinking systemically in a shrinking world. *Infectious Diseases of Poverty* 1, 5.

Butler, C.D. 2014a. Famine, hunger, society and climate change. In: Butler, C.D. (ed.) *Climate Change and Global Health*. CABI, Wallingford, UK, 124–34. Available (open access) at: www.cabi.org/openresources/42659, accessed 5 January 2015.

Butler, C.D. 2014b. Food, water and climate change. In: Freedman, B. (ed.) *Global Environmental Change*. Springer, Netherlands, 630–47.

Butler, C.D. (ed.) 2014c. *Climate Change and Global Health*. CABI, Wallingford, UK.

Butler, C.D. (2015). Revised hunger estimates accelerate apparent progress towards the MDG hunger target *Global Food Security* 5(6): 19–24.

Califano, J. 1981. *Governing America*. Simon and Schuster, New York, USA.

Campbell, M., Cleland, J., Ezeh, A. & Prata, N. 2007. Return of the population growth factor. *Science* 315, 1501–2.

Carolan, M. 2012. The food and human security index: rethinking food security and growth. *International Journal of Sociology of Agriculture and Food* 19, 176–200.

Cooper, A.S., 2015. Why would the Saudis deliberately crash the oil markets? Simple: to undermine Tehran. *Foreign Policy* foreignpolicy.com/2014/12/18/why-would-the-saudis-crash-oil-markets-iran/, accessed 30 March 2015.

Cordell, D., Drangert, J.-O. & White, S. 2009. The story of phosphorus: global food security and food for thought. *Global Environmental Change* 19, 292–305.

de Vries, S.C., van de Ven, G.W.J., van Ittersum, M.K. & Giller, K.E. 2010. Resource use efficiency and environmental performance of nine major biofuel crops, processed by first-generation conversion techniques. *Biomass and Bioenergy* 34, 588–601.

Easterling, W.E., Aggarwal, P.K., Batima, P., Brander, K.M., Erda, L., Howden, S.M., et al. 2007. Food, fibre and forest products. In: Parry, M.L., Canziani, O.F., Palutikof, J.P., van der Linden, P. & Hanson, C.E. (eds) *Climate Change 2007: Impacts, Adaptation and Vulnerability. Contribution of Working Group II to the Fourth Assessment Report of the Intergovernmental Panel on Climate Change*. Cambridge University Press, Cambridge, UK, 273–313.

Ehrlich, P.R., 1968. *The Population Bomb*. Ballantyne, London, UK.

Ehrlich, P.R. & Ehrlich, A.H. 2013. Can a collapse of global civilization be avoided? *Proceedings of the Royal Society B: Biological Sciences* 280.

Ejeta, G. 2010. African Green Revolution needn't be a mirage. *Science* 327, 831–2.

FAO (Food and Agricultural Organization) 2012. *The State of Food Insecurity in the World 2012*. FAO, Rome, Italy.

FAO 2013. *The State of Food and Agriculture*. FAO, Rome, Italy.

FAO 2014. *The State of Food Insecurity in the World 2014*. FAO, Rome, Italy.

Finkle, J.L. & Crane, B. 1985. Ideology and politics at Mexico City: the United States at the 1984 International Conference on Population. *Population and Development Review* 11, 1–28.

Freire, P., 1970. Pedagogy of the Oppressed. Herder and Herder, New York, USA; 40th anniversary edition, Continuum, www.pedagogyoftheoppressed.com, accessed 30 March 2015.

Garnett, T., Appleby, M.C., Balmford, A., Bateman, I.J., Benton, T.G., Bloomer, P., et al. 2013. Sustainable intensification in agriculture: premises and policies. *Science* 341, 33–4.

Godfray, H.C.J., Beddington, J.R., Crute, I.R., Haddad, L., Lawrence, D., Muir, J.F., et al. 2010. Food security: the challenge of feeding 9 billion people. *Science* 327, 812–8.

Goldsmith, E. & Hildyard, N. 1991. World agriculture: toward 2000, FAO's plan to feed the world. *The Ecologist* 21, 81–92.

Grassini, P., Thorburn, J., Burr, C. & Cassman, K.G. 2011. High-yield irrigated maize in the Western U.S. corn belt: I. On-farm yield, yield potential, and impact of agronomic practices. *Field Crops Research* 120, 142–52.

Grove, R.H., 1998. Global impact of the 1789-93 El Niño. *Nature* 393, 318–9.

Gunn, G.C. 2011. The Great Vietnamese Famine of 1944–45 revisited. Available at: naosite.lb.nagasaki-u.ac.jp/dspace/bitstream/10069/25151/1/toasia52_81.pdf, accessed 20 April 2014.

Hansen, J., Kharecha, P., Sato, M., Masson-Delmotte, V., Ackerman, F., Beerling, D.J., et al. 2013. Assessing 'dangerous climate change': required reduction of carbon emissions to protect young people, future generations and nature. *PLoS ONE* 8, e81648.

Heinberg, R. 2014. The oil price crash of 2014. Post Carbon Institute. www.postcarbon.org/the-oil-price-crash-of-2014/ March 30, 2015.

Horton, R. 2008. Maternal and child undernutrition: an urgent opportunity. *The Lancet* 371, 179.

Institution of Mechanical Engineers 2013. *Global Food; Waste Not, Want Not*. www.imeche.org/knowledge/themes/environment/global-food, accessed 30 March 2015.

Kelley, C.P., Mohtadi, S., Cane, M.A., Seager, R. & Kushnir, Y., 2015. Climate change in the Fertile Crescent and implications of the recent Syrian drought. *Proceedings of the National Academy of Sciences (USA)*112: 3241–6.

Lappé, F.M. & Collins, J. 1971. *Diet for a Small Planet*. Institute for Food and Development Policy, San Francisco, California, USA.

Lappé, F.M., Clapp, J., Anderson, M., Lockwood, R., Forster, T., Nierenberg, D., et al. 2013. *Framing Hunger*. Small Planet Institute, Cambridge, Massachusetts, USA, WhyHunger, New York City, USA, Institute for Agriculture and Trade Policy, Minneapolis, Minnesota, USA, Food & Water Watch, Washington, DC, USA, Canada, Ottawa, ETC Group, Canada, Terra Nuova, Rome, Italy.

Liverani, M., Waage, J., Barnett, T., Pfeiffer, D.U., Rushton, J., Rudge, J.W., et al. 2013. Understanding and managing zoonotic risk in the new livestock industries. *Environmental Health Perspectives* 121, 873–7.

Long, S.P., Ainsworth, E.A., Leakey, A.D.B., Nösberger, J. & Ort, D.R., 2006. Food for thought: lower-than-expected crop yield stimulation with rising CO_2 concentrations. *Science* 312, 1918–21.

Mallory, W.H. 1926. *China: Land of Famine*. American Geographical Society, New York, USA.

McMichael, A.J. 1993. *Planetary Overload. Global Environmental Change and the Health of the Human Species*. Cambridge University Press, Cambridge, UK.

McMichael, A.J. & Butler, C.D. 2011. Promoting global population health while constraining the environmental footprint. *Annual Review of Public Health* 32, 179–97.

McMichael, A.J., Powles, J., Butler, C.D. & Uauy, R. 2007. Food, livestock production, energy, climate change and health. *The Lancet* 370, 1253–63.

McMichael A.J., Butler C.D. & Dixon, J. 2015. Climate change, food systems and population health risks in their eco-social context *Public Health*. doi: dx.doi.org/10.1016/j.puhe.2014.11.013.

Maxwell, D., Haan, N., Gelsdorf, K. & Dawe, D. 2012. The 2011–12 famine in Somalia: introduction to the special edition. *Global Food Security* 1, 1–4.

Michaux, S., 2014. The coming radical change in mining practice. In: J. Goldie and K. Betts (eds.), *Sustainable Futures: Linking Population, Resources and the Environment*. CSIRO Press, Collingwood, Vic, Australia, 73–84.

Monbiot, G. 2008. Population growth is a threat. But it pales against the greed of the rich. *The Guardian*. www.theguardian.com/commentisfree/2008/jan/29/politics.greenpolitics, accessed 30 March 2015.

Moran, M. 2014. Is Saudi Arabia trying to cripple American fracking? Foreign Policy. foreignpolicy.com/2014/12/23/is-saudi-arabia-trying-to-cripple-american-fracking-oil-iran/, accessed 30 March 2015.

Motesharrei, S., Rivas, J. & Kalnay, E. 2014. Human and nature dynamics (HANDY): modeling inequality and use of resources in the collapse or sustainability of societies. *Ecological Economics* 101, 90–102.

Murray, J. & King, D. 2012. Climate policy: oil's tipping point has passed. *Nature* 481, 433–5.

Naugler, C. 2008. Hemochromatosis: a Neolithic adaptation to cereal grain diets. *Medical Hypotheses* 70, 691–2.

Peters, G.P., Andrew, R.M., Boden, T., Canadell, J.G., Ciais, P., Quéré, C.L., et al. 2013. The challenge to keep global warming below 2°C. *Nature Climate Change* 3, 4–6.

Pogge, T. 2004. The first United Nations Millennium Development Goal: a cause for celebration? *Journal of Human Development* 5, 377–97.

Porter, J.R., Xie, L., Challinor, A.J., Cochrane, K., Howden, S.M., Iqbal, M.M., et al. 2014. Food security and food production systems. In: *Climate Change 2014: Impacts, Adaptation, and Vulnerability*. Part A: Global and Sectoral Aspects. Contribution of Working Group II to the Fifth Assessment Report of the Intergovernmental Panel on Climate Change [Field, C.B., Barros, V.R., Dokken, D.J., Mach, K.J., Mastrandrea, M.D., Bilir, T.E., Chatterjee, M., Ebi, K.L., Estrada, Y.O., Genova, R.C., Girma, B., Kissel, E.S., Levy, A.N., MacCracken, S., Mastrandrea, P.R. & White, L.L. (eds)]. Cambridge University Press, Cambridge, United Kingdom and New York, NY, USA, 485–533.

Rahman, M. 2006. Indian leader likens caste system to apartheid regime. *The Guardian*, 28 December 2006. www.theguardian.com/world/2006/dec/28/india.mainsection, accessed 30 March 2015.

Ray, D.K., Mueller, N.D., West, P.C. & Foley, J.A. 2013. Yield trends are insufficient to double global crop production by 2050. *PLoS ONE* 8, e66428.

Royal Society 2012. *People and Planet*. The Royal Society, London, UK.

Sainath, P. 1996. *Everybody Loves a Good Drought: Stories from India's Poorest Districts*. Penguin, New Delhi, India.

Sen A.K. 1981 Poverty and Famines: An Essay on Entitlement and Deprivation. Clarendon Press, Oxford, UK, New Delhi, India.

Séralini, G.-E., Mesnage, R., Clair, E., Gress, S., de Vendômois, J. & Cellier, D. 2011. Genetically modified crops safety assessments: present limits and possible improvements. *Environmental Sciences Europe* 23, 1–10.

Sheehy, J.E., Peng, S., Dobermann, A., Mitchell, P.L., Ferrera, A., Yang, J., et al. 2004. Fantastic yields in the system of rice intensification: fact or fallacy? *Field Crops Research* 88, 1–8.

Sheeran, J. 2011. Preventing hunger: sustainability not aid. *Nature* 479, 469–70.

Shiva, V. 1991. *The Violence of the Green Revolution. Third World Agriculture, Ecology and Politics*. Third World Network and with ZED Books, London, UK.

Staples, A.L.S. 2003. To win the peace: the Food and Agriculture Organization, Sir John Boyd Orr, and the World Food Board proposals. *Peace & Change* 28, 495–523.

Steinbrecker, R. 1996. From green to gene evolution. The environmental risks of genetically engineered crops. *The Ecologist* 26, 273–81.

Steinfeld, H., Gerber, P., Wassenaar, T., Castel, V., Rosales, M. & de Haan, C., 2006. Livestock's Long Shadow, FAO, Rome, Italy.

Tainter, J.A. 1988. *The Collapse of Complex Societies*. Cambridge University Press, Cambridge, UK.

Turner, G.M. 2008. A comparison of the limits to growth with 30 years of reality. *Global Environmental Change* 18, 397–411.

Victora, C.G., Adair, L., Fall, C., Hallal, P.C., Martorell, R., Richter, L., et al. 2008. Maternal and child undernutrition 2: maternal and child undernutrition: consequences for adult health and human capital. *The Lancet* 371, 340–57.

Vidal, J. 2013. Typhoon Haiyan: what really alarms Filipinos is the rich world ignoring climate change. *The Guardian*. www.theguardian.com/commentisfree/2013/nov/08/typhoon-haiyan-rich-ignore-climate-change, accessed 30 March 2015.

Wood, G.D.A. 2014. *Tambora: The Eruption that Changed the World*. Princeton University Press, Princeton, New Jersey, USA.

World Bank 2012. *Turn Down the Heat: Why a 4 Degree Celsius Warmer World Must be Avoided*. The World Bank, Washington, DC, USA.

REPRINT F

Social and Cultural Perspectives

BASIL HETZEL AND ANTHONY J. MCMICHAEL

Hetzel, B. & McMichael, A.J. 1987. *The LS Factor: Lifestyle and Health*. Penguin Australia, Melbourne, Australia, pp. 10–25.

Pages: 287 to 306

Reprinted with permission from Penguin Australia, with our thanks.

2

Social and Cultural Perspectives

Awareness of the connection between health and lifestyle has increased greatly over the past two decades. In developed countries, this awareness has arisen in the light of findings from medical research since about 1960. Examples of lifestyle factors that have been studied extensively include diet, alcohol consumption, cigarette smoking, physical activity, sexuality and reproductive behaviour. Collectively, these personal behaviours are now thought to be related to about three-quarters of the premature illness and death that occurs in contemporary Western populations.

The idea that health is related to lifestyle is not new. The Greeks and Romans recognised that health and disease reflected the conditions of living. Hygeia, the Greek goddess of health, represented the view that 'health is the natural order of things and a positive attribute to which men are entitled if they govern their lives wisely.' The Greeks considered that medicine's function was to discover the natural laws by which human beings ensured 'a healthy mind and a healthy body'.

There is a strong social dimension to health – the health of the individual is very much dependent on both the physical and social environment.

In the Third World rural communities, a high prevalence of infectious disease, particularly bowel and respiratory infection, reflects poor sanitation, overcrowding and inadequate nutrition. The urban communities of Europe in the nineteenth and early twentieth centuries and Asian cities now beginning to industrialise also suffer from a high prevalance of infectious disease, again

'Health is the natural order of things and a positive attribute to which people are entitled if they govern their lives wisely.' Greek view of health

associated with poor sanitation, overcrowding and inadequate nutrition.

Modern metropolitan communities in the West, which have proceeded a long way on the path of industrialisation and now have reasonably good sanitation and better housing, have developed a sedentary lifestyle with access to plenty of high-energy foods, alcohol and cigarettes. These communities have a quite different pattern of health problems – characterised by coronary heart disease, stroke, certain forms of cancer, and other chronic (especially respiratory and digestive) conditions related to cigarette smoking and alcohol consumption. These differences are demonstrated clearly in figure 2.1, which shows the changing profile of mortality in Australia and New Zealand during this century.

It is this latter pattern of health problems that is the concern of this book. These diseases are non-infectious in contrast to the infectious diseases, which were the major problem until about 1940 in Western countries, and are still the main concern of Third World countries today. These late twentieth-century diseases are related to personal behaviour which in turn is conditioned by social and cultural factors. In the case of the once dominant infectious diseases, the personal factor is overwhelmed by the importance of the physical environment.

HEALTH : DEFINITIONS AND COMMUNITY ATTITUDES

The World Health Organization has defined health as 'a state of physical, mental and social wellbeing and not merely the absence of disease or infirmity'. This refers to a general and positive state of health – an ideal which is attractive and important to everyone, but which is difficult to study in contrast to the more clearly defined specific disease states. Indeed, the WHO definition has been

Figure 2.1: Changes in distribution of major causes of death, Australia 1910–83, and New Zealand 1900–78

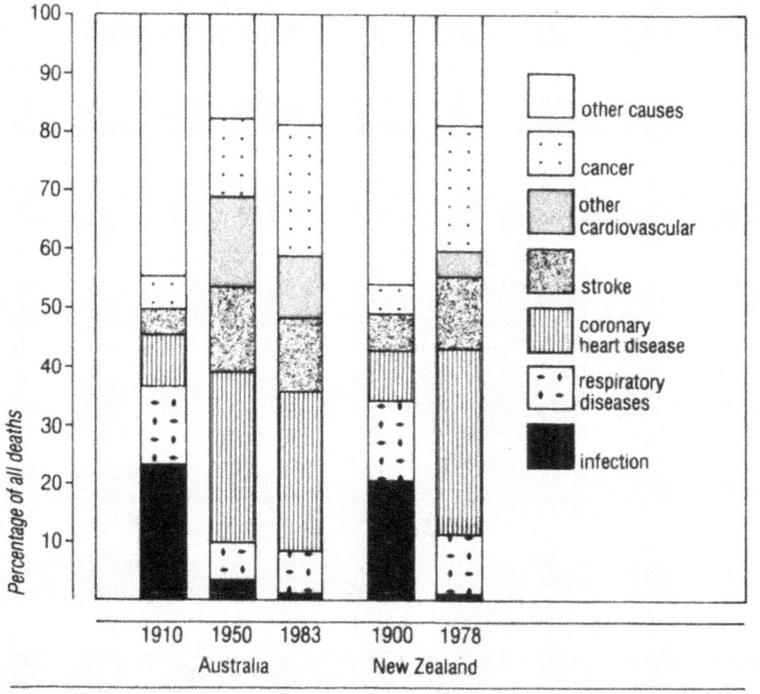

The fall in deaths due to infection and rise in deaths due to coronary heart disease is shown.

Source: data from the Australian Bureau of Statistics and New Zealand National Health Statistics Centre

criticised because it has not been readily translated into useful and measurable goals.

It is of interest to know just what Australians' current attitudes to health are. A survey was carried out in 1985 by the Better Health Commission (appointed by the Minister of Health in early 1985).[1] 1266 persons aged fourteen years and over (a random sample from all of Australia) were asked (in a formal interview at home) what 'health' meant to them as individuals.

Their responses were fairly evenly distributed over the four listed available answers: health was described as 'being free from illness' by 26 per cent, as 'feeling well and being able to cope' by 25 per cent, as 'being physically fit and active' by 31 per cent, and as 'being able to do the things one tries to do' by 18 per cent. Men and people from rural areas were much more likely to choose the latter two, action-oriented, answers. Women's answers in particular, emphasised the importance of 'being able to cope' (31 per cent versus 18 per cent of men), especially in the child-rearing age range, 18-39 years (34 per cent).

Respondents were then asked how much control they had over their own health. Only 10 per cent considered that they had 'little' or 'almost no' control, 24 per cent said they had 'some' control, and a majority (70 per cent of women and 61 per cent of men) said they had either a 'lot of' control or 'almost complete' control. While neither age nor income bore any clear-cut relationship to the response, the subject's amount of formal education did. Twenty per cent of people reporting little or almost no control had no secondary education, 10 per cent had 1–3 years, 8 per cent 4–6 years of secondary education, and 5 per cent had tertiary education. The corresponding proportions reporting a 'lot of control' or 'almost complete control' were 60, 62, 65 and 77 per cent.

When asked to select which six changes would most improve their future health, 18 per cent said 'better diet', 26 per cent said 'more exercise', 17 per cent said 'stop or reduce smoking', 3 per cent said 'reduce alcohol consumption', 12 per cent said 'cope better with stress', and 23 per cent said that no change was needed. Men and women gave similar answers; slightly more men referred to smoking and alcohol, while slightly more women referred to diet and exercise.

Respondents were then asked why they had not made the specified change. Approximately one-quarter said they were too lazy and another quarter said they had no time; 17 per cent said it was too hard, 12 per cent said they were unsure how to go about it, 10 per cent were not convinced it was worthwhile, and 9 per cent said they lacked the facilities, money, or social support.

When asked to pick out the lifestyle or behaviour pattern responsible for the most health problems in Australia, 25 per cent nominated alcohol abuse, 23 per cent the abuse of legal or illegal drugs, and 23 per cent poor diet. Insufficient exercise was nominated by 14 per cent, while 13 per cent considered smoking was the main health problem.

Finally, respondents were asked to state their main source of information about health and lifestyle. The orthodox health professionals (doctors and nurses) are the most frequently cited sources; women also report obtaining much information from magazines. Reliance upon the print media is positively correlated with educational attainment, whereas reliance upon doctors and nurses is strongly inversely related to education.

When asked to identify the behaviour pattern responsible for most health problems in Australia, 25% of respondents nominated alcohol abuse, 23% the abuse of legal or illegal drugs, 23% poor diet, 14% insufficient exercise, 13% smoking.

This information is of great interest. Most important is the awareness of a majority that they had considerable control over their own health. In other words they accepted some degree of personal responsibility for their health. This is a prime focus for the preventive approach that is advocated in this book, entailing the sharing of responsibility between individual and community.

PIONEERING STUDIES

The importance of behavioural factors to health has been indicated by investigations that have been carried out by Lester Breslow and his colleagues in the Human Population Laboratory in California.[2] In one study which extended over fifteen years, mortality was examined in relation to a 'health practice' score derived from seven basic health-related behaviours or habits:

- Never smoke cigarettes
- Regular physical activity
- Moderate or no use of alcohol
- 7-8 hours sleep regularly
- Maintaining proper weight
- Eating breakfast
- Not eating between meals

An initial survey of health habits was carried out in 6928 adults in 1965. The first follow-up was carried out in 1970, a second in 1974. The health practice scores (1–7) determined in 1974 revealed little change as compared to 1965: those with a low score in 1965 usually maintained their low score in 1974. (The average score was 4.9 for both the 1965 and 1974 survey.)

A man aged 45 who observed six or seven of the seven health practices had a life expectancy of about 11 years more than one who observed three or less.

The results of the 1974 follow-up indicated clearly that as the health practice score increased so did the age-adjusted mortality rate fall. Men following seven health practices had a mortality rate only 28 per cent of that of men following zero to three health practices. Women following seven health practices had a mortality rate only 43 per cent of that of women with a score of 0–3. This inverse trend of mortality in relation to health practice was shown clearly for cancer, cardiovascular diseases and all other causes in men. In women the trend was evident for total cardiovascular disease, but not for cancer or all other causes. This meant that a man aged forty-five observing six or seven of these health practices had a life expectancy of about eleven years more than that of a forty-five year old man with a health practice score of 3 or less.

Another aspect of lifestyle examined by the Human Population Laboratory in California was the social network – a measure of social connections in the form of marriage, contacts with close friends and relatives, and membership of community groups. The age-adjusted mortality in the most isolated men was 2.3 times higher than in men with strong social connections; among women the difference was 2.8 times. These differences could not be explained by the presence of pre-existing disease or other risk factors. The differences in mortality were apparent with coronary heart disease, stroke and cancer.

The importance of social support in relation to health has also been shown in a cross-cultural perspective in studies of Japanese migrants to California and Hawaii. A series of 3809 Japanese-Americans in California were classified according to the degree to which they retained a traditional Japanese culture. The most traditional group of Japanese-Americans had a coronary heart disease prevalence rate similar to that observed in Japan. By contrast, the group that had undergone most change towards Western culture had a three- to five-fold excess in prevalence of coronary heart disease. This difference in rate between the groups of Japanese-Americans could only partially be accounted for by difference in diet or smoking or other known risk factors.

It was suggested that the features of traditional Japanese cultural-community ties, group cohesion and social stability were important in protecting the Japanese from coronary heart disease. The contrast between this pattern and the strongly individualistic American emphasis on geographic mobility and ambition may be significant in relation to coronary heart disease.

These several studies indicate the relevance of personal behaviour and social factors to health status. People with high risk health practices and weak social networks do not live so long. These associations were found to be independent of age, sex, socioeconomic status, and initial physical health.

HEALTH AND LIFESTYLE ACROSS CULTURES

It is instructive to consider health and lifestyle from the perspective of human cultural evolution. By reference to various historical stages, we can see that lifestyle is part of the dynamic relationship between humans and their environment, including other humans, the plants, and the animals, and the physical environment on which all living beings depend. 'Ecosystem' refers to the dynamic equilibrium between all these various components. Changes in any component can affect the other components – an obvious example is the effect of Western communities on the physical environment as they have proceeded to clear vast forests in order to plant crops for agriculture. Massive soil erosion then follows because of loss of the permanent holding structure for the soil. This in turn affects the future of agriculture, and can threaten the food supply.

The three major ecosystems in human history have been: the

hunter/gatherer ecosystem; the peasant agricultural ecosystem; the affluent industrial ecosystem.

The hunter/gatherer ecosystem

The hunter/gatherer ecosystem has existed for 30 000–50 000 years. Typically, the men do the hunting while the women collect the plant foods. There are a number of these hunter/gatherer groups still surviving today – they include the Australian Aborigines and the Kung Bushmen of Africa (north-west Botswana). The supply of meat is intermittent so that the diet is essentially vegetarian (for this reason, some anthropologists prefer the term gatherer/hunter). Meat, when available, is lean game meat, which has about one-fifth the saturated fat content of meat from domesticated animals.

Survival in the desert was dependent on careful restriction of numbers so that mobility was preserved – only the fittest could survive. The desirability of few (and small) babies is obvious and infanticide was practised. Contraception was achieved by a reduced frequency of menstrual cycles due to the combination of marginal nutrition, physically strenuous lifestyle, and prolonged non-nutritive suckling, which would go on for four or five years. Cause of death was likely to be by starvation, injury or infection or a combination of these. The small size of the nomad communities (up to thirty) precluded significant childhood epidemics, which awaited the arrival of the white man. However, boils, eye and intestinal infections are frequent. The danger of starvation is always present for the hunter/gatherer.

Data on the diet of the Australian Aborigines are available from Arnhem Land in 1960 and from Central Australia in 1971.[3] The diet mainly consists of various edible seeds – supplemented by snake, lizards and mice which were described as reasonably plentiful. On the coast, fish were also available. The desert-dwelling Aborigines when first seen by the nineteenth-century explorers impressed them with their fitness – they looked like well-trained athletes, which indeed they were. Mature height was within the normal European range but the Aborigines had a lighter, lean body frame quite different to the modern urban Australian. More recent studies of blood mineral and vitamin levels revealed a normal range and haemoglobin was normal indicating there was no anaemia due

Studies of Aborigines in South Australia reveal that cardiovascular diseases and obesity develop as a Western lifestyle is increasingly adopted.

to iron deficiency. Blood pressure has been found to be low as late as 1975 and the blood cholesterol was also low (relative to Caucasian Australians). There was no evidence of cardiovascular disease at post-mortem.

It is of great importance that recent studies of Aborigines in South Australia reveal the development of vascular diseases (coronary heart disease, hypertension, diabetes mellitus) and obesity in association with increasing adoption of the Western lifestyle. The rates for these disorders were lower in the less urbanised reserves (Ernabella and Yalata), compared to the more urbanised (Point Pearce, Koonibba) indicating the relevance of lifestyle including particularly diet and physical activity.[4]

The peasant agricultural ecosystem

The growing of crops and domestication of animals appeared first in the Mesopotamian region between 9000 and 8000 BC. Agriculture provided the base for the great ancient civilisations of China, Egypt, classical Greece, and the Mayans. The highland village of Papua New Guinea provides a good example of the early peasant agricultural ecosystem. The village groups vary in size from 20 to 200, mostly living on the hills and mountains surrounded by their gardens on land cleared from the jungle by fire. Their food is almost entirely root vegetables – taro, sweet potato and yam. Pig once every one to two years would be a great luxury.

The supply of food in this ecosystem is much more reliable than in the hunter/gatherer ecosystem. However, reliance on a single crop presents an ever-present danger of starvation due to crop failure, and can lead to specific deficiency diseases, which the diverse diet of the hunter/gatherer would avoid.

Such deficiency diseases are more likely to occur in children because of their low social status and the extra nutrients required for growth. Examples are iron deficiency causing anaemia, and iodine deficiency causing endemic goitre and endemic cretinism (brain damage); both conditions are very common in Papua New Guinea, and are also common throughout Asia (China, India, Indonesia). Vitamin A deficiency causing blindness due to softening of the cornea of the eye (keratomalacia) and Vitamin B (thiamine) deficiency due to removal of the husk of the rice by milling also occur.

Another problem is deficiency of protein in children, because it may not be possible for them to eat enough of the root vegetable to ensure an adequate intake due either to lack of availability or indigestibility. The sweet potato which was introduced about 350 years ago grows at higher altitudes than the taro or yam so that settled communities extended from altitudes of 2100 metres up to 2700 metres. But the protein content is low in the sweet potato and it is very susceptible to frosts.

Studies of the diet taken by the people of Murapin in the Western Highlands in the 1970s revealed that sweet potato supplied over 90 per cent of the food, carbohydrate provided 94.6 per cent of the energy with fat only 2.4 per cent and protein 3 per cent. (In Australia, as we shall see later, the figures would be approximately 48 per cent (carbohydrate), 40 per cent (fat), 12 per cent (protein).) The protein intake was 34g per day for males and 27g per day for females (compared with Australian and European figures of 150–200g per day).

Growth in height was not completed until the age of 18 years in females and 24 years in the case of males (compared with 15 years and 17 years in Australian school children). This difference reflects the difference in protein intake.[5]

Cardiovascular disease is virtually unknown in the Highland communities but has begun to appear in the indigenous community living in Port Moresby where European foods are readily available and a sedentary lifestyle is much more prevalent.

The affluent industrial ecosystem

The industrial revolution dating from the eighteenth century in Europe, which moved with an accelerated pace through the nineteenth century, has led to an unprecedented degree of affluence in the Western world in the latter half of the twentieth century. One effect of industrialisation has been the development of large cities with populations in millions (Sydney and Melbourne now have populations of three million each, while much bigger cities exist elsewhere – Tokyo, Sao Paulo, New York, London). All the indications are that these cities will increase further in size.

A big city is itself an ecosystem with a metabolism requiring air, food, water from its environment and excreting waste products into its environment. Appropriate provision has to be made for these functions to provide the basis for a healthy lifestyle for its inhabitants.[6]

Lifestyle in large cities is very different from that of the rural world in preceding centuries. There is only limited space available for living, including recreation, while there is a much greater number of casual human contacts than ever before, which allows the transmission of respiratory infection on a scale never before known. Big city life promotes a sedentary way of life which is reinforced by television and mass spectator sport, public transport and the private motor car. There is increasing pressure of time, with tension as appointments and deadlines have to be kept by white-collar populations of administrators, clerks and professionals of all sorts; other pressures and tensions occur in the mechanised factory production line. Such tensions are associated with the smoking of cigarettes, the drinking of alcohol and the taking of various drugs and 'tonics' prescribed and unprescribed, including vitamin and mineral supplements.

Family life is characterised by small nuclear families composed of parents and children, in contrast to the large extended families of most parts of the rural world. One in three marriages in Australia ends in divorce; one in eight children is being raised by a single parent. Children are exposed to long hours of television, as an alternative to longer contact with parents. The mother is likely to be working outside the home with pressure on time for conversation, food preparation and general care of the family, in contrast to the former rural lifestyle. Fathers generally have not compensated by assuming greater involvement with family life. Reproduction is controlled efficiently with modern methods of contraception. The ageing grandparents are likely to be living some distance from the nuclear family and therefore not nearly so readily available for support, advice and recreation. There has also been a loss of religious belief which provided support and authority for control of behaviour in previous generations. These aspects of contemporary Western life, entailing diminution of social support networks and of a sense of personal purpose and control, are discussed further in chapter 10.

There has been a big change in diet with much greater availability of processed foods of high-energy content – sugar and fat – in contrast to the higher complex carbohydrate content in previous centuries from staple cereals of wheat, with a much higher fibre content. This changed food supply has resulted from a more efficient agriculture, and food industry, with the production of dairy products, meat and processed food, on a scale never before known. The development of larger-scale food multi-nationals incorporating agriculture with the marketing and distribution of food has accelerated this process. The relation of this changed diet to health forms a major topic for discussion in this book. There is now a large body of evidence pointing to the relevance of diet to the twentieth-century epidemic diseases of cardiovascular disease, diabetes mellitus, hypertension, and certain forms of cancer.

THE DEVELOPMENT OF LIFESTYLE

The development of lifestyle is a social phenomenon, beginning in childhood in the setting of family, friends and cultural background. The parents are a very important influence – especially the mother in many societies. The infant learns first from the parents in many different cultural settings. There are great differences between cultures – demand feeding with absence of toilet training is characteristic of the Hindu culture; in Germany a strict control is enforced; in Japan children are seldom punished and mothers are renowned for their patience; distant relationships are characteristic of the Kibbutz in Israel and the crèches of the People's Republic of China, associated with a full working life for both parents.

There is today in developed countries a greater variation in parental relations than previously. Marriage followed by divorce is more common and many other types of relationships occur and are often transient compared to traditional marriage. This means that children do not have the same parental figures for as long as they did in previous generations. Many school teachers are well aware of the association of 'problem children' with troubled family backgrounds.

In these circumstances the role of media, especially television, becomes more significant than otherwise. Children are commonly spending 20-30 hours a week with television (either direct broadcast or video recorder) and its impact is likely to be greater in the absence of stronger and more caring parental figures. The American College of Pediatrics has expressed concern about the 'gimme syndrome' which has been developed partly as a result of television advertisements. Many of these advertisements are concerned with foods and so aim to influence the lifestyle of children. Television has been described as the 'third parent'.

During childhood, extending from the age of five to twelve years, children usually learn to manage their environment and impulses, which is an essential prelude to adolescence. They learn to concentrate and achieve at work and play and to socialise. At school they are no longer the centre of attention, as in the limited family, but are in a group situation requiring conformity and imposing some competition. They discover themselves through contact with others outside the family circle. So the child's orientation and lifestyle moves from that of the family to that of the outside world. The influence of television on this process has not yet been adequately studied.

In adolescence, the peer group becomes a very important influence on lifestyle. There is a very strong feeling of seeking identity and achieving it through the peer group. Adolescence entails a striving for emotional independence from the parents, a search for stable, intimate relationships, often culminating in marriage, career choice, and the attainment of some philosophy of life or religious belief. In the past these major landmarks have often been achieved by the age of twenty years in developed countries, and together constitute what Erik Erikson has called 'identity'. Many adolescents do not in fact achieve this personal identity for many reasons – including an inadequate home background and a greater range of choices available today than ever before. In this setting, the use of drugs including alcohol and cigarettes may be seen to offer an opportunity for quick achievement of self-identity –

certainly often a way of flaunting independence from parents.

The high level of alcohol and cigarette consumption by adolescents has become a matter of great concern in many developed countries and will be discussed further in chapters 6 and 7. The probability is that such patterns will persist into adult life. Obviously the advertising industry believes this, and so has paid special attention to the trainee consumers of this age period.

In Australia, one brand of cigarette associated with promotion by one particular television personality, Paul Hogan, had become very popular among adolescents. It is of interest that a public health activist group – Action on Smoking and Health (ASH) – was successful in securing a court injunction leading to the banning of television appearances by Paul Hogan because of contravention of the voluntary code controlling advertisements directed to adolescents. There is also a voluntary code covering advertisements of alcoholic beverages. As this code has evolved, advertisements directed to adolescents that were passed as acceptable ten years ago are no longer considered acceptable. However, the sponsorship of sports heroes and major sporting events by alcohol and tobacco companies, although specifically condemned by the Senate Select Committee of Social Welfare in its 1977 report on *Drug Taking in Australia,* has become an influential, albeit indirect, form of advertising.

Television offers new possibilities for education and the enrichment of life. It could also be a major resource for promoting a healthy lifestyle. Its control should not be left to the market place.

There is a quiet evolution proceeding in these matters which recognises the hazards to adolescent lifestyle from the media. The same applies to adults but they are less susceptible than are adolescents. Health education programs, aimed at promoting a healthy lifestyle among adolescents, have not been very successful so far, but we shall be considering some new initiatives in chapter 11.

The impact of television on the behaviour of younger age groups requires much more investigation. Initial studies in the USA, investigating the relationship of television to violence, attempted to minimise the impact. More recent investigations have taken a different view. Experiments are now proceeding in the USA with a 7–9 pm 'family hour' from which violence and sex have been largely banished.

The availability of television offers new possibilities for education and the enrichment of human life. It is also a major resource for promoting a healthy lifestyle. Its control should not be left solely to the market place, although as indicated later, the market place is sensitive to a better-educated consumer.

The overall impression that emerges from this brief review of the development of lifestyle is its plasticity and flexibility. There is plenty of evidence indicating that lifestyle can be modified in the interests of better health. This clearly involves both individual and social aspects which will be considered in subsequent chapters.

CHANGES IN HEALTH OVER THE LAST CENTURY

Data available from Australia and other industrialised countries show how health has improved over the past century.[7] One basic indication is by the measurement of life expectancy. The change of life expectancy at birth for both sexes over the period 1930–83 in Australia is shown in figure 2.2.

Three phases can be distinguished. In *the first phase* there was a long period of increase of life expectancy; this occurred progressively from the 1880s to 1950. The increase is similar for both men and women, and antedated most of the modern advances in medical treatment. This better health status is attributed mainly to improvements in the food supply, housing and control of sanitation. The advent of antibiotics during the 1940s made a late, and small, contribution.

In *the second phase,* dating from 1950 until 1970, there is a relative plateau indicating little increase. This is particularly true of men, so that the difference between men and women has become greater than it was before. This relative plateau has been due to the epidemics of coronary heart disease (which accounts for 30 per cent of deaths), followed by cancer (20 per cent) and stroke (13 per cent), bronchitis, emphysema and asthma (4.1 per cent) and motor

2 Social and Cultural Perspectives

1 A.J. McMichael, 'The Better Health Commission' in *Proceedings of Annual Conference ANZSERCH/APHA Inc.: Progress on Health for all Australia, New Zealand, the Region, the World,* 1986, pp. 116–32.
2 L.F. Berkman & L. Breslow, *Health and Ways of Living, The Alameda County Study,* Oxford University Press, New York, 1983.
3(i) R. Gould, *Yiwara: Foragers of the Australian Desert,* Collins, Sydney, 1970. This book tells the story of the life of a nomad Aboriginal tribe from personal observation and participation.
(ii) B.S. Hetzel & H. J. Frith (eds), *The Nutrition of Aborigines in Relation to the Ecosystem of Central Australia,* CSIRO, Melbourne, 1978. This book reviews the evidence about the lifestyle and diet of Aborigines before and since the coming of the white man.
4 F.M. Edwards, P.H. Wise, D.W. Thomas, J.B. Murchland & R.J. Craig, 'Blood pressure and electrocardiographic findings in the South Australian Aborigines', *Australia and New Zealand Journal of Medicine,* vol. 6, 1976, pp. 197–205. This reference documents the high rate of cardiovascular disease in Aborigines.
5 P.F. Sinnett & H.M. Whyte, 'Papua New Guinea' in *Western Diseases: Their Emergence and Prevention* (H.C. Trowell & D.P. Burkitt, eds), Edward Arnold, London, 1981, p.171. This book on Western diseases collects data on the recent changes in the pattern of diseases in many countries particularly in relation to diet. It provides a fascinating store of information.
6 B.S. Hetzel, *Health and Australian Society,* 3rd edition, Penguin, Ringwood, 1980. This book gives a general view of health and the health care system in Australia.
7 Life expectancy data. Australian data are published annually in the report of the Director-General of Health, Canberra. A published compilation *Perspectives on Health* by the South Australian Health Commission (1985) provides a useful collection of available data and charts on all aspects of mortality and morbidity with primary reference to South Australia.
8 National Heart Foundation, *Risk Factor Prevalence Survey,* no.1 (1980), Canberra, 1982. More recent data are provided by the 1983 survey (no. 2).
9 A.J. Dobson, R.W. Gibberd, S.R. Leeder & D.L. O'Connell, 'Occupational differences in ischemic heart disease mortality and risk factors in Australia', *American Journal of Epidemiology,* vol. 122, 1985, pp. 283–90.
10 A.A. Congalton, *Status and Prestige in Australia,* Cheshire, Melbourne, 1969, Appendix B, pp. 143.
11 A.J. McMichael, 'Social class (as estimated by occupational prestige)

and mortality in Australian males in the 1970s', *Community Health Studies*, vol. 9, 1985, pp. 220–30.
12 D.R. Dunt, 'Recent mortality trends in the adult Australian population and its principal ethnic groupings', *Community Health Studies*, vol. 6, 1982, pp. 217–22.

3 Diet: Fatted Calves or Loaves and Fishes

1 D.P. Burkitt & H.C. Trowell (eds), *Refined Carbohydrate Foods and Disease: Some Implications of Dietary Fibre*, Academic Press, New York, 1975.
2 B.S. Hetzel & H.J. Frith (eds), *The Nutrition of Aborigines in Relation to the Ecosystem of Central Australia*, CSIRO, Melbourne, 1978.
3 K.I. Baghurst & S.J. Record, 'Intake and sources in selected Australian sub-populations of dietary constituents implicated in the etiology of chronic disease', *Journal of Food Nutrition*, vol. 40, 1983, pp. 1–15; this reference provides detailed information on the Australian diet. A general review – *The Assessment of Nutritional Status* (B.S. Hetzel & K.I. Baghurst, eds) – is to be found in volume 3 of Transactions of the Menzies Foundation, 1981.
4 US Senate Select Committee on Nutrition and Human Needs, *Dietary Goals for the United States*, US GPO Washington DC, 1977. This is the famous 'McGovern Committee' which first popularised the idea of dietary goals in the Western world. The committee was intitially concerned with the food supply of underprivileged groups in the USA but soon became aware of the major problem of overnutrition.
5 Food and Agriculture Organisation, *Dietary Fats and Oils in Human Nutrition*, Report of an expert consultation jointly organised by FAO and WHO, Rome, September 1977; FAO, Rome, 1978. These regular FAO reports are an important source of international data on food and nutrition.
6 A. Worsley & D. Crawford, 'Australian dietary supplementation practices: health and dietary supplements', *Medical Journal of Australia*, vol. 140, 1984, pp. 579–83.
7 G.A. Bray, 'Obesity, definition, diagrams and disadvantages', *Medical Journal of Australia*, vol. 142, 1985, Supplement, 1 April, 1985. This is an excellent review – in the same supplement there are other good review articles on the other aspects of obesity.
8(i) W.A. Langsford, 'A food and nutrition policy', *Food Nutrition Notes and Reviews*, vol. 36, 1979, pp. 100–3; this is the first formal statement of the dietary guidelines by the Commonwealth Department of Health.
(ii) A useful series of articles on the development of dietary guidelines and their implications for food industry and agriculture are published in *Food*

END OF REPRINT F

Social and Cultural Perspectives

BASIL HETZEL AND ANTHONY J. MCMICHAEL

15

ECO-NUTRITION, ECOSYSTEMS AND HEALTH

Reflections and Aspirations

MARK L. WAHLQVIST

Abstract

Our generation has had the privilege and opportunity to appreciate scientifically the ecosystems that we have occupied, transformed or left alone. Now we, with them, face an unprecedented crisis brought about from the rather short 150,000 years or so presence on Earth of our own so-called 'species'. The concept of 'self' and 'species', and its health, is now challenged by our science, by new concepts of bio-communication and by the known fragility of our ecology. But, our journey from childhood to later life with family, friends and colleagues, as health-care professionals, knowledge workers, teachers and citizens, may yet be one of an optimistic future, if we act locally under a global vision.

Personal Reflections

Reflections and aspirations in celebration of Tony McMichael's career and contributions are bound to be rewarding. Our lives had been entwined in several ways. With my late wife, Dr Soo Sien Huang, we were medical students together at Adelaide University. We moved to Melbourne at about the same time, with a similar sociopolitical mindedness. Tony and his wife, Judy, lived with us in Parkville, Tony as President of the National Union of University Students and me as a National Heart Foundation Fellow and tutor at Melbourne University and St Vincent's Hospital. We worked together in the evenings and on weekends in a then depressed district of Melbourne as General Practitioners, where families often slept in cold warehouses and universal health insurance was yet to arrive.

Basil Hetzel, who had been our Professor of Medicine in Adelaide, moved to Monash University as its Foundation Professor of Social and Preventive Medicine. I had kept in touch with him and brokered an arrangement whereby Tony could do a PhD with Basil. In due course, we both left Melbourne for overseas destinations. Ultimately, we teamed up again in the field of migrant health when the Division of Human Nutrition was created in Adelaide, with Basil Hetzel as Chief. I was appointed Foundation Professor of Human Nutrition at Deakin University.

I doubt that we understood where this was leading. But, there was a new synergy when Tony distilled his planetary health concept in 1993 (McMichael, 1993) and I began in the late 1980s to gather the evidence for biodiversity and food variety as integrated ecohealth pathways (Wahlqvist et al., 1989; Wilcox et al., 1990) critically affecting human history (Wahlqvist, 1992) and eventually formulating the concept of eco-nutrition in 1998 (Wahlqvist and Specht, 1998). Now and again, we shared a platform to corroborate these socio-scientific passions. When, as President of the International Union of Nutritional Science, I commissioned the New Nutrition Science initiative for integration between the biomedical, societal and environmental sciences, Tony was surely involved (Beauman et al., 2005; Wahlqvist, 2005; Cannon and Leitzmann, 2006). And so it is that I now reflect and hope.

Eco-nutrition for Food and Human Security

Eco-nutrition conceptualises how we and other living things can acquire the nutrients we need to optimise our well-being, health and lifespan in ways that are sustainable and respectful of the animate and inanimate. The sense of connectedness and the need for diversity now, in the past and in the future, characterise eco-nutrition. Wahlqvist and Specht argue that eco-nutrition 'is the most critical conjunction of all the sciences for human survival, health and well-being' (Wahlqvist and Specht, 1998).

These authors identified ways in which biodiversity might contribute to successful eco-nutrition, which included an obligate varied food supply for human health; a range of diverse food sources as security against natural disaster, climate change and pestilence; a rich source of medicinals, many as yet unknown; ecosystem buffers against invasive plants and animals, and of pathogens and toxins; and a 'spiritual' value in diversity and ecosystems with mental health benefit and the feeling of 'belonging to the landscape'. Seasons would add diversity and vigour (Wahlqvist and Specht, 1998).

Because of the complex inputs into food and nutrition systems, they provide an opportunity to mitigate or amplify the risks posed by finite water, non-renewable energy, fertiliser, health, education and fiscal resources (Wahlqvist et al., 2012). These resource limitations are at the root of most human conflict. Therefore, greater emphasis on an ecological approach to food security should go some way to improve human security at large, while being attentive to planetary health. Expressly, it would seem time for the traditional security community to commit to ecosystem services as defined by the UN system.

Connected Communities and Households: Food-based Systems

We are members of families, households and communities. We are conceived, born, raised, toil, reproduce, age and die as social and environmental creatures with varying degrees of health. Only for a few or in small part will health differentials be genetically determined in the Mendelian sense. This means that how locality and life-course intersect could be expected to be the principal determinants of health patterns, especially those that are seasonally, diurnally, nutritionally and microbiologically related. This situation merits an eco-nutritional nomenclature rather than the clichéd terminology of 'communicable' and 'chronic disease' (Wahlqvist, 2002).

There is increasing potential for communities to connect digitally in cyberspace and generate new problem-defining and solving strategies. In turn, this could revitalise what have come to be known as FBDGs (food-based dietary guidelines), which were formalised in Cyprus in 1995 by a joint WHO–FAO working party, with the intention of enabling food and nutrition policies to be locally and culturally relevant and sustainable (Wahlqvist, 2009).

The Health of Species and Ecosystems

It is now evident that the boundaries between species are blurred in newly understood ways. First, our microbiome in gut, on skin, in the reproductive tract and more is greater than 90 per cent of our genome, and it is prokaryotic (has no nuclei) with an arbitrary interface with the environment. Second, environmental factors alter gene expression within each generation and intergenerationally, by epigenetic and non-RNA-producing DNA surveillance. Third, it seems possible that plant food micro-RNA or oligonucleotides, as in rice, can be assimilated in humans and alter, at least in a small fashion, metabolic phenotype (Zhang et al., 2012). Fourth, human endocrine systems are inadequate without food and environmental inputs and connections for which phytoestrogens are a good example (Wilcox et al., 1990). We are part of our ecosystem(s). Fifth, our very presence and gait activates soil microorganisms beneath our feet by bio-communication; these microorganisms network our presence to distant sites – the nature of our ecology still largely escapes us, even though it disappears in dust clouds of 'development' (Witzany, 2010).

The rate of biodiverse ecosystem loss is rising rapidly, and with this loss we lose ourselves, since these systems are part of us. Our future health depends on how well we manage our ecology.

Aspirations

When we were health care professional students, we lived in a time of war in Indochina, of student revolt, of reformist folk songs, of protest against racism and much grievance over the establishment. Then things went relatively quiet (notably on university campuses) and prosperous in the developed world, while billions went hungry and remained poor in the rest of the world, and also at home in the developed world, too.

Now, we face much greater crises of human and planetary security. My grandchildren will most probably have no choice but to eat a more parlous and less safe diet, even if advances in agricultural and food technology make the progress we expect. The well resourced will still be more likely to survive, even as natural disasters increase with climate change. We vaguely knew it could happen, some of us more clearly than others. Time has since been lost.

So, what can we do? Identification with our locale, its food, health and cognate systems should help us to act locally while we think and advocate globally. It is not too late! By 2050, the world's population should be in decline and the planet may begin to recover. Along mountain trails inaccessible for months in Taiwan, after the devastating Morakot typhoon of August 2009, plants and animals rarely seen began to reappear in the absence of humans. It is sobering to realise that not all of the world's ecosystems are in need of our 'species' for their management! They can and do, indeed, take care of themselves!

Tony McMichael was all of a problem identifier, risk assessor and solution seeker in the quest for favourable and sustainable health ecology, beginning from intense engagement in student affairs and thereafter ever more global (McMichael, 1972; McMichael, 2012; Liverani et al., 2013; The Conversation 2014).

References

Beauman, C., Cannon, G., Elmadfa, I., Glasauer, P., Hoffmann, I., Keller, M., et al. 2005. The principles, definition and dimensions of the new nutrition science. *Public Health Nutrition* 8, 695–8.

Cannon, G. & Leitzmann, C. 2006. The new nutrition science project. *Scandinavian Journal of Food and Nutrition* 50, 5–12.

Conversation, The. *Profile A.J. McMichael* Available at: theconversation.com/profiles/anthony-mcmichael-56/profile_bio, accessed 21 January 2015.

McMichael, A.J. 1972. *Student Mental Health: An Epidemiological Approach.* PhD thesis, Monash University, Victoria, Australia.

McMichael, A.J. 1993. *Planetary Overload: Global Environmental Change and the Health of the Human Species.* Cambridge University Press, Cambridge, UK.

McMichael, A.J. 2012. Insights from past millennia into climatic impacts on human health and survival. *Proceedings of the National Academy of Sciences (USA)* 109, 4730–7.

Wahlqvist, M.L. 1992. Critical nutrition events in human history. *Asia Pacific Journal of Clinical Nutrition* 1, 101–5.

Wahlqvist, M.L. 2002. Chronic disease prevention: a life-cycle approach which takes account of the environmental impact and opportunities of food, nutrition and public health policies – the rationale for an eco-nutritional disease nomenclature. *Asia Pacific Journal of Clinical Nutrition* 11, S759–S762.

Wahlqvist, M.L. 2005. The new nutrition science: sustainability and development. *Public Health Nutrition* 8, 766–72.

Wahlqvist, M.L. 2009. Connected community and household food-based strategy (CCH-FBS): its importance for health, food safety, sustainability and security in diverse localities. *Ecology of Food and Nutrition* 48, 457–81.

Wahlqvist, M.L. & Specht, R.L. 1998. Food variety and biodiversity: econutrition. *Asia Pacific Journal of Clinical Nutrition* 7, 314–9.

Wahlqvist, M.L., Lo, C.S. & Myers, K.A. 1989. Food variety is associated with less macrovascular disease in those with Type II diabetes and their healthy controls. *Journal of the American College of Nutrition* 8, 515–23.

Wahlqvist, M.L., McKay, J., Chang, Y.C. & Chiu, Y.W. 2012. Rethinking the food security debate in Asia: some missing ecological and health dimensions and solutions. *Food Security* 4, 657–70.

Wilcox, G., Wahlqvist, M.L., Burger, H.G. & Medley, G. 1990. Oestrogenic effects of plant foods in postmenopausal women. *BMJ* 301, 905–6.

Witzany, G. 2010. Uniform categorization of biocommunication in bacteria, fungi and plants. *World Journal of Biological Chemistry* 1, 160–80.

Zhang, L., Hou, D., Chen, X., Li, D., Zhu, L., Zhang, Y., et al. 2012. Exogenous plant MIR168a specifically targets mammalian LDLRAP1: evidence of cross-kingdom regulation by microRNA. *Cell Research* 22, 107–26.

16

REVISITING THE 'URBAN BIAS' AND ITS RELATIONSHIP TO FOOD SECURITY

JANE DIXON AND PHILIP MCMICHAEL

Abstract

Accentuating both damaging environmental change and food insecurity, we focus on the dynamics between national development policies and food systems. Using Lipton's 'urban bias' hypothesis, we position citizen-consumers as a pre-eminent socio-political force facilitated by the urban–rural power relations underpinning the food system. Urban consumers particularly benefit from industrial food systems through cheap food and from cheap manufacturing and service sector labour, released as rural populations become marginal to agricultural productivity gains. Consequently, many cities overflow with redundant workers, while rural areas contain impoverished, insecure agrarian populations often tied to global supermarket supply chains. For these populations, food security can be elusive. While Lipton's argument applied to three and more decades ago, his hypothesis that policies favour urban populations when policies pursuing economic growth are based on a presumed 'natural' coupling between rural outmigration and urban manufacturing jobs could apply more contemporaneously. We apply key urban bias concepts to the unfolding of events in Thailand, detecting conditional support for the hypothesis. We conclude by canvassing food system actions to counter the urban bias with a more ecological view of urban–rural interdependencies linked to sustainable food production and consumption.

Introduction

> The world is at a turning point as for the first time in human history the urban population is today larger than the rural population. However, poverty has still overwhelmingly a rural face and the rural economy and society still perform a vital part in the development process and in people's well-being. (Kay, 2009, p. 103)

For more than 25 years, Tony McMichael examined population health, including nutritional health, impacts of lifestyle changes and widespread, escalating and deepening environmental change. He was particularly concerned with the health consequences of affluent lifestyles and the environmentally unsustainable nature of the international spread of industrial and meat-based diets (Hetzel and McMichael, 1989; McMichael, 2005a; McMichael et al., 2007).

Underlying the diffusion of industrial foods is the global retailing revolution (Burch et al., 2013), whereby supermarket diets for the majority world (middle and working classes) converge on a narrowing base of staple grains, increasing consumption of animal protein, edible oils, salt and sugar and declining dietary fibre as consumption of brand-name processed foods rises. These combined changes contribute to an increasing prevalence of (non-communicable) dietary diseases (Hawkes, 2008).

In this chapter, we argue that rural producers have been rendered redundant as a result of the industrialisation of agriculture in world regions classified as 'developed'. Further, the model of industrial agriculture has since been exported to post-colonial regions in the form of Green Revolution technologies (Patel, 2013), universalising urbanism as the desired or naturalised end point of an international 'development project' (McMichael, 1996). In the post-World War II development era, this outcome gave rise to the concept of 'urban bias' (Lipton, 1977), which focused on the political privileging of cities over the countryside. For our purposes, this concept anticipated a more profound discounting of the centrality of agriculture to human sustainability.

We argue further that urbanisation has incubated a global process of supermarketisation, concentrated populations no longer producing their own food, and reconstituted them as 'consumers' (Dixon and Isaacs, 2013). Here, the retailing revolution has not simply displaced local food systems, but now governs consumption patterns associated with urbanism: anonymised and monetised exchange and the commercial construction of value, including authoritative dietary 'knowledge' (Dixon, 2009). Such knowledge is the construct of an industrial food system that is not only global but also one that steadily undermines the lay science of the remaining rural producers; and the possibility of retaining diverse farm systems that restore and preserve ecological cycles is lost (McMichael, 2013). In these terms, then, 'urban bias' represents a long-term threat to human health and planetary sustainability.

Valorising the Urban

In 2007, UN-Habitat declared the urban millennium to have arrived. At that point, cities housed a majority of the world's population, which added to their already formidable political status gained over centuries through providing the seat of government, vast stocks of finance capital and entrepreneurial zeal, cheap wage labour to underpin industrialisation, and diverse cultural forms and relative tolerance. With the symbolic, political and economic re-ascension of the city over the last half a century, a simultaneous decline in attention to rural spaces and peoples has been under way, in line with the ever-diminishing contribution of rural productivity to Gross National Product (GNP). In both developed and developing countries, there are now many fewer rural people than in the past, and those who remain are typically poorer, less educated, less healthy and less potent at the ballot box and in policy development. As Kay observes in the opening quote, the contribution of rural populations to national development is being denied.

Reinforcing the political and symbolic elevation of cities has been economic geography's declaration that the urban–rural binary is redundant, with the appropriate unit for any spatial planning or policy focus being 'city regions' (Jones and Corbridge, 2010), especially where food is concerned (Marsden, 2012).

In addition, 'feeding the city' from within peri-urban boundaries has become a fashionable topic for urban ecologists, agri-food, climate change and development researchers.[1] However, championing the food security potential of urban agriculture obscures the fact that for almost half of the world's population, which continues to reside in rural spaces, their food production activities are essential for their own food security. It also denies the various estimates of urban population dependence on smallholder food provisioning for most of their food requirements: the Erosion, Technology, Concentration NGO (ETC, 2009) estimates that 'peasants' produce 70 per cent of the world's food, while Public Citizen and the food sovereignty movement claim an even higher percentage is peasant produced: 'Family farm- and peasant-based production for domestic purposes is responsible for approximately 90 per cent of the

1 'The FAO (2007) estimates that as many as 200 million urban residents produce food, representing about 15 per cent of total world food output' (Jones and Corbridge, 2010, p. 8).

world's food production, much of which does not even pass through markets' (Public Citizen, available at: www.citizen.org/documents/wtofood.pdf. See also: ag-transition.org/?p=1769).

Our concern is that the political and cultural reframing of cities as the vital engines of development exacerbates food insecurity and unsustainable food systems. According to the UN Special Rapporteur on the Right to Food, the ongoing adoption of public policies consolidating urban privilege contributes to food insecurity through a spiral of loss of farmer livelihoods and productive landscapes (de Schutter and Sepulveda, 2012).

This dynamic pivots on the 'cheap food regime' (Rosset, 2006), with two key consequences. On the one hand, the cheap food regime steadily undermines the food security of rural producers with imports of artificially cheapened foodstuffs, displacing some into urban slums, and compromising a diverse smallholder foundation that, given support, may steward the land. Further, the cheap food regime has enabled a universal 'supermarketisation', involving rising proportions of unhealthy processed foods, now accounting for over 80 per cent of the world food trade, and rising rates of obesity (Hawkes et al., 2010).

So, how has this situation arisen? And, how do these dynamics contribute to food insecurity?

'Urban Bias' Theory/Hypothesis

In 1977, development economist, Michael Lipton, outlined his 'theory' on urban bias to explain why, under conditions of economic development, 'poor people stay poor'. The theory was based on a multi-country comparison of data – from 63 less-developed countries (LDCs) and nine now-developed countries (NDCs) – describing the situation a few years either side of 1970, 10–30 years after their recent growth acceleration.

Lipton measured urban–rural disparity by calculating the ratio of non-agricultural to agricultural income per person, and found that in the NDCs the disparity was typically lower. Robert Bates, World Bank political economist, explained this outcome to be due in part to governments in poor countries 'tend[ing] to intervene in markets in ways that impose a tax on agriculture, while governments in richer nations would tend to intervene in ways that confer subsidies on farmers' (Bates, 1993, p. 221). This geopolitical variation in farm to non-farm resource transfer policy had two effects: developed country farmers had an incentive to improve productivity, while farmers in developing countries were faced with financial disincentives; and within developing countries, farm household incomes were much lower than non-farm household incomes, resulting in urban–rural inequalities and rural poverty (Anderson, 2010, p. 23). Thus, developing country farmers were being penalised by the policies of their own governments, as well as by the policies of other agricultural producing nations, with any gains from their farming labour and other inputs accruing disproportionately to those whom Lipton referred to as 'urban classes'. Moreover, the taxes on agricultural producers were used to subsidise imported goods (often through currency overvaluation that also harmed farm exports), particularly those deemed essential to establish a more industrial future. This 'price twist' mechanism 'turns prices against a rural group' (Lipton 1984, p. 158).

Based on the analyses, Lipton defined urban bias (UB) as 'the tendency of public authorities and private persons to allocate, and their disposition to justify, for large urban areas, proportions of developmental or welfare-generating resources in excess of any reasonable norm of either efficiency or well-being' (Lipton, 1977, p. 43). Two of the most important welfare-generating resources were identified as cheap food and urban infrastructures – public transport, water, etc – typically financed through agricultural export revenues. With healthier, fitter populations and vastly superior infrastructures, urban citizens could devote themselves to generating even greater personal wealth and wealth for their nations.

In essence, rural people were being parasitised by urban populations, who benefitted disproportionately from both the consumption of cheap foods and urban infrastructures. This form of urban population appeasement had the effect of deepening inequalities between rural and urban areas. Lipton argued that UB was responsible for the growth in undernutrition in countries that were spectacularly improving their income per person (in the period 1950 to the early 1970s). Referring to Brazil between 1960 and 1970, for example, real income per person increased 37 per cent, while the levels of the poorer half of the population increased by just 1 per cent. As income per person grew, the poor spent 55–80 per cent of any extra income on food, while the rising working and middle class spent a much smaller share of 20–30 per cent (generally on varying their diets and simplifying cooking).

Numerous criticisms have been levelled at the theory, especially in relation to the difficulty in making urban and rural distinctions (see Kay, 2009); Lipton's idiosyncratic interpretation of class (Byres, 1979; Kay, 2006); and in generalisability across countries. In revisiting his original work, Lipton (1984) reframed the UB as a testable hypothesis, agreeing that in-depth, historical process case studies were required. His hypothesis received endorsement from an analysis of sub-Saharan Africa, where governments were described as using agricultural commodity boards as taxation revenue raisers, redistributing the income to urban populations to avoid food riots or coups (Bates, 1993; Jones and

Corbridge, 2010). However, this reappraisal did not deter development economists and economic geographers from further critical engagement (see special issue of *Journal of Development Studies* 1993, Vol. 29(4); Jones and Corbridge, 2010), especially on the point that the UB theory ignored 'the urban penalty', namely the plight of the urban poor as underemployed rural people flooded into cities, often with worse health and prosperity than those they left behind.[2]

While recognising the urban penalty, those denying the UB paradoxically proceed to argue that there are good development grounds for an urban, synonymous with industrial development, bias in terms of:

1. The livelihood opportunities afforded by urban employment in the face of de-agrarianisation, as well as the cross-sectoral livelihood strategies created by urban–rural economic zones or 'city regions';
2. The economic benefits, according to urban scale, of concentrating services and goods in cities;
3. The importance in terms of justice to individuals and to national economies of removing obstacles to mobility, even though urban problems (crime, disease) follow neglect of the countryside;
4. Important instances of agricultural demand-led industrialisation, which can be pro-rural (Jones and Corbridge, 2010).

However, there is an alternative way of interpreting the flow of rural people to cities and the 'opportunities' awaiting them. Mobility and migration become key mechanisms to avoid rural immiseration in the face of declining terms of trade, climate change and other obstacles to improving productivity. Not only do rural people have little choice in their actions, but also the argument about a natural coupling between rural outmigration and urban manufacturing jobs as economies grow is rarely the case (McMichael, 2009) – unless there is strong state shepherding of the twin processes, as with Taiwan and South Korea (Kay, 2009).

De-agrarianisation and the Contribution of Urban Bias to Food Insecurity – Now and into the Future

As Lipton and his critics have noted, UB and urban penalty go hand in hand. Where they differ is in describing the beneficiaries, with the critics believing that rural people are pulled rather than pushed out of agriculture. Others argue

2 In a point overlooked by his critics, Lipton (1993, p. 231) had argued that: 'extreme relative rural deprivation of health and educational services in most LDCs risks accelerating urban drift, and hence congestion (with increasing marginal external costs, ultimately unsustainable fiscally or environmentally); curtails services for the neediest and reduces overall returns to those services ...'.

that anti-agricultural forces are at work and that systematic discrimination against the rural economy operates, expressed as 'de-agrarianisation' (Bryceson, 2004). This process has resulted in a steady growth of urban slums, where more than one in every seven humans now lives (UN-Habitat, 2003). For example, by 2015 the number of rural dispossessed in India will equal twice the population of the UK, France and Germany combined (Sharma, 2007). Mike Davis (2006) suggests that this 'planet of slums' phenomenon stems from the *decoupling* of urbanisation and industrialisation. The decoupling (as slum catalyst) can be explained only by the greater rate of deterioration of the rural economy than of growth of the urban economy, where according to the International Labour Organization, informal sectors now equal 51 per cent in Latin America, 65 per cent in Asia and 72 per cent in sub-Saharan Africa (Boyd, 2006).

Deterioration of the rural economy reflects an identification of urbanism with modernism; in effect, an ontologically determined UB. Related to this discursive positioning, technologies of scale have allowed food production to be converted over (modern) time from slave plantations to agroindustrial estates, consolidating the power of corporations rather than family farms. Complementing the discriminatory effects of agroindustrialisation on smallholder farming culture has been a long-term challenge from the disposal of highly subsidised staple foods (mainly grains) from the global north into southern markets. This began with US Public Law 480 in 1954, disposing of surplus wheat at concessional prices as food aid to client states on the Cold War perimeter (Friedmann, 1982), extending into a rivalry between the USA and the European Union to capture Third World markets through surplus food 'dumping' by the later 1970s and into the present day; a process which intensified following new rules established at the inception of the World Trade Organization (WTO) in 1995 to open markets to agricultural trade (McMichael, 2005b). This is a clear illustration of Lipton's 'price twists', which may no longer operate within developing countries but which operate globally under the protection of the WTO.

Meanwhile, under the dictates of structural adjustment policies elaborated by the International Monetary Fund and the World Bank, states in the global south have been compelled to reduce supports for their farm sectors (e.g. rural credit, marketing boards, subsidies); and, as the Bank itself acknowledged in its 2008 *World Development Report* (the first annual report to address the agricultural sector in 25 years): structural adjustment has 'dismantled the elaborate system of public agencies providing farmers with access to land, credit, insurance, inputs and cooperative organization' (World Bank, 2008, p. 138).

As above, the early development model encouraged taxation of agriculture and the process of industrialisation via 'unlimited supplies of labour' (Lewis, 1954), naturalising rural outmigration. During the 1990s, the FAO estimated that between 20 and 30 million smallholders were displaced, and food prices reached their lowest level in 150 years (Anonymous, 1999; Madeley, 2000). The international peasant movement, La Vía Campesina (2000), noted: 'the massive movement of food around the world is forcing the increased movement of people'. Despite the rise in net farm incomes where the tax on food exports had been removed, the World Bank estimated that three-quarters of the world's poor resided in farm households (Anderson, 2010).

Access to cheap labour, whether enslaved or dispossessed, with rising sources of fossil fuel, has enabled the industrialisation of farming on increasingly concentrated tracts of land, supplying larger and larger amounts of primary products to feed machines and urban populations. The resulting rift in the human–nature metabolism has not only deprived farm soils (and food products) of natural nutrients, as rural migrants deposit night soil in urban areas and mixed farming patterns decline with the specialisation of livestock farming, but also farming and local ecological knowledge is lost, only to be replaced by commercial agro-inputs (hybrid seeds, inorganic fertilisers, agrochemicals), converting farming into an increasingly toxic industrial economic sector (Schneider and McMichael, 2010). From another angle, modern urbanism has grown via an extractive relationship with the countryside, colonised by industrial technologies involving 'biophysical override' as modern agriculture has required commercial inputs to substitute for displaced ecological processes (Weis, 2007). The Green Revolution is a paradigmatic example of urban extraction insofar as it introduces external technologies to amplify delivery of staple crops to urban residents, displacing local rural (leafy green-based) diets, privileging larger farmers, introducing herbicides and pesticides and undermining the ecological base in the long run (Patel, 2013).

As Dorward (2013, p. 44) has recently argued:

> food prices, agricultural worker productivity, and global threats to supply/demand balances are fundamental long-term development issues. Not only are they critically important for poorer children's and adult food security, health and physical and mental development, they affect the global economy and the welfare of rich nations and people.

For Dorward, a primary mechanism for delivering food security for urban and rural people alike involves lower food prices, made possible by increased rural labour productivity, which, with the appropriate technological investments, can require fewer workers released from the drudgery that is so often associated with peasant and smallholder agriculture. However, we remain concerned about the social, political and health consequences of this development trajectory, particularly for the remaining rural producers and the growing numbers of rural to urban low-paid factory and service sector workers.

Applying the Urban Bias Hypothesis to Thailand

All protagonists to the UB debate agree that national case studies are required to determine the context-specific features by which groups benefit from public resource allocations, and especially transfers between agricultural producer communities and urban consumer communities. Space precludes any substantial case study development, but using key concepts of the UB approach – price twists to support export agriculture and industrial imports; government support for cheap food alongside urbanisation and industrialisation; deploying agricultural commodity revenues to underwrite social and infrastructure policies that disproportionately favour urban populations; leaving food supply research and development to the private sector – we present material on the role of rice production in Thailand's national development, and a nuanced understanding of UB.

Now classified as an upper-middle-income country, Thailand described itself up until recently as an agrarian society and even now 40 per cent of the population resides in rural areas. The nation entered the 20th century as a major rice exporting nation (Johnston, 1981), and in the period between the 1850s and 1930s, the land under rice cultivation almost quadrupled, with agricultural exports growing over many years at an annual average of 6 per cent (Resnick, 1970). During these years, rice production was undertaken by peasant farmers and private entrepreneurs, who were encouraged by government investments in agricultural infrastructure, especially canals. During the 1940s and 1950s, a rice export tax was introduced, and this, along with the earlier reduction of tariffs for foreign traders, inserted price twist mechanisms into national development. Simultaneously, government policies kept domestic food prices low (Goss and Burch, 2001), and the value of rice export earnings meant that there was no push to move people out of agriculture into the cities. This started to change from the 1960s, once the limits of further agricultural land developments had been reached, and rice export revenues started to fall relative to other agricultural commodities (Siamwalla, 1996). Despite agricultural export taxes being eliminated in the mid-1980s, and the more recent introduction of the rice mortgage scheme to guarantee farm prices for rice stocks – for Lipton, such financial supports of farmers to compete on world markets resembles developed world agricultural subsidies – Thailand's rice farmers now have among the lowest productivity levels in the Southeast Asian region (IRRI, 2013). This may, in part, be due to a marked decline in government investment in agriculture, post Green Revolution (Walker, 2012). While the deteriorating terms of trade have seen Bangkok and some regional cities grow rapidly, the steady flow of people into urban centres slowed for some years after the 1998 Asian Financial Crisis and the 2009–10 Global Financial Crisis, since urban unemployment was high.

In the last 30 years, there has been a marked shift within the agri-food sector, between primary and secondary production. Food processing, led in part by the Thai agri-business conglomerate, Charoen Pokphand, backed by a raft of government policies keen to consolidate Thailand's role as the leading southern hemisphere food exporter (enshrined in policy as Kitchen to the World and/or known as 'Asia's supermarket'), means that the manufacture and domestic sale, and export, of processed foods now account for greater revenues than primary production. The relative power of giant food manufacturers, which includes domestic and global supermarket chains with their home-brand product portfolios, has also meant that farmers are no longer self-employed but have become contracted labourers to the corporations, and hence highly vulnerable to any changes in corporate supply chain strategies. Thailand leads the world in terms of relative numbers of contract farmers, who are now at a higher risk of poverty and food insecurity than other Thais (Jitsuchon and Siamwalla, 2009). Other contributors to lower farm incomes are low levels of government investment in agricultural productivity (Walker, 2012), and the despoliation of farming lands and aquatic environments, alongside urban encroachment on fertile plains, making food yield increases problematic (Amekawa, 2010; Dorward, 2013). For Thai rural producers locked into free trade agreements and corporate supply chains, difficult choices follow: invest their own capital in agricultural productivity gains while continuing to receive low returns for supplying the cheapest food possible, move to the cities in the hope of a higher-income occupation, or engage in seasonal migration in order to keep household income streams flowing.

While Thailand, in the century following the 1850s, illustrates the operations of UB in terms of price twists, agricultural revenues underwriting industrial sector expansion, a lack of public investment in agricultural research and the growth in the production of processed foods, or 'rich men's foods', to use a phrase from Lipton, a less straightforward reading of UB is required in relation to social infrastructural investments in rural and urban areas. In the last 20 years, successive governments have instituted what could be considered pro-rural policies, particularly in terms of easier lines of credit being made available to small farmers and a higher proportion of primary health-service providers than exists in Bangkok (Yiengprugsawan et al., 2010). Another populist policy, the universal health insurance scheme, is also considered to be a pro-poor policy assisting poor urban and rural citizens alike. These policy outcomes are due to (i) the long-time potency at the ballot box of rural Thais, coupled with government fears of their pro-communist sympathies during the 1970s and 1980s (Goss and Burch, 2001); and (ii) significant levels of civil society activism, often with the support of the military (Meesomboonpoonsuk, 2013). Nevertheless, despite rapid economic growth over 60 years, regional income disparities have been widening, and the infant mortality rate has been widening between urban and rural areas (Yiengprugsawan et al., 2010). Further, for those aged 15–39 who remain in rural areas, their incomes and education are likely to decline significantly compared to their urban counterparts (Lim et al., 2009).

Thus, it is difficult to declare Thai governments to be pro-urban and anti-rural. Rather, in common with many OECD nations, they are pursuing economic policies that cede power to corporations and to a form of neoliberal capitalist development. Global corporations and free trade agreements, Kay (2009) suggests, lie behind the fate of rural areas more than any systematic UB. However, the end result could well prove Lipton correct: without greater government attention to rural development as central to national development, the food and nutrition security prospects for poor rural and urban Thais alike look elusive. In Thailand, as elsewhere (Mei and Shao, 2011), the emphasis on cheap food appears not to be the answer to sustainable national development, given that it is both a recipe for rural producer poverty and for diet-related diseases with the cheapest food generally being processed food made available by modern retailers, including supermarkets (Banwell et al., 2013; Kelly et al., 2015). It is the supermarkets and hypermarkets that so appeal to a Thai urban middle-class notion of modernity (Isaacs, 2009).

Countering Urban Bias

Global agri-food systems are coming under greater scrutiny from different quarters: food security and human rights, public health and ecosystem health. In the midst of the recent global food crisis, the UN- and World Bank-sponsored International Assessment of Agricultural Science and Technology for Development (2008) expressed a deepening international scientific and development practitioner consensus that sustaining Earth and its peoples requires massive support for agroecological methods that have been shown in recent studies to be equally productive, less energy-intensive, restorative, resilient and carbon-sequestering, and stabilising of rural cultures and healthy diets (e.g. FAO, 2002; Pretty et al., 2003; Badgley et al., 2007). To date, these have been the methods practised primarily by the smallholders who have left farming.

Within Thailand, a self-sufficiency movement vies with the Kitchen to the World approach to food security. Supported by government, the 'Sufficiency Economy' (SE) is a response to the wide-scale poverty that arose in the late 1980s, and it 'aims to encourage people to develop self discipline in consumption' as well as to be more self-reliant through cooperative production (Seubsman et al., 2013, pp. 57–58). The model incorporates agroecology principles including discouraging pesticide use and encouraging diverse cropping and organic agriculture. It is concerned to help rural producers adapt to emerging market opportunities and to secure long-term agricultural futures through environmental restoration. However, a study undertaken in Thailand's poorest Isan region showed that while a majority of villagers had become self-sufficient in food through participating in the SE programme, had low levels of debt and high levels of life satisfaction, they wanted more for their children; in particular, the educational opportunities that were available in cities (Seubsman et al., 2013). This understandable predisposition reinforces the urban bias of modernity.

The Thai example is a valiant attempt to create a place for non- or less socially and environmentally exploitative food systems. For the sake of food system resilience (which requires diverse production approaches, scales of farming and food crops), there is a place for large and small rural producers practising agroecology. At present, rural areas in many nations are acting as sinks for urban waste, and they generate the clean air and pure water needed by the cities for their sustenance. Lack of recognition of the role that rural populations play in 'cleaning up' urban environments penalises them in another way; yet this contribution to the environmental commons could create opportunities for employment based on novel technologies, public investment and new income streams, and strengthen awareness of urban–rural interdependencies.

Conclusion

From our perspective, urban bias continues to operate; both as anti-agricultural bias or as corporate industrial agricultural bias, and as an ontological framing of modernity and progress. Current scholarship concerning food security policy, in all countries, needs to re-situate policy formulations in a new ontology recognising farming and food as essential to planetary and human health. The point is that our social and political theories arose in an ecological vacuum, so to speak, with urbanity as the measure of progress.

Ecological interdependencies have been ignored, with the rural seen simply as a source of labour and products. Thus, capitalist modernity has converted agriculture into an economic sector, alongside of, and serving, the manufacturing sector with foods for processing and as an outlet for industrial agri-inputs to override biophysical processes (Weis, 2007). Losing sight of our earthly foundations has thus privileged the 'urban' over the 'rural', de-naturalised food and agriculture and enabled markets (and their corporate and retailing agents) to shape social diets, often at the expense of public health.

We recommend restoring a healthier, reciprocal relation between urban and rural, requiring policies that eschew urban (developmentalist) bias, revaluing farming as an ecological act, and as such as a source of healthy food. Suitable policies should encourage urban–rural solidarity in pursuit of sustainable land use and preservation of food cultures. Some concrete proposals would include redirecting energy subsidies into rebuilding rural infrastructure (including extension services to support rather than replace farming knowledge), providing incentives for ecosystem stewardship (taxing those who use the rural sinks), shortening supply chains (localising/farmers' markets) and, where producers depend on export markets, supporting fair trade. Finally, prioritising domestic food security as a democratic and sustainable alternative to the current WTO agro-export regime is a significant step towards reuniting urban complexes with their rural foundations.

Acknowledgements

The authors would like to thank Andrew Dorward and Cris Kay for stimulating discussions regarding Urban Bias theory. We also thank Matthew Kelly for alerting us to relevant references in relation to Thai agriculture.

References

Amekawa, Y. 2010. Rethinking sustainable agriculture in Thailand: a governance perspective. *Journal of Sustainable Agriculture* 34, 389–416.

Anderson, K. 2010. Krueger/Schiff/Valdes Revisited. Agricultural price and trade policy reform in developing countries since 1960. *Policy Research Working Paper 5165*. The World Bank Development Research Group.

Anonymous. 1999. Finance and economics: A raw deal for commodities, *The Economist*, April 17, 75–6.

Badgley, C., Moghtader, J., Quintero, E., Zakem, E., Chappell, M.J., Aviles-Vazquez, K., et al. 2007. Organic agriculture and the global food supply. *Renewable Agriculture and Food Systems* 22, 86–108.

Banwell, C., Dixon, J., Seubsman, S., Pangsap, S. & Kelly, M. 2013. Evolving food retail environments in Thailand and implications for the health and nutrition transition. *Public Health Nutrition* 16(4), 608–15.

Bates, R. 1993. 'Urban bias': a fresh look. *Journal of Development Studies* 29, 219–28.

Boyd, R. 2006. Labour's response to the informalization of work in the current restructuring of global capitalism: China, South Korea and South Africa. *Canadian Journal of Development Studies* 27, 487–502.

Bryceson, D. 2004. Agrarian vista or vortex? African rural livelihood policies. *Review of African Political Economy* 102, 617–29.

Burch, D., Dixon, J. & Lawrence, G. 2013. Introduction to symposium on the changing role of supermarkets in global supply chains: from seedling to supermarket: agri-food supply chains in transition. *Agriculture & Human Values*, doi:10.1007/s10460-012-9410-x.

Byres, T. 1979. Of neo-populist pipe dreams: Daedalus in the Third World and the myth of urban bias. *The Journal of Peasant Studies* 6, 210–40.

Davis, M. 2006. *Planet of Slums*. Verso, London, UK.

de Schutter, O. & Sepulveda, M. 2012. Underwriting the poor. A global fund for social protection. Briefing Note 7, UN Special Rapporteur on the right to food, Geneva, Switzerland.

Dixon, J. 2009. From the imperial to the empty calorie: how nutrition relations underpin food regime transitions. *Agriculture and Human Values* 26, 321–31.

Dixon, J. & Isaacs, B. 2013. Why sustainable and 'nutritionally correct' foods are not on the local agenda: Western Sydney, the moral arts of everyday life and public policy. *Food Policy* 43, 67–76.

Doward, A. 2013. Agricultural labour productivity, food prices and sustainable development and indicators. *Food Policy* 39, 40–50.

ETC (Erosion, Technology, Concentration) 2009. Who will feed us? ETC Group Communiqué, 102 (November). Available at: www.etcgroup.org, accessed 5 March 2015.

FAO (Food and Agriculture Organization) 2002. *Organic Agriculture, Environment and Food Security*. FAO, Rome.

Friedmann, H. 1982. The political economy of food: the rise and fall of the postwar international food order. *American Journal of Sociology* 88, 248–86.

Goss, J. & Burch, D. 2001. From agricultural modernisation to agri-food globalisation: the waning of national development in Thailand. *Third World Quarterly* 22(6), 969–86.

Hawkes, C. 2008. Dietary implications of supermarket development: a global perspective. *Development Policy Review* 26, 657–92.

Hawkes, C., Blouin, C., Henson, S., Drager, N. & Dubé, L. (eds) 2010. *Trade, Food, Diet and Health: Perspectives and Policy Options*. Wiley Blackwell, Oxford, UK.

Hetzel, B. & McMichael, A.J. 1989. *The LS Factor: Lifestyle and Health*. Penguin Books, Melbourne, VIC, Australia.

International Assessment of Agricultural Science and Technology for Development 2008. Summary for decision makers of the Global Report. International Assessment of Agricultural Knowledge, Science and Technology for Development, www.unep.org/dewa/assessments/ecosystems/iaastd/tabid/105853/default.aspx, accessed 20 March 2015.

IRRI (International Rice Research Institute) 2013. World Rice Statistics. Available at: ricestat.irri.org:8080/wrs2, accessed 20 November 2013.

Isaacs, B. 2009. Imagining Thailand in European hypermarkets: new class-based consumption in Chiang Mai's 'cruise ships'. *Asia Pacific Journal of Anthropology* 10(4), 348–63.

Jitsuchon, S. & Siamwalla, A. 2009. Economic shocks and the vulnerable in Thailand: case study of rising food and fuel prices. Discussion Paper for UNICEF. Available at: www.childimpact.unicef-irc.org/documents/view/id/102/lang/en, accessed 15 December 2014.

Johnston, D. 1981. Rice cultivation in Thailand: the development of an export economy by indigenous capital and labour. *Modern Asian Studies* 15(1), 107–26.

Jones, A. & Corbridge, S. 2010. The continuing debate about urban bias: the thesis, its critics, its influence and its implications for poverty-reduction strategies. *Progress in Development Studies* 10, doi:10.1177/146499340901000101.

Kay, C. 2006. Rural poverty and development strategies in Latin America. *Journal of Agrarian Change* 6, 455–508.

Kay, C. 2009. Development strategies and rural development: exploring synergies, eradicating poverty. *The Journal of Peasant Studies* 36, 103–37.

Kelly, M., Seubsman, S., Banwell, C., Dixon, J. & Sleigh, A. 2015. Traditional, modern or mixed? Perspectives on social, economic and health impacts of evolving food retail in Thailand. *Agriculture and Human Values*, epub ahead of print, doi:10.1007/s10460-014-9561-z.

La Vía Campesina 2000. Declaration of the International Meeting of the Landless in San Pedro Sula, Honduras. July. Available at: viacampesina.org/en/index.php/main-issues-mainmenu-27/agrarian-reform-mainmenu-36/73-declaration-international-meeting-landless-in-san-pedro-sula-honduras, accessed 2 March 2015.

Lewis, W.A. 1954. Economic development with unlimited supplies of labour. *The Manchester School* May, 400–49.

Lim, L.-Y., Kjellstrom, T., Sleigh, A., Khamman, S., Seubsman, S., Dixon, J., et al. 2009. Associations between urbanisation and components of the health-risk transition in Thailand. A descriptive study of 87,100 Thai adults. *Global Health Action* 2, doi:10.3042/gha.v5210.1914, 1–13.

Lipton, M. 1977. Why Poor People Stay Poor: Urban Bias in World Development. Temple Smith, London, UK.

Lipton, M. 1984. Urban bias revisited. *Journal of Development Studies* 20, 139–66.

Lipton, M. 1993. Urban bias: of consequences, classes and causality. *Journal of Development Studies* 29, 220–48.

McMichael, A.J. 2005a. Integrating nutrition with ecology: balancing the health of humans and biosphere. *Public Health Nutrition* 8, 706–15.

McMichael, A.J., Powles, J., Butler, C.D. & Uauy, R. 2007. Food, livestock production, energy, climate change, and health. *The Lancet* 370, 1253–63.

McMichael, P. 1996. *Development and Social Change. A Global Perspective*. Sage, Thousand Oaks, California, USA.

McMichael, P. 2005b. Global development and the corporate food regime. In: Buttel, F.H. & McMichael, P. (eds) *New Directions in the Sociology of Global Development*. Elsevier, Amsterdam, 269–303.

McMichael, P. 2009. Banking on agriculture: a review of the World Development Report. *Journal of Agrarian Change* 9, 235–46.

McMichael, P. 2013. *Food Regimes and Agrarian Questions*. Fernwood, Halifax, Canada.

Madeley, J. 2000. *Hungry for Trade*. Zed Books, London, UK.

Marsden, T. 2012. Third natures? Reconstituting space through place-making strategies for sustainability. *International Journal of the Sociology of Agriculture and Food* 19(2), 257–74.

Meesomboonpoonsuk, S. 2013. Urban bias and civil unrest in contemporary Thailand. Paper delivered to the Annual Conference of Development Studies. Fernwood, Halifax, Canada. Available at: ics.nccu.edu.tw/ced/admin/data/PANEL-A/A9.2.pdf, accessed 26 February 2015.

Mei, L. & Shao, D. 2011. Too cheap hurt farmers, too expensive hurt customers: the changing impacts of supermarkets on Chinese agro-food markets. *Millenial Asia* 2(1), 43–64.

Patel, R. 2013. The long green revolution. *The Journal of Peasant Studies* 40, 1–63.

Pretty, J., Morison, J. & Hine, R. 2003. Reducing food poverty by increasing agricultural sustainability in developing countries. *Agriculture, Ecosystems and Environment* 95, 217–34.

Resnick, S. 1970. The decline of rural industry under export expansion: a comparison among Burma, Philippines and Thailand, 1870–1938. *The Journal of Economic History* 30(1), 51–73.

Rosset, P. 2006. *Food is Different. Why We Must Get the WTO Out of Agriculture*. Fernwood Publishing, Halifax, Nova Scotia, Canada.

Schneider, M. & McMichael, P. 2010. Deepening, and repairing, the metabolic rift. *The Journal of Peasant Studies* 37, 461–84.

Sharma, D. 2007. Displacing farmers: India will have 400 million refugees. Share the World's Resources. Available at: www.stwr.net/content/view/1999/37, accessed 2 March 2015.

Seubsman, S., Kelly, M. & Sleigh, A. 2013. The Sufficiency Economy and community sustainability in rural northeastern Thailand. *Asian Culture and History* 5(2), 57–65.

Siamwalla, S. 1996. Thai agriculture: from engine of growth to sunset status. *Thai Development Research Institute Quarterly Review* 11(4), 3–10.

UN-Habitat 2003. The Challenge of Slums. Global Report on Human Settlements. Earthscan, London, UK.

Walker, A. 2012. *Thailand's Political Peasants: Power in the Modern Rural Economy*. University of Wisconsin Press, Madison, Wisconsin, USA.

Weis, T. 2007. The Global Food Economy. The Battle for the Future of Farming. Zed Books, London, UK.

World Bank 2008. *World Development Report*. World Bank, Washington, DC, USA.

Yiengprugsawan, V., Carmichael, G., Lim, L., Seubsman, S. & Sleigh, A. 2010. Has universal health insurance reduced urban–rural inequalities in health service use in Thailand? *Health and Place* 16(5), 1030–7.

PART 5

CLIMATE CHANGE AND HEALTH

REPRINT G

Global Warming, Ecological Disruption and Human Health: The Penny Drops

ANTHONY J. MCMICHAEL

McMichael, A.J. 1991. Global warming, ecological disruption and human health: the penny drops. *Medical Journal of Australia* 154, 499 501.

Pages: 333 to 338

LEADING ARTICLES

Global warming, ecological disruption and human health: the penny drops

The environment debate is warming up. Tussles between conservationists, industrialists, unions and politicians over environmental policies and strategies are commonplace. The foci of concern are economics, aesthetics, preservation of amenity, and protection of foliage, fur, feathers and fins.

A late — but hugely important — entrant to the debate is the health lobby. In the longer-term (and admittedly anthropocentric) view of macroenvironmental degradation, the "bottom line" will be dominated by adverse effects upon human health and survival.

In July 1990, the Federal Government issued a draft Discussion Paper on "ecologically sustainable development".[1] The Public Health Association of Australia, and others, protested that this document displayed no awareness that environmental degradation endangers population health — despite the Prime Minister's earlier proclamation that: "The environment ultimately sustains all life . . . Ultimately, environmental destruction means not only plant and animal destruction but also the end of humanity."[2]

Just as someone on the Prime Minister's staff understands that ecosystems are life-support systems, so the "ecologically sustainable development" debate must recognise that the health of any species, including ours, cannot exist apart from its ecosystem. Good health is the living manifestation of a species' biological compatibility with its ecosystem. We will not understand the intimate connection between environment and population health while we continue to think in environmental rather than ecological terms and talk of damage to the environment "out there".

At the risk of digressing from the main stimulus for this editorial — the paper by Ewan and colleagues on the potential health impact of climate change on page 554 of this issue of the Journal — we must understand clearly the evolutionary perspective on environment and health. Otherwise our policy responses will continue to be trivial and irrelevant.

Of billions of planets, Earth may be one of the few that can support "life". Confluence of the basic conditions for complex organic life — including temperature, atmosphere, water and protection from ultraviolet irradiation — is a huge statistical improbability. For the first billion years of Earth's four-billion-year existence, as a globule of cosmic condensate, the elements and simple molecules remained in lifeless form. Then, by chance, simple organic molecules with the power of self-replication arose within the primordial sludge. That was "it"; once a self-replicating molecule had formed, its progeny inexorably became dominant among the ingredients in the sludge. As further accidental advances in the self-replication process conferred added advantage, more complex life-forms emerged.

Early life existed in an anaerobic (oxygen-free) environment. Because Earth was exposed to the sun's unfiltered ultraviolet radiation (UVR) — injurious to complex molecules — early life was confined to the oceans. Over subsequent millenia, oxygen, a waste product of primitive chlorophyll-using aquatic plants, accumulated in the atmosphere. The UVR converted some of this oxygen into an ozone layer which then, about 400 000 years ago, allowed life-forms to venture on to dry land, protected from that same UVR.

A myriad species came and went as the planet's environment underwent slow but ceaseless change. The impartial process of natural selection sifted through the chance offerings, discarding most, favouring some. The survival of each successful species depended on a finely tuned compatibility with the prevailing ecosystem.

During the dinosaurs' massive dynasty early mammals emerged. Among later mammals came the primates and hominids, and then — in the last ten-thousandth of the planet's history (the last 10 seconds on the 24-hour clock) — the human species. This was a big-brained, tool-using species with complex communications, self-consciousness, awareness of death, and a learned ability to dominate and change the very environment that had shaped its own biological evolution. Puny in impact at first, humanity with its recent development of burgeoning populations, energy-intensive technology and consumerism has caused massive changes to the environment. Global ecosystems are today coming under threat from a resident species. This is a "first" in Earth's history; it is a dramatic development. We must understand its enormous public health implications.

To argue that humans are adaptable and already live in varied environments — and could therefore cope with a hotter world — is to miss the point. Those currently habitable environments exist within a supportive ecological framework, entailing stable weather patterns, an interdependent fabric of diverse plant and animal life, healthy soils and access to water. If significant global warming occurs — and an historically unprecedented rise of at least 2°-3°C is likely within the next century[2-6] — then the ecological framework will begin to disintegrate.

The Second World Climate Conference (November 1990) reviewed the impending consequences of global warming and the need for urgent multilateral action. Uncertainties and imprecision in the predictions are rife — and unavoidable — but there is little residual doubt about the need for immediate action. The Report of the Intergovernmental Panel on Climate Change, the centrepiece of that Conference, says:

> The most vulnerable human settlements are those especially exposed to natural hazards . . . In coastal lowlands such as in Bangladesh, China and Egypt as well as in small island nations, inundation due to sea-level rise and storm surges could lead to significant movements of people. Major health impacts are possible, especially in large urban areas owing to changes in the availability of water and food and increased health problems due to heat stress and spreading of infections. Changes in precipitation and temperature could radically alter the patterns of vector-borne and viral diseases by shifting them to higher latitudes, thus putting large populations at risk. As similar events have in the past, these changes could initiate large migrations of people, leading over a number of years

> to severe disruptions of settlement patterns and social instability in some areas. . . . Global warming and increased ultraviolet radiation resulting from depletion of stratospheric ozone may produce adverse impacts on air quality such as increases in ground-level ozone in some polluted urban areas.[6]

In Australia, the greenhouse effect has received top media billing. Other health-endangering ecological disruptions in Australia include stratospheric ozone depletion and land degradation through soil erosion and salination. Globally, adverse health effects will result from acid rain; loss of biodiversity; and cumulative contamination of food and water with toxic agents. The influential United States-based Worldwatch Institute said recently:

> Every major indication shows a deterioration in the Earth's natural systems. Forests are shrinking, deserts expanding, croplands are losing topsoil, the ozone layer continues to thin, greenhouse gases are accumulating, the number of plant and animals species drops, and biological damage from air pollution and acid rain spreads.[7]

Increasingly, the available data support these claims.

Given these ominous trends, the commissioning by the National Health and Medical Research Council (NHMRC) of a review of the health consequences of long-term climate change is a welcome step forward. This review, conducted during 1990, resulted in a report to the November (1990) Council meeting of the NHMRC.[8] The principal findings are summarised by Ewan et al. in this issue. Two categories of health consequences are discussed: increases in existing problems (heat waves, cyclones, spread of arboviruses, air pollutants, etc.), and new threats to health (disrupted food supply, social upheaval, mental stress, reintroduction of malaria, etc.).

The paper emphasises the substantial uncertainty of those predictions, and makes clear the urgent need for a more systematic approach to research, surveillance and policy development. It also emphasises that, at least initially, the greatest impact upon health will be in the socially and politically marginalised groups.

Because of criticisms of the thrust of the abovementioned Discussion Paper on "ecologically sustainable development", the Federal Government is redoing the exercise — and has urged that account be taken of public health impact. An NHMRC Working Party is preparing health impact guidelines for the nine environment-perturbing activities (mining, agriculture, tourism, etc.) that constitute the framework of the exercise. It must be stressed that adverse health impact is not an incidental byproduct of ecological damage, to be casually dealt with in footnotes — it is the central consequence.

It is important that the NHMRC now develops a capacity for evaluating the health impact of macroenvironmental change and for providing policy advice to government. Effective working relations should be established between the NHMRC, the Australian Health Ministers Advisory Council, and the ANZ Environmental Council (i.e., environment ministers), in order that a multisectoral strategy may be developed for tackling the health impact of global and regional environmental changes. These Australian initiatives will need to be part of, and should accord with, multilateral international strategies that address the real roots of the problem; 20% reductions in carbon emissions by 2005 will slow up the greenhouse process, but to actually stop it we have to substantially curtail our society's addiction to fossil fuel.[3,6] We have built a societal edifice which depends on "cheap" energy — acquired at well below its true environmental cost.

The Federal Government, in consultation with the States, plans an Environmental Protection Agency. Bureaucratic territorialism must be put aside; we need a multisectoral approach to the larger problems of ecological disruption — in addition to the management of localised environmental toxicity problems. The health sector must lift its gaze to bigger, ecological, horizons. This will require a radical extension of the public health agenda, new forms of professional training in environmental health, a preparedness to base policy advice upon predictions and best guesses (as opposed to empirical data), and an ability to collaborate with unfamiliar disciplines (e.g., climatology and ecology).

We must understand our vulnerability; the world does not owe us a living, and our boisterous and expansionist occupancy of the ecological niche into which our hominid forebears evolved is now rebounding upon us. *Homo sapiens* could even become an endangered species later next century.

This is an entirely unprecedented type of public health problem — and it requires us to anticipate the future. The struggle for species survival has always been conducted in the present tense: survival today means reproductive success tomorrow. However, we now find that we must act in relation to this planet's future. That is a tall order. Although we have acquired, through evolution, a capacity to respond ("fight or flight") to immediate hazards, we have not been phylogenetically programmed to act in relation to the non-immediate future.[9]

Relatedly, our society is preoccupied with immediate "needs" — consumer goods, economic growth and physical security. The health of the economy is a more politically compelling issue than is the long-term health of the human population. The landmark United Nations-commissioned Brundtland Report,[10] now a prime template for governmental policy review around the world, itself manifests this recurring blind spot in our social agenda. "Health impact" is the missing chapter in Brundtland.

One major difficulty in assessing health impact is that we cannot foresee all the health consequences of environmental deterioration. This applies in particular to "exposures" for which we have yet had no prior experience — e.g., thinning of the ozone layer. Hence, estimation of health impact must be by extrapolation from related circumstances or by application of theory. This makes for a basic distinction between traditional environmental health problems and today's macroenvironmental problems. The former category allows observation of the health impact of some localised pollution problem and then pre-empting its recurrence elsewhere. With problems of global scope we do not have that luxury.

Another important distinction is between toxic pollutants and "non-toxic" factors that disrupt ecosystems. Sulphur dioxide, nitrogen oxides and heavy metals cause direct biological insult. Much of our traditional environmental health concern has been over such noxious factors. By contrast, factors like carbon dioxide, methane, chlorofluorocarbons and salt (in groundwater) are not toxins; yet they now portend disruption to life-support systems. This disruption will have indirect, longer-term effects upon our health via adverse effects on other animal and plant species in the food supply chain. For example, acidification of waterways contaminates and kills aquatic life. Increased UVR exposure can reduce crop yields and weaken microbial activity in soils.

These macroenvironmental problems will challenge our basic value system. What do we really mean by "standard of living"? How should we value material consumption against other things (such as good health) that contribute to the quality of life? Do we recognise the environmentally destructive nature of conventional short-term economic thinking, with its inbuilt discounting of the future?

We must consider ways of reorganising society according to ecological principles that ensure a sustainable — and healthy — environment.[11] The "Greens" propose a circular "conserver" economy, with maximum recycling and use of renewable sources of materials and energy. The gross national product (GNP), measuring throughput in the consumer economy, was never intended as an indicator of human well-being. Used that way, the GNP leads to ecologically bizarre accounting; the Exxon Valdez oil spill boosted the GNP of Alaska. An ecologically sustainable economy would measure success via real-life indicators such as population health, and quality of air, water and food, maintenance of biodiversity, and reduced use of non-renewable resources.

Good health requires a health-sustaining environment. If "ecologically sustainable development" policies do not ensure the population's health, then they make nonsense of the word "ecological". For three billion years ecology has been about health and survival; for several recent years it has been misconstrued as being about other ephemeral societal goals. The paper by Ewan et al. will promote the inclusion of health as a primary criterion in the environment debate; it will help to bring us back to Earth.

A J McMichael
Professor of Occupational and Environmental Health
Department of Community Medicine
University of Adelaide

1. Department of Prime Minister and Cabinet. Ecologically sustainable development. A Commonwealth discussion paper, June 1990. Canberra: AGPS, 1990.
2. Hawke RJL. Our country our future: statement on the environment. Canberra: AGPS, 1989.
3. Lowe I. Living in the greenhouse. Newham, Victoria: Scribe, 1989.
4. World Health Organization. Environment and Health: the European Charter and commentary. Geneva: WHO, 1989. (WHO regional publication. European series, no. 35.)
5. World Health Organization. Potential health effects of climate change. Report of WHO Task Group, WHO/PEP/90/10. Geneva: WHO, 1990.
6. Intergovernmental Panel on Climate Change. IPCC first assessment report. Volume I. Geneva: World Meteorological Organization, 1990.
7. Brown L. Editorial. Worldwatch 1990; 3(4): 2.
8. Ewan C, Bryant EA, Calvert GD. Health implications of long term climate change. Volumes 1 and 2. Discussion document commissioned by NHMRC. Canberra: Department of Community Services and Health, 1990.
9. Ornstein R, Ehrlich P. New world, new mind. London: Methuen, 1989.
10. World Commission on Environment and Development. Our common future. Oxford: Oxford University Press, 1987.
11. Boyden S, Dovers S, Shirlow M. The biosphere under threat: ecological realities and Australia's opportunities. Melbourne: Oxford University Press, 1990.

END OF REPRINT G

Global Warming, Ecological Disruption and Human Health: The Penny Drops

ANTHONY J. MCMICHAEL

17

FRAGILE PARADISE

Health and Climate Change in the South Pacific

LACHLAN MCIVER AND ELIZABETH HANNA

Abstract

Island countries of the South Pacific are among the most vulnerable in the world to the effects of climate change, including the likely detrimental impacts on health. In general, the burden of these impacts falls disproportionately to particular subsectors of the population, such as the socio-economically deprived, certain occupational groups, those with pre-existing illnesses and residents of areas of high exposure to climate-related phenomena such as floods, droughts and sea level rise. Thus, climate change has the potential to exacerbate social and health inequalities further. As part of a suite of adaptations integrated across sectors, protection of Pacific Island communities from climate change-related health threats requires an evidence-based approach that incorporates a context-based assessment of vulnerability.

Pioneering work by McMichael and colleagues in the 1990s and early 2000s provided templates for performing assessments of vulnerability and compiling plans for adaptation to protect human health from the effects of climate change. This chapter reviews the inclusion of the human health dimension in the climate change impact and adaptation research landscape. We summarise the mixed methods approaches employed to assess climate change and health vulnerabilities and adaptation opportunities in the Pacific region. Results of these assessments are provided, key themes are identified and we map the planned direction of health adaptation to climate change in the Pacific.

Background

While it may seem, to some, that the scientific community's interest in and concern about the changing global climate is a relatively recent phenomenon, the reality is radically different. The concurrent rise in post-Industrial Revolution global greenhouse gas emissions and increasing ambient temperatures has been occurring for more than two centuries, and the causal link between the two was first hypothesised in the 19th century, when Arrhenius recognised the relationship between atmospheric carbon dioxide concentrations and the temperature at the Earth's surface (Arrhenius, 1896), building on earlier work that explored the effect of gases and vapour on radiation and heat (Tyndall, 1861).

In the late 1980s, the World Health Organization (WHO) convened a working group to consider the health impacts of the climate change scenarios developed in 1987 by the World Meteorological Organization (WMO) and the United Nations Environment Programme (UNEP). These scenarios included the possibility of warming air and sea surface temperatures, rising seas and increasing variability and impacts of extreme weather events such as floods, droughts and storms (WMO and UNEP, 1988). The resulting WHO report, entitled 'Potential health effects of climatic change', considered both 'direct' impacts, such as heat-related morbidity and mortality, as well as 'indirect' effects, including the impacts on crops and nutrition, communicable diseases such as those spread by vectors (e.g. malaria, schistosomiasis, lymphatic filariasis) and those related to water quality (e.g. diarrhoeal illness) (WHO, 1990). This early, speculative work has been expanded and refined over recent years, with much of that led by McMichael, who continued to update and improve upon his own conceptual models of the pathways and impacts of climate change on health to incorporate contemporary evidence and reflect the evolution of our understanding of the issues.

The Intergovernmental Panel on Climate Change (IPCC) was convened in 1988, and issued its first report in 1990. Within three years, WHO was collaborating with WMO and UNEP in a series of consultations that culminated in the publication of the seminal work, *Climate Change and Human Health*, in 1996. This book laid out the established and potential links between climate variables and the climate-sensitive determinants of health and disease (McMichael et al., 1996). It expanded on the original list of diseases of concern in the context of climate change and laid the epidemiological foundation for investigation of the current and, more importantly, future impacts of climate change on health. In so doing, the authors explained the methodological challenges involved in estimating climate change-attributable impacts and burdens of disease, based on multiple scenarios and layers of uncertainties. It was a pioneering work of public health research, and its authors were breaking new scientific ground in the exploration of the link between a healthy human population and a healthy planet. The book's first editor was Tony McMichael.

McMichael and a group of close colleagues (including Andy Haines, Jonathan Patz, Diarmid Campbell-Lendrum, Sari Kovats, Carlos Corvalán, Alistair Woodward, Simon Hales, Kris Ebi and Yasushi Honda) published a series of subsequent papers and texts in the late 1990s and early 2000s that undertook the difficult dual tasks of estimating the attribution of climate change causality to the global burden of disease and suggesting strategies to manage these climate change-related threats to health. Assistance with this venture came in the form of the establishment of a small unit within WHO's Environmental Health team in its Geneva headquarters and research support provided by the London School of Hygiene and Tropical Medicine.

Of the most significant achievements of this group during that period were the compilation of chapters on the potential risks of climate change to human population health for the Second (1996) and Third (2001) Assessment Reports of the IPCC. While the focus was still primarily on the direct health effects of heat and hydrometeorological disasters and the indirect impacts on communicable diseases and malnutrition, by the time of the Third Assessment Report there was growing recognition of the unique vulnerabilities of certain regions (e.g. low-lying island communities) and populations (e.g. developing countries, the socio-economically deprived) (IPCC, 2001). Terms such as 'adaptive capacity' were coined, defined and used to explain both natural and social phenomena in the climate change context.

In 2003, McMichael and colleagues compiled another pivotal work, commissioned by WHO, WMO and UNEP, entitled *Climate Change and Human Health – Risks and Responses* (McMichael et al., 2003b). One of the most widely referenced texts on the topic ever since, this book built on the growing body of literature describing the pathways by which climate change affected health and, for the first time, quantified the estimated global burden of disease due to climate change (as part of WHO's 'Comparative Quantification of Health Risks' project in 2000) and reviewed and synthesised the attempts by a number of countries to assess the health impacts of climate change at a national level. The global climate change-attributable burden of disease at that time (using 2000 as a baseline) was estimated at approximately 150,000 deaths per year (McMichael et al., 2004), a figure which included the results of regional assessments, including the Oceania risk assessment, led by McMichael (McMichael et al., 2003b).

This burgeoning regional focus prompted the Western Pacific Regional Office (WPRO) of WHO to compile a 'Regional Framework for Action to Protect Human Health from the Effects of Climate Change in the Asia Pacific Region'.

This important document mandated WHO to support member countries in the region to assess their vulnerabilities to the health impacts of climate change and develop national strategies and plans to manage those risks (WHO, 2008). The health ministers in the Pacific region responded at their biennial meeting in Madang, Papua New Guinea, in 2009, with the resultant 'Madang Commitment', laying out a series of recommendations related to planning, coordination, implementation and health system strengthening in the context of climate change and health adaptations in the Pacific (WHO, 2009).

It is important to note that, while these may have been the first policy documents from the health sector specifically addressing the health impacts of climate change in the Pacific region, these issues had been considered in many Pacific island countries (PICs) as part of their early work on climate change adaptation. Much of this had been taking place since the early 1990s, often in the absence of significant inputs from the health sector. As part of their Initial National Communications to the United Nations Framework Convention on Climate Change (UNFCCC) (mostly submitted in the mid- to late 2000s), several countries in the region noted the potential for climate change to impact on health, despite the limited level of understanding of those effects at the time.

Also in the late 2000s, the Australian government embarked on an ambitious programme of technical support for PICs in the area of climate science via the Australian Bureau of Meteorology (BOM) and the Commonwealth Scientific and Industrial Research Organisation (CSIRO). Originally called the Pacific Climate Change Science Program (now the Pacific–Australia Climate Change Science and Adaptation Program), this project included among its key outputs a series of country reports outlining historical climate trends and climate change forecasts for the 21st century in the key areas of temperature, rainfall, sea level rise, ocean acidification and extreme weather events (BOM and CSIRO, 2011).

These regional projects, guidelines and mandates provided the launching pad for another ambitious WHO initiative. Commencing in 2010 and completed in 2012, this project saw WHO assisting 11 PICs in conducting climate change and health vulnerability assessments and adaptation plans, culminating in National Climate Change and Health Action Plans (or variations thereof) for each of these countries in this most vulnerable of regions.

The following sections summarise the methods employed for – and the results of – these assessments and plans and, in doing so, highlight key knowledge gaps, challenges and opportunities related to the protection of human health from climate change in the South Pacific.

Methods

The 11 PICs involved in WHO climate change and health project (Federated States of Micronesia, Republic of the Marshall Islands, Palau, Vanuatu, Solomon Islands, Nauru, Kiribati, Tonga, Niue, Cook Islands and Tuvalu) were divided into three groups, based on broadly geo-cultural lines. Each of these three groups was supported by a team of WHO consultants throughout a three-phase project over two years.

The first phase involved inception workshops, which brought together the country representatives and consultants to review the current state of knowledge on climate change and health and discuss vulnerabilities and approaches appropriate to each country. The second phase saw the consultant teams visit each of the countries for further stakeholder consultations – across government and non-government agencies, including community representatives and the private sector – as well as examination of the available local data on climate and climate-sensitive diseases. In the final phase, during return visits to each country, WHO teams assisted the country teams in drafting National Climate Change and Health Action Plans (NCCHAPs), reflecting each country's key vulnerabilities and adaptation priorities with respect to the country-specific health impacts of climate change.

The process and outcomes described above, while broadly similar across the 11 countries, were nevertheless unique for each country, reflecting the preferred methodological approach and expertise of the consultant groups, the availability of climate and health data (or, more often, the lack thereof) and the particular priorities of the stakeholders and climate change and health teams within each country.

The project in each PIC incorporated, to varying degrees, the separate elements of vulnerability assessments recommended by WHO (Kovats et al., 2003; Campbell-Lendrum and Woodruff, 2007) and others, including a modified Health Impact Assessment (HIA) approach appropriate to climate change and health (Nelson, 2003; Brown et al., 2011), as well as quantitative estimations of the climate health–disease relationship (Campbell-Lendrum and Woodruff, 2006).

A common and recurring theme throughout this process was the imperative to consider the specific needs of vulnerable groups (such as young children, the elderly, those in poverty, those with pre-existing illnesses and disabilities, those in certain geographic locations – coastal villages, for example – and people engaged in certain occupations, such as fishing, agriculture or construction). Thus, in the context of health systems strengthening related to climate change adaptation, issues of equity and access are cross-cutting and of paramount importance, reflecting yet another area in which McMichael made his mark

(Friel et al., 2008; Patz et al., 2008). It is worth highlighting at this point, the irony of inequity in the context of climate change in the Pacific (and other developing countries around the world), vis-à-vis the fact that PICs have contributed the least of almost any country to the problem of greenhouse gas emissions but will be among those countries and communities hit hardest by a changing climate.

A strong feature of carrying out this work in PICs was its qualitative element, achieved by engagement with stakeholders in a series of consultations in each country. This was particularly important, given the very small populations in question (Tuvalu and Nauru vie for the title of the world's smallest independent country, with Tuvalu's population hovering around 10,000; Niue, in free association with New Zealand, has a population of approximately 1,500), under-resourced health systems and health professional capacities stretched to the extreme. While in many cases health data were incomplete, of poor quality, or missing altogether, the relevance and urgency of the challenge is widely acknowledged. Health-sector colleagues and other stakeholders proved willing to engage in the discussions, debates and consensus building that ultimately resulted in assessments and plans that were strong on qualitative inputs, albeit weak quantitatively. This characteristic of the PIC project, where precision was lacking and uncertainty large, meant that the adaptation planning process tended towards a 'no-regrets' approach, consistent with that recommended for smaller and/or developing countries and weaker health systems (Wardekker et al., 2012).

Results

The results of the vulnerability assessments in the 11 above-mentioned countries are summarised in Table 17.1 (McIver, 2012).

Table 17.1 Priority climate-sensitive health risks in Pacific Island countries.

Country	Main climate-sensitive issues
Cook Islands	Dengue fever, diarrhoeal disease
Federated States of Micronesia	Water- and mosquito-borne diseases, malnutrition
Fiji	Dengue fever, typhoid fever, leptospirosis, diarrhoeal disease
Kiribati	Food (safety, security, food-borne diseases), water (safety, security, water-borne diseases) and vector-borne diseases
Nauru	Air quality, food security, non-communicable diseases (NCDs)

Country	Main climate-sensitive issues
Niue	Vector-borne diseases, ciguatera, diarrhoeal disease, respiratory disease, heat-related illness, NCDs, trauma from extreme weather events
Palau	Vector-borne diseases, zoonotic infections, gastroenteritis, respiratory disease, NCDs, trauma from extreme weather events, mental health issues
Republic of the Marshall Islands	Food-, water- and vector-borne (dengue) diseases, respiratory diseases, malnutrition
Solomon Islands	Vector-borne diseases (malaria), respiratory diseases
Tonga	Diarrhoeal diseases, vector-borne diseases (dengue), food security/nutrition, NCDs, injuries and deaths from extreme weather events
Tuvalu	Diarrhoeal disease, respiratory disease, compromised food security and impacts on NCDs
Vanuatu	Food- and water-borne diseases

Source: McIver, 2012.

The priority adaptation strategies for each PIC, outlined in their respective NCCHAPs, relate directly to their key vulnerabilities. Broadly speaking, a holistic but pragmatic approach was taken to the adaptation planning process, with countries strongly favouring adaptation strategies that were feasible – recognising technical capacity limitations and financial constraints – in the context of grossly under-resourced health systems and multiple, often competing, health priorities.

Adaptation strategies were considered under a number of different categories, listed below with examples of specific activities under each category:

- Legislative/Regulatory
  - Reviewing building codes and standards to ensure adequate resilience to hydrometeorological disasters
- Public Education/Communication
  - Developing health promotion materials regarding food safety and protection against water-borne diseases under warmer conditions
- Surveillance/Monitoring
  - Expanding and enhancing 'syndromic surveillance' for key climate-sensitive diseases such as diarrhoeal illness and dengue fever
- Ecosystem Intervention
  - Carrying out regular community clean-up activities targeting mosquito breeding sites (e.g. pots, puddles, tins, tyres, coconut shells)

- Infrastructure/Development
  - Retrofitting schools, aged care facilities and public buildings with adequate ventilation and/or air conditioning
- Technological/Engineering
  - Procuring appropriate laboratory equipment for food testing, water monitoring and mosquito identification
- Medical Intervention
  - Refining clinical case definitions for climate-sensitive diseases; stockpiling appropriate medications and supplies for extreme weather events
- Research/Further Information
  - Collecting, collating, synthesising and analysing health data in relation to historical climate variability, with a view to estimating future country-specific, climate change-attributable burdens of disease.

Discussion

As can be seen from Table 17.1, the majority of the climate change and health priorities identified in the PICs largely reflect the long-held concerns of experts in the field: issues such as increasing incidence of food-, water- and vector-borne diseases; the health impacts of heat extremes and natural disasters; and mental health stressors have all been included in earlier conceptual models.

One important area of emerging concern – and a climate change exposure-impact pathway largely missing from the conceptual models to date – is the potential for climate change to exacerbate the existing and rapidly increasing burden of non-communicable diseases (NCDs). NCDs were among the top priorities in terms of climate change and health in several PICs, and many participants in the vulnerability assessment and adaptation planning process around the Pacific were firm in their opinion that climate change would lead to a worsening of the NCD 'crisis'.

The literature on climate change impacts on NCDs is scant; once again, one of the most significant contributions to the topic – a paper that focuses on the pathways between extreme weather events and acute exacerbations of existing disease; adaptation and development opportunities; and the potential for 'co-benefits' (see below) – has been made by a group that included the indefatigable Tony McMichael (Friel et al., 2011).

Island countries in the Pacific region have among the highest rates of obesity and NCDs such as hypertension, dyslipidaemia and type 2 diabetes in the world (WHO, 2011a). Concern about this trend has led some countries to take extraordinary measures, such as the government of Palau declaring a state of emergency in an attempt to access a wider range of resources to tackle the problem. At least some PICs see climate change as a potential additional driver of NCD risk; for example, by further worsening the conditions for domestic agriculture (due to increasing temperatures, variable rainfall, salinisation of soil and other factors) and by decreasing one's willingness or ability to exercise or perform outdoor work in hotter and/or wetter conditions.

An extensive recent online discussion forum on the topic of climate change impacts on NCDs in the Pacific, moderated by WHO, to which more than 30 prominent stakeholders and community members from a wide range of PICs and backgrounds contributed, found that four key themes emerged in relation to potential solutions to the problem: community education, legislation and government regulation, improved food security (e.g. the propagation of drought- and salt-resistant traditional staples such as taro and cassava) and further research.

Another area in which the Pacific may be unique in terms of the timing and/or nature of climate change impacts on health relates to the combined geographic and demographic vulnerabilities of PICs. In 2000, McMichael and Beaglehole (2000) pointed out the contemporary convergence of globalisation, environmental change and the gradual transition from a world where infectious diseases were the predominant burden of ill health to the new world of NCDs. This transition is taking place, apace, in Pacific atoll nations.

Kiribati and the Marshall Islands provide alarming examples of this confluence of social and environmental determinants of ill health, where NCDs such as diabetes coexist with overcrowding and high rates of smoking – all major risk factors for tuberculosis transmission in these two high-prevalence countries (Clark et al., 2002; Alisjahbana et al., 2007; Lin et al., 2007; Baker et al., 2008; Jeon and Murray, 2008). There is a real and concerning possibility that, in these tiny, very low-lying countries with high population densities, climate change phenomena – in particular, sea level rise – may contribute to the burden of diseases such as tuberculosis by additional forcing of population pressures and NCDs.

Despite these risks, and the challenges of implementing effective adaptations for climate change and health in very small countries with limited capacity in many areas, there are some causes for optimism and examples of innovation and progress in PICs. Some of these examples include:

- Mainstreaming: Palau merged its climate change and health team within a larger Pacific Adaptation to Climate Change project, ensuring that health issues were considered in community awareness surveys and adaptation activities such as experimenting with climate-resistant crops and fish and clam aquaculture.

- Infrastructure and health systems development: Kiribati's NCCHAP has been reviewed extensively and implementation of this Plan, which focuses on building environmental health capacity (via direct investment in physical resources as well as training and programme support), is the main objective of a well-funded climate change adaptation project coordinated by the Office of the President, with external donor and technical assistance.
- Research: Fiji is one of seven countries participating in a global climate change and health adaptation pilot project aimed at using climate information for disease early warning systems and improving the abilities of health professionals and communities to manage climate-sensitive health hazards.
- All-hazards planning: Tonga, the Marshall Islands and the Cook Islands have opted to combine plans for climate change adaptation with disaster risk reduction in Joint National Action Plans (JNAPs), thus opening up additional avenues for funding and technical support to manage the threats presented by extreme weather events such as cyclones, floods, droughts and storm surges, which almost certainly will all be affected by climate change.

Finally, and somewhat paradoxically, given the negligible contribution of PICs to the problem of climate change itself, it is clear that these countries have a substantial amount to gain from the potential 'co-benefits' of mitigation strategies, such as increasing the use of active and public transport over motorised vehicles and increasing physical activity in the pursuit of fishing and farming (noting that the loss of the latter skills, particularly in younger generations, is an oft-heard lament in the Pacific) (Ganten et al., 2010).

Conclusion

Most of the scenario-based predictions of climate change impacts pertain to the 21st century; many focus on what our world will look like in the year 2100. Over the past 25 years, Tony McMichael was instrumental in shaping, thinking and guiding research and policy priorities related to the health impacts of climate change. His intellectual footprints can be seen in most, if not all, significant works on the topic; his name dominates reference lists of scholarly publications on climate change and human health. To the end of his long and productive life, he continued to supervise research, analyse data and publish on these issues. Much of his work is of critical significance to climate change and health in the island countries of the South Pacific, including a very recent review of the health aspects of climate change-related migration, co-authored by two generations of McMichaels (McMichael et al., 2012).

Given the vogue for basing future climate scenarios around 2100, it is poignant to note that there are now babies and small children alive today who may still be alive in 2100. What world will they see? By that time, some PICs may be uninhabitable, or at least unrecognisable, from the effects of climate change. What will that mean for the health – physical, emotional, spiritual and mental – as well as the nationhood and identity of the most vulnerable communities in the South Pacific?

While climate change represents one of the most significant challenges to development in small island countries in the 21st century, it also provides a unique opportunity to build resilience in the health sector, address health inequities and pilot new approaches to health protection and improvement, for the betterment of communities in the Pacific and around the world.

References

Alisjahbana, B., Sahiratmadja, E., Nelwan, E.J., Purwa, A.M., Ahmad, Y., Ottenhoff, T.H.M., et al. 2007. The effect of type 2 diabetes mellitus on the presentation and treatment response of pulmonary tuberculosis. *Clinical Infectious Diseases* 45, 428–35.

Arrhenius, S. 1896. On the influence of carbonic acid in the air upon the temperature of the ground. *Philosophical Magazine and Journal of Science* 5, 237–76.

Baker, M., Das, D., Venugopal, K. & Howden-Chapman, P. 2008. Tuberculosis associated with household crowding in a developed country. *Journal of Epidemiology and Community Health* 62, 715–21.

BOM (Bureau of Meteorology) and CSIRO, 2011. *Climate Change in the Pacific: Scientific Assessment and New Research*. Volume 1: Regional Overview. Volume 2: Country Reports, Melbourne, VIC, Australia.

Brown, H.L., Proust, K., Spickett, J. & Capon, A. 2011. The potential role of health impact assessment in tackling the complexity of climate change adaptation for health. *Health Promotion Journal of Australia* 22, S48–S53.

Campbell-Lendrum, D. & Woodruff, R. 2006. Comparative risk assessment of the burden of disease from climate change. *Environmental Health Perspectives* 114, 1935–41.

Campbell-Lendrum D. & Woodruff R. 2007. Climate change: quantifying the health impact at national and local levels. Editors, Prüss-Üstün A, Corvalán C. WHO Environmental Burden of Disease Series No. 14. World Health Organization, Geneva, Switzerland, 5–55.

Clark, M., Riben, P. & Nowgesic, E. 2002. The association of housing density, isolation and tuberculosis in Canadian First Nations communities. *International Journal of Epidemiology* 31, 940–5.

Friel, S., Marmot, M., McMichael, A.J., Kjellstrom, T. & Vågerö, D. 2008. Global health equity and climate stabilisation: a common agenda. *The Lancet* 372, 1677–83.

Friel, S., Bowen, K., Campbell-Lendrum, D., Frumkin, H., McMichael, A.J. & Rasanathan, K. 2011. Climate change, noncommunicable diseases, and development: the relationships and common policy opportunities. *Annual Review of Public Health* 32, 133–47.

Ganten, D., Haines, A. & Souhami, R. 2010. Health co-benefits of policies to tackle climate change. *The Lancet* 376, 1802–4.

Intergovernmental Panel on Climate Change (IPCC) 2001. *Climate Change 2001: Third Assessment Report, Impacts, Adaptations and Vulnerability of Climate Change* (McCarthy J.J., Canianai O.F., Leary, N.A., Dokken, D.J., White, K.S. (eds)). Cambridge University Press, Cambridge, UK.

Jeon, C.Y. & Murray, M.B. 2008. Diabetes mellitus increases the risk of active tuberculosis: a systematic review of 13 observational studies. *PLoS Medicine* 5, e152.

Kovats, R.S., Ebi, K., Menne, B., Campbell-Lendrum, D., Canziani, O.F., Githeko, A., et al. 2003. *Methods of Assessing Human Health Vulnerability and Public Health Adaptation to Climate Change*. WHO, Health Canada, UNEP, WMO, Copenhagen, Denmark. Available at: researchonline.lshtm.ac.uk/14942, accessed 31 December 2013.

Lin, H.-H., Ezzati, M. & Murray, M. 2007. Tobacco smoke, indoor air pollution and tuberculosis: a systematic review and meta-analysis. *PLoS Medicine* 4, e20.

McIver, L. 2012. Climate change and health in the Pacific: cause for concern; opportunities for adaptation. *Inform'Action* (the Bulletin of the Secretariat for the Pacific Community), 36, 3–6.

McMichael, A.J. & Beaglehole, R. 2000. The changing global context of public health. *The Lancet* 356, 495–9.

McMichael, A.J., Haines, A., Slooff, R. & Kovats, S. (eds) 1996. *Climate Change and Human Health*. World Health Organization, Geneva, Switzerland.

McMichael, A.J., Campbell-Lendrum, D.H., Corvalán, C.F., Ebi, K.L., Githeko, A., Scheraga, J.D., et al. (eds) 2003. *Climate Change and Human Health – Risks and Responses*. World Health Organization (WHO), World Meteorological Organization (WMO), United Nations Environment Programme (UNEP), Geneva, Switzerland.

McMichael, A.J., Campbell-Lendrum, D., Kovats, S., Edwards, S., Wilkinson, P., Wilson, T., et al. 2004. Global climate change. In: Ezzati, M., Lopez, A., Rodgers, A. & Mathers, C. (eds) *Comparative Quantification of Health Risks: Global and Regional Burden of Disease due to Selected Major Risk Factors*. World Health Organization, Geneva. Switzerland, 1543–649.

McMichael A.J., Woodruff R.E., Hales S. 2006. Climate change and human health: present and future risks. *The Lancet*. 367: 859–69.

McMichael, C., Barnett, J. & McMichael, A.J. 2012. An ill wind? Climate change, migration, and health. *Environmental Health Perspectives* 120, 646–54.

Nelson, D. 2003. Health impact assessment of climate change in Bangladesh. *Environmental Impact Assessment Review* 23, 323–41.

Patz, J., Campbell-Lendrum, D., Gibbs, H. & Woodruff, R. 2008. Health impact assessment of global climate change: expanding on comparative risk assessment approaches for policy making. *Annual Review of Public Health* 29, 27–39.

Tyndall, J. 1861. On the absorption and radiation of heat by gases and vapours, and on the physical connection. *Philosophical Magazine* 22, 277–302.

Wardekker, J.A., de Jong, A., van Bree, L., Turkenburg, W.C. & van der Sluijs, J.P. 2012. Health risks of climate change: an assessment of uncertainties and its implications for adaptation policies. *Environmental Health* 11, 67 10.1186/1476-069X-11-67.

WHO 1990. Potential Health Effects of Climatic Change – Report of a WHO Task Group. WHO, Geneva, Switzerland.

WHO 2008. Regional Framework for Action to Protect Human Health from the Effects of Climate Change in the Asia Pacific Region. WHO Western Pacific Regional Office, Manila, The Philippines.

WHO & Secretariat for the Pacific Community 2009. *Madang Commitment*. WHO, Geneva, Switzerland.

WHO 2011. Non-communicable Diseases Country Profiles 2011. WHO, Geneva, Switzerland.

WMO & UNEP 1988. Developing policies for responding to climatic change – a summary of the discussions and recommendations of the workshops held in Villach (28 September–2 October 1987) and Bellagio (9–13 October 1987) under the auspices of the Beijer Institute, Stockholm, Sweden (WMO/TD – 225, April 1988).

18

FROM SOCIAL REFORM TO SOCIAL TRANSFORMATION

Human Ecological Systems and Adaptation to a More Hostile Climate

HILARY BAMBRICK AND STEFANO MONCADA

Abstract

Improving public health frequently involves bringing about societal change. Increasingly large-scale and complex problems such as climate change pose significant threats to human health and impel re-conceptualisation of environment–human interrelationships, affording them the complexity they deserve and the opportunity to think 'ecologically'. Large-scale problems often trigger a large-scale response, but these attempted solutions may be slow to materialise, a poor fit to the local context, unsustainable and are often poorly evaluated. There is also a place for locally relevant community-managed activities, aimed not only at reducing adverse health impacts caused by the very large problem of climate change but also by improving other determinants of environmental health and poverty. One such potential case, in Ethiopia, is described.

Introduction

Since its very early days, successful public health has been a vehicle for social reform, driving fundamental changes to the human environment in order to understand and improve health, and to address inequalities. Much of what we think of as 'public health' could equally be called 'environmental health'. It recognises the importance of *context* to the capacity for a population to be healthy. It strives to make our surroundings conducive to better health, optimising benefits for the population at large by making changes to the settings in which we go about our daily lives. The domain of public – or environmental – health, then, is very broad. It does not take an individualistic, curative, short-term, market-driven approach but is more concerned with disease prevention on a mass-scale and with long-term benefits to health and well-being. By definition, it is a progressive movement, arising from a core concern for social justice.

Over time, the type of exposure of interest to public health researchers and advocates has evolved, from solely 'miasmic' concerns to biological and then chemical and physical agents, and also, more recently, to embrace systemic environmental change. Biological agents – bacteria, viruses (though not identified as such at the time) – were the primary domain of the early public health movement, bringing about profound changes to water distribution and sanitation infrastructure. Chemical and physical agents, largely by-products of industry, then became of increasing concern with economic development. Vehicle emissions, pesticide residues and chemical waste are now all subject to legislation and control, though, like sanitation, this achievement has been greatest in more developed countries.

For much of the past 150 years, this focus on biological and chemical agents was appropriate, given the expanding knowledge of their associations with health. In hindsight, these problems appear relatively simple and well-defined, confined in time and space to readily describable and mechanistically straightforward causal chains. They frequently have linear dose–response relationships, or a definable risk threshold, and clear, observable benefits arising from action taken to minimise exposure. A traditionally scientific reductionist approach may be appropriate in these circumstances in order to identify specific agents responsible for ill health and to intervene to reduce exposure.

The Next Public Health Challenge: Eroding Civilisation's Life-Support Mechanisms

In contrast, and more recently, we have come to realise the significance of a third type of exposure, in that contemporary and substantial threats to human health are now resulting from large-scale disruptions to our life-supporting ecosystems. These involve changes that occur on a very large scale over space and time, affecting environmental stability, productivity, regenerative and waste-absorptive capacities and biodiversity. These systemic changes are shaped by complex social, political and economic drivers. Their associated health outcomes are more difficult to identify, measure and act upon than exposure to the simple causative agents described previously. A key example of such a large-scale and potentially intractable threat is anthropogenic climate change (Martens and McMichael, 2002).

Studying the health impacts of systemic environmental change requires new methodological approaches. Measurement of exposure at the community or broader population level is more appropriate (and feasible) than at the individual level, which is difficult to quantify. The challenge is to think 'ecologically', paying special attention to interconnectivity while recognising that associations may be indirect, non-linear and multidirectional. At the same time, it is essential not to lose sight of what is happening at the scale at which people actually live.

Tackling the consequences of climate change thus requires a kind of revolutionary thinking and revolutionary action, including in public health and epidemiology. After two decades of research effort into the potential health impacts of climate change, we are still developing a comprehensive understanding of what some of these impacts might be, let alone what we can do about them. We know, for example, that people die when temperatures are unusually hot, especially if they are older, unwell and socially isolated (Harlan et al., 2012). Mathematical and empirical modelling tell us that, up to a certain point and as long as humidity is sufficient, an increase in ambient temperature promotes the transmission of vector-borne diseases through its effects on vector survival and behaviour, as well as on pathogen replication (Jetten and Focks, 1997; Patz et al., 1998; Hales et al., 2002; Rogers et al., 2006). While such parameters determine whether or not a disease *can* occur, we know that the economic status of a country affects the intensity of transmission or even whether a certain disease *does* occur, given suitable parameters. We can therefore surmise that social and economic conditions will determine to a large extent how climate change will affect health, so that certain countries or particular groups of people are more vulnerable than others. Countries that have limited capacity to cope with existing climate-associated health risks are unlikely to have the resources to plan for and manage future risks. Populations with an already heavy burden of disease are particularly vulnerable; chronic obesity-related disease increases risk of death or ill health during periods of high temperatures, for example. These chronic non-communicable diseases are prevalent in many of the more developed countries such as the USA and Australia, and are an emergent problem in many least-developed countries (LDCs), such as Fiji and Samoa in the Pacific.

Yet, health-impacts modelling with regard to climate change has, to date, accounted only for changes to average climatic conditions over average populations, with little consideration of specific vulnerabilities, including impacts on elderly, migrant or indigenous groups in more developed countries or among those living in extreme poverty in LDCs. Neither has modelling attempted to quantify extreme events that may be outside previous experience and that, with expected increases in climate variability, are precisely the type about which we are being warned. Nevertheless, the evidence that climate change has adverse consequences for population health is very strong (McMichael et al., 2005).

The Need for Transformational Thinking

Climate change is an unprecedented, systemic problem, and successful adaptation to minimise its human health impacts requires transformative thinking. This means moving beyond the social reform of early public health interventions that dealt with discrete, localised and measurable problems, towards changing the way we think about and relate to the environment. Fundamentally, it means seeing ourselves as part of the human ecological system rather than as something outside of or disconnected from it. This is the type of thinking pioneered by Tony McMichael and argued so persuasively in *Planetary Overload* (McMichael, 1993). Transformation for adaptation means changing our expectations about how we live, our relationships with the environment and, importantly, even our social, economic and political structures. But adaptation activities, when they do occur, tend to focus only on the short-term and can therefore be maladaptive. We are not fixing the system or thinking 'big' enough, and may even be creating problems for the future through accidently introducing practices that are maladaptive.

Often, there is a problem with institutions failing to recognise the nature and scale of the changes, as well as calibrating the responses. This is particularly true when funding opportunities look at adaptation mostly as a technological-based response to future climate change conditions, *de facto*, excluding the option of reducing countries' vulnerabilities to foster adaptation and improve health (Klein, 2008). This is a significant hurdle for small island developing states (SIDS) in particular. When developing one of its infrastructure projects following the implementation of its National Adaptation Programs of Action, Tuvalu was given funding only for the part of the project that would tackle the 'additional' costs due to adaptation, leaving the burden of financing the 'baseline' infrastructure of that project to Tuvalu's poor finances (Ayers and Huq, 2009). As a result, the project could not start until the proper cofinance could be found, effectively delaying Tuvalu's adaptation needs.

While climate change is a global problem, the global machinery that should be mitigating it through emission reductions is clunky, unconvinced, unwilling and, even with the best of intentions, slow. All may not be lost just yet; success in dealing with global environmental crises has occurred before; for example, in mobilising action for environmental (and human health) benefit with the worldwide ban on chlorofluorocarbons under the 1989 Montreal Protocol and the nearly completed phasing out of leaded petrol.

Often, however, transformation begins at a smaller scale. The 'Transition Town' movement (www.transitionnetwork.org) commenced in the UK in 2003. The movement is about taking practical steps to advance local sustainability, largely by shifting from large-scale commercial production and supply to more local production. The movement aims to achieve low-carbon local economies and to adapt to changing climate independently from government and corporate decision making. It works to increase resilience by creating deliberate redundancy in the system through reliance on multiple, small-scale local producers. Diversification in production and supply, community self-reliance and independence are also key characteristics.

These changes are occurring in well-resourced and well-informed communities that probably will not suffer greatly under climate change, at least in the next few decades. Relatively speaking, they are well-buffered by economic and social resources and have populations in reasonably good health; also, the climate impacts in such temperate regions may be less severe, though recent events such as flooding and storm surges in the UK suggest even wealthy temperate nations may be affected. But the poorest populations in the poorest countries have far fewer resources to deal with climate change.

The appropriate scale is important when considering the impacts in any population. Problems that occur and are important at a community level may be overlooked in large-scale models. Absence of data can be partially compensated for by interpolation over large geographic areas, but this can miss local issues altogether. This problem is particularly marked in developing countries, where the capacity to collect or analyse health and environmental data is often low, and sometimes virtually absent.

Improving the Evaluation of Adaptation

The evaluation of adaptation interventions, both prospective and in place, is both commonly missing and urgently needed. Such evaluation could quantify benefits (or their absence), improving the evidentiary basis for policy and action. Qualitative methods can also tease out relevant problems and can be used to develop feasible solutions. Mistakes in adaptation no doubt occur. Comprehensive evaluation means that not only could successful programmes be replicated but also that unintended harmful consequences of health adaptation actions could be spotted and minimised. If research on climate change-related health impacts and vulnerability remains underdeveloped, then research on the health impacts of *adaptation*, whether in rich or poor countries, is positively embryonic.

The Principles of Successful Adaptation in Low-Income Settings

Despite the considerable barriers to understanding impacts, implementing adaptation activities and evaluating these interventions, locally driven, small-scale adaptation activities are emerging in less wealthy parts of the world. Interventions that are likely to be most successful are those that bring multiple benefits to community health and economy, those that are developed through consultation and those where the community has ownership of the activity and responsibility for its ongoing management. One such adaptation intervention that fits these criteria is the building of biogas digester systems in poor urban communities to provide sanitation and fuel for cooking. The benefits of such biogas systems include the enhancement of long-term adaptive capacity and an overall improvement of key public health indicators and socio-economic attributes (Moncada et al., 2014).

A Health-promoting Technology in Ethiopia of Benefit for Climate Mitigation and Adaptation

Poor sanitation is a major cause of chronic diarrhoea, contributing to undernutrition and ill health, especially among children (Fenn et al., 2012). It can also be associated with trachoma, including in Ethiopia (Golovaty et al., 2009). The use of wood and charcoal as cooking fuel leads to high levels of indoor pollution and local deforestation, and is associated with respiratory disease (Po et al., 2011) and otitis media (Amusa et al., 2005). Wood and charcoal take time and money to procure.

A community-managed biogas digester system, costing approximately US$32,000 (costs that include a 25 cubic metre digester, four bio-latrines, a communal kitchen, a water point, sewerage system, environmental sanitation material and training, personnel cost and monitoring and evaluation), was installed as part of an official development assistance intervention financed by the Maltese government within the internationally funded initiative FAST-START.[1]

1 This initiative was agreed during the Conference of the Parties (COP 15) held in December 2009 in Copenhagen, where developed countries pledged to provide new and additional resources for the period 2010–12, with the intention to implement projects on climate change mitigation and adaptation.

This research project aimed to contribute to climate change mitigation by reducing reliance on both fossil fuels and firewood, and also to improve long-term climate change adaptive capacity in an informal (poor) community of 200 households (approximately 700 people) in the southern Ethiopian city of Shashemene, about 240 km from the capital, Addis Ababa. Such communities are especially vulnerable to climate change because of extreme poverty, a marginally productive and highly variable climate (Figure 18.1), little infrastructure and a heavy burden of existing health problems.

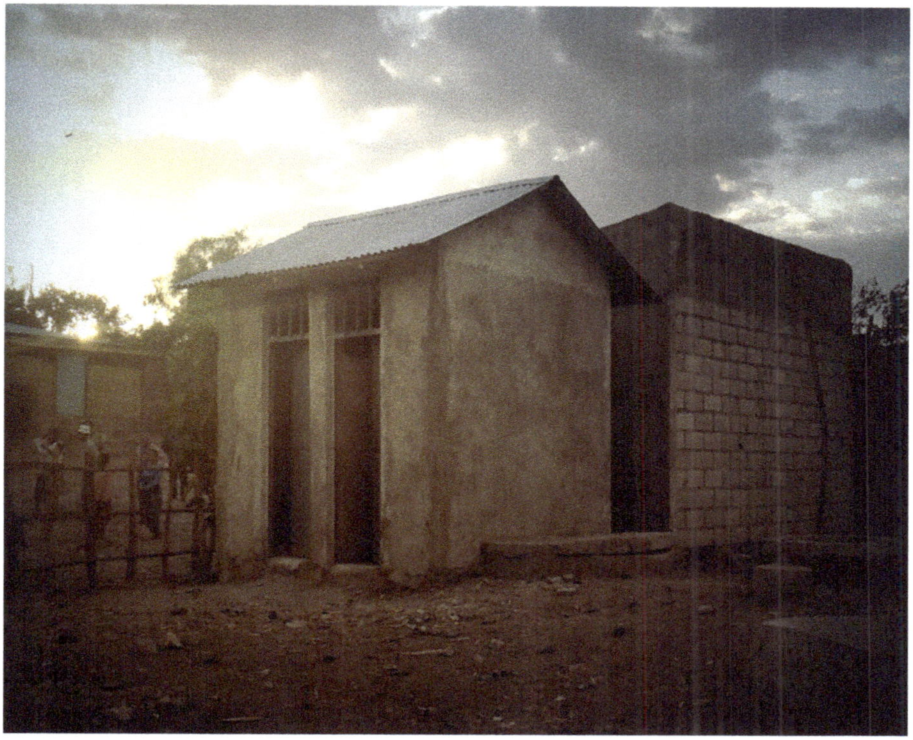

Figure 18.1 The biogas compound. The foreground building contains the latrines and the adjacent building is the community kitchen.
Source: Hilary Bambrick.

The biogas digester system, constructed by using locally resourced material and employing local companies, installed in the community takes the form of a simple four-cubicle latrine, from which methane gas produced by the waste is collected and piped into an adjacent community kitchen (Figure 18.2). The kitchen has four gas hotplates (Figure 18.3) and two clay plates for cooking the staple food, *injera*, a fermented flat bread made from the highly nutritious grain called *tef*. The slurry from the biogas system is also collected for use on the community garden. Goat and cattle manure is also collected from within the community and added to the system, contributing to the facility's output while managing waste better. The provision of piped (treated) town water is also part of the facility intended to replace the use of water from the polluted local river.

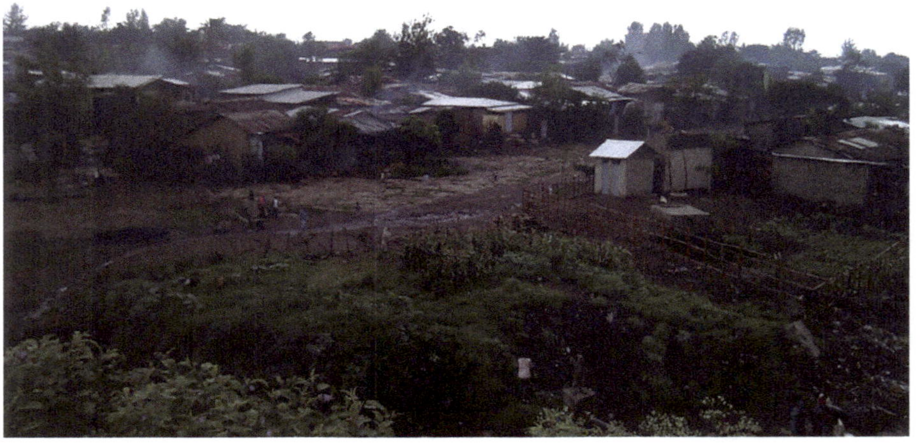

Figure 18.2 The community towards the end of the wet season, September 2012, looking east from the main road over the river.
Source: Stefano Moncada.

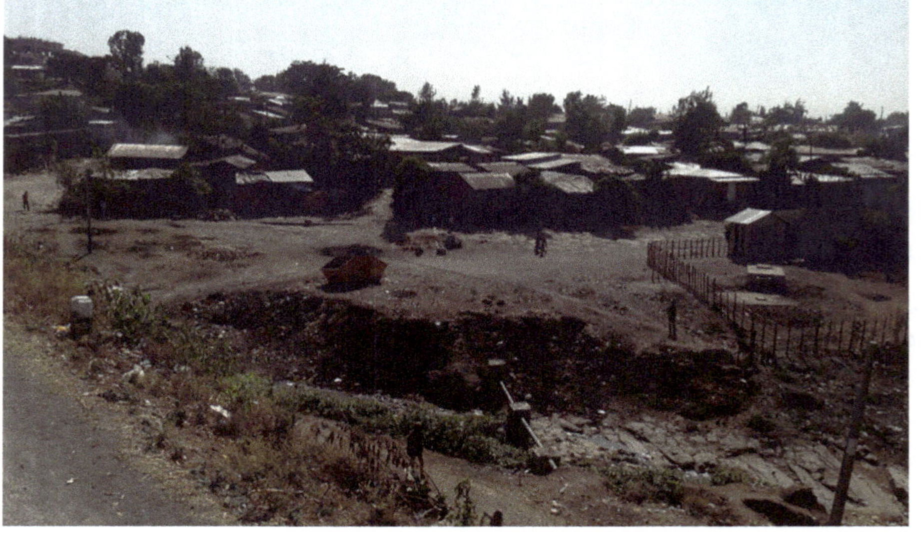

Figure 18.3 The community during the dry season, February 2013.
Source: Stefano Moncada.

The facility was built in close consultation with the community, is managed by the community and provides a source of communal income. Use of the latrine and kitchen is free for all members of the community but a small fee is charged for use of the water (20 Ethiopian cents per 20-litre container, approximately 1 US cent). Custodianship of the system and responsibility for its upkeep is held by an elected community-user committee, which is led by the head male elder.

This small, relatively simple facility is expected to bring multiple benefits to the community, including a reduction in typhoid and other diarrhoeal episodes (which will, in the longer term, lead to improved growth and health outcomes for children) and reduced respiratory and other illnesses associated with indoor air pollution, such as otitis media and eye disease. Other benefits to household economy and community functioning are also anticipated, generating synergistic improvements to health and well-being. These include less time and money spent on collecting cooking fuel and water, and enhanced economic productivity due to fewer illnesses. The local environment will also benefit, with the loss of fewer trees and improved outdoor air quality. Climate change mitigation through reduced greenhouse gas production by the community has the potential to be scaled-up in Ethiopia, with planned support from its government. Importantly, this project addresses a locally identified need. The facilities are community managed. This local relevance and sense of ownership will increase the likelihood that it will be sustained.

Evaluation of this project involves a pre-intervention survey (undertaken) and three or more follow-up surveys, involving all households in the community, to be undertaken four and 12 months after the biogas system becomes operational. These surveys will ask detailed questions on individual's health and sanitation practices, household socio-economic indicators, time use and economic resources. The post-intervention surveys will identify which households are using the new facilities and how they are being used, enabling comparison of health and other outcomes according to 'exposure' to the intervention. Preliminary results show a significant uptake in use of the new facilities, as well as improved public health-related behaviour, such as the reduced use of the polluted rivers, both for defecation and as a source of water for drinking and cooking, with an increased used of piped treated water (Moncada et al., 2014).

Some key community characteristics garnered through the baseline survey include a mean household size of 3.6 people, mean age of 23 and mean household income of US$1.56 per day. Participants were identified as being from 13 different ethnic groups. Most were identified as being Orthodox Christian or Protestant, with a minority being Muslim or Catholic. Most participants had a primary school education, with 21 per cent having a secondary and 4 per cent a tertiary education. A non-trivial fraction of those with a primary school education are likely to be illiterate (Bambrick et al., 2015).

Before the intervention, approximately two-thirds of households used a shared or private pit for a toilet, and approximately one-quarter practised open defecation in or near the river. Notable health problems included malaria, typhoid, anaemia, trachoma and tuberculosis, while eye conditions, gastrointestinal disease, otitis media and acute and chronic respiratory conditions represented the greatest cause of sick days.

In addition to the quantitative data collection through the household survey, the study also uses participatory rural appraisal methods (Chambers, 1994). These involve in-depth focus group discussions with women and men from the community to identify the ways in which climate – especially climate variability – affects their daily life and their strategies for coping with climate-associated risks. This information, along with the data gathered through the surveys, will help to develop adaptation further; to guide future development interventions that are locally relevant, feasible and sustainable.

Planned systematic evaluation studies such as the one just described are all very well for deliberate formal adaptation interventions, but it is likely that many climate adaptation actions will be *ad hoc*, informal and context specific, and will arise in response to a perceived immediate threat. Documentation and monitoring of such activities, when they occur and when possible, will be useful to avert or minimise any adverse unintended consequences.

Conclusion: Local Adaptation for a Global Problem

While climate change poses challenges to human health that are unprecedented in scale and complexity, attempts to adapt to minimise adverse health outcomes will occur at varying scales: large-scale, government-reliant and small-scale, community-driven. Other informal adaptive responses to climate change may arise independently, and even set trends, perhaps spreading via social media and mobile telephony. At any scale, and whether formal or informal, successful adaptation will require greater understanding of the human ecological system so as not to attempt to impose change without due consideration of interconnectivity, feedback and non-linearity. Opportunities to maximise community co-benefits (i.e. other positive outcomes such as reduced obesity-related chronic diseases or improved income security) should be given priority, if they appear more cost-effective.

We still await multilateral government action to deal with the global problem of climate change. While the support of governments and large corporations remains necessary (especially in taking action to limit the amount of warming caused by greenhouse gas emissions), multiple implementation of successful small-scale, locally appropriate adaptation activities driven by communities is also vital. Enough of these could restrict the health consequences arising from anthropogenic climate change to a manageable scale. And, as we believe this project in Ethiopia will demonstrate, many such projects will also deliver short- as well as long-term economic and health benefits.

Acknowledgements

The Shashemene biogas project is a collaboration between KOPIN (Kooperazzjoni Internazzjonali), WCDO (Women and Children Development Organization Ethiopia), the Institute for European Studies at the University of Malta and the Centre for Health Research at the University of Western Sydney. Involved in project implementation and evaluation are Kassahun Ararso, Melaku Hailu Marie Briguglio, Sarah Mallia, Adriana Grech, Eyob Lalensa, Tesfahun Bekele, Berket Mola, Zegeye H. Michael, Zelalem Tarekegn, Muluwork Gemechu, William Grech and Dominik Kalweit.

References

Amusa, Y.B., Ijadunola, I.K. & Onayade, O.O. 2005. Epidemiology of otitis media in a local tropical African population. *West African Journal of Medicine* 24, 227–30.

Ayers, J.M. & Huq, S. 2009. Supporting adaptation to climate change: what role for Official Development Assistance? *Development Policy Review* 27, 675–92.

Bambrick, H., Moncada, S. & Briguglio, M. 2015. Climate change and health vulnerability in informal urban settlements in the Ethiopian Rift Valley. Environmental Research Letters 10(5) doi: 10.1088/1748-9326/10/5/054014.

Chambers, R., 1994. The origins and practice of participatory rural appraisals. World Development 22(7): 953–69.

Fenn, B., Bulti, A.T., Nduna, T., Duffield, A. & Watson, F. 2012. An evaluation of an operations research project to reduce childhood stunting in a food-insecure area in Ethiopia. Public Health Nutrition 15(9): 1746–54.

Golovaty, I., Jones, L., Gelaye, B., Tilahun, M., Belete, H., Kumie, A., et al. 2009. Access to water source, latrine facilities and other risk factors of active trachoma in Ankober, Ethiopia. *PloS One* 4, e6702.

Hales, S., de Wet, N., Maindonald, J. & Woodward, A. 2002. Potential effect of population and climate changes on global distribution of dengue fever: an empirical model. *The Lancet* 360, 830–34.

Harlan, S.L., Declet-Barreto, J.H., Stefanov, W.L. & Petitti, D.B. 2012. Neighborhood effects on heat deaths: social and environmental predictors of vulnerability in Maricopa County, Arizona. *Environmental Health Perspectives*. 121(2): 197–204.

Jetten, T.H. & Focks, D.A. 1997. Potential changes in the distribution of dengue transmission under climate warming. *American Journal of Tropical Medicine and Hygiene* 57, 285–97.

Klein, R.J.T. 2008. Mainstreaming climate adaptation into development policies and programmes: a European perspective. In: *European Parliament, Financing Climate Change Policies in Developing Countries*. European Parliament, PE 408.546 IP/A/ CLIP/A/CLIM/ST/2008-13, Brussels, Belgium.

McMichael, A.J. 1993. *Planetary Overload: Global Environmental Change and the Health of the Human Species*. Cambridge University Press, Cambridge, UK.

McMichael, A.J., Woodruff, R.E. & Hales, S. 2005. Climate change and human health: present and future risks. *The Lancet* 367, 859–69.

Martens, W.J.M. & McMichael, A.J. (eds) 2002. *Environmental Change, Climate and Health: Issues and Research Methods*. Cambridge University Press, Cambridge, UK.

Moncada, S., Bambrick, H. & Briguglio, M. 2014. Enhancing Local Adaptive Capacity in Informal Urban Settlements in Ethiopia. *Adaptation Futures. Third International Climate Change Adaptation Conference*. Fortaleza, Brazil May 2014.

Patz, J.A., Martens, W.J., Focks, D.A. & Jetten, T.H. 1998. Dengue fever epidemic potential as projected by general circulation models of global climate change. *Environmental Health Perspectives* 106, 147–53.

Po, J.Y., FitzGerald, J.M. & Carlsten, C. 2011. Respiratory disease associated with solid biomass fuel exposure in rural women and children: systematic review and meta-analysis. *Thorax* 66, 232–39.

Rogers, D.J., Wilson, A.J., Hay, S.I. & Graham, A.J. 2006. The global distribution of yellow fever and dengue. *Advances in Parasitology* 62, 181–220.

19

CLIMATE CHANGE, HEALTH AND WELL-BEING IN INDIGENOUS AUSTRALIA

DONNA GREEN AND LEANNE WEBB

Abstract

The *National Adaptation Research Plan for Human Health*, the Intergovernmental Panel on Climate Change's *Fourth Assessment Report* and Garnaut's *Climate Change Review* all identify Indigenous Australians as disproportionately vulnerable to adverse health impacts from climate change. These statements are based on the reasonable assumption that significantly socio-economically disadvantaged people will have less capacity to adapt to anthropogenic climate change. There is, however, very limited quantitative analysis of this relationship that could be used to substantiate these claims. The two projects outlined in this chapter address this issue by detailing studies undertaken in Australia to investigate how climate impacts the morbidity and psychosocial health of Indigenous people. This research aims to provide decision makers with clear and robust policy-relevant evidence that identifies the connections between climate and the health and well-being of Indigenous people living in the tropical north of Australia.

Introduction

To readers of this volume, it would come as no surprise that Tony McMichael was always at the forefront of strategic research on the relationship between human health and climate. Our first experience of his leadership in this area came during a presentation he gave at a meeting of Indigenous Elders and scientists in 2006, where he discussed the indirect health impacts of climate change in northern Australia (McMichael, 2006). Five years later, he had further developed his model, presenting some novel dimensions at the International Congress of Biometeorology (McMichael, 2011).

Cultural and Psychosocial Health Dimensions of Climate Change

One frequently overlooked area that Tony identified in this latter presentation was that of the 'community morale and mental health disorders' likely to be exacerbated through a number of complex mediated processes resulting from various climate impacts. Concern over this research area has been given much less attention than the more 'visible' (i.e. physical) impacts of climate change on human health, although the implications of these more insidious impacts have significant ramifications for at least one specific subpopulation in Australia (Baker et al., 2001; Hunter, 2009; Australian Institute of Health and Welfare (AIHW), 2011; Doherty and Clayton, 2011).

Indigenous people living in rural and remote Australia have close attachments to their country[1] (Altman and Kerins, 2012). Despite the 'best' efforts of colonisation, the cultural link between Indigenous people and their country has, for large areas of the continent, remained strong (Carson et al., 2007; Campbell et al., 2011). What has been weakened by the work of missionaries and government intervention over the last two to three generations is the maintenance of their 'country' and, by inference, the cultural responsibility of 'looking after' their ancestors that comes with the practice of this 'people on country' interaction (Baker et al., 2001).

In the past two decades, the 'healthy country, healthy people' literature has pointed to the multiple co-benefits of strengthening the connections between people and place (Burgess et al., 2009; Biddle, 2011). If cultural practice is to be maintained properly, its transmission needs to occur *on the country* and from Traditional Owners to younger generations (Reid, 1992; Altman and Kerins, 2012).

In addition, when Traditional Owners are able to manage their country properly, by burning, hunting and performing ceremony, there is a significant psychological benefit (Rose, 1992, in Carson et al., 2007). That is to say, when the country has people looking after it, it is no longer considered 'wild' (Parry, 2007). For Indigenous Australians, 'wild' or unmanaged country, that which is overgrown and depopulated, is a source of shame or embarrassment for those who have a cultural obligation to look after it. This view of managing landscapes sits in sharp relief to the colonial perception of untouched 'wilderness' areas, where the very desolation of the landscape is itself a source of beauty.

1 'Country' is a term much preferred by Aboriginals to 'land'. Though much Aboriginal territory has been colonised, at least the most common word in English which expresses some of the values of that territory has been adapted, allowing a partial reclamation.

Climate change is most likely to complicate this established relationship between people and place in a range of ways. Although Indigenous people have been living in a changing natural environment for thousands of years, these shifts have tended to be more gradual than the climate change impacts projected to occur in the next two to three generations (Parry, 2007; Galloway McLean, 2010). Indeed, some of these biophysical impacts on Indigenous managed land and sea country have already been documented: coastal areas have been threatened with more frequent and/or severe inundation (Green et al., 2010b), saltwater intrusion has occurred in wetland systems (Kakadu National Park, 2007; Green et al., 2009) and erosion of areas of special cultural significance have all been documented in the peer-reviewed literature, as well as via less traditional methods, such as video recordings (Ameyali, 2009).

Subtle impacts are occurring at the species level in response to climate change. For Indigenous communities that maintain cultural practices dependent on specific plants and animals, a change in flowering times, animal behaviour or species' ranges has important implications for their ability to hunt or harvest specific bush foods (Green et al., 2010a). Previously associated species' behaviours are being 'de-linked', so that, for example, the timing of hunting or foraging for a specific animal due to the visual cue of the behaviour of another animal, or the flowering of a specific plant, is being disrupted (Green et al., 2010a). When these processes are associated with cultural practice, a disruption in culture is a likely result – as has already been documented in other Indigenous communities around the world (see, for example, Turner and Clifton, 2009).

Within this context, we brought together a multidisciplinary team to carry out two distinct but related research projects to explore these issues further. Using different approaches appropriate to each research question, we wanted to explore both the quantitative and qualitative dimensions to this issue. The rest of this chapter outlines how we shaped these projects, and the preliminary results we have obtained.

Qualitative Environmental Change and Health and Well-being Project

The first research project takes a qualitative approach to explore how the health and well-being of an Indigenous community might be affected by climate impacts, and what strategies might best be engaged to build the community's resilience to these impacts. Specifically, this research examines connections between the health of Indigenous individuals and the health of their community, their culture and their country.

To explore these possible psychosocial impacts of climate change on Indigenous Australians living in remote areas, we drew on the Indigenous research methods (IRM) approach (see Sherwood, 2010, for details on this process). This approach suggests that the research project be guided by the partner Indigenous community to establish their initial set of priorities and concerns for the research to respond to.

Another facet of this project is to show whether cultural practice and knowledge of their country still remain with these Elders. If this is the case, then it would be reasonable to design climate adaptation policies for this region that would encourage the return to living in and working on the country and the reinvestment in families returning to live for some of the year on outstations, where their connection to the country can continue to be strengthened. This research explores the proposition that taking people back on the country, and allowing the transfer of cultural knowledge between generations to occur, facilitates cultural resilience. With this mechanism to strengthen cultural practice, we test the hypothesis that resilience to environmental changes, such as those brought about by climate change, will also be strengthened.

Through developing a collaborative research partnership with *Aak Puul Ngantam*, an Aboriginal owned and run organisation based in Aurukun, on the west side of Cape York, Queensland, the project design was finalised and approved by its steering committee in 2012. The steering committee considered the research important to the community because of the need to factor climate adaptation strategies into their new economic development plan. It was also seen as an approach to strengthen their work on cultural resilience to make the community more sustainable by encouraging community members to take more trips out of Aurukun and back on to their traditional country.

This project was directed by the committee to work directly with Wik and Kugu Traditional Owners via the use of video recording, so that people could have a visual and audio record that they could keep for themselves and also use as a cultural record to enable material to be passed down to younger family members. This process follows the oral tradition of Indigenous societies, and the methods engaged in this project have international precedent (Willox et al., 2012). There was a clear direction from the steering committee that people wanted to return to their country in order to be able to speak about it, and so the logistics were organised to bring people out for short trips away from the Aurukun community to facilitate this process.

On the first trip, we worked with three Traditional Owners, who were taken out with an anthropologist who had worked with them in the mid-1970s and with whom they had spent a great deal of time. On each occasion, we worked in a different setting. With one artist, we spent time documenting the collection of traditional materials for weaving and painting. This recording occurred just outside of the main town area of Aurukun, and at the arts centre. The second recording took place at Waakacham, an area known for good geese hunting. To get to this location, we travelled by boat, and on the way, we discussed the environmental changes that this Elder observed along the riverbanks. We spent time discussing burning strategies and the damage caused to the country by feral pigs, while the rangers who had accompanied us went geese hunting. The final recording was taken of an Elder discussing his country and remembering, and singing, songs associated with it, although we were not able on that occasion to be able to travel to his country due to the overgrown state of the land between it and Aurukun. From these three recordings, it was clear that there remained a good level of knowledge about songs for these regions, and that the Elders were very keen on returning to their country to be able to carry out cultural activities there on future trips.

On the second trip, three Elders were again taken out with the anthropologist. This trip took people back to country near the Kendall River (see Figure 19.1), which they had not seen for years, including for one Elder, a trip back to the country where he had been born but had not visited since that time. The trip also allowed opportunities for people to remember times spent on the country when they were younger and events that had happened there, which was triggered by seeing specific plants, animals and features in the landscape. Some areas of the country were considered to have become overgrown and wild, and so were burned during our time working there. In other places, the Elders noted that there had been significant shifts in the landscape features, from changes in the composition of mangroves and trees, to the location of sandbanks and dunes. Feral pigs had also caused a great deal of environmental damage in many areas. Due to the overgrowth of weeds that had occurred in many of these regions, people had effectively been prevented from spending significant, if any, time back on their country. On this second trip, the use of a helicopter was essential, as we had to get over land that had roads which had become inaccessible or were non-existent (as people previously would have walked through these regions). The perspective from the air gave the Elders an opportunity to see how various places had become overgrown, the damage that had been caused by feral animals and which areas of the land were in need of being burned.

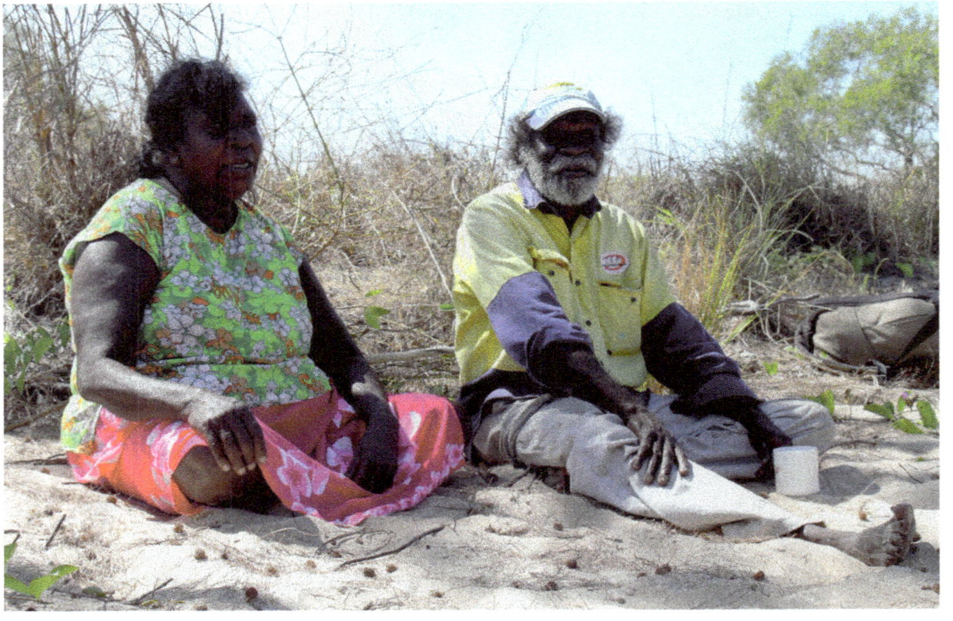

Figure 19.1 Mavis Ngallametta and Stuart Korkaktain discussing the management of their country, Kendal River, Cape York.
Source: Donna Green.

Over eight hours of material was recorded from these trips. Much of this material documents Traditional Owners' experiences in going back to their country, and their thoughts and feelings about how it has changed since their last visit. It records songs connected to place, and cultural activities carried out there. From these recordings, we will spend time working with the Elders to explore how people's perceptions of ecosystems have changed. This approach is taken in order to understand better what environmental change is likely to cause distress, and therefore what activities might be considered important to mitigate this problem.

These two trips back to country were considered a great success, with people keen to return to their land for a longer period during the following dry season, and to bring some of their children with them so that specific cultural knowledge could be transmitted to the younger generation. This return trip was carried out in the dry season of 2013, and the researchers collaborated with the school in order that some of this cultural transmission work could be incorporated into the children's activities.

Other potential benefits from this research work were identified by the collaboration. For example, the new federal climate change policy could provide employment opportunities to reconnect Elders with their land via burning and feral animal management programmes. Ranger programmes are now providing real employment opportunities over thousands of hectares, and these programmes must operate under the direction of Traditional Owners to ensure that the correct protocols are followed to burn and manage country (Green and Minchin, 2012). One relatively new initiative is that of carbon management; that is, the controlled burning of dry land savannah in mosaic patterns in the cooler earlier months. In this way, less carbon dioxide is emitted through uncontrolled late-season burns, which have a much greater fuel load available to them (Barnsley, 2008). Through projects such as this, it is anticipated that Australia's greenhouse gas emissions can be reduced (Parry, 2007). A carbon management project that would fit within this federal climate change policy is currently under consideration by the Elders of this community.

Quantitative Health and Climate Project

The quantitative dimension of this work was carried out in a separate research project. This project was designed to investigate whether we could establish a climate–health link that might have disproportionate impacts on Indigenous Australians (Webb et al., 2014). We used epidemiological methods to analyse observed admission rates for cardiovascular disease over a 20-year period (1992–2011) from the five public hospitals in the Northern Territory. Admissions made on very hot, very cold and 'other' days were quantified. These days are defined as the fifth and 95th percentile of observed maximum temperature (Tmax °C), minimum temperature (Tmin °C) and wet bulb globe temperature (WBGT °C) (Steadman, 1994). Results were assessed separately for the Indigenous and the non-Indigenous community, younger and older age groups and males and females.

The rationale behind this assessment relates to the fact that, on most measures of health, Indigenous Australians fare much worse than non-Indigenous Australians, including experiencing significantly higher rates of chronic diseases and hospitalisations (Pink and Allbon, 2008) and lower life expectancy (Hill et al., 2007). Despite this, an investigation as to whether there could be a connection between the rates of hospitalisations of Indigenous Australians for specific diseases and the climate in which they live has not occurred.

Because the study population is spread over a very large area, and influenced by greatly varying climatic conditions, it was necessary to break the admissions data into similar 'exposure' groups by aligning the residence data with the closest weather station (see Webb et al., 2014, for a detailed description of the method employed to create the subregions in the study).

The analysis focused on cardiovascular disease, the largest contributor to the disparity in the health of Indigenous and non-Indigenous people (Penm, 2008). Further, the association between cardiovascular disease and environmental conditions has already been established for some regions in Australia (Khalaj et al., 2010; Loughnan et al., 2008, 2010a, 2010b).

Two of the more common cardiovascular diseases were studied. Ischaemic heart disease (IHD) (ICD9 410–414, ICD10 I20–I25) is the major cardiovascular disease diagnosis in the Northern Territory region (Pink and Allbon, 2008) and is characterised by a reduced blood supply to the heart muscle. Symptoms of IHD include angina, characteristic chest pain on exertion and decreased exercise tolerance. Heart failure (ICD9 428, ICD10 I50), the other disease studied, occurs where the heart is unable to provide sufficient pump action to maintain blood flow to meet the body's requirements (McMurray and Pfeffer, 2005). Heart failure is 1.7 times more prevalent in Indigenous compared to non-Indigenous Australians (Penm, 2008).

It is interesting to note the different rates for the various cohorts, showing that the major disparity in admission rates is found in the younger population (25 to 64 years), with the contrast in the admission rate for the older group less striking. In fact, older non-Indigenous males have higher rates of admission than their Indigenous counterparts (Webb et al., 2014). Notably, for most of the study groupings, males are admitted at higher rates than females.

The sensitivity in daily admissions data to climatic 'extremes' varied by disease group, age category and sex. These are described by 'rate ratios'. Rate ratios are rates for 'very hot' and 'very cold' periods divided by the rates for the 'non-extreme' periods, with numbers greater than one associated with increased rates and numbers less than one with decreased rates.

In the 25- to 64-year-old cohort, a significant 17 per cent increase in admission rates for IHD was detected in the Indigenous population on very hot days. In particular, Indigenous females (32 per cent increase, $P < 0.05$) were most affected by higher maximum temperatures. No strong temperature response was noted for heart failure admissions in the younger group. We proposed ambient heat would not be a direct cause of the increased rates of IHD in the Indigenous females, but would increase physiological stress and, given other pre-existing health issues, the heat impact would be compounded.

We found a contrasting response to climatic conditions compared with the younger group. In general, for older people, an increased rate of admissions was observed in response to cold conditions, with a reduction in admissions on very hot days. The most notable increase was found in the older male population. This tendency was also apparent for females being admitted for heart failure.

This finding is consistent with other studies showing the positive influence of cold temperatures on rates of admission for heart conditions (McGregor, 2001; Abrignani et al., 2009).

In cold conditions, the primary autonomic defences are vasoconstriction and shivering (Sessler, 2009). The cold sensitivity response derives from a combination of cardiorespiratory response, blood clotting, renal and immune effects. These increase heart rate and blood pressure, while reducing cardiac muscle contractility, deplete blood volume and increase blood viscosity (Keatinge et al., 1984; Pozos and Danzl, 2001). Cold conditions may have a stronger influence on increasing morbidity associated with heart failure, compared to IHD, because of the extra effort for the heart to pump around more viscous, higher-pressure blood. It is interesting to note that in the older population, on hotter days there is a tendency towards lower admissions for heart failure.

This epidemiological assessment indicates that projected climate change may exacerbate recently documented disparities in cardiovascular disease outcomes for Indigenous and non-Indigenous populations (Vos et al., 2009). This is because an increase in the frequency of hot days and a decrease in the frequency of cold days, as projected (Alexander and Arblaster, 2009), will possibly cause increased admissions for IHD in younger Indigenous people and reduced admissions in older populations.

Overall, rates of hospitalisation were found to be higher for older people compared to younger people, Indigenous people compared to non-Indigenous people and males compared to females. In general, the younger (25 to 64 years) Indigenous population has a tendency to higher rates of admissions on very hot days and the older (65+) non-Indigenous male population have higher rates of admission on very cold days.

In the absence of adaptation activities, this analysis suggests that climate change is likely to have greater adverse health effects – at least for cardiovascular-related events – in the Indigenous compared to non-Indigenous population, with the increase in heat-related admissions in the younger population most likely to outweigh the reduction to rates of admission in older Indigenous people, especially from a burden of disease perspective.

From this work to date, our initial conclusions are that increasingly disproportionate impacts on the health of the Indigenous population living in the Northern Territory may result from projected climate changes. Further analysis on other non-communicable diseases and climate thresholds will be assessed prior to making broader policy recommendations. Due to the success of this investigation into cardiovascular responses to climate, the next phase of this research will investigate whether there is also a link between respiratory admissions and climate.

References

Abrignani, M.G., Corrao, S., Biondo, G.B., Renda, N., Braschi, A., Novo, G., et al. 2009. Influence of climatic variables on acute myocardial infarction hospital admissions. *International Journal of Cardiology* 137(2), 123–9.

Alexander, L.V. & Arblaster, J.M. 2009. Assessing trends in observed and modelled climate extremes over Australia in relation to future projections. *International Journal of Climatology* 29, 417–35.

Altman, J. & Kerins, S. 2012. *People on Country, Vital Landscapes, Indigenous Futures*. The Federation Press, Canberra, ACT, Australia.

Ameyali, R. 2009. Sea level rise in Kowanyama. Available at: ourworld.unu.edu/en/sea-level-rise-in-kowanyama, accessed 27 January 2015.

Australian Institute of Health and Welfare (AIHW) 2011. *Australia's Welfare 2011*. AIHW, Canberra, Australia.

Baker, R., Davies, J. & Young, E. 2001. *Working on Country: Contemporary Indigenous Management of Australia's Lands and Coastal Regions*. Oxford University Press, Oxford, UK.

Barnsley, I. 2008. *Emissions Trading, Carbon Financing and Indigenous Peoples*. UNU-IAS, Japan.

Biddle, N. 2011. Measures of Indigenous wellbeing and their determinants across the lifecourse. CAEPR Lecture series. The Australian National University, Canberra, ACT, Australia.

Burgess, C., Johnston, F., Berry, H., McDonnell, J., Yibarbuk, D., Gunabarra, C., et al. 2009. Healthy country, healthy people: the relationship between Indigenous health status and 'caring for country'. *Medical Journal of Australia* 190, 567–72.

Campbell, D., Burgess, C., Garnett, S. & Wakerman, J. 2011. Potential primary health care savings for chronic disease care associated with Australian Aboriginal involvement in land management. *Health Policy* 99, 83–9.

Carson, B., Dunbar, T., Chenhall, R. & Bailie, R. (eds) 2007. *Social Determinants of Indigenous Health*. Allen and Unwin, Sydney, NSW, Australia.

Doherty, T. & Clayton, S. 2011. The psychological impacts of global climate change. *American Psychologist* 66 (4), 265–76.

Galloway McLean, K. 2010. *Advance Guard: Climate Change Impacts, Adaptation, Mitigation and Indigenous Peoples*. Australia, United Nations University – Traditional Knowledge Initiative, Darwin, NT, Australia.

Green, D. & Minchin, L. 2012. The co-benefits of carbon management on country. *Nature Climate Change* 2, 641–3.

Green, D., Jackson, S. & Morrison, J. 2009. *Risks from Climate Change to Indigenous Communities in the Tropical North of Australia*. Department of Climate Change, Canberra, ACT, Australia.

Green, D., Alexander, L., Mclnnes, K., Church, J., Nicholls, N. & White, N. 2010a. An assessment of climate change impacts and adaptation for the Torres Strait Islands, Australia. *Climatic Change* 102, 405–33.

Green, D., Billy, J. & Tapim, A. 2010b. Indigenous Australians' knowledge of weather and climate. *Climatic Change* 100, 337–54.

Hill, K., Barker, B. & Vos, T. 2007. Excess Indigenous mortality: are Indigenous Australians more severely disadvantaged than other Indigenous populations? *International Journal of Epidemiology* 36, 580–9.

Hunter, E. 2009. 'Radical hope' and rain: climate change and the mental health of Indigenous residents of northern Australia. *Australasian Psychiatry* 17, 445–52.

Kakadu National Park 2007. Management Plan 2007–2014. Board of Management (Director of National Parks, Northern Territory), Kakadu, NT, Australia.

Keatinge, W., Coleshaw, S., Cotter, F., Mattock, M., Murphy, M. & Chelliah, R. 1984. Increases in platelet and red cell counts, blood viscosity, and arterial pressure during mild surface cooling: factors in mortality from coronary and cerebral thrombosis in winter. *BMJ* 289, 1405–8.

Khalaj, B., Lloyd, G., Sheppeard, V. & Dear, K. 2010. The health impacts of heat waves in five regions of New South Wales, Australia: a case-only analysis. *International Archives of Occupational and Environmental Health* 83, 833–42.

Loughnan, M., Nicholls, N. & Tapper, N. 2008. Demographic, seasonal, and spatial differences in acute myocardial infarction admissions to hospital in Melbourne Australia. *International Journal of Health Geographics* 7, 42 doi:10.1186/1476-072X-7-42.

Loughnan, M.E., Nicholls, N. & Tapper, N.J. 2010a. The effects of summer temperature, age and socioeconomic circumstance on Acute Myocardial Infarction admissions in Melbourne, Australia. *International Journal of Health Geographics* 9, 41. www.ij-healthgeographics.com/content/9/1/41.

Loughnan, M.E., Nicholls, N. & Tapper, N.J. 2010b. When the heat is on: threshold temperatures for AMI admissions to hospital in Melbourne Australia. *Applied Geography* 30 (1), 63–9.

McGregor, G. 2001. The meteorological sensitivity of ischaemic heart disease mortality events in Birmingham, UK. *International Journal of Biometeorology* 45, 133–42.

McMichael, A.J. 2006. Climate change and risks to health in remote Indigenous communities. Sharing Knowledge: A Workshop on Climate Change Impacts and Adaptation Strategies for Northern Australian Indigenous Communities. Darwin, Australia. Available at: www.sharingknowledge.net.au, accessed 27 January 2015.

McMichael, A.J. 2011. Climate and health (Keynote address). 19th International Congress of Biometeorology, Auckland, New Zealand.

McMurray, J.J.V. & Pfeffer, M.A. 2005. Heart failure. *The Lancet* 365, 1877–89.

Parry, M.L. (ed.) 2007. *Climate Change 2007: Impacts, Adaptation and Vulnerability: Working Group I Contribution to the Fourth Assessment Report of the IPCC*. Cambridge University Press, Cambridge, UK.

Penm, E. 2008. Cardiovascular disease and its associated risk factors in Aboriginal and Torres Strait Islander peoples 2004–05. *Cardiovascular Disease Series No. 29*. AIHW, Canberra, ACT, Australia.

Pink, B. & Allbon, P. 2008. *The Health and Welfare of Australia's Aboriginal and Torres Strait Islander Peoples*. Australian Bureau of Statistics, Australian Institute of Health and Welfare, Canberra, ACT, Australia.

Pozos, R.S. & Danzl, D. 2001. Human physiological responses to cold stress and hypothermia. In: Pandoff, P. & Burr, M. (eds) *Medical Aspects of Harsh Environments Vol 1*. Department of the Army, Washington, DC, USA, 351–82.

Reid, J. 1992. *Body, Land and Spirit: Health and Healing in Aboriginal Society*. University Queensland Press, Brisbane, QLD, Australia.

Rose, D. (ed.) 1992. *Dingo Makes Us Human: Life and Land in an Australian Aboriginal Culture*. Cambridge University Press, Cambridge, UK.

Sessler, D.I. 2009. Thermoregulatory defense mechanisms. *Critical Care Medicine* 37, S203–S210.

Sherwood, J. 2010. *Do No Harm: Decolonising Aboriginal Health Research*. PhD thesis, University of New South Wales, Sydney, NSW, Australia.

Steadman, R.G. 1994. Norms of apparent temperature in Australia. *Australian Meteorological Magazine* 43, 1–16.

Turner, N. & Clifton, H. 2009. 'It's so different today': climate change and Indigenous lifeways in British Columbia, Canada. *Global Environmental Change* 19, 180–90.

Vos, T., Barker, B., Begg, S., Stanley, L. & Lopez, A.D. 2009. Burden of disease and injury in Aboriginal and Torres Strait Islander peoples: the Indigenous health gap. *International Journal of Epidemiology* 38, 470–7.

Webb, L., Bambrick, H., Tait, P., Green, D. & Alexander, L. 2013. Effect of ambient temperature on Australian Northern Territory public hospital admissions for cardiovascular disease among Indigenous and non-Indigenous populations. *International Journal of Environmental Research and Public Health*, 11 (2), 1942–59.

Willox, A., Harper, S. & Edge, V. 2012. Storytelling in a digital age: digital storytelling as an emerging narrative method for preserving and promoting indigenous oral wisdom. *Qualitative Research* 13, 127–47.

20

THE SOCIOCULTURAL CONTEXT OF CLIMATE CHANGE ADAPTATION IN AUSTRALIA, WITH A FOCUS ON HOT WEATHER

CATHY BANWELL, JANE DIXON, HILARY BAMBRICK
FERNE EDWARDS AND TORD KJELLSTROM

Abstract

In this chapter, we draw inspiration from Tony McMichael's research on the implications of climate change for human health and well-being and his exhortations to pay attention to the big picture. As a consequence, we use historical and contemporary materials to reflect on how Australia's cultural history has contributed to the development of our somewhat relaxed attitudes and practices in relation to increasingly hot weather and climate change. We consider the historical experiences of European settlers who arrived from the northern hemisphere with little understanding of hot weather and attempted to impose themselves on a foreign landscape. They developed a stoic approach to hot weather; something to be endured, if they were to survive. Over time, a more compromising attitude has developed as Australians gradually, and partially, adapt their clothing, behaviour, housing and location of residence to cope with the bodily discomforts of heat. Now they rely on techno-fixes, such as air conditioning, to manage hot weather, with unhelpful implications for climate change mitigation. Instead of relying on individual behaviour change, we nominate three policy domains where action is urgently required.

Introduction

Neither a complaint nor a boast, 'It's a scorcher!', is a common Australian summertime vernacular. In this chapter, we describe how cultural approaches that favour 'techno-fixes' at the household level have evolved in response to hot weather in Australia. We then proceed to describe them in terms of inadequate adaptive responses to climate change. We consider as a contextual narrative how these approaches have evolved from the historical experiences of European settlers who arrived from the northern hemisphere with little physical or psychological understanding of hot weather and attempted to impose themselves on a foreign landscape. They developed a stoic approach to hot weather; something to be endured, if they were to survive. Over time, a more compromising attitude has developed as Australians gradually, and partially, adapt their clothing, behaviour, housing and location of residence to cope with the bodily discomforts of heat.

Tony McMichael's research, over several decades, provided inspiration and guidance in analysing the nature of Australia's limited response to climate change science. First, he drew attention to the implications of climate change for human health and well-being and considered everyday responses to changed climatic conditions to be inadequate (McMichael, 1993, 2009). Second, he exhorted researchers not only to focus on proximate and measurable risk factors but also to consider their context, 'the big picture' (McMichael, 1999) – a point we return to in the conclusion.

In this chapter, we use historical and contemporary materials to provide context, reflecting on how Australia's cultural history influences our responses to future challenges posed by increasing numbers of heatwaves and droughts as the ramifications of a changing climate unfold. We argue that somewhat 'lazy' attitudes and related practices can be seen in our modern responses to hot weather; with unhelpful implications for climate change mitigation. Instead of relying on individual behaviour change, we nominate three policy domains where action is urgently required.

The Impact of Heatwaves

Typically during summer over much of Australia, consistently hot weather can last for several days, and even for weeks. Heatwaves (usually defined as daily maximum temperatures above 35°C for three or more consecutive days) cause significant human health impacts for the elderly, people on medication, the very young, the poor and Indigenous communities (Climate Commission, 2013). Certain respiratory and cardiovascular conditions increase the risk of morbidity and mortality during and immediately following very hot days (Vaneckova and Bambrick, 2013), particularly for people with a mental disorder or those who have at least one cardiac risk factor (Hansen et al., 2008a, 2008b).

According to the Australian Bureau of Meteorology and the Commonwealth Government (2009), heatwaves have actually accounted for more deaths in Australia than any other natural hazard. Findings from modelling studies that investigate the links between climate change and health (Hennessy et al., 2007; Kjellstrom and Weaver, 2009; McMichael et al., 2009) show that heatwaves are potentially one of the most damaging side effects of global warming, especially in a 'hot' country such as Australia, where the death rate from heatwaves may triple by 2100 in all Australian cities (Barlow, 2008).

With more frequent and intense heatwaves brought on by climate change, increasing numbers of Australians will be affected. This situation will require greater public health and medical attention, which, in turn, will be costly and resource-demanding. Heatwaves, especially as they become increasingly extreme, lead to loss of life and property through bushfires, and also place additional strain on infrastructure such as water, transport and electricity, causing a possible rise in social disturbance and instigating systemic economic flow-on effects to the retail industry, ecosystem services and tourism. For example, unexpected complications of the 2009 Melbourne heatwave included a full morgue, overworked hospital staff and limited resources, power loss to more than 6000 homes, heat-stricken wildlife, communication blockages and public transport breakdowns as railway tracks buckled (*Progress Leader*, 2009; *Whittlesea Leader*, 2009). The effects of extreme heat impact other species, too: in 2000, an unexpected impact of the Adelaide and Brisbane heatwaves was the substantial number of deaths of pigs, poultry and bees (Harris and Hooper, 2000; Nicholson, 2000).

While the effects of heat on mortality have now long been studied (e.g. Smoyer, 1998), there are still significant gaps in the study of the social experience of heat. Some research has been conducted into the social science of disasters (Klinenberg, 2002; Fothergill and Peek, 2004), but there has been little social research into the everyday aspects that contribute to such situations. This paucity of data could be attributed to research not yet published, a lack of social research into the experiences of hazard scenarios or the concentrated focus on the USA and Europe rather than on Australia or on developing countries.

Furthermore, the invisible and silent nature of heatwaves – as one of the most underrated and least-studied natural phenomena – needs to be unpacked because, once their initial impact is digested, they fade very quickly into the background. The deadly 1995 Chicago heatwave 'was forgotten as soon as the temperatures fell' (Klinenberg, 2002). Klinenberg's work is one of the few pieces of research to have examined the human experience and the sociocultural dimensions of heatwaves.

In essence, heatwaves cannot be categorised as a conventional environmental health hazard to be handled by public health departments. Their cumulative effect is to weaken life-support systems that underpin the survival of all species, requiring whole-of-government and whole-of-society responses. As the science of weather patterns becomes more settled, the research focus should shift to sociocultural studies as a basis both for preventive health campaigns (avoiding heatstroke and stress) and, more important, for strategies to strengthen engagement by civil society in policy advocacy to act to slow climate change.

How Hot Weather has Shaped the Australian Psyche

> To the fierce sun of Australia, which tempers men as fire tempers steel; to the gracious sun of Australia, which makes nature teem with bounty; to the glowing sun of Australia, which warms the heart, enkindles the eye, ruddies the cheek, this in the tribute. (Fox, 1927)

The image of Australia is divided between pre- and post-European settlement – a world once inhabited solely by Aboriginal peoples suddenly transitioning in 1788 with the arrival of the fair-skinned British. It is not possible, in this short chapter, to do justice to the knowledge of, and adaptation to, the Australian climate demonstrated by Australia's first inhabitants, which was disrupted by the arrival of European settlers. Instead, we focus on the latter arrivals, who became enshrined in tales of the Aussie Bushman, Battler and the bronzed Sunbather. These cultural stereotypes were influenced strongly by the Australian landscape and climate, with the harsh, untamed, sun-drenched and isolating environment of the Outback contributing to the development of the Australian psyche as masculine, stoic, tough and quietly courageous. Hence, heat and the sun scorching the Earth, drying the ground and baking the skin is a consistent narrative contributing to, and sedimenting, the development of a particular Australian character. It is a narrative replete with health risks, as highlighted below.

The Outback, the desert, the bush and the red heart

The Australian bush, and the Outback, with an associated hot and harsh climate, was encountered by early settlers, and it helped form the contemporary Australian psyche. For well over a century, the Australian climate has been described as having irregular, uncertain and sporadic seasons in a threatening, alienating, endless and unrelenting landscape. Ranken (1874) pronounced the climate to be 'not only niggardly on the whole, it is a most capricious tyrant, destroying at uncertain intervals what it has reared in a few milder seasons'. Terminologies of drought differ between Europe and Australia, where the former defines drought as 'a period of a few days or weeks in which not a drop of rain falls', whereas in Australia drought becomes 'a period of months or years during which little rain falls and the country gets burnt up, grass and water disappear, crops become worthless and sheep and cattle die' (Sherratt, 2005, p. 6). In their first test, and as a matter of survival, European pioneers strove to adapt their agriculture and pastoralism to what was regarded as one of the driest continents on Earth. Even the lusher parts of Australia were drier and more climatically variable than most European landscapes, and the first settlers saw Australia in terms of opposites, pitting nature against civilised, wild versus tamed, opportunity versus anxiety and masculine versus feminine (Sherratt, 2005).

The obvious discomfort of Europeans on Australian soil led some to question if, indeed, they should be there at all. Foster Fraser believed that pioneer Australians 'lacked vim' and 'showed signs of having been drained by their climate' (cited in Walker, 2005, p. 94). Sunstroke, leading to madness for the colonial white male, became a prominent concern in the late 1800s. In the 1870s, 16 per cent of the male patients in the Yarra Bend asylum were diagnosed as 'sunstruck', awarding the Victorian colony the 'most unenviable position of being the maddest place in the world' (Foster, 1981). Boucher (2004) likens this malady within the medical discourse of the time as a consequence of white, middle-class, male, protestant bodies being out of place within the Australian environment and climate.

> The sunstroke of Port Philip [causes] many deaths among the white population … the thin skull of the European is unduly exposed to solar rays … during the hot season in this climate … Another distressing effect of Sunstroke, not infrequent in Victoria, is Insanity. (Mackin, 1856)

In view of this situation, it was suggested that, rather than trying to fight the climatic conditions, people from similarly tropical climes should be introduced to the north to populate the region. In response, the settlers of the time acted to make Australian conditions work for them, and hence began a campaign to embrace and celebrate the resilient persona of the Australian Battler. In one account, C. E. W. Bean described the qualities of the Australian character as forged in the battle against the elements, with progress won by an ongoing confrontation with nature. 'The Australian is always fighting something. In the bush it is drought, fires, unbroken horses and cattle' (Bean cited in Walker, 2005, p. 4). The ensuing typical Australian humour, too, was sculpted out of the harsh weather as dry and full of irony with 'a stoical acceptance of hardship; shrewd practicality; and sheer, sardonic bloody-mindedness' (Willey, 1988, p. 158). Portrayals of the Australian bush and its impact on new arrivals alternated from the realistic to the romantic, exemplified by its two key protagonists A. B. Banjo Patterson and Henry Lawson, with one describing Australia as 'benign and bountiful' and the other as a harsh destination that strips away civilisation for people to discover something within themselves (Radio National Hindsight, 2007).

From Europeans trapped under a blazing sun in the dry Australian bush came a strong impulse to control nature, including the weather. The result was a series of scientific fixes, or 'silver bullets', including irrigation systems, dams, bores, the planting of forests and even the seeding of clouds (see Home, 2005). Rather than engaging with, or embedding themselves within, the Australian continent and climate, European colonialists tried to impose familiar features from their homelands (Lowe, 2005); such that D. H. Lawrence observed:

> A grey, strange spirit, and the people that are here are not really here: only like ducks that swim on the surface of a lake. But the country has a fourth dimension and the white people float like shadows on the surface. (D. H. Lawrence cited in Drew, 1994, p. 36)

This disconnect between the Australian landscape and its inhabitants – serving also to disconnect humans from nature – has created what Symons (2007), in his discussion of the Australian diet, describes as 'picnicking' atop Australia's surface. In a dramatic break from their previous lived experience, newly arrived Europeans could dispatch with a peasant existence, which involved growing food for themselves and a small number of households. They leapfrogged to becoming farmers and pastoralists, producing agriculture on a large scale, with the help of irrigation and later with fossil fuel inputs, 'riding the sheep's back' to prosperity for themselves and their nation. In so doing, they contributed to feeding their colonial masters, and to the present situation where pastoral agriculture makes a major contribution to Australia's greenhouse carbon and methane emissions a topic central to Tony McMichael's research on the multiple links between food systems, climate change and population health (McMichael et al., 2007).

City life, beach and sun worship

Despite the Outback mythology, Australia is one of the most urbanised countries in the world, with 89 per cent of its population living along the coast in or near its six state capital cities (Bambrick et al., 2011). Therefore, city, not desert, has arguably become most representative of the Australian identity. As more Australians have moved from the bush to urban centres, the stoic Aussie Battler has become supplanted in city settings. Traditionally equated with conquering Outback conditions, the Aussie Battler is now more likely to be seen lying prone on a city or peri-urban beach after a week spent in the office or factory.

Indeed, visiting an Australian beach for health, relaxation and to escape the heat forms another rich vein in the Australian psyche. The Australian coast has a long history of habitation, serving as a healthy holiday destination since the era of the First Settlers, where the combination of sea breeze and sun acted as a cure-all and as a place for renewal. At the beach, the Australian heat was seen as energising, and the 'new Australians' ability to adapt and endure beach conditions made them bolder, adventurous and more resilient' (Walker, 2005, p. 97). The sun as a source of pleasure and revitalisation became fully realised in the surf culture that flourished on waves of consumerism and bikini contests in the 1920s and 1930s. The beach, and surfing in particular, became the urban equivalent to Australia's frontier, and the surf lifesaver became the new urban hero after the war. Maxwell (cited in Huntsman, 2001, p. 199) sums up lifesaving clubs as fostering 'a spirit of selflessness, of chivalry, such as is found in no other sporting movement in all the world today, not counting the cost when a life is for the saving'. Surfing heroics were also well expressed by Fox:

> Australian surfing is not a matter of tip-toeing over wet sands and through shallow pools. It is standing up to great breakers of ocean water, champagned to foam as they break their crests; and giving to the meeting body mighty thumps, massaging and bracing the muscles delightfully. (Fox, 1927, pp. 101–2)

Rodwell (1999) describes this surf culture in terms of eugenics, with the sun's rays improving the physical attributes of both men and women. Similarly, Professor H. G. Chapman, in his 1928 address at the Australasian Association for the Advancement of Science Congress, calls Australians 'sun-worshippers' and states that 'not only in height, weight and build, but also in chemical composition and in nutrition was the Australian changing from his British forefathers. One factor that acted all over Australia in producing persons more fitted to live in Australia was sunshine' (Chapman, 1928). It was almost half a century later before it was recognised that the sun produced adverse health effects, such as skin cancers, with McMichael again providing early calls to examine the links between these health outcomes and climate change (McMichael, 1993).

Australian Adaptations to Hot Weather

Over the two centuries of European settlement, Australians have adapted their dwellings to cope with hot weather, using three particular strategies; the veranda, the air conditioner and water-thirsty gardens. The ubiquitous Australian veranda, adopted from British India, symbolises Australians' relationship to place, weather and their own cultural ambivalence towards heat. Drew (1994) uses the veranda as a metaphor to analyse the implications on the Australian identity for living on the edge or periphery of the continent looking out to sea. The pattern of space created by the veranda and repeated by verandaways (a passage of linked verandas from adjoining buildings) reveals 'how Australians have responded to the physical presence of Australia' (Drew, 1994, p. 11). It represents a transitional zone between indoor and outdoor living.

The veranda was 'tacked on' to existing European-style buildings from the time of colonisation, providing a lived-in passage that also acted as a protective barrier against harsh sun and rain while harnessing sea breezes. Australians, in fact, have revealed a preference to 'live outside their homes' (Huntsman, 2001, p. 182), reflected by the cultural value they attach to active outdoor pursuits of sport, the beach and the outdoor kitchen in the form of the barbecue. Rather than internalising their moral or intellectual dilemmas, the Aussie Battler has been described as getting 'on with the business of surviving'. Philip Drew, in his book, *The Coast Dwellers*, expresses this national propensity to the great outdoors as 'Australia is a verandah country inhabited by a verandah people' (Drew, 1994, p. 21).

Supplanting this enculturated 'fringe behaviour' are new technologies to replace older approaches to climate adaptation. The two most common are home air conditioning and climate-controlled cars. Modern houses are being designed without eves or verandas, and may have sealed windows to suit air conditioning better. Before air conditioning, people used their verandas. They 'created opportunities for casual observations and social exchange, and people would eat, play and sleep outside' (Shove, 2003, p. 45). In contrast, air conditioning has privatised comfort, drawing people from their social networks on the verandas back inside their homes. People would also employ their own techniques to regulate the temperature, such as a liberal use of water for cooling: whether a bowl of water in front of a window or old fan, damp cloths on the back of the neck, garden sprinklers or sitting in a water-filled container. They would evaluate personally what they considered to be comfortable, displaying an achievement of personal skill and climatic awareness (Shove, 2003).

The arrival of new technologies has allowed modern Australian families to adapt to heat in different, albeit more climate damaging, ways. They can turn on air conditioning at home or jump into climate-controlled cars to drive to cooler destinations, such as the beach, country streams, waterholes or rivers, or to hide out in air-conditioned shopping malls, cinemas or libraries. They can call up fast-food deliveries instead of home-meal preparation on the hottest of days, further increasing the consumption of fossil fuels and their associated emissions (Banwell et al., 2012). Stoicism has given way to energy consumption in the name of comfort, but both are lazy responses and have the same negative impact on the climate. As Hamilton has noted, modern Australians' desire to climate-proof their lives

> is an extension of human attempts to control the natural world and its impacts on us, and this is transforming our psyches in profound ways. ... we harden ourselves against the effects of Nature's unexpected forces, and our relationship to the natural world is transformed. (Hamilton, 2005, p. 191)

Rather than supporting stronger and more costly household energy- and water-saving measures, Australians have recently voted in a government that campaigned on abolishing the Department of Climate Change and on repealing carbon pricing in favour of so-called 'direct action' on the climate. While it is still unclear what this means, it appears to signal a voluntary code to deal with non-renewable energy production and consumption. It frames the problems of the environment and climate in terms of negotiable, and easy, solutions. It situates the national response in terms of the national psyche, as forged through a relative abundance of natural resources and an easy-going national psyche. This lazy and laissez-faire approach was evidenced by the behaviour of citizens during the 2009 Melbourne heatwave in the suburb of Boroondara. The four public swimming pools increased in use by 90 per cent compared to the same time the previous year, and trips to aquatic centres proved very popular (Rollins, 1997; *Progress Leader*, 2009). Likewise, a DVD shop manager said his store was extremely busy as customers stocked up on videos and DVDs for the hot weather (*Whittlesea Leader*, 2009). Others spent their hot days purchasing acquired technologies and tastes to keep them cool – air conditioners, fans and other cooling appliances 'walked out the door' as stores experienced a spike in sales of ice, water, ice cream and cold drinks, such as beer (Norrie, 2002; Chambers and Minchin, 2003; *Illawarra Mercury*, 2003).

Yet, these adaptations in no way address the problem of heat and heat-related illness and death. The extreme case of possible statewide energy failure occurred in summer 2004, in Western Australia, leading the Western Power company to ban the use of energy-hungry air conditioners in homes and offices, effectively ordering a shutdown of all industry. To endorse this behaviour change, Western Power threatened to fine residents A$1000 and businesses A$10,000 for non-compliance (Martin et al., 2004). Nevertheless, the following year, *The Australian* reported that 'more than 100,000 new household air conditioners have been installed in Western Australia' (Wilson, 2005, p. 2).

There is a final irony to the Australian laconic approach to climate change adaptation: 'move away'. Heat can be an important factor leading to some people moving to entirely new locations. Australians who relocate to more temperate climes include those who 'downshift', 'sea or tree change' or, specifically for the elderly, become part of the 'grey nomad' phenomenon, escaping the cold in winter and the heat in summer. In *The Big Shift*, Salt documents a sizeable population shift from the cities to non-metropolitan coastal towns (Salt, 2001). According to 2001 census data, 3.9 million people live in provincial coastal Australia with allegiance to neither city nor bush (Salt, 2001).

These sea-changers consist predominantly of retirees, alternative lifestylers, people who conduct business over the Internet, people with low incomes who cannot afford appropriate housing in city centres, periodic tourists and gentrifiers (people who buy and renovate houses to sell for profit). Their motivations are varied, but the benefits of temperate weather are certainly factored into these relocations (Murphy, 2002). The recognition of this population shift and corresponding impact on coastal communities led to the national government establishment in 2004 of a National Sea Change Taskforce to represent the interests of coastal councils and communities experiencing the effects of rapid growth and development (Gurran and Blakely, 2007). Since then, these same councils have been alerted to the potential loss of coastline due to sea level rise associated with climate change, with some state governments overriding local government planning permissions for development on their most valuable ocean-hugging lands.

Conclusions

The Australian character has been shaped by myriad landscapes morphing from the Aussie (rural) Battler to sportsman to surfer to lifesaver, all based on inhabiting (adapting to) and taming the natural environment and weather 'elements'. As rising tides consume Australia's shorelines and as increasingly erratic weather tears at the landscape, the Australian island will become hotter, drier and smaller. The historical influences of the stoic Australian psyche may foster a more recent state of denial or laziness, slowing the uptake of green technologies, policies and action, even as Australians become increasingly reliant on air conditioning to micromanage their hot weather. Whether Australians, as The Climate Institute suggests they should in their paper, *Towards a Climate Strategy for Australian Agriculture* (2009, p. 5), take hot weather seriously enough to transit to a low-carbon country currently appears an increasingly doubtful proposition.

Indeed, climate change has become a more, rather than less, politically contested area in Australia over the last decade, contributing to the need to understand what McMichael refers to as the 'big picture'. And, the 'big picture' embraces the cultural and social contexts that have influenced, and continue to influence, experiences and understandings of the impact of climate change. If we are correct about the weight of history, then leaving the response to heatwaves to individual behaviour change is self-defeating. What we propose are three 'lifestyle' policy domains that urgently require action because they change the calculus of choices available. They are higher non-renewable energy and water costs; built environment designs that are less reliant on electric air conditioners and more reliant on urban greening for cooling; and mass transit options to make car travel less attractive. Each of these policy alternatives has equity considerations and will require increases to minimum wages and pensions to offset the impacts on lower-income households. However, given that lower socio-economic groups are more exposed to heat effects, the equity dimensions to climate change policy cannot be avoided. We are not arguing that community lifestyle change is adequate to the task of slowing climate change and we endorse non-voluntary action to change the energy, materials and water-use behaviour of Australian businesses and governments. However, whole-of-community lifestyle change is an increasingly urgent task, as the growing impact of climate change on Australian weather conditions will generate enough floods, droughts, fires and heatwaves to test even the most resilient of Australians.

References

Bambrick, H.J., Capon, A.G., Barnett, G.B., Beaty, R.M. & Burton, A.J. 2011. Climate change and health in the urban environment: adaptation opportunities in Australian cities. *Asia Pacific Journal of Public Health* 23, 67–79.

Banwell, C., Dixon, J., Bambrick, H., Edwards, F., Kjellstrom, T. 2012. Socio-cultural reflections on heat in Australia with implications for health and climate change adaptation. *Global Health Action* 5, 19277, dx.doi.org/10.3402/gha.v5i0.19277.

Barlow, G. 2008. Nurses feel impact of climate change. *Australian Nursing Review* 15, 24–7.

Boucher, L. 2004 Masculinity gone mad: settler colonialism, medical discourse and the white body in late nineteenth-century Victoria. *Lillith* 13, 51–67.

Chambers, T. & Minchin, L. 2003. How the heat is taking its toll (and how we're coping). *The Sunday Age*, Melbourne, VIC, 2 February 2003.

Chapman, H.G. 1928. Science Congress: Sun-Worshippers: The Typical Australian. Address by Professor H. G. Chapman.

Climate Commission 2011. The Critical Decade: Climate Change and Health www.climatecouncil.org.au/uploads/1bb6887d6f8cacd5d844fc30b0857931.pdf, accessed 4 July 2015.

Commonwealth Government. 2009 Protecting human health and safety during severe and extreme heat events. www.pwc.com.au/industry/government/assets/extreme-heat-events-nov11.pdf.

Drew, P. 1994. *The Coast Dwellers*. Penguin Books Australia, Ringwood, VIC, Australia.

Foster, S.G. 1981. Imperfect Victorians: insanity in Victoria in 1888, Australia 1888. *Bulletin,* 8, 97–116.

Fothergill, A. & Peek, L. 2004. Poverty and disasters in the United States: a review of recent sociological findings. *Natural Hazards* 32, 89–110.

Fox, F. 1927. *Australia*. A. & C. Black Ltd, London, UK.

Gurran, N. & Blakely, E. 2007. Suffer a sea change? Contrasting perspectives towards urban policy and migration in coastal Australia. *Australian Geographer* 38, 113–31.

Hamilton, C. 2005. Social psychology of climate change. In: Sherratt, T., Griffith, T. & Robin, L. (eds) *A Change in the Weather: Climate and Culture in Australia*. National Museum of Australia Press, Canberra, ACT, Australia, 187–95.

Hansen, A., Bi, P., Nitschke, M., Ryan, P., Pisaniello, D. & Tucker, G. 2008a. The effect of heat waves on mental health in a temperate Australian city. *Environmental Health Perspectives* 116, 1369–75.

Hansen, A., Bi, P., Ryan, P., Nitschke, M., Pisaniello, D. & Tucker, G. 2008b. The effect of heat waves on hospital admissions for renal disease in a temperate city of Australia. *International Journal of Epidemiology* 37, 1359–65.

Harris, S. & Hooper, B. 2000. Surviving in a sunburnt country. *Adelaide Advertiser*, SA, 12 January 2000, 19.

Hennessy, K., Fitzharris, B., Bates, N., Harvey, S., Howden, L., Hughes, J., et al. 2007. Chapter 11. Australia and New Zealand. *Climate Change 2007: Impacts, Adaptation and Vulnerability. Contribution of Working Group II to the Fourth Assessment. Report of the Intergovernmental Panel on Climate Change*. 507–40. IPCC, Geneva, Switzerland.

Home, R.W. 2005. Rainmaking in CSIRO: the science and politicis of climate modification. In: Sharratt, T., Griffith, T. & Robin, L. (eds) *A Change in the Weather: Climate and Culture in Australia*. National Museum of Australia Press, Canberra, Australia, 66–79.

Huntsman, L. 2001 *Sand in our Souls. The Beach in Australian History*. Melbourne University Press, Melbourne, Australia.

Illawarra Mercury, Wollongong, NSW. 2003. Perth roasts in heat wave, 11 March 2003.

Kjellstrom, T. & Weaver, H. 2009. Climate change and health: impacts, vulnerability, adaptation and mitigation. *New South Wales Public Health Bulletin* 20, 5–9.

Klinenberg, E. 2002. *Heat Wave: A Social Autopsy of Disaster in Chicago.* University of Chicago Press, Chicago, Illinois, USA.

Lowe, I. 2005. Solar energy. In: Sherratt, T., Griffith, T. & Robin, L. (eds) *A Change in the Weather: Climate and Culture in Australia.* National Museum of Australia Press, Canberra, Australia, 116–25.

Mackin, C.T. 1856. Sunstroke or coup de soleil: its causes, consequences and pathology. *Australian Medical Journal* 5, 85–6.

McMichael, A.J. 1993. *Planetary Overload: Global Environmental Change and the Health of the Human Species.* Cambridge University Press, Cambridge, UK.

McMichael, A.J. 1999. Prisoners of the proximate: loosening the constraints on epidemiology in an age of change *American Journal of Epidemiology* 149, 887–97.

McMichael, A.J., Powles, J., Butler, C.D., Uauy, R.. 2007. Food, livestock production, energy, climate change, and health. *The Lancet* 370, 1253–63.

McMichael, A.J., Neira, M., Bertollini, R., Campbell-Lendrum, D. & Hales, S. 2009. Climate change: a time of need and opportunity for the health sector. *The Lancet* 374, 2123–5.

Martin, B., Pennels, S. & Adshead, G. 2004. WA faces shutdown in new power crises – power orders what you can't do. *The West Australian,* 18 February 2004.

Murphy, P. 2002. Sea change: re-inventing rural and regional Australia. *Transformations* 2, 1–12.

Nicholson, S. 2000. Heatwave plays havoc with lives. *The Australian,* 29 January 2000, 44.

Norrie, J. 2002. Heatwave has valley sizzling. *Newcastle Herald,* NSW, 20 March 2002.

Progress Leader, VIC. 2009. Heat wave pushes people's temperatures up. 3 February 2009.

Radio National Hindsight 2007. *The Australian Landscape – The Long Hot Summer – Heat.* Directed by Radio National Hindsight.

Ranken, W.H.L. 1874. *The Dominion of Australia: An Account of its Foundation*. Chapman and Hall, London, UK.

Rodwell, G. 1999. The sense of victorious struggle; the eugenic dynamic in Australian popular surf-culture, 1900–1950. *Journal of Australian Studies* 23, 56–63.

Rollins, A. 1997. Last time it was this hot, ball gowns were beachwear. *Sunday Age*, 23 February, 1997.

Salt, B. 2001. *The Big Shift: Welcome to the Third Australian Culture*. Hardie Grant, Melbourne, VIC, Australia.

Sherratt, T. 2005. Human elements. In: Sherratt, T., Griffith, T. & Robin, L. (eds) *A Change in the Weather: Climate and Culture in Australia*. National Museum of Australia Press, Canberra, Australia, 1–17.

Shove, E. 2003. *Comfort, Cleanliness and Convenience. The Social Organisation of Normality*. Berg, Oxford, UK & New York, NY, USA.

Smoyer, K. 1998. A comparative analysis of heat waves and associated mortality in St Louis, Missouri – 1980 and 1995. *International Journal of Biometeorology* 42, 44–50.

Symons, M. 2007. *One Continuous Picnic. A Gastronomic History of Australia*, 2nd edition. Melbourne University Press, Melbourne, VIC, Australia.

The Climate Change Institute 2009 *Towards a climate strategy for Australian agriculture* www.climateinstitute.org.au/verve/_resources/towards_climate_friendly_ag_policy_brief.pdf.

Vaneckova, P. & Bambrick, H. 2013. Cause-specific hospital admissions on hot days in Sydney, Australia. *PLoS ONE*, doi:10.1371/journal.pone.0055459.

Walker, D. 2005. The curse of the tropics. In: Sherratt, T., Griffith, T. & Robin, L. (eds) *A Change in the Weather: Climate and Culture in Australia*. National Museum of Australia Press, Canberra, ACT, Australia, 92–101.

Whittlesea Leader, Preston, VIC. 2009. City wilts in heat. 4 February 2009.

Willey, K. 1988. A hard, dry humour for a hard, dry land. In: Burgmann, V. & Lee, J. (eds) *Constructing a Culture. A People's History of Australia since 1788*. McPhee Gribble Publisher, Fitzroy, VIC, Australia, 156–69.

Wilson, N. 2005. Aircon boom a power risk for Gallop. *The Australian*, 11 January 2005.

21

ARCHIVED NEWSPAPER REPORTS AS A COMPLEMENTARY SOURCE OF EPIDEMIOLOGICAL DATA FOR RESEARCH INTO CLIMATE CHANGE ADAPTATION

Alberta, Canada, 1960–2000

COLIN L. SOSKOLNE, JUSTINE D. A. KLAVER-KIBRIA
KAREN M. MCDONALD, DONALD W. SPADY, J. PETER ROTHE,
KAREN SMOYER TOMIC, KAILA-LEA CLARKE AND GIAN S. JHANGRI

Abstract

The impact of weather extremes on population health can be studied using descriptive information about pre- and post-event circumstances. Yet, descriptive data are not typically recorded in administrative databases used in quantitative health research by epidemiologists. This chapter introduces, describes and validates a method for using newspaper reports to complement traditional epidemiological data sources for research on climate change impacts.

As per the innovative methods and systems-based approaches advanced by Anthony (Tony) J. McMichael in his research across a broad array of epidemiological enquiry, our method development focuses on four areas by combining qualitative and quantitative methods: first, selecting and extracting information regarding extreme weather-related events and extreme weather-related disasters, and linking them to the appropriate newspapers; second, creating a content analysis framework (CAF) and extracting factual health data (i.e. manifest content) and its implied meaning (i.e. latent content) from newspaper reports; third, verifying the factual health-related data found in newspaper reports; and, fourth, corroborating the number of deaths cited in mortality data.

Our research supports the use of newspaper reports related to extreme weather as a complementary source of contextual epidemiological data when assessing climate-related health impacts to support more traditional epidemiological research in health and social policy.

Introduction

Human health and well-being are linked closely to social, cultural, economic and physical environments, which in turn are shaped and sustained principally by the forces of nature and human action.

The Fourth Assessment Report of the Intergovernmental Panel on Climate Change (IPCC, 2007) states that over recent decades the frequency and severity of extreme weather events have increased, reflecting a trend towards global heating (Hansen, 2009) and more systemic and extreme climate disruption (Lovelock, 2009; Rockström et al., 2009). These changes have profound implications for life-sustaining habitats.

Extreme weather can disturb lives, livelihoods and physical and societal infrastructure profoundly. Direct health effects of extreme weather include injury, illness, significant human stress and mortality. Indirect health impacts include damage to local health services and civic infrastructure, disruption of community and economic functioning, and displacement of people (McMichael et al., 2003; Patz et al., 2005; Confalonieri et al., 2007; Berry et al., 2008; Lemmen et al., 2008; Costello et al., 2009).

Epidemiologists could help lessen the harms described above by assessing how communities cope with weather disasters, their emergency services and infrastructure, and local public health and social services. Understanding the nature and consequences of the direct and indirect effects of climatic disruptions is essential for developing effective risk assessments and policies for action and adaptation (Ebi et al., 2006; Berry et al., 2008).

In this chapter, we describe an innovative method (and its validation) for obtaining direct and indirect health impacts by using newspaper reports of the community impacts of and the responses to local extreme weather disasters. Such innovation is characteristic of Tony McMichael's approach to public health challenges.

Aims and Objectives

We designed this study to assess (i) if newspaper reports could provide useful information for planning responses to weather events; and (ii) if qualitative methods applied to these data could be an effective analytic tool (Brown, 2003; Scammell, 2010).

Newspaper reports describe how significant weather events affect a community, plus they describe how community infrastructure and services have been affected; such qualitative data are normally not incorporated into quantitative epidemiologic analysis employing administrative databases. We evaluated and used data derived from newspaper reports to assess the impact of historical extreme weather events and disasters on Alberta's population from 1960 to 2000. Such data could assist epidemiologists and health planners to gain insight into community responses to disasters associated with extreme weather and thus improve community disaster policy and planning initiatives.

Throughout this chapter, disasters are defined by the Canadian Disaster Database (CDD), and have specific criteria for inclusion. Extreme weather events, on the other hand, are calculated statistically using Environment Canada's daily meteorological records as being outside of a community's normal range of weather intensity, but do not meet the criteria for a disaster (both described below in the section headed Methodological Development). Unless specified, both 'extreme weather events' and 'disasters' are called collectively 'extreme weather'.

Why newspapers?

Newspapers provide situational information (e.g. loss of critical infrastructure such as power during a heatwave) that could exacerbate negative health outcomes of populations affected by extreme weather. Such information is commonly unavailable in administrative databases. Newspaper reports often describe the number of individuals affected, including health outcomes, socio-economic conditions, infrastructure damage and other relevant contextual details of importance to public health. They also describe interviews on how the event and outcomes were experienced by locals.

The peer-reviewed literature using newspaper reports investigates mainly specific health issues; e.g. the media's role in risk perception or in public health education. While newspapers commonly report research findings on health issues (e.g. Bubela and Caulfield, 2004), they are rarely used as a data source for health research. Consequently, valuable information may be missed.

Three relevant peer-reviewed studies combined disaster incidence with newspaper resources. Carley et al. (1998) found that most incidents in Britain went unreported in the health literature. Palecki et al. (2001) documented that, aside from mortality, newspapers reported additional impacts from heatwaves in the USA that would be inaccessible from secondary data sources (e.g. power losses, water shortages). Most recently, Stephens et al. (2007) demonstrated that newspaper reports of deaths in New Orleans after Hurricane Katrina were consistent with state-level vital statistics data. Thus, newspapers may help planners to anticipate the potential health and social consequences of future disasters.

Reporters describe the facts surrounding an event, editors set the tone and headline writers capture the essence. However, even 'objective' news reports reflect societal contexts and priorities, and the only 'peer review' is editorial oversight (Lowrey et al., 2007; Mogil, 2008). Therefore, our analytical approach includes a secondary level of enquiry. As described in the content analysis framework (CAF) below, we identified manifest and latent knowledge dimensions found within our newspaper reports, permitting exploration of their complementary nature for epidemiological assessments.

While mainstream reports should reflect a balanced perspective, editorials focus on issues and are often subjective (Fiske and Hartley, 2003). We wanted to gather contextual information, not editorial opinion, thus editorials were ignored.

Content analysis of newspaper reports

Media analysis is a rich source of public health information and is more commonly being used for analysis (Wilson et al., 2005; Kennedy et al., 2006; Renzulli et al., 2006; Barnes et al., 2008). While the latter three studies examined newspaper reports, their analyses focused on a single event; we consider the value of newspaper reports over extended periods and multiple events.

Human adaptation to climate change requires a multidimensional community response plan to decrease harms associated with future extreme weather. Therefore, researching the effects of climate change on human health would benefit from a mixed methods approach, because many dimensions of human society are affected. While some health consequences are described quantitatively by epidemiology, we argue that qualitative newspaper data will assist human adaptation to climate change. The data types are complementary and, used together, they can enrich the policy debate.

A newspaper report provides two forms of qualitative information: 'manifest content' (factual) and 'latent content' (hidden, institutional, interest driven) (Merton, 1949). According to critical communication theory (Rothe, 1993), extracting and analysing both types of content using media analysis should liberate the reader from institutional influence. Indeed, Foucault and Rivière (1982) consider manifest information as insufficient, and we should focus on what influences the manifest, i.e. the report's 'latent content'.

Consistent with critical communication theory and qualitative research, we constructed a framework to address both manifest and latent contents in newspaper reports. In so doing, we make certain assumptions:

- As scientists we pursue truth. The media do not portray truth, but an ideological perspective on reality.
- The media, as an institution, mediates information flow. Our task as analysts is to deconstruct mediation rules.
- Information processed into knowledge is powerful. The analyst's role is to sensitise the reader regarding the underlying ideology behind a newspaper report.

The above assumptions serve as the platform used in our CAF described below.

Methodological Development

Our approach used both quantitative and qualitative methods. We created a database combining quantitative weather data and administrative mortality data sources together with qualitative newspaper reports on 'extreme weather'.

We used the CDD (Public Safety Canada, 2007) to select disasters (drought, heatwaves and coldwaves, snowstorms, forest fires and floods/rainstorms), and used Environment Canada's daily meteorological records to identify extreme weather events (i.e. heat, cold, rain and snow). Tornadoes and hailstorms were excluded because, at the time, their association with climate change was unclear. We then selected and extracted reports from the newspapers of the community affected.

Finally, we developed a CAF to organise, code and assess health-related information reported in the selected newspapers. The accuracy of the reported health information was verified through various secondary data sources and the number of deaths cited in newsprint was compared to mortality data.

Disasters

A 'disaster' (Public Safety Canada, 2007) includes events meeting at least one of the following criteria:

- 10 or more people killed
- 100 or more people affected, injured, evacuated or homeless
- an appeal for national/international assistance
- historical significance
- significant damage or interruption of normal processes, such that the community affected cannot recover independently.

From the CDD, we identified 70 disasters across Alberta between 1960 and 2000; 19 drought and 51 non-drought disasters.

The CDD states the location of an extreme event. The newspaper used relating to each event was determined using four approaches:

- If the CDD identified an exact location, then the local community newspaper (usually published weekly) and the nearest daily newspaper were selected for investigation.
- If several communities were in the affected area, we investigated one or two randomly selected community newspapers and the nearest daily.
- If the CDD provided only a region, e.g. the Pembina River basin, then the 'Rand McNally Alberta Provincial Map' (2000) was used to determine communities in the area; from these, one or two local newspapers were selected randomly along with the nearest daily.
- Several extreme events, particularly drought, had prairie- or Canada-wide effects. For these events, all community newspapers associated with Alberta meteorological weather stations were identified. The province was then divided into three regions: north (seven communities), central (23) and south (25). One community was chosen randomly from each region. Since most community newspapers were weeklies, we selected the *Edmonton Journal* to provide a daily perspective reflecting provincial concerns. Edmonton was the most central major city and the capital of Alberta and was deemed most likely to cover provincial news.

The 40-year period (1960–2000) searched in newspapers for disasters adhered to the following search criteria:

- For dailies, we searched the duration of the event and two weeks beyond its end date.
- For weeklies, we searched for at least four weeks beyond the event end date.

- If the event was associated with only a weekly, we searched the weekly paper and the nearest city with a daily newspaper according to the rules outlined above.
- For droughts, the periods searched were modified so as to maintain a manageable scope and to address the fact that droughts had long-term effects and broad geographical ranges. Only months during which droughts had their most severe effects were searched, i.e. May–September, inclusive.

Of the original 70 disasters, 27 were unsearchable. Table 21.1 depicts the number of types of events identified in the CDD that were investigated originally and also the final number of disasters (by type) studied. For the remaining 43 disasters, 801 newspaper reports were analysed (Table 21.2).

Table 21.1 Number of each disaster type in the Canadian Disaster Database from 1960 through 2000 compared to the number of disasters analysed in this study.

Disaster type	Number of disasters in the CDD	Number of disasters with newspaper reports that were investigated	Reason for exclusion (*n* = number excluded)
Floods	30	15	Overlapping disasters, vague dates and/or location (*n* = 15)
Cold	7	6	Vague dates and/or location (*n* = 1)
Snow	5	3	Vague dates and/or location (*n* = 2)
Fire	5	2	Vague dates and/or location, on a provincial border (*n* = 3)
Heat	1	0	Overlapping disasters (drought and flood) (*n* = 1)
Storms	3	2[a]	Possible mistake in date, no reports found, vague dates and/or location (*n* = 3)
Drought	19	17	Possible mistake in database, prairie-wide event, larger problems in Saskatchewan (*n* = 2)
Total	70	45[a]	(*n* = 27)

[a] Storms were later eliminated due to low numbers, lowering the total to 43.

Source: Authors' work.

Table 21.2 Ratio of number of archived newspaper reports to weather-related disasters, Alberta, 1960–2000.

Disaster type	Number of reports found in archives	Number of discrete events	Ratio
Drought	137	17	8.1:1
Flooding	436	15	29.0:1
Cold	92	6	15.3:1
Snow	72	3	24.0:1
Fire	64	2	32.0:1
Total	801	43	18.6:1

Source: Authors' work.

Extreme weather events

Extreme weather lies outside a locale's normal range of weather intensity and is, therefore, uncommon. Although often destructive, this is not always the case (Francis and Hengeveld, 1998). We defined an 'extreme weather event' using upper and lower percentiles for respective types of local weather (heat, cold, snow and rain), as described below and in more detail in Soskolne et al. (2004).

Extreme weather events were extracted from the daily meteorological records provided by Environment Canada. For data to be entered into the Environment Canada Climate Archive (www.climate.weatheroffice.gc.ca/prods_servs/normals_documentation_e.html#appendixa), they must meet the World Meteorological Organization data collection and archival standards; i.e. over 84 per cent of data must be recorded for any acceptable climate station. There were 1211 stations in Alberta that had potentially usable weather data. A criterion of '30 years or more' of observable data is required to establish climate norms for a local area; thus, only those stations with 30+ years of consistent daily weather records having at least four measured variables (specifically including temperature and precipitation) were considered. This reduced the number of 'useful' stations from 1211 to 102.

Communities selected for analysis had to be associated with a regular (daily or weekly) newspaper for the entire study period. Communities with more than one weather station had only one station included. Fifty-one communities met our final criteria. For extreme weather events, our analysis was limited to newspaper searches that extended to three days beyond each extreme weather event for dailies and to two weeks beyond the event for weeklies.

Extraction and assessment of health data

We used the CAF to determine the categories under which media reports would be analysed. The CAF reflected media analysis principles inspired by phenomenology and critical theory (Rothe, 2000). It used reasoning that depended on both deduction (categories were predefined or logical) and induction (categories were validated through a pilot study analysis of reports).

Qualitative researchers tend to look only at manifest meaning. In our framework, we considered both manifest and latent meaning, allowing us to establish the extent of any power relationships. Our CAF let us determine how newspaper reports demonstrated power relationships by examining the practices, techniques and procedures used in the reporting process. In doing so, we recorded how the reports were shaped, using the textual processes that underlaid the shaping of those reports (i.e. latent content), as well as the factual (i.e. manifest) content into one database.

The *manifest content variables* include descriptor and health-related variables. The descriptors included the newspaper studied and the location(s) and dates of the disaster. Health-related variables included advanced warning and preparedness, response, direct and indirect health outcomes, long-term solutions, mitigation or adaptation and additional information (for example, information about vulnerable segments of society).

Latent content variables included language use (the tone, metaphors, vernacular used in the report), forms of knowledge (political, economic, technical), explicitly stated beliefs and credibility of sources (who is quoted, why?; is the source credible?), case building, emphasis or ideology of the report (what is the key message?) and social relationships and social responsibility for the event (reports of consensus or conflict between major players).

We used the CAF to extract qualitatively and code numerically the information found in newspaper reports (Soskolne et al., 2004) and to show the ability of narrative reports in linking extreme weather events to health and well-being. Pilot studies were conducted to investigate the validity of the framework itself, to explore whether it could capture the required data and the reliability of newspaper search criteria.

The reliability of data abstraction was assessed by two raters, each independently examining a single sample of 150 newspaper reports, covering various events. They abstracted data on ten different aspects of each event, such as language use and advance warning, assigning codes to each. Because each newspaper report might have had several possible outcomes, the rater chose the dominant aspect first. We used Cohen's Kappa to assess interrater reliability. Once determined, each report was evaluated by a single researcher using the CAF.

We verified factual health outcomes conveyed in newspaper reports by comparing five extreme events with secondary sources (see Appendix housed at www.colinsoskolne.com/documents/Supplemental-Published-Information.pdf). Further, we verified death counts to compare newspaper-reported numbers of deaths associated with three extreme weather events using newspaper reports against administrative mortality data from Statistics Canada as the benchmark. We found that both direct and indirect health outcomes were verifiable and that deaths could be readily verified for larger numbers, but not for smaller numbers.

This chapter focuses on the methods associated with using newspapers in epidemiological research. While some preliminary analysis has been completed (see Soskolne et al., 2004), this has yet to be formally analysed and published.

For the initial analysis of the manifest content variables, the data regarding health-related risks was consolidated into three categories: direct health effects, indirect health effects and contextual information. Direct effects include injury, death or illness. Indirect health effects include other determinants influencing people's health negatively, such as energy and other service losses, infrastructure damage, water contamination and vulnerability of certain populations. Contextual information describes factors that contribute to health threats caused by extreme events and includes circumstances surrounding a particular event that can exacerbate its effects (e.g. a multi-year drought). Data from these three categories assist public health professionals as they plan and manage health risks associated with extreme events. This information also helped verify the accuracy of the data collected in the manifest content variables.

Applications and Discussion

In this chapter, we focus on the methods employed to determine the usefulness of newspaper reports for epidemiological enquiry. With an overall Kappa of 0.88, and Kappas ranging from 0.62 to 0.93 for individual aspects, the final CAF had a high degree of reliability.

An interesting observation from our study is the irregular ratio of the number of reports to disaster type in the following order of public interest: fire, floods, snow, cold and drought (Table 21.2). In Mogil (2008), 'the newsworthy factor' in reporting is recognised. This shows that, consistent with the observation by Mogil (2008), weather disasters need to be considered in context, such as their nature, degree of severity, economic costs and numbers of people affected.

Public policy

The type of data found in our analysis – descriptive, latent or health-related – could help formulate public policy regarding climate change adaptation. For example, past impacts could help assess the potential health and social consequences of future extreme weather, because the ways in which they were managed successfully could be incorporated into future response plans.

Individuals, organisations and institutions affected and responding to extreme weather include government departments, community committees, businesses, emergency responders, volunteer groups and community representatives. The contextual information revealed in newspaper reports, and not found in administrative data sources, may assist these groups to identify potential partners to help respond to future local extreme events. It may also help identify and coordinate their respective roles for future events. The database lends itself to future enquiry into the latent content dimensions of extreme weather. Future analysis of the latent content would be helpful.

Social planning

Our newspaper analysis demonstrated a broad range of health impacts and human experiences that could occur during extreme weather. These events, as noted in newspaper reports, can create intense psychological distress, health concerns, financial ruin, social upheaval and spiritual doubt.

Given the IPCC (2007) observation that extreme weather phenomena will become more common and more severe, preparing for effective adaptation measures is all the more critical. Thus, use of any data providing locally relevant contextual information to help develop adaptation measures, such as archived newspaper reports on past extreme weather experience, is recommended.

Although very resource-intensive, building the CAF was a valuable and successful exercise. The use of CAFs can provide a valuable tool in any epidemiological study where social context is relevant. Outside the scope of our analysis, a separate CAF could be constructed to examine how disasters and extreme weather events are editorialised in different media outlets. This approach would help determine social, cultural and political dimensions to a greater degree than from newspaper reports alone.

Limitations

Extracting disasters from the CDD and extreme events from Environment Canada meteorological records was straightforward in that they were both administrative data resources. However, extracting newspaper reports from various archives, plus coding the reports, took far more resources than anticipated, mainly because of the time needed to search and code reports. Searching for newspaper reports in the archives was onerous; older records were of poorer quality, had smaller font sizes and were not indexed, and thus required manual searching. Incomplete library collections, short library hours and relocations added to the difficult task. Coding reports required a technician to scan them, convert the scanned reports to text and then edit the textual reports for accuracy. The researcher would read all reports, determine their relevance and then code each. It is likely that this intensive use of resources will decline with electronic media and searchable databases.

Although newspaper representations of the investigated events appeared to be accurate, they might be biased or incomplete. Newspapers have clear limitations, partly because other relevant events could be occurring but not reported. The tendency of newspapers to report other people's opinions suggests that there could be unreported facts. What is reported may or may not assign all factors equal representation, possibly due to editorial policy. Major newspapers, like the *Edmonton Journal*, may more likely print national press accounts of disasters; thus reflecting the interests of large mainstream press agencies in their news coverage. Further, as editorial policy changes over time at the various newspapers, their reporting likely would require regular verification and cross-referencing with other sources.

Finally, while print news media provide a novel source for epidemiological research, the advent of electronic media may change the reliability and integrity of using future news reports. For retrospective events, archived newspaper reports have demonstrably reliable contextual sources. For future events, E-media could make such work more efficient, but (i) assessing the reliability of electronic news reports is essential, and caution, as with any data source, needs to be exercised when selecting sources; and (ii) electronic data storage and access may pose problems because such data sometimes are ephemeral.

In summary, we report two major methodological lessons learned regarding the use of newspapers as a data source for linking extreme weather events to health impacts. They are:

- Newspaper-based research takes longer than expected. There are usually more data than anticipated and older reports are more difficult to obtain and review.
- Formal training programmes should be created to guide archive researchers in meeting the challenges associated with newspaper research.

Advantages

The complementary aspects of (usually qualitative) newspaper-derived data will enrich data obtained from (usually quantitative) epidemiological data sources concerning climate change. Policymakers will find helpful the contextual aspects derived from newspaper reports. While newspapers could stand alone as a data source, the combination of both qualitative and quantitative data, by providing the context for traditional epidemiological data, will better inform policymaking.

We do not suggest that newspaper-based data eclipse traditionally obtained epidemiological data, but we do demonstrate that newspapers can be valuable complementary sources. The mixed methods approach provides complementary and context/content derivable insights, and may point to areas of potential research interest. Therefore, access to archived newspaper reports should be considered whenever insights are sought to address a complex health issue. This study is consistent with the holistic and systems-based approaches so characteristic of Tony McMichael's many contributions.

Conclusions

We conclude that newspaper reports can be used as a source of complementary epidemiological data. The method described here may be applicable in other contexts. Because data collected from newspaper reports reflect local conditions, any lessons learned should be generalised with caution. We encourage the use of such data in much the same way that case reports act as leads to more rigorous, higher-level investigation.

Our CAF is reliable and serves as a model for others to conduct similar research. Using newspapers to achieve our objectives provides a perspective on the direct and indirect impacts of extreme weather in a prairie region. Using mortality data and secondary sources, we could verify the majority of health data found in newspaper reports, as also demonstrated by Stephens et al. (2007).

We conclude that newspaper reports are a reliable source of contextual data surrounding extreme events. Our study advances a method that is pioneering and, applied elsewhere, may well be valuable for informing public policymakers, emergency preparedness teams and health and infrastructure planners at the local, regional and national levels when developing adaptation strategies. Clearly, extreme weather events are multifactorial in both origin and effects, such that any analysis should reflect a systems-based approach.

Acknowledgements

A 2002–04 funding award from Health Canada's Health Policy Research Program (HPRP # 6795-15-2001/4400013) made this work possible. Robyn Hyde-Lay, Alexander Affleck and Tyler Daignault contributed to data extraction and computerisation. From the Canadian Federal Government, Environment Canada and Statistics Canada provided essential data. Anonymous reviewers helped in refining earlier drafts.

References

Barnes, M.D., Hanson, C.L., Novilla, L.M., Meacham, A.T., McIntyre, E. & Erickson, B.C. 2008. Analysis of media agenda setting during and after Hurricane Katrina: implications for emergency preparedness, disaster response, and disaster policy. *American Journal of Public Health* 98, 604–10.

Berry, P., McBean, G. & Séguin, J. 2008. Vulnerabilities to natural hazards and extreme weather. In: Séguin, J. (ed.) *Human Health in a Changing Climate: A Canadian Assessment of Vulnerabilities and Adaptive Capacity.* Health Canada, Ottawa Ontario, Canada, 44–111.

Brown, P. 2003. Qualitative methods in environmental health research. *Environmental Health Perspectives* 111, 1789–98.

Bubela, T.M. & Caulfield, T.A. 2004. Do the print media 'hype' genetic research? A comparison of newspaper stories and peer reviewed research papers. *Canadian Medical Journal Association* 170, 1399–407.

Carley, S., Mackway-Jones, K. & Donnan, K. 1998. Major incidents in Britain over the past 28 years: the case for the centralized reporting of major incidents. *Journal of Epidemiology and Community Health* 52, 392–8.

Confalonieri, U., Menne, B., Akhtar, R., Ebi, K.L., Hauengue, M., Kovats, R.S., et al. 2007. Human health. In: Parry, M.L., Canziani, O.F., Palutikof, J.P., van der Linden, P.J. & Hanson, C.E. (eds) *Climate Change 2007: Impacts, Adaptation and Vulnerability. Contribution of Working Group II to the Fourth Assessment Report of the Intergovernmental Panel on Climate Change.* Cambridge University Press, Cambridge, UK, 391–431.

Costello, A., Abbas, M., Allen, A., Ball, S., Bell, S., Bellamy, R., et al. 2009. Managing the health effects of climate change. *The Lancet* 373, 1693–733.

Ebi, K.L., Burton, I. & Menne, B. 2006. Policy implications for climate change-related health risks. In: Menne, B. & Ebi, K.L. (eds) *Climate Change and Adaptation Strategies for Human Health*. Steinkopff Verlag, on behalf of the World Health Organization Regional Office for Europe, Darmstadt, Germany, 297–344.

Fiske, J. & Hartley, J. 2003. *Reading Television*. Methuen, London, UK.

Foucault, M.I. & Rivière, P. 1982. *Having Slaughtered My Mother, My Sister, and My Brother ...: a Case of Parricide in the 19th Century*. University of Nebraska Press, Lincoln, Nebraska, USA.

Francis, D. & Hengeveld, H. 1998. *Extreme Weather and Climate Change*. Environment Canada, Ottawa, Ontario, Canada.

Hansen, J. 2009. *Storms of my Grandchildren*. Bloomsbury, New York, USA.

Intergovernmental Panel on Climate Change (IPCC) 2007. Summary for policymakers. In: Solomon, S., Qin, D., Manning, M., Chen, Z., Marquis, M., et al. (eds) *Climate Change 2007: The Physical Science Basis. Working Group I Contribution to the IPCC Fourth Assessment Report*. Cambridge University Press, Cambridge, UK, 1–18.

Kennedy, J.F., Trethewy, C. & Anderson, K. 2006. Content analysis of Australian newspaper portrayals of emergency medicine. *Emergency Medicine Australasia* 18, 118–24.

Lemmen, D.S., Warren, F.J., Lacroix, J. & Bush, E. 2008. *From Impacts to Adaptation: Canada in a Changing Climate 2007*. Government of Canada, Ottawa, Canada.

Lovelock, J. 2009. *The Vanishing Face of Gaia, A Final Warning*. Allen Lane, London, UK.

Lowrey, W., Evans, W., Gower, K.K., Robinson, J.A., Ginter, P.M., McCormick, L.C., et al. 2007. Effective media communication of disasters: pressing problems and recommendations. *BMC Public Health* 7, 97, doi:10.1186/1471-2458-7-97.

McMichael, A.J., Campbell-Lendrum, D.H., Corvalán, C.F., Ebi, K.L., Githeko, A., Scheraga, J.D., et al. 2003. *Climate Change and Human Health: Risks and Responses*. World Health Organization, Geneva, Switzerland.

Merton, R.K. 1949. Manifest and latent functions in social theory and social structure. In: Merton, R.K. *Social Theory and Social Structure; Toward the Codification of Social Theory and Research*. Free Press, New York, USA, 73–138.

Mogil, H.M. 2008. Is the weather really getting worse? *Weatherwise*, 61, 46–52.

Palecki, M.A., Changnon, S.A. & Kunkel, K.E. 2001. The nature and impacts of the July 1999 heat wave in the Midwestern United States: learning from the lessons of 1995. *Bulletin of the American Meteorological Society* 82, 1353–67.

Patz, J.A., Campbell-Lendrum, D., Holloway, T. & Foley, J.A. 2005. Impact of regional climate change on human health. *Nature* 438, 310–7.

Public Safety Canada. 2007. Canadian Disaster Database. Available at: www.publicsafety.gc.ca/cnt/rsrcs/cndn-dsstr-dtbs/index-eng.aspx, accessed 4 July 2015.

Rand McNally. 2000. *Alberta Provincial Map*. Rand McNally Canada Inc, Ontario Canada.

Renzulli, D.R., Mebane, F. & Sieff, E. 2006. News coverage analyses of mental health services immediately after September 11, 2001. *Psychiatric Services* 57, 1339–41.

Rockström, J., Steffen, W., Noone, K., Persson, Å.F., Chapin F.S., Lambin, E.F., et al. 2009. A safe operating space for humanity. *Nature* 461, 472–5.

Rothe, J.P. 1993. Critical evaluation of educational software from a social perspective: uncovering hidden assumptions. In: Hlynka, D. & Belland, J.C., (eds) *Paradigms Regained: the Uses of Illuminative, Semiotic and Post-modern Criticism as Modes of Inquiry in Educational Technology*. Educational Technology Publications, Englewood Cliffs, New Jersey, USA, 367–85.

Rothe, J.P. 2000. *Undertaking Qualitative Research: Concepts and Cases in Injury, Health and Social Life*. University of Alberta Press, Edmonton, Alberta, Canada.

Scammell, M.K. 2010. Qualitative environmental health research: an analysis of the literature, 1991–2008. *Environmental Health Perspectives* 118, 1146–54.

Soskolne, C.L., Tomic, K.E.S., McDonald, K.M., Rothe, J.P., Spady, D.W. & Klaver, J.D.A. 2004. *Climate Change, Extreme Weather Events and Health Effects in Alberta* (485 pages). Final Report to Health Canada's Health Policy Research Program (#6795-15-2001/4400013).

Stephens, K.U. Sr, Grew, D., Chin, K., Kadetz, P., Greenough, P.G., Burkle Jnr, F.M., et al. 2007. Excess mortality in the aftermath of Hurricane Katrina: a preliminary report. *Disaster Medicine and Public Health Preparedness* 1, 15–20.

Wilson, N., McIntyre, M., McDonald, M., Tanner, H., Hart, K., Tomlinson, R., et al. 2005. Communication and health protection issues arising from a flooding emergency. *Prehospital and Disaster Medicine* 20, 193–6.

22

HEALTH CO-BENEFITS OF CLIMATE CHANGE MITIGATION POLICIES

ANDY HAINES

Abstract

Policies to reduce greenhouse gas emissions in a number of sectors can result in ancillary (co-benefits) for health. In the case of electricity generation, for example, reduced combustion of coal would result in lowered fine particulate air pollution. Improved housing insulation with efficient ventilation systems can reduce indoor air pollution while also reducing exposure to heat and cold extremes. In low-income settings, improved efficiency cookstoves can reduce black carbon emissions and other climate-active pollutants while reducing exposure to hazardous indoor air pollution. Urban transport policies that support active travel and access to affordable public transport can increase physical activity and reduce air pollution. Increased fruit and vegetable consumption and reduced consumption of animal products (particularly from ruminants) in high-consuming populations can improve health and reduce greenhouse gas (GHG) emissions. Finally, addressing reproductive health rights in countries where the need for modern contraception is not fully met can improve the prospects for child and maternal survival and ultimately reduce GHG emissions. Taking into account the value of the health gains and other co-benefits of policies to mitigate climate change can help to offset the costs of such policies and make them more acceptable to decision makers.

Background

Current trends of inequitable and unsustainable development, which are largely responsible for many of the environmental threats now confronting us, are related directly or indirectly to many risk factors responsible for major causes of ill health, particularly non-communicable diseases (NCDs). These now account for over half of the world's disease burden. This chapter illustrates linkages between health and policies in a number of sectors responsible for large emissions of greenhouse gases (GHG) or short-lived, climate-active pollutants such as black carbon. It also makes the case that appropriately designed policies to reduce emissions, and thus mitigate climate change, can improve health in the near term, over and above the improvements from reducing the probability of dangerous climate change. First, as this book is for a Festschrift, I document the early years of my collaboration with Tony McMichael.

My Collaboration with Tony McMichael

As mentioned in the introduction of this volume (Chapter 1), Tony had left the London School of Hygiene and Tropical Medicine by the time I was appointed Dean in December 2000. However, I was well aware of Tony's work and influence in relation to climate change and health. We had collaborated extensively on these issues since 1993, first in a paper (part of a pioneering special series in *The Lancet* on global change and health) that we wrote with the late Paul Epstein (Haines et al., 1993). Later, we contributed to the second and third Intergovernmental Panel on Climate Change (IPCC) reports, which were the first to include chapters on health, each of which was led by McMichael (McMichael et al., 1996; McMichael et al., 2001).

Tony and I also co-edited (including with Sari Kovats) the first book to assemble systematically the evidence on climate change and health (McMichael et al., 1996) and wrote several other co-authored papers on climate and health from the late 1990s (Haines and McMichael, 1997; McMichael and Haines, 1997; Haines et al., 2000). Tony's wide influence extended well beyond climate change, of course, as this book illustrates.

Electricity Generation

The combustion of fossil fuels for electricity generation, particularly coal, is responsible for a substantial proportion of air pollution due to fine particulates, notably in countries such as India and China. In general, as societies develop, exposure of populations to outdoor air pollution rises at first, then decreases as more effective particulate pollution controls are implemented and other sources of energy or more efficient technologies are used, particularly for electricity generation and transportation. This phenomenon is well illustrated in the case of London, the original 'Big Smoke', as exemplified by the Great Smog of 1952 (Bell et al., 2004) and subsequent clean air legislation. However, there is increasing appreciation that the switch to alternative means of power generation (and more efficient vehicles) does not fully address the challenge of fine particulate air pollution, which remains at unacceptably high levels today, even in many high-income countries, with the accompaniment of large, and in some cases increasing, emissions of greenhouse gases.

Overall, currently, exposure to ambient (outdoor) particulate matter is estimated to be responsible for around 3.2 million premature deaths per year worldwide (Lim et al., 2012). Recent World Health Organization (WHO) estimates (WHO, 2014a) suggest the burden may be even higher, at around 3.7 million premature deaths.

Household Environment

Additionally, in low-income countries, exposure to high levels of household air pollution due to inefficient combustion of solid fuels – biomass or coal – is responsible for major contributions to the burden of disease (e.g. lower respiratory tract infections, chronic obstructive pulmonary disease and ischaemic heart disease (IHD)), and is also associated with substantial emissions of short-lived climate pollutants such as black carbon. Overall, household air pollution is estimated to be responsible for around 3.5 million premature deaths per year (Lim et al., 2012), or even higher according to recent WHO estimates of 4.3 million per annum (WHO, 2014b), with some overlap between both categories as household sources contribute to ambient exposure, particularly in urban settings.

In high- and middle-income countries, the household environment can contribute to ill health in various ways, including mould and damp, indoor air pollutants such as radon and environmental tobacco smoke, and exposure to cold and/or heat (Wilkinson et al., 2009). Household environments can also pose fire risks at all levels of development, but particularly where open fires are used. Poor design and maintenance has resulted in the construction of many dwellings that use energy inefficiently because of heat loss (or gain) due to inadequate insulation and/or ventilation control. This can contribute to uncomfortable or harmful indoor temperatures, fuel poverty and the emission of large amounts of GHGs, where the energy source is from the combustion of fossil fuels.

Food and Agriculture

The agriculture sector is responsible for 10–12 per cent of global GHG emissions (an additional 6–17 per cent if land-use change is included). Of the non-land-use emissions from this sector, around 80 per cent are due to livestock, particularly as the result of methane emissions from ruminants such as cows and sheep

(Steinfeld et al., 2006). The demand for animal products is increasing as populations become more affluent, and is driving forest clearance in some parts of the world. At a time when freshwater supplies are diminishing in many regions, animal products also contain large amounts of embedded water.

The global food production system is focused increasingly on promoting the consumption of refined, energy-dense food containing substantial amounts of saturated fats from animal sources and refined carbohydrates. At the same time, recent estimates suggest that inadequate consumption of fruit and vegetables is responsible for large burdens of disease such as some types of cancer and IHD (Lim et al., 2012). Replacing some animal source saturated fat by increased dietary intake of unsaturated fats (largely from liquid vegetable oils) can also reduce IHD risk (Hooper et al., 2011). Consumption of red and processed meat is associated with increased risk of colon and rectal cancer, diabetes and, in the case of the latter, IHD.

Urban Transport

Around 3.2 million premature deaths a year are thought to be related to physical inactivity (Lim et al., 2012), partly because of the growth in motorised transport, particularly private cars. Low levels of physical activity have been found consistently to increase the risk of seven conditions – diabetes, IHD, cerebrovascular disease, breast and large bowel cancer, Alzheimer's disease and depression (Woodcock et al., 2009). Road transport is responsible for a growing proportion of GHG emissions, as well as contributing substantially to urban air pollution, particularly due to fine particulates from diesel engines. Road injuries are responsible for nearly 1.3 million deaths a year, particularly of pedestrians and cyclists.

Addressing Reproductive Health Needs

Reducing population growth can bring direct and indirect benefits to health and to the environment through improved child survival and reduced maternal mortality, and by alleviating pressures on land use. In low-income countries, this will have limited effects on GHG emissions in the near term, but it could have substantial effects in the long term, particularly if poor populations adopt Western lifestyles in large numbers (O'Neill et al., 2012). Population growth has slowed in many parts of the world but remains high in parts of sub-Saharan Africa, with projections suggesting a world population of around 10 billion before the end of this century. The unmet need for contraception is as high as 30 per cent in some sub-Saharan African countries. Funding for family planning on a per capita basis has fallen over the last decade in virtually all recipient nations. Population growth in high resource use economies could also have an important impact on future GHG emissions. For example, the population of the USA will rise from just over 300 million in 2010 to up to 458 million in 2050, depending on migration levels (Ortman and Guarneri).

Measuring Progress Towards Sustainable Development Using Indicators that Link Health with Development Policies

Access to information about sector policies and their associated health risks and impacts through the integrated indicators of health, development and environment and through the systematic health impact assessment of policies is key to improving global governance for sustainable development, as well as to raising public awareness and the accountability of decision makers. It will be critical to take such an approach when considering the Sustainable Development Goals that will come into operation following the Millennium Development Goals (MDGs), which are supposed to be achieved by the end of 2015. These goals and their associated indicators might include, for example, levels of ambient particulate air pollution and access to clean sources of household energy, the proportion of journeys by public transport and active travel in cities, consumption of diets that are both healthy and low in GHG emissions (Dora et al., 2015).

Co-benefits to Health of Environmentally Sustainable Policies in Different Sectors

It is increasingly recognised that there are health co-benefits (i.e. ancillary benefits) from policies to reduce GHG emissions (Haines et al., 2009). These health co-benefits can reduce the costs to health-care systems and can increase labour productivity. The economic benefits arising from health co-benefits can partly or wholly offset the costs of implementing low greenhouse gas emission strategies, depending on the sector, the assumptions made and the socio-economic context (Jensen et al., 2013).

Some low GHG emission technologies may, however, have adverse health effects; for example, the growth of biofuels that compete for land for food crops may increase food prices (FAO, 2013), and the emission reductions from some types of biofuels (e.g. maize alcohol) have been challenged. Excessively 'tight' buildings can increase indoor air pollution. Overall, however, health can be improved through more efficient use of energy in housing, with benefits exceeding the costs of insulation, provided adequate ventilation is maintained (Wilkinson et al., 2009). Each potential GHG mitigation strategy should be assessed on a case-by-case basis.

In developing countries, new stove technologies can reduce indoor air pollution, and lower fuel consumption as well as the risk of acute respiratory infections in children, chronic obstructive pulmonary disease and IHD (Wilkinson et al., 2009). More efficient stoves save time needed for cooking and time and energy collecting wood, and thus also lower the risk of violence, particularly against women for whom collecting fuel is a potential risk.

Transportation policies have a great potential to prevent NCDs, especially in rapidly growing cities that face large increases in motor vehicles. Greater reliance on public transport systems and walking and cycling reduces air pollution and noise, promotes physical activity and can potentially lessen traffic injuries. These policies also give access to goods and services to the poor and to women, children and the elderly, who rarely own a private vehicle. Longitudinal studies show that people in Copenhagen (Andersen et al., 2000) and Shanghai (Matthews et al., 2007) who cycle to work regularly have 30 per cent lower all-cause mortality than those who do not. Transport interventions and urban planning are among the most effective interventions to promote physical activity.

Shifting away from the combustion of coal for electricity generation will reduce GHG emissions and deaths associated with fine particulate air pollution, particularly in developing countries (Markandya et al., 2009).

Shindell and colleagues (2012) identified 14 measures targeting methane and black carbon emissions that would reduce projected global mean warming ~0.5°C by 2050. These strategies would avoid 0.7–4.7 million annual premature deaths from outdoor air pollution and improve agricultural productivity. The estimated value of the benefits significantly exceeded the typical marginal abatement costs.

Increasing the consumption of fruit, vegetables and unsaturated fat, together with reducing animal product consumption (particularly from ruminants) in high-consuming countries, could benefit health and reduce greenhouse gas emissions (McMichael et al., 2007; Friel et al., 2009), as well the pressure on land for growing animal feed stocks.

Stern (2010) has suggested that the cost of holding concentrations of GHGs below 500 parts per million CO_2e[1] are around 2 per cent of global gross domestic product (GDP),but could be considerably less if technological progress was rapid. According to his analysis, the benefits of early action as a result of averting some of the adverse effects of climate change on the world economy outweigh the costs. The health and other co-benefits of these policies, which will in many cases be felt in the relatively near term, provide an added incentive for their implementation.

Currently, energy subsidies for fossil fuels amount to US$1.9 trillion (2.5 per cent of global GDP) on a post-tax basis – which also factors in the negative externalities from energy consumption. Removing these subsidies would lead to an estimated 13 per cent reduction in CO_2 emissions and reduce inequalities (International Monetary Fund, 2013).

With new and emerging 'clean' technologies, increased energy efficiency and the implementation of policies to reduce inequities and promote healthier lifestyles, there is the potential for greatly improved health worldwide at much lower levels of environmental impact than today.

References

Andersen, L.B., Schnohr, P., Schroll, M. & Hein, H.O. 2000. All-cause mortality associated with physical activity during leisure time, work, sports, and cycling to work. *Archives of Internal Medicine* 160, 1621–8.

Bell, M.L., Davis, D.L. & Fletcher, A. 2004. A retrospective assessment of mortality from the London smog episode of 1952; the role of influenza and pollution. *Environmental Health Perspectives* 112, 6–8.

Dora, C., Haines, A., Balbus, J., Fletcher, E., Adair-Rohani, H., et al. 2015. Indicators linking health and sustainability in the post 2015 development agenda. *The Lancet* 385, 380–91.

FAO 2013. Biofuels and food security. A Report by a High Level Panel of Experts on Food Security and Nutrition June 2013. Available at: www.fao.org/fileadmin/user_upload/hlpe/hlpe_documents/HLPE_Reports/HLPE-Report-5_Biofuels_and_food_security.pdf, accessed 23 March 2014.

1 CO_2equivalent (CO_2e) is an aggregate measure of the main GHGs (e.g. CO_2 and methane) in CO_2e 'units', which reflects their global warming potential over a given period. The concept has limitations, for example, because of the wide range of residence times in the atmosphere of different GHGs and short-lived climate pollutants, but is nevertheless widely used.

Friel, S., Dangour, A.D., Garnett, T., Lock, K., Chalabi, Z., Roberts, I., et al. 2009. Public health benefits of strategies to reduce greenhouse-gas emissions: food and agriculture. *The Lancet* 374, 2016–25.

Haines, A. & McMichael, A.J. 1997. Climate change and health: implications for research, monitoring, and policy. *BMJ* 315, 870–4.

Haines, A., Epstein, P.R. & McMichael, A.J. 1993. Global health watch: monitoring impacts of environmental change. *The Lancet* 342, 1464–9.

Haines, A., McMichael, A.J. & Epstein, P.R. 2000. Global climate change and health. *Canadian Medical Association Journal* 163, 729–34.

Haines, A., McMichael, A.J., Smith, K.R., Roberts, I., Woodcock, J., Markandya, A., et al. 2009. Public health effects of strategies to reduce greenhouse-gas emissions: overview and implications for policy makers. *The Lancet* 374, 2104–14.

Hooper, L., Summerbell, C.D., Higgins, J.P.T., Thompson, R.L., Clements, G., Capps, N., et al. 2011. Reduced or modified dietary fat for preventing cardiovascular disease. *The Cochrane Database of Systematic Reviews* 7, CD002137.

International Monetary Fund. 2013. Energy Subsidy Reform: Lessons and Implications. January 2013. Available at: www.imf.org/external/np/pp/eng/2013/012813.pdf, accessed 23 March 2014.

Jensen, H., Keogh-Brown, M., Smith, R., Chalabi, Z., Dangour, A., Davies, M., et al. 2013. The importance of health co-benefits in macroeconomic assessments of UK greenhouse gas emission reduction strategies. *Climatic Change* 121, 223–37.

Lim, S.S., Vos, T., Flaxman, A.D., Danaei, G., Shibuya, K., Adair-Rohani, H., et al. 2012. A comparative risk assessment of burden of disease and injury attributable to 67 risk factors and risk factor clusters in 21 regions, 1990–2010: a systematic analysis for the Global Burden of Disease Study 2010. *The Lancet* 380, 2224–60.

McMichael, A.J. & Haines, A. 1997. Global climate change: the potential effects on health. *BMJ* 315, 805–9.

McMichael, A.J., Ando, M., Carcavallo, R., Epstein, P., Haines, A., Jendritzky, G., et al. 1996. Human population health. In: Watson, R.T., Zinyowera, M.C. & Moss, R.H. (eds) *Climate Change 1995, Impacts, Adaptations and Mitigation of Climate Change: Scientific Technical Analyses. Contribution of*

Working Group II to the Second Assessment Report of the Intergovernmental Panel on Climate Change. Cambridge University Press, Cambridge, UK, New York USA, 561–84.

McMichael, A.J., Haines, A., Slooff, R. & Kovats, S. (eds) 1996. *Climate Change and Human Health*. World Health Organization, Geneva, Switzerland.

McMichael, A.J., Githeko, A., Akhtar, R., Carcavallo, R., Gubler, D., Haines, A., et al. 2001. Human health. In: McCarthy, J., Canziani, O.F., Leary, N., Dokken, D.J. & White, K.S. (eds) *Climate Change 2001; Impact, Adaptation and Vulnerability. Contribution of Working Group II to the Third Assessment Report of the Intergovernmental Panel on Climate Change*. Intergovernmental Panel on Climate Change, Cambridge, UK, New York USA, 451–86.

McMichael, A.J., Powles, J., Butler, C.D. & Uauy, R. 2007. Food, livestock production, energy, climate change and health. *The Lancet* 370, 1253–63.

Markandya, A., Armstrong, B.G., Hales, S., Chiabai, A., Criqui, P., Mima, S., et al. 2009. Public health benefits of strategies to reduce greenhouse-gas emissions: low-carbon electricity generation. *The Lancet* 374, 2006–15.

Matthews, C.E., Jurj, A.L., Shu, X.-O., Li, H.-L., Yang, G., Li, Q., et al. 2007. Influence of exercise, walking, cycling, and overall non-exercise physical activity on mortality in Chinese women. *American Journal of Epidemiology* 165, 1343–50.

O'Neill, B.C., Liddle, B., Jiang, L., Smith, K.R., Pachauri, S., Dalton, M., et al. 2012. Demographic change and greenhouse gas emissions. *The Lancet* 380, 157–64.

Ortman, J.M. & Guarneri, C.E. United States Population Projections 2000–2050. Available at: www.census.gov/population/projections/files/analytical-document09.pdf, accessed 21 March 2014. CD002137.

Shindell, D., Kuylenstierna, J.C.I., Vignati, E., van Dingenen, R., Amann, M., Klimont, Z., et al. 2012. Simultaneously mitigating near-term climate change and improving human health and food security. *Science* 335, 183–8.

Steinfeld, H., Gerber, P., Wassenaar, T., Castel, V., Rosales, M. & de Haan, C. 2006. *Livestock's Long Shadow*. FAO, Rome, Italy.

Stern, N.A. 2010. *Blueprint for a Safer Planet*. Vintage Books, London, UK.

WHO 2014a. Ambient (outdoor) air quality and health. Fact sheet No 313, updated March 2014. World Health Organization, Geneva, Switzerland. Available at: www.who.int/mediacentre/factsheets/fs313/en, accessed 15 April 2014.

WHO 2014b. Household air pollution and health 2014. Fact sheet No 292, updated March 2014. World Health Organization, Geneva, Switzerland. Available at: www.who.int/mediacentre/factsheets/fs292/en, accessed 15 April 2014.

Wilkinson, P., Smith, K.R., Davies, M., Adair, H., Armstrong, B.G., Barrett, M., et al. 2009. Public health benefits of strategies to reduce greenhouse-gas emissions: household energy. *The Lancet* 374, 1917–29.

Woodcock, J., Edwards, P., Tonne, C., Armstrong, B.G., Ashiru, O., Banister, D., et al. 2009. Public health benefits of strategies to reduce greenhouse-gas emissions: urban land transport. *The Lancet* 374, 1930–43.

23

FROM GRASS ROOTS TO GOVERNMENT

The Role of Social Connections and Integrated Policy Responses to Support Our Path to Health in a Sustainable World

KATHRYN BOWEN

Abstract

Strong action on climate change is moving at a very slow pace globally. Are workers in the field really making a worthwhile difference to the health issues brought about by climate change? If we are not, what are the reasons for this lack of progress and how do we better address the impact of climate change on both local and global health issues? This chapter shifts from outlining the problems with the lack of action on climate and health to proposing ways by which we can galvanise attention and promote appropriate action. We can progress action on climate change and reducing its ill effects on human health by using a two-pronged approach: (i) by highlighting and encouraging basic human positive attributes, such as being connected with one's community and recognising the finite nature of our resources; and (ii) by framing health and sustainability as an integral part of poverty-reduction strategies and national development plans. These two mechanisms may provide an approach by which we can synergise broader-based support by communities for meaningful action on the promotion of sustainability and the development of an active ongoing working partnership with grass-roots groups as well as national- and international-level organisations.

Introduction

I first came across Professor McMichael's work when I was assisting the Australian Greens develop their climate change and human health policy in the run-up to a federal election. I was at an intersection in my public health career; I felt that my choices were either to continue working on specific public health issues such as HIV, mental health and women's health, or to follow my instinct to move away from public health and work in the environmental sustainability arena. On coming across Tony's work, I realised that public health and sustainability dovetailed in a very powerful way. I was inspired by what Tony was doing. His passion for his work was clear in his writing, and this encouraged me to consider the possibility of combining both public health and sustainability, which was incredibly exciting. This brief chapter reminds us of some basic solutions that may contribute to supporting and respecting our natural environment, with clear positive repercussions for us as humans.

Two Approaches and Two Solutions

Plenty of evidence pointing to environmental change, and the impact this has on global health, has been articulated by other authors in this book. Thus, this chapter expands on ways, such as the support of social connectedness and cooperation, that can propel our efforts to actually change the way that we, as humans, support our Earth. And this, in turn, may mean that the Earth might be able to continue to support us. This thinking is in line with the Gaia theory. The first solution that I propose is the importance of encouraging basic positive human attributes, such as being connected with one's community and recognising the finite nature of our resources. The second solution that I propose is a strategic approach by which we can address global environmental change (particularly climate change) in the most vulnerable populations, which is often in developing contexts. This entails the linking of climate change activities and funding with national policies, including health policies, National Development Plans (NDPs), disaster reduction policies and Poverty Reduction Strategy Papers (PRSPs).

A recent straw poll carried out in early 2013 by *The Guardian* newspaper in the UK asked 50 readers and public figures to indicate ways by which we might extricate ourselves from the dire predicament brought about by an impending global warming of more than 2° Celsius. While all of the solutions proposed made sense in terms of making a change that benefitted the planet, many were just too unrealistic to be useful, such as fomenting mass protest (which has not mobilised any change to this point), mobilising as if on a war footing (requires impetus from within government) and ending lobbyists' influence on government (again requiring government cooperation and will to act, both of which are currently sorely lacking). The theme that came through most often in the 50 responses was the importance of building community resilience, commonly through measures that increased social capital, such as knowing your neighbours and pulling together on shared tasks. This is a commendable and potentially feasible option; the question now is what is the best way to go about doing this. Should it be mandated by government or should the impetus come from the grass roots? Or, is it indeed an 'either/or' scenario?

Social Connectivity

The ability to withstand the gathering stresses from global environmental changes requires a combination of physical, financial and intellectual resources and preparedness. It also requires strong social cohesion, social connectedness and human cooperation. These unifying forces are commonly referred to as social capital. I suggest that a prerequisite for establishing sufficient social capital to protect both our immediate environment and our planet as a whole is to actively promote an increasing respect for the natural environment.

The importance of developing an increased respect for the natural environment is illustrated by research connecting children with their natural environment. The more exposure children of a young age have to their natural environment (parks, reserves, bush, beach, lakes and so on), the greater their appreciation and understanding of the need to protect and preserve these environments (Sobel, 1990).

The perceived lack of children's connection to nature has resulted in the formation of various groups that seek to re-establish this link. These began in the USA, and have also recently commenced in at least one city in Australia. It is somewhat ironic that extolling the virtues of connecting a child with nature nowadays seems to require structured sessions in a controlled and somewhat artificial environment. The existence of these groups highlights the emerging reality that children's engagement and enthusiasm for the natural environment does not seem to occur quite as spontaneously as before the advent of the electronic age; children now seem much more connected to electronic devices than to each other and their natural environment.

The husbanding of social capital needs to operate in tandem with the establishment of a connection to nature to help preserve and sustain our natural environment. The concept of social capital is rooted in antiquity, but usage of the term is recent (Putnam, 1995). Despite competing definitions of the term, there is general agreement that it can be considered as the capacity of a population to work harmoniously as a self-organising unit, in which many individuals cooperate but in which no single person, or even group, controls all activities. Instead of having control imposed from the top down, self-organising groups generally function well because participants both apply and acquire norms and customs that inform and influence behaviour from their milieu; their parents, families, schools, the media and, more recently, from a plethora of informed correspondents on Internet blogs (e.g. Rough, 1996). Two of the chief protagonists often cited in the social capital literature – Putnam and Bourdieu – display differences in their conceptual approaches to social capital (e.g. Bourdieu, 1986; Putnam, 1995). One main difference between the two is Bourdieu's emphasis on individual connections that foster greater connectivity between these individuals versus Putnam's approach on connectivity that has benefits on a broader scale, such as within communities as a whole (Portes, 1998).

In relation to this greater emphasis on communities that Putnam adopts, the quality of the social capital within a community has been suggested as a measure of its potential for adopting a cooperative approach to addressing local problems (Fukuyama, 2001; Pilkington, 2002). Groups with lower amounts of social capital are likely to exhibit a lower degree of trust between members of the group. Communication is likely to be impeded, due to factors such as differences in language, dialect, tone of speech and even nuances of body language. Trade is also likely to be less efficient, due, for example, to an increased need for mediators and agents, such as lawyers and contracts. Weak controls on individuals or groups who attempt to appropriate a share of produce which is disproportionate to their contribution) can reduce the morale and productivity of those individuals and groups who are highly motivated to build community cohesiveness (Ohtsuki et al., 2009).

Cohesive societies are more likely to be able to build and retain the many other forms of wealth (Arrow et al., 2004) that contribute to human well-being (Butler et al., 2003). Such societies are also more likely to respond to and withstand pressures that threaten well-being, including global environmental change (such as climate change). Of course, social cohesion alone does not provide a simple solution for increasing the overall wealth of a community; this also requires access to other forms of capital and raw material, especially environmental resources, appropriate financing and technological knowledge. In this way, social capital should not be seen as an unreservedly positive concept, but rather as a key ingredient in a recipe that must also consider issues including broader socio-economic reform (Tittensor, 2007).

Despite such reservations about the concept of social capital and the importance of understanding the broader policy settings, there is a growing interest in social capital and its potential impact for affecting collective action. This is particularly evident in research into sustainable renewable natural resource institutions (Rudd, 2000; Sobels et al., 2001; Walters, 2002; Adger, 2003). For example, Pretty and Ward (2001) identified that where social capital was well developed, local groups with locally developed rules and sanctions were able to make more of existing resources than individuals working alone or in competition. Social institutions that are based on trust and reciprocity and agreed norms and rules for behaviour can mediate private action such as overuse and underinvestment in natural capital (Pretty and Ward, 2001).

Adger (2003) notes that benefits accrue out of building trust and cooperation between the state, its bureaucracy and wider society when addressing the issue of climate change adaptation. One is that there is a useful synergism to be gained from an alliance of community social capital and inclusive decision-making institutions to promote the sustainability and legitimacy of any adaptation strategy. The second is that adaptation processes that are community initiated and based on social capital can shift the perception of climate change from being an insoluble global problem to that of a local problem that may, in fact, be at least partially solvable.

Alongside strengthening community connectivity sits the second suggested solution to increasing our pace of change to prevent further environmental degradation and to improve population health simultaneously. This solution needs only a short explanation. It does not rely on or introduce theory, nor is it particularly controversial. It is more specifically around supporting health in this era of climate change, but with an awareness of the co-benefits of action (both mitigation and adaptation) on both environmental and health outcomes. It is proposed that health and sustainability issues are framed as an integral part of (i) health policies; (ii) disaster reduction policies; (iii) poverty reduction strategies; and (iv) NDPs. The latter two types are common to least-developed countries. All these policies and plans are often developed in isolation from one another, but this is particularly the case for health policies. It is vital that the aims of health policies are integrated into the others, as this will force the understanding of health impacts that are as a result of global environmental change. Progress is being made to integrate these policies with each other, as often this integration is demanded by donors in order for activities to be funded. Additional regulation would further support this progress. Learning from the lessons of the Health in All Policies (HiAP) process and outcomes would also be useful here, as one way to assist the strengthening of a holistic approach to health, development and sustainability policies. HiAP incorporates health impacts into the policy development processes of all sectors and government agencies, creating an integrated policy response across the whole of government (Kickbusch, 2008). This approach is generally regarded as a useful and important step towards improving health equity and is being implemented in many settings, including Australia (South Australia) (Kickbusch, 2008).

Conclusion

In conclusion, there are at least two means by which we can support our efforts to protect our natural environment while supporting our human health; by encouraging (i) the social connections that can spur on individual and hence community action, as well as (ii) ensuring environmental change issues and their health impacts are considered in an integrated manner across more segments of government policy. If we can focus on these two elements of grass-roots and government change, we can hopefully see some quicker, and lasting, progress.

References

Adger, N.W. 2003. Social capital, collective action, and adaptation to climate change. *Economic Geography* 79, 387–404.

Arrow, K., Dasgupta, P., Goulder, L., Daily, G., Ehrlich, P., Heal, G., et al. 2004. Are we consuming too much? *Journal of Economic Perspectives* 18, 147–72.

Bourdieu, P. The forms of capital. In: John G. Richardson (ed.): *Handbook of Theory and Research for the Sociology of Education*. New York: Greenwood Press 1986, 241–258.

Butler, C.D., Chambers, R., Chopra, K., Dasgupta, P., Duraiappah, A., Kumar, P., et al. 2003. *Ecosystems and Human Well-being. A Framework for Assessment. Millennium Ecosystem Assessment*. Island Press, Washington, DC, USA, 71–84.

Fukuyama, F. 2001. Social capital, civil society and development. *Third World Quarterly* 22, 7–20.

Kickbusch, I. 2008. *Healthy Societies: Addressing 21st Century Health Challenges*. Department of Premier and Cabinet, Adelaide, SA, Australia.

Ohtsuki, H., Iwasa, Y. & Nowak, M.A. 2009. Indirect reciprocity provides only a narrow margin of efficiency for costly punishment. *Nature* 457, 79–82.

Pilkington, P. 2002. Social capital and health: measuring and understanding social capital at a local level could help to tackle health inequalities more effectively. *Journal of Public Health* 22, 7–20.

Portes, A. 1998. Social capital: its origins and applications in modern sociology. *Annual Review of Sociology* 24, 1–24.

Pretty, J. & Ward, H. 2001. Social capital and the environment. *World Development* 29, 209–227.

Putnam, R.D. 1995. Bowling alone: America's declining social capital. *Journal of Democracy* 6, 65–78.

Rough, J. 1996. The Wisdom Council and responsible leadership. *Journal for Quality and Participation* 19, 74–9.

Rudd, M.A. 2000. Live long and prosper: collective action, social capital and social vision. *Ecological Economics* 34, 131–44.

Sobel, D. 1990. A place in the world: adults' memories of childhood's special places. *Children's Environments Quarterly* 7, 5–12.

Sobels, J., Curtis, A. & Stewart, L. 2001. The role of Landcare group networks in rural Australia: exploring the contribution of social capital. *Journal of Rural Studies* 17, 265–76.

Tittensor, D. 2007. Social capital and public policy – the current challenge facing the Victorian government. *The Australian Journal of Public Administration* 66, 512–8.

Walters, W. 2002. Social capital and political sociology: re-imagining politics? *Sociology* 36, 377–97.

PART 6

ECOSYSTEM CHANGE, INFECTIOUS DISEASES AND WELL-BEING

REPRINT H

Social and Environmental Risk Factors in the Emergence of Infectious Diseases

ROBIN A. WEISS AND ANTHONY J. MCMICHAEL

Weiss, R.A. & McMichael, A.J. 2004. Social and environmental risk factors in the emergence of infectious diseases. *Nature Medicine* 10(12), S70–S76.

Pages: 431 to 440

nature medicine

Social and environmental risk factors in the emergence of infectious diseases

Robin A Weiss[1] & Anthony J McMichael[2]

Fifty years ago, the age-old scourge of infectious disease was receding in the developed world in response to improved public health measures, while the advent of antibiotics, better vaccines, insecticides and improved surveillance held the promise of eradicating residual problems. By the late twentieth century, however, an increase in the emergence and re-emergence of infectious diseases was evident in many parts of the world. This upturn looms as the fourth major transition in human–microbe relationships since the advent of agriculture around 10,000 years ago. About 30 new diseases have been identified, including Legionnaires' disease, human immunodeficiency virus (HIV)/acquired immune deficiency syndrome (AIDS), hepatitis C, bovine spongiform encephalopathy (BSE)/variant Creutzfeldt-Jakob disease (vCJD), Nipah virus, several viral hemorrhagic fevers and, most recently, severe acute respiratory syndrome (SARS) and avian influenza. The emergence of these diseases, and resurgence of old ones like tuberculosis and cholera, reflects various changes in human ecology: rural-to-urban migration resulting in high-density peri-urban slums; increasing long-distance mobility and trade; the social disruption of war and conflict; changes in personal behavior; and, increasingly, human-induced global changes, including widespread forest clearance and climate change. Political ignorance, denial and obduracy (as with HIV/AIDS) further compound the risks. The use and misuse of medical technology also pose risks, such as drug-resistant microbes and contaminated equipment or biological medicines. A better understanding of the evolving social dynamics of emerging infectious diseases ought to help us to anticipate and hopefully ameliorate current and future risks.

Popular writing on emerging infectious diseases resounds with dire warnings about the threat of modern 'plagues' and losing the 'war against microbes.' This adversarial language obscures the fact that most of the microbial world is either neutral toward, or supportive of, human well-being and survival. Indeed, we would not survive long without commensal microbes such as the beneficial strains of *Escherichia coli* in our gut. That aside, the study of emerging infections is more than a passing fad. The recent rate of identification of such infections, the impact of the SARS outbreak, the devastation caused by AIDS, and the ever-present threat of a new influenza pandemic indicate that we cannot control our disease destiny. Nor are emerging infections unique to humans; the Irish potato famine in 1845 and the English foot-and-mouth disease epidemic in 2001 underscore the consequences for human societies of disease emergence in crops and livestock.

Emerging infectious diseases in humans comprise the following: first, established diseases undergoing increased incidence or geographic spread, for example, Tuberculosis and Dengue fever; second, newly discovered infections causing known diseases, for example, hepatitis C and *Helicobacter pylori*; and third, newly emerged diseases, for example, HIV/AIDS and SARS.

This Perspective will discuss the human ecology of both the (apparently) new and re-emerging diseases.

The demography of infectious disease

Interest in infectious disease has itself recently re-emerged. In 1972, Burnet and White commented, "The most likely forecast about the future of infectious disease is that it will be very dull. There may be some wholly unexpected emergence of a new and dangerous infectious disease, but nothing of the sort has marked the past fifty years"[1]. Today, we may criticize the short-sightedness of our mentors' generation, yet in demographic terms they were essentially correct because the proportion of deaths from infectious disease has fallen throughout the twentieth century[2,3] (**Fig. 1**).

Humankind currently faces neither apocalyptic extinction nor even a population reduction such as occurred in Europe during the Black Death of the fourteenth century. Rather, overpopulation in relation to environmental resources remains a more pressing problem in many developing countries, where poor economic and social conditions go hand-in-hand with infectious disease. In industrializing countries during the nineteenth century, a major reduction in enteric infections was achieved by separating drinking water from sewage—an environmental change that probably saved more lives than all the twentieth century vaccines and antibiotics together. Today, however, the growth of shanty towns without sanitation around the megalopolis cities of Asia, Africa and South America is recreating similar conditions, and in the past 40 years cholera has made a remarkable re-emergence through its longest ever (seventh) pandemic[4].

In most countries, life expectancy has risen over the past 50 years[5] (**Fig. 2**). The most important exception is those regions where HIV infection is rife. Moreover, during the past 15 years, falling living standards in some African countries and the breakdown of public health

[1]Wohl Virion Centre, Division of Infection and Immunity, University College London, W1T 4JF, UK [2]National Centre for Epidemiology and Population Health, The Australian National University, Canberra, ACT 0200, Australia. Correspondence should be addressed to R.A.W. (r.weiss@ucl.ac.uk) or A.J.M. (tony.mcmichael@anu.edu.au).

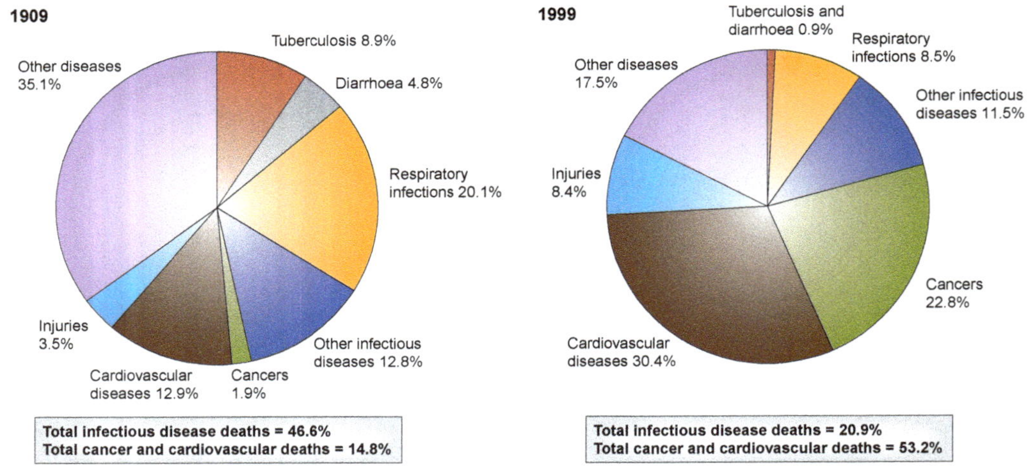

Figure 1 Proportions of total deaths from major cause-of-death categories, 1909 and 1999, in Chile[2]. This country illustrates the full transition from developing to developed status during the twentieth century.

infrastructure in ex-Soviet nations has aided the re-emergence of transmissible diseases like tuberculosis[4,6]. Further, severe outbreaks such as the 1918–1919 influenza A pandemic temporarily reversed the decline of deaths caused by infectious disease. The 50 million estimated deaths from that pandemic[7] represented about 2% of the global population at that time, and is twice as many as the cumulative AIDS mortality of the past 20 years. The next influenza pandemic may be just around the corner, and may spread even faster[8], if access to appropriate vaccines and drug treatment is not available[9,10].

For other newly emerging infections that make headlines, such as SARS, Ebola or vCJD, it is important to keep a sense of demographic proportion. Placing these emerging infections on a 'Richter' scale of human mortality (**Box 1**) shows that they elicit scarcely detectable

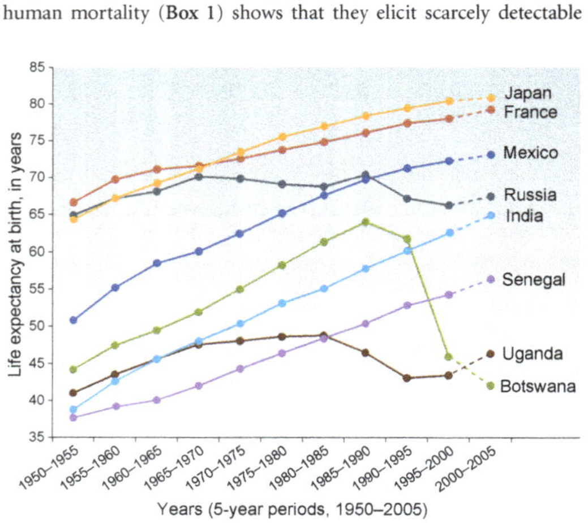

Figure 2 Changes in life expectancy at birth for both sexes in eight representative countries during the last 55 years[5].

minor tremors in numbers of fatalities — despite the fear they invoke. We do not know, however, which one might leap to the top of the scale like HIV has done; indeed, it may be a completely unknown agent, as the SARS coronavirus was two years ago. A major challenge is to predict which infection presages the next big quake, hopefully allowing preventive action.

Emerging infectious diseases, past and present

Like any other animal or plant species, humans have been prone to infection by pathogens throughout their evolutionary history. Such ancient infections by helminth and protozoan parasites, bacteria, fungi and viruses are endemic, eliciting a range of effects from a heavy burden of disease (*e.g.*, malaria) to being essentially commensal in immunocompetent hosts (*e.g.*, most types of herpesvirus and papilloma virus). Other infections depend on an animal reservoir for their maintenance; their infection of humans may be pathogenic, but it has little part in the evolving ecology of the microbe or parasite. An estimated 61% of the 1,415 species of infectious organisms known to be pathogenic in humans are transmitted by animals[11], for which the human represents a dead-end host. Occasionally, however, a zoonotic infection adapts to human-to-human transmission and diversifies away from its animal origin. Epidemic diseases are generally caused by infections that are directly transmissible between humans. HIV is a recent example of a long line of human infections initiated by a switch of host species, stretching back to the origins of measles and smallpox.

Free-living microbes may also find a human niche that suits their lifestyle, such as the lung for *Legionella pneumophila* and the gut for *Vibrio cholerae*. Legionnaires' disease, first recognized in Philadelphia in 1976, is the environmental equivalent of a zoonosis. It is seldom passed directly from person to person but it was human ingenuity in designing warm, aerated, humid 'artificial lungs' called air-conditioning systems that allowed the microbe to proliferate and become an opportunistic colonizer of the human lung. Cholera, which was unknown beyond the Ganges delta before it spread widely in Asia and the Middle East during the period 1815–1825, at around that time

BOX 1 NATURAL WEAPONS OF MASS DESTRUCTION PLACED ON A 'RICHTER' SCALE[52,53].

The values are approximate global death rates for the year 2003, taken from the World Health Organization (WHO) and other sources. HBV and HCV, hepatitis B and C viruses; RSV, respiratory syncytial virus; HPV, human papilloma viruses; vCJD, variant Creutzfeldt-Jakob disease.

Two major, novel causes of mortality top the list: cigarette smoking and HIV infection; they emerged in the twentieth century and continue to increase in many developing countries. Among the chronic and re-emerging infections, malaria and tuberculosis are near the top, so it becomes apparent why there is a need for the Global Fund for Malaria, Tuberculosis and AIDS. Accidental injuries, particularly road deaths, continue to rise, with 85% occurring in developing countries[54]. Although 2003 was the year of the SARS outbreak[52,55], less than 1,000 people actually died as a result of SARS coronavirus infection despite the collateral damage to daily life, psychological well-being and economic activity in the affected cities.

This Richter scale represents a snapshot in time. Twenty years ago, HIV was three logs further down the scale, whereas polio was three logs higher. Fifty years ago, malaria was finally eradicated from Europe, where it had formerly been widespread, including in England (Shakespeare's 'ague'). Bacterial respiratory diseases used to have a more important role in human mortality and, despite concern over multi-resistance to antibiotics[40,56], the situation is considerably better than in the era before the advent of antibiotics. Common bacterial infections of childhood, such as diphtheria and whooping cough, have become rarities in the developed world, largely through vaccination. Viral diseases have similarly been reduced. Thanks to effective immunization policies of the WHO, smallpox was eradicated in 1977; polio and measles viruses, which have no animal reservoir, may soon be eliminated in the same way.

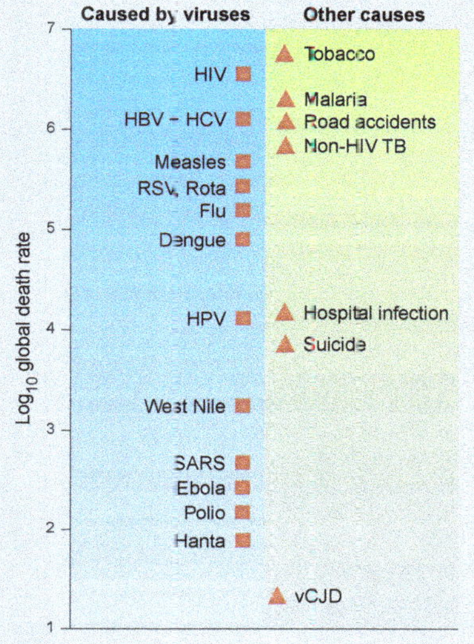

horizontally acquired a toxin gene and other factors in a genetic package that helped it to colonize the gut; the resultant diarrhea aids dispersal of the microbe[12,13].

Human society has undergone a series of major transitions that has affected our pattern of infectious disease acquisition and dissemination[4]. These transitions illustrate the interrelationship between environmental, social and behavioral influences on the emergence and subsequent spread of infectious disease. Some infections were acquired when our australopithecine ancestors left their arboreal habitat to live in the savannah. This ecological change included exposure to new species of mosquito and tick as vectors for infection. After the emergence of *Homo sapiens*, the eventual migration of neolithic hunter-gatherers out of Africa 50,000 to 100,000 years ago exposed them to new infections in distant regions.

The first major transition of prehistoric/early historic times gave rise to the epidemic, or 'crowd,' infections. This change must have started in the millennia following the advent of agriculture—from around 10,000 years ago—as agriculturally based society developed larger, denser populations. The domestication of livestock and the rich dividends available in human settlements to other animals (*e.g.*, rodents, dogs and various insects) provided further opportunities for pathogens to move between species. Sometimes such a pathogen (or a mutant strain thereof) would have been well suited to humans as a new host species, and, if human numbers were adequate, could therefore persist indefinitely as a human infection. Thus, measles emerged about 7,000 years ago, probably from rindepest of cattle, and diverged to become an exclusively human infection when population size and density became sufficient to maintain the virus without an animal reservoir. Similarly, smallpox became epidemic about 4,000 years ago, possibly evolving from camelpox, its closest phylogenetic relative.

The next two transitions were primarily to do with great extensions in the spread of infectious diseases, entering distant populations as 'new infections.' Thus, the second historical transition occurred in Classical times as large Eurasian civilizations came into commercial and military contact. They inadvertently exchanged their pools of infections, and vectors such as rats and fleas, across the Mediterranean basin, the Middle East, India and China. The plague of Athens in 430 BCE during the Peloponnesian war vividly described by Thucidides may represent the first report of typhus. This Rickettsial infection is transmitted from rats to humans and thence among louse-ridden humans. Typhus frequently accompanies human conflict and deprivation, as seen in a recent outbreak among Rwandan refugees in Burundi[14]. The Justinian plague of 542 CE devastated the eastern Mediterranean region and probably extended as far as China[15] like the Black Death 800 years later (and both are attributable to *Yersinia pestis*[16]).

The third historical transition accompanied the era of worldwide exploration and colonization by Europeans from circa 1500 CE onward. A contemporary account by one of Hernan Cortes' fellow conquistadors, Bernal Diaz, recalls that they might well have failed to overthrow the mighty Aztec empire had they not been aided by a raging epidemic. This was possibly a combination of smallpox and measles, both wholly unknown to the New World population. Curiously, the Columbian exchange was unidirectional regarding infectious diseases; the one contentious possible exception being syphilis. The New World is believed to have had substantially fewer human zoonotic infections[15,17], and vector-borne infections like Chagas' disease did not travel in the absence of an appropriate vector.

Two centuries later, Captain Cook unwittingly repeated the decimation of indigenous peoples through syphilis, measles and tuberculosis in many of the Pacific islands, whereas Lord Jeffrey Amherst deliberately attempted to spread smallpox among 'hostile' Native Americans, one of the better documented cases of germ warfare[18]. The transmission dynamics of infections in naive populations is markedly different from those in which the majority of adults are immune[19]. Onboard *The Beagle*, Charles Darwin observed with his customary acuity, "Wherever the European has trod, death seems to pursue the aboriginal ...Most of the diseases have been introduced by ships and what renders this fact remarkable is that there might be no appearance of the disease among the crew which conveyed this destructive importation."

Today we are living through the fourth historical transition of globalization. Urbanization, dense and usually impoverished peri-urban settlements, social upheaval, air travel, long-distance trade, technological developments, land clearance and climate change all influence the risks of infectious disease emergence and spread. Although some of the apparent increase in infectious disease may be attributable to better diagnostic methods and surveillance, there seems little doubt that more incidents are occurring, and have the potential to spread more widely than 50 years ago, as outbreaks and spread of infections like Nipah virus and SARS would not have passed unnoticed.

Environment and emerging infectious diseases

As humans encroach further into previously uncultivated environments, new contacts between wild fauna and humans and their livestock increases the risk of cross-species infection[20]. This process will only diminish as wild species become rarer and eventually endangered, like the great apes today. An example of such contact followed the establishment of piggeries close to the tropical forest in northern Malaysia, where, in 1998, the Nipah virus first crossed over from fruit bats (flying foxes, *Pteropus* spp.) to pigs and thence to pig farmers[21]. Destruction of natural forest has also encouraged fruit bats to relocate nearer human habitation, like the large colony in the botanic gardens in the heart of Sydney. Indeed, in 1997, Hendra, a related paramyxovirus of Australian fruit bats[22], fatally infected a veterinarian examining a sick horse.

Rodents continue to be sources of re-emerging infections, as witnessed in the 1990s with hantaviruses in the United States. Rodent-borne hantavirus is prevalent in agricultural systems in South America and East Asia, in arid grasslands in North America and elsewhere. In mid-1993, an unexpected outbreak of acute, sometimes fatal, respiratory disease occurred in humans in the southwestern United States[23]. This 'hantavirus pulmonary syndrome' was caused by a previously unrecognized virus, maintained primarily within the native deer-mouse, and transmitted through excreta. The 1991–1992 El Niño event, with unseasonal heavy summer rains and a proliferation of piñon nuts, hugely amplified local rodent populations which led to the 1993 outbreak[23,24]. In South America, there have been several outbreaks of hantavirus and arenavirus infections linked to forest clearance and the growth of rodent populations in the new grasslands[4].

Habitat destruction is not the only cause of increased human infection, however. Dengue virus is extending its range and prevalence because its mosquito vector breeds rapidly in the urban environment[25]. In the United States, nature conservation and increased woodland in the eastern states has led to the emergence of Lyme disease. This disease is caused by a tick-borne spirochete and the presence of tick-infested deer near suburban homes leads to ticks residing on bushes adjacent to baseball diamonds and gardens.

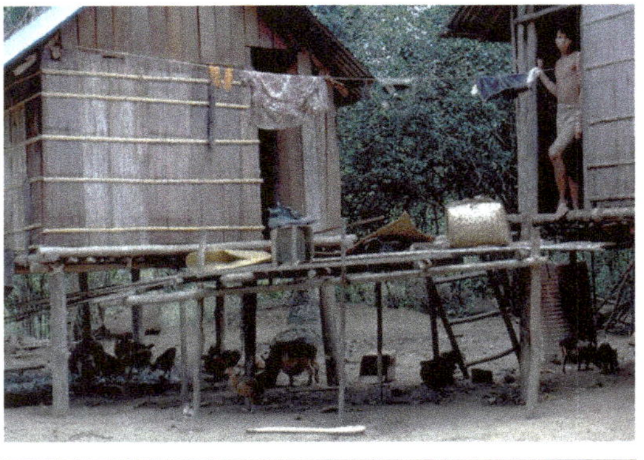

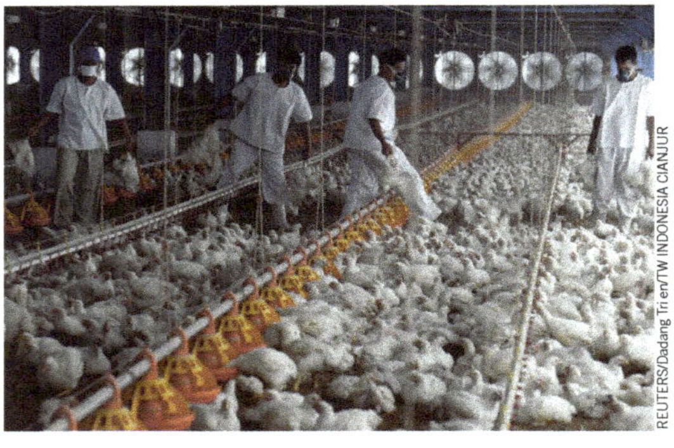

Figure 3 The changing pattern of farming in South East Asia. Top, traditional mixed homestead; bottom, intensive single-species industry. (Top photo courtesy of R.A. Weiss)

Food-borne infections

Intensification of production of meat and meat products has led to new infections[26]. Most notorious is vCJD in the UK arising from consumption of contaminated food products of cattle affected by BSE[27]. BSE, or 'mad cow disease,' emerged in British cattle in 1986 because of industrialized cannibalism, whereby rendered neural tissue and bone meal from slaughtered cattle were recycled into cattle feed, as well as into pies and hamburgers for human consumption[28]. Originally, infectious prions from scrapie in sheep were the suspected source, but it now seems more likely that it arose from a bovine with sporadic prion disease. The extent of the human epidemic remains unclear. Although natural transmission is unsustainable ($R_0 < 1$ in both cattle and humans), there are concerns that vCJD might be transmissible through blood transfusions[29]. Without effective diagnostic tests for presymptomatic vCJD infection, this situation is extremely unfortunate.

Other recently emergent food-borne infections include *E. coli* O157:H7, which is harmless to cattle but toxic to humans, and *Salmonella enteriditis* in chickens. Better hygiene in abattoirs, butchers and domestic kitchens can greatly reduce the incidence of infection. In theory, closed and intensive farming of a single species should reduce the risk of cross-species infection (**Fig. 3**). But it also allows large-scale epidemics to emerge, as seen recently for avian influenza strains in southeast Asia and the Netherlands[8,30].

Ancient dietary taboos, such as those of Hindus, Muslims and Jews regarding pork as unclean, doubtless had their roots in protection from infectious disease. Today, an increasing demand for consumption of exotic and wild animals raises new risks of infectious diseases such as SARS (**Box 2**).

Transmissibility and globalization

Changing patterns of human behavior and ecology affect two distinct steps in the emergence of new infectious disease. The first is an

BOX 2 BUSHMEAT AND LIVE ANIMAL MARKETS

"If there is any conceivable way a germ can travel from one species to another, some microbe will find it," wrote William McNeill in his classic text *Plagues and Peoples*[15]. For millennia, small farmsteads accommodated mixed species living closely with humans—goats, pigs, cattle, ducks, geese, chickens and perhaps a water buffalo or a donkey—and exchanged infections. When species are raised separately but are sold together, the opportunity for cross-infection moves from the farm to the marketplace. The 1997 outbreak of avian influenza in Hong Kong occurred in mixed markets, where live chickens, quail and ducks were stacked together in close quarters with humans. The H5N1 virus that emerged may have been derived by recombination between those of different avian hosts[8]. After 1997, mixed species were separated into different areas of the markets. But this year's H5N1 virus is spreading among intensively reared chickens across southeast Asia.

The increasing predilection for meat of exotic species has exacerbated the risk of exposure to infections not previously encountered, and this situation probably triggered the SARS epidemic[55]. Although we are still not sure of the natural reservoir species of SARS coronavirus, the live markets and restaurants in Guangzhong sold small carnivores, and several species of civet cat, racoon dog and ferret badger captured in China, Laos, Vietnam and Thailand, were brought into close proximity[57]. Clearly, some of the palm civet cats were infected with SARS-related viruses, but it is less clear whether they represent the original source species. There is a danger in incriminating the wrong species; if the true reservoir resides in the rodent prey of these carnivores, then culling the predators may be counterproductive. Stopping the exotic meat trade altogether would seem to be a simple solution to prevent the reappearance of SARS, but once the taste for it has been established, that may prove no more practical than attempting to prohibit the tobacco trade.

In Africa, bushmeat also poses a serious problem for emerging infectious diseases, as well as for nature conservation. Sick animals may be more easily captured. For example, 21 human deaths owing to Ebola virus infection ensued from the butchering of a single chimpanzee[58]. HIV has crossed from chimpanzees to humans on at least three occasions, and a higher number of zoonotic events from sooty mangabeys are indicated for HIV-2 (ref. 32). Whether these cross-species infections arose from butchering the animals or from keeping them as pets is unknown, but a recent survey of primate hunters in Africa showed that they are susceptible, like handlers of primates in captivity, to infection (though not disease) from foamy retroviruses[59].

The escalating intercontinental trade in exotic pets can lead to unexpected infectious disease outbreaks. The United States has only recently imposed more stringent regulations and quarantine following cases of monkeypox in humans and in prairie dogs introduced by rodents imported from Africa as pets[60].

increased opportunity for animal-to-human infection to occur owing to greater exposure, which may be necessary but not sufficient to lead to the emergence of a new human infection. The second step is the opportunity for onward transmission once a person has become infected. For each novel epidemic, such as the 1918–1919 influenza pandemic or AIDS, there are probably thousands of failed transfers.

Some infections simply do not take in the new host. Innate host-specific restrictions on viral replication have recently become evident for primate lentiviruses[31], which may explain why certain species that harbor simian immunodeficiency virus, but not others more commonly in contact with humans, gave rise to HIV-1 and HIV-2. Even in the case of HIV-1, only one pedigree of three independent chimpanzee-to-human crossover events[32] has given rise to the AIDS pandemic, whereas the other two smolder as poorly transmissible infections.

Fatal pathogenesis is not necessarily coupled with infectiousness[12], which is evident for H5N1 avian influenza in humans[9]. But genetic reassortment between avian and human influenza viruses could easily give rise to a new, rapidly spreading strain[8]. A poorly infectious pathogen may not spread at all from the index case, as is usual with rabies, or may only infect close contacts and soon peter out, as seen with Lassa fever and Ebola virus. SARS nearly became self-sustaining but was brought under control. Some of the most insidious infections are those with long, silent incubation periods during which the person is infectious. These emerge surreptitiously so that when the new disease is eventually recognized, as AIDS was in 1981, the infection has already spread far beyond control.

Like the ships of centuries past, the speed of modern air travel works wonders for the dispersal of infectious diseases. SARS was eventually constrained by quarantine and strict adherence to infection control guidelines in hospitals, but not before it quickly traveled from Guangzhong to Hong Kong and on to Toronto. If Ebola broke out in a city with a busy international airport, it might also travel across continents in a similar manner. Brockmann[33] has modeled how rapidly such infections can move once they reach a major airport hub; closing the hubs becomes an immediate imperative. We cannot be sure what the initial vector was for the arrival of West Nile virus into North America in 1999: a migratory bird blown off course, an infected human with a valid air ticket or a stowaway mosquito on a similar flight. Whatever the means of entry and early colonization of crows in New York, it has taken less than four years to reach the Pacific coast[25]. Thus, West Nile virus has found a new reservoir in American birds, just as yellow fever virus reached New World primates 350 years earlier.

Social and economic conditions, behavioral changes and geopolitical instability

Microbes frequently capitalize on situations of ecological, biological and social disturbance. Biologically weakened and vulnerable populations—especially if also socially disordered and living in circumstances of privation, unhygienic conditions and close contact—are susceptible to microbial colonization. The severity of the bubonic plague (Black Death) in mid-fourteenth-century Europe seems to have reflected the nutritional and impoverishment consequences of several preceding decades of unusually cold and wet weather with crop failures compounding the incipient destabilization of the hierarchical feudal system.

Many of the rapid and marked changes in human social ecology in recent decades have altered the probabilities of infectious disease emergence and transmission. These changes include increases in population size and density, urbanization, persistent poverty (especially in the expanding peri-urban slums), the increased number and movement of political, economic and environmental refugees, conflict and warfare. Political ignorance, denial and obduracy often compound the risk of infectious disease transmission—as has been tragically observed with HIV/AIDS in parts of Africa, where widespread poverty, a culture of female disempowerment and political instability further exacerbate the problem[34,35]. But we have little understanding of why the prevalence of HIV infection varies so greatly between cities in sub-Saharan Africa[36].

The urban environment has only recently become the dominant human habitat. Urbanism typically leads to a breakdown in traditional family and social structures, and entails greater personal mobility and extended and changeable social networks. These features, along with access to modern contraception, have facilitated a diversity of sexual contacts and, hence, the spread of sexually transmitted diseases[37]. This risk is further amplified by the growth in sex tourism in today's internationally mobile world, which capitalizes on the desperation and ignorance of poverty, combined with exploitative behaviors, in developing countries. More generally, cities often function as highways for 'microbial traffic'[38]. Rapid urbanization boosts certain well established infectious diseases, such as childhood pneumonia, diarrhea, tuberculosis and dengue, and facilitates dissemination of various 'emerging' diseases—as occurred for SARS in the high-rise housing of Hong Kong. Crowded and dilapidated public housing can potentiate infectious disease transmission through drug abuse and sexually transmitted infections[39].

Nosocomial and iatrogenic infections

Technological advances in medicine and public health can also inadvertently promote the emergence and spread of infectious disease. It has become commonplace to quip that you go to the hospital at the peril of acquiring an intractable nosocomial infection such as methicillin-resistant *Staphylococcus aureus*[40], and such infections killed around 40 times as many people as SARS did in 2003 (**Box 1**). Multidrug-resistant tuberculosis has also become a major problem, and, paradoxically, regions with health programs that reduced wild-type tuberculosis strains can develop into 'hot zones' for multidrug-resistant tuberculosis[41].

By far the most effective medical vector of infectious disease has been the syringe and needle. Drucker *et al.*[42] have charted the massive increase in the use of injecting equipment over the past 100 years. Individuals with hemophilia treated with pooled clotting factors became almost universally infected with hepatitis B and C viruses before diagnostic screening tests were developed. Over 20% of such affected individuals also became infected with HIV[43], and more recently, transmission of West Nile virus by blood transfusion and by organ transplantation has been reported[44,45]. The use of contaminated needles among intravenous drug users has had similar consequences. Infectious diseases have also been amplified by the use of nonsterile medical injections in developing countries[42]. Egypt has the highest prevalence of hepatitis C infection in the world because of the use and reuse of syringes and needles in an earlier public health campaign to reduce bilharzia by medication given by injection. The transmission of CJD through contaminated surgical instruments is another example of iatrogenic spread of infection[29].

Biological medicines produced from animal-cell substrates present an inherent potential hazard for introducing new infections. Great care must be taken to ensure that live attenuated vaccines grown in animal cells or eggs are devoid of pathogens; for example, several early batches of live and inactivated polio vaccine unwittingly contained live SV40 virus, a polyoma virus of macaques. After SV40 was discovered in 1960, polio vaccine production shifted to virus propagation in primary kidney cells of African green monkeys. These cultures were free of SV40 but possibly contained SIVagm, a relative of HIV that fortunately does not infect humans[31]. The irony of the SV40 story is that the United States Food and Drug Administration prohibited the use of well known, permanent cell lines demonstrably free of adventitious infectious agents, for fear that such immortalized cells might exert oncogenic properties on the vaccine. There is no epidemiological evidence of increased tumor incidence in those populations who are known to have received SV40-contaminated polio vaccine. But there have been a number of recent claims of an association of SV40 DNA sequences in a variety of human malignancies[46], although these findings remain controversial[47].

The ultimate medical means of introducing animal viruses into humans is xenotransplantation. The implantation of animal cells or tissues into immunosuppressed individuals seems to be a perfectly designed way to encourage cross-species infection. It is astonishing that trials were started without much thought about the consequences for potentially emerging pathogens, for example, porcine retroviruses[48]. The generation of genetically modified knockout or transgenic animals to prevent hyperacute rejection of donor tissues may exacerbate the infection hazard[49,50]. Happily, there is no evidence so far of retrovirus infection in individuals who were exposed to living pig cells[50], and clinical xenotransplantation is now stringently regulated; so it seems all the more extraordinary that cellular therapies with fetal lamb cells and extracts continue to be practiced with impunity in alternative medicine clinics in Europe and the Far East.

Conclusions and prospects

Novel infectious diseases can emerge in any part of the world at any time. HIV and Ebola came out of Africa, avian influenza and SARS from China, Nipah virus from Malaysia, BSE/vCJD from the UK and hantavirus pulmonary syndrome from the Americas. It is difficult to predict what new disease will come next or where it will appear, but changing ecological conditions and novel human-animal contacts will be useful clues as to which horizons require scanning with most scrutiny. We must expect the unexpected.

As a codicil, another factor that needs to be taken into account is the potential impact of the HIV pandemic on the emergence of other infectious diseases[51]. We already know that persons with AIDS act as 'superspreaders' of tuberculosis, and we can only speculate what course the SARS outbreak might have taken had someone incubating the disease flown to Durban rather than Toronto[52]. People with AIDS may persistently harbor infections that would otherwise be transient, and this could hamper the eradication of measles and polio. Multivalent *Pneumococcus* vaccines are ineffective in HIV-infected people with $CD4^+$ lymphocyte levels below 200/μl, whereas live 'attenuated' vaccines such as vaccinia can cause virulent disease in the immunocompromised host. Immunodeficient persons living at high density could also be the seed-bed for microorganisms that are initially ill adapted to human infection to evolve into transmissible human pathogens. Thus, an infection from a zoonotic or environmental source—for example, the *Mycobacterium avium intracellulare* complex—could conceivably emerge as the tuberculosis of the twenty-first century, although direct transmission between individuals with AIDS of such opportunistic infections have not been documented so far.

We shall give Girolamo Frascatoro the last word on emerging and re-emerging infectious diseases by quoting from his treatise *De Contagione*, published almost 450 years ago, "There will come yet other new and unusual ailments in the course of time. And this disease [syphilis] will pass way, but it later will be born again and be seen by our descendents."

ACKNOWLEDGMENTS

We are grateful to M. E. Chamberland, H. W. Jaffe and S. Leff for critically reading the manuscript.

COMPETING INTERESTS STATEMENT
The authors declare that they have no competing financial interests.

1. Burnet, F.M. & White, D. *Natural History of Infectious Disease* (Cambridge Univ. Press, Cambridge, 1972).
2. McMichael, A.J. *Human Frontiers, Environments and Disease. Past patterns, uncertain futures* (Cambridge Univ. Press, Cambridge, 2001).
3. Morens, D.M., Folkers, G.K. & Fauci, A.S. The challenge of emerging and re-emerging infectious diseases. *Nature* **430**, 242–249 (2004).
4. McMichael, A.J. Environmental and social influences on emerging infectious diseases: past, present and future. *Philos. Trans. R. Soc. Lond. B. Biol. Sci.* **359**, 1049–1058 (2004).
5. McMichael, A.J., McKee, M., Shkolnikov, V. & Valkonen, T. Mortality trends and setbacks: global convergence or divergence? *Lancet* **363**, 1155–1159 (2004).
6. Garrett, L. *Betrayal of Trust: the Collapse of Global Public Health* (Hyperion, New York, 2000).
7. Johnson, N.P. & Mueller, J. Updating the accounts: global mortality of the 1918–1920 "Spanish" influenza pandemic. *Bull. Hist. Med.* **76**, 105–115 (2002).
8. Webby, R., Hoffmann, E. & Webster, R. Molecular constraints to interspecies transmission of viral pathogens. *Nat. Med.* **10**, S77–S81 (2004).
9. Palese, P. Influenza: old and new threats. *Nat. Med.* **10**, S82–S87 (2004).
10. De Clercq, E. Antivirals and antiviral strategies. *Nat. Rev. Microbiol.* **2**, 704–720 (2004).
11. Taylor, L.H., Latham, S.M. & Woolhouse, M.E. Risk factors for human disease emergence. *Philos. Trans. R. Soc. Lond. B. Biol. Sci.* **356**, 983–939 (2001).
12. Weiss, R.A. Virulence and pathogenesis. *Trends Microbiol.* **10**, 314–317 (2002).
13. Speck, R.S. Cholera. in *The Cambridge World History of Human Disease* (ed. Kiple, K.F.) 642–647 (Cambridge Univ. Press, Cambridge, 1993).
14. Raoult, D. *et al.* Jail fever (epidemic typhus) outbreak in Burundi. *Emerg. Infect. Dis.* **3**, 357–360 (1997).
15. McNeill, W.H. *Plagues and Peoples* (Penguin, London, 1976).
16. Drancourt, M. *et al.* Genotyping, orientalis-like *Yersinia pestis*, and plague pandemics. *Emerg. Infect. Dis.* **10**, 1585–1592 (2004).
17. Diamond, J. *Guns, Germs and Steel. A Short History of Everybody for the Last 13,000 Years* (Jonathan Cape, London, 1997).
18. Duffy, J. Smallpox and the Indians in the American colonies. *Bull. Hist. Med.* **25**, 324–341 (1951).
19. Anderson, R.M. & May, R.M. *Infectious Diseases of Humans: Dynamics and Control* (Oxford Univ. Press, 1992).
20. Patz, J.A. *et al.* Unhealthy landscapes: Policy recommendations on land use change and infectious disease emergence. *Environ. Health. Perspect.* **112**, 1092–1098 (2004).
21. Chua, K.B. *et al.* Fatal encephalitis due to Nipah virus among pig-farmers in Malaysia. *Lancet* **354**, 1257–1259 (1999).
22. Halpin, K., Young, P.L., Field, H. & Mackenzie, J.S. Newly discovered viruses of flying foxes. *Vet. Microbiol.* **68**, 83–87 (1999).
23. Parmenter, R., Brunt, J., Moore, D. & Ernest, S. The hantavirus epidemic in the southwest: rodent population dynamics and the implications for transmission of hantavirus-associated adult respiratory distress syndrome (HARDS) in the four corners region. *Sevilleta LTER Publ. (University of New Mexico)* **41**, 1–44 (1993).
24. Engelthaler, D.M. *et al.* Climatic and environmental patterns associated with hantavirus pulmonary syndrome, Four Corners region, United States. *Emerg. Infect. Dis.* **5**, 87–94 (1999).
25. MacKenzie, J.S., Gubler, D.J. & Petersen, L.R. Emerging flaviviruses: the spread and resurgence of Japanese encephalitis, West Nile and dengue viruses. *Nat. Med.* **10**, S98–S109 (2004).
26. Frenzen, F.D. Deaths due to unknown foodborne agents. *Emerg. Infect. Dis.* **10**, 1536–1543 (2004).
27. Will, R.G. *et al.* A new variant of Creutzfeldt-Jakob disease in the UK. *Lancet* **347**, 921–925 (1996).
28. Schwartz, M. *How the Cows Turned Mad* (University of California Press, London, 2003).
29. Wilson, K. & Ricketts, M.N. Transfusion transmission of vCJD: a crisis avoided? *Lancet* **364**, 477–479 (2004).
30. Koopmans, M. *et al.* Transmission of H7N7 avian influenza A virus to human beings during a large outbreak in commercial poultry farms in the Netherlands. *Lancet* **363**, 587–593 (2004).
31. Lee, K. & KewalRamani, V.N. In defense of the cell: TRIM5α interception of mammalian retroviruses. *Proc. Natl. Acad. Sci. USA* **101**, 10496–10497 (2004).
32. Hahn, B.H., Shaw, G.M., De Cock, K.M. & Sharp, P.M. AIDS as a zoonosis: scientific and public health implications. *Science* **287**, 607–614 (2000).
33. Brockmann, D. Dynamics of epidemics spread across airline networks. in *SARS: A Case Study in Emerging Infections* (eds. McLean, A.R., May, R., Pattison, J.R. & Weiss, R.A.) (Oxford Univ. Press, Oxford, 2005).
34. Caldwell, J.C. Rethinking the African AIDS epidemic. *Popul. Dev. Rev.* **26**, 117–135 (2000).
35. Butler, C. HIV and AIDS, poverty, and causation. *Lancet* **356**, 1445–1446 (2000).
36. Auvert, B. *et al.* Ecological and individual level analysis of risk factors for HIV infection in four urban populations in sub-Saharan Africa with different levels of HIV infection. *AIDS* **15** Suppl 4, S15–S30 (2001).
37. Johnson, A.M. *et al.* Sexual behaviour in Britain: partnerships, practices, and HIV risk behaviours. *Lancet* **358**, 1835–1842 (2001).
38. Morse, S.S. Factors in the emergence of infectious diseases. *Emerg. Infect. Dis.* **1**, 7–15 (1995).
39. Cohen, A. Urban unfinished business. *Int. J. Environ. Health Res.* **13**, S29–S36 (2003).
40. Tiemersma, D.W. *et al.* Methicillin-resistant *Staphylococcus aureus* in Europe, 1999–2002. *Emerg. Infect. Dis.* **10**, 1627–1634 (2004).
41. Blower, S.M. & Chou, T. Modeling the emergence of the 'hot zones': tuberculosis and the amplification dynamics of drug resistance. *Nat. Med.* **10**, 1111–1116 (2004).
42. Drucker, E., Alcabes, P.G. & Marx, P.A. The injection century: massive unsterile injections and the emergence of human pathogens. *Lancet* **358**, 1989–1992 (2001).
43. Darby, S.C. *et al.* Mortality before and after HIV infection in the complete UK population of haemophiliacs. *Nature* **377**, 79–82 (1995).
44. Pealer, L.N. *et al.* Transmission of West Nile virus through blood transfusion in the United States in 2002. *N. Engl. J. Med.* **349**, 1236–1245 (2003).
45. Iwamoto, M. *et al.* Transmission of West Nile virus from an organ donor to four transplant recipients. *N. Engl. J. Med.* **348**, 2196–2203 (2003).
46. Butel, J.S. & Lednicky, J.A. Cell and molecular biology of simian virus 40: implications for human infections and disease. *J. Natl. Cancer. Inst.* **91**, 119–134 (1999).
47. zur Hausen, H. SV40 in human cancers—an endless tale? *Int. J. Cancer.* **107**, 687 (2003).
48. Patience, C., Takeuchi, Y. & Weiss, R.A. Infection of human cells by an endogenous retrovirus of pigs. *Nat. Med.* **3**, 282–286 (1997).
49. Weiss, R.A. Transgenic pigs and virus adaptation. *Nature* **391**, 327–328 (1998).
50. Magre, S. *et al.* Reduced sensitivity to human serum inactivation of enveloped viruses produced by pig cells transgenic for human CD55 or deficient for the galactosyl-α(1–3) galactosyl epitope. *J. Virol.* **78**, 5812–5819 (2004).
51. Weiss, R.A. Gulliver's travels in HIVland. *Nature* **410**, 963–967 (2001).
52. Weiss, R.A. & McLean, A.R. What have we learnt from SARS? *Philos. Trans. R. Soc. Lond. B. Biol. Sci.* **359**, 1137–1140 (2004).
53. Hale, P. *et al.* Mission now possible for AIDS fund. *Nature* **412**, 271–272 (2001).
54. Perel, P., McGuire, M., Eapen, K. & Ferraro, A. Research on preventing road traffic injuries in developing countries is needed. *BMJ* **328**, 895 (2004).
55. Peiris, J.S.M., Guan, Y. & Yuen, K.Y. Severe acute respiratory syndrome. *Nat. Med.* **10**, S88–S97 (2004).
56. Levy, S.B. & Marshall, B. Antimicrobial resistance worldwide: causes, challenges and responses. *Nat. Med.* **10**, S122–S129 (2004).
57. Bell, D., Roberton, S. & Hunter, P.R. Animal origins of SARS coronavirus: possible links with the international trade in small carnivores. *Philos. Trans. R. Soc. Lond. B. Biol. Sci.* **359**, 1107–1114 (2004).
58. Mahy, B.W.J. Zoonoses and haemorrhagic fever. in *Safety of Biological Products Prepared from Mammalian Cell Culture. Dev. Biol. Stand.* **93** (eds. Brown, F., Griffiths, E., Horaud, F. & Petricciani, J.C.) 31–36 (Karger, Basel, 1998).
59. Wolfe, N.D. *et al.* Naturally acquired simian retrovirus infections in central African hunters. *Lancet* **363**, 932–927 (2004).
60. Di Giulio, D.B. & Eckburg, P.B. Human monkeypox: an emerging zoonosis. *Lancet Infect. Dis.* **4**, 15–25 (2004).

END OF REPRINT H

Social and Environmental Risk Factors in the Emergence of Infectious Diseases

ROBIN A. WEISS AND ANTHONY J. MCMICHAEL

24

CLIMATE CHANGE, ROSS RIVER VIRUS AND BIODIVERSITY

PHILIP WEINSTEIN AND PENG BI

Abstract

Infection with the Australian Ross River virus (RRV) results in rash, fever and rheumatic symptoms lasting several weeks, with epidemics strongly influenced by climatic variables that impact mosquito biology. The disease can be contextualised in terms of broader issues of resource overutilisation that leads to the degradation of ecosystems, with biodiversity loss potentially contributing to the emergence of the disease. The possible ecological linkage mechanisms between biodiversity loss and RRV infection are discussed and research needs in the area are highlighted.

Background

Tony McMichael's 1993 book, *Planetary Overload*, introduced ecological approaches to public health researchers and epidemiologists. The concept of carrying capacity was presented in such a way as to make many of these researchers rethink their approaches to a variety of pathogens, including RRV.

Ross River Virus

This Australian arbovirus (arthropod-borne virus) causes symptomatic infection in up to 5,000 people per annum, resulting in rash, fever and rheumatic symptoms lasting several weeks. Epidemics were first described in the late 1920s (Nimmo, 1928), and the ecology and distribution of RRV is now known to be determined by climatic variables that impact mosquito biology, including temperature and rainfall (for a review, see Russell, 2002).

Until *Planetary Overload* (McMichael, 1993), the ecology of RRV and other vector-borne diseases had not been contextualised in terms of the broader issues of resource overutilisation that leads to the degradation of ecosystems. Anthropogenic climate change is prominent among the 'ecosystem services' (*sensu* Millennium Ecosystem Assessment, 2005) that are lost when resource utilisation exceeds carrying capacity, and several of McMichael's students and colleagues studied the relationships between climate and RRV (e.g. Tong et al., 1998; McMichael et al., 2003).

The ecological context of RRV transmission has been considered (Weinstein, 1997; Jardine et al., 2011), and the disease has been used to illustrate the importance of responding to the research challenges presented by the Millennium Ecosystem Assessment (MEA) (Weinstein, 2005). The MEA highlighted the significant loss in biodiversity that has resulted from 'planetary overload' and, importantly, ties adverse human health outcomes to that loss.

We suggest that the relationship between climate change, RRV and biodiversity loss remains under-researched and now should be prioritised. Carver et al. (2010) describe the role of biodiversity (predators and competitors) in suppressing the potential dominance of an RRV vector mosquito in an area in Western Australia affected by both decreasing rainfall and deforestation. In the study area, the combined effects of climate change and biodiversity loss may be synergistic because rainfall is inadequate to wash away saline surface water; residual brackish water pools then provide habitat for the salt-tolerant vector, *Aedes camptorhynchus*, which survives there better than do its competitors. Consequently, the 'emergence' of RRV infection is potentially facilitated. An additional layer of complexity is added to this analysis if one takes into account the populations of natural reservoir hosts for RRV, which may also be affected adversely by climate change. In other systems, a loss of potential host biodiversity has been shown to enhance disease transmission (Ostfeld and Keesing, 2000), perhaps because the 'dilution effect' provided by poorer reservoir species is lost. Conversely, a biologically sterile environment provides little opportunity for vector-borne disease transmission, but is hardly an attractive alternative. The possible relationship between climate change and reservoir biodiversity remains unstudied for RRV and, clearly, together with land use, has the potential to affect the future disease burden.

Other mechanisms by which climate change and biodiversity loss could interact to affect vector mosquitoes and disease ecology include changed water temperature and nutrient depletion in standing water (O'Reilly et al., 2003); seasonality and phenological disruption between predators and prey (Saino et al., 2011); and, the frequency and intensity of extreme weather events affecting species composition (Willig and Walker, 1999).

Conclusions Relating to Ross River Virus as a Model

Ross River virus may provide a case study for climate change and biodiversity loss interactions and effects on vector-borne disease (Figure 24.1). In keeping with the thrust of *Planetary Overload,* such research would ideally lead to recommendations for interventions that provide benefits for both a healthy ecosystem and healthy human populations concurrently.

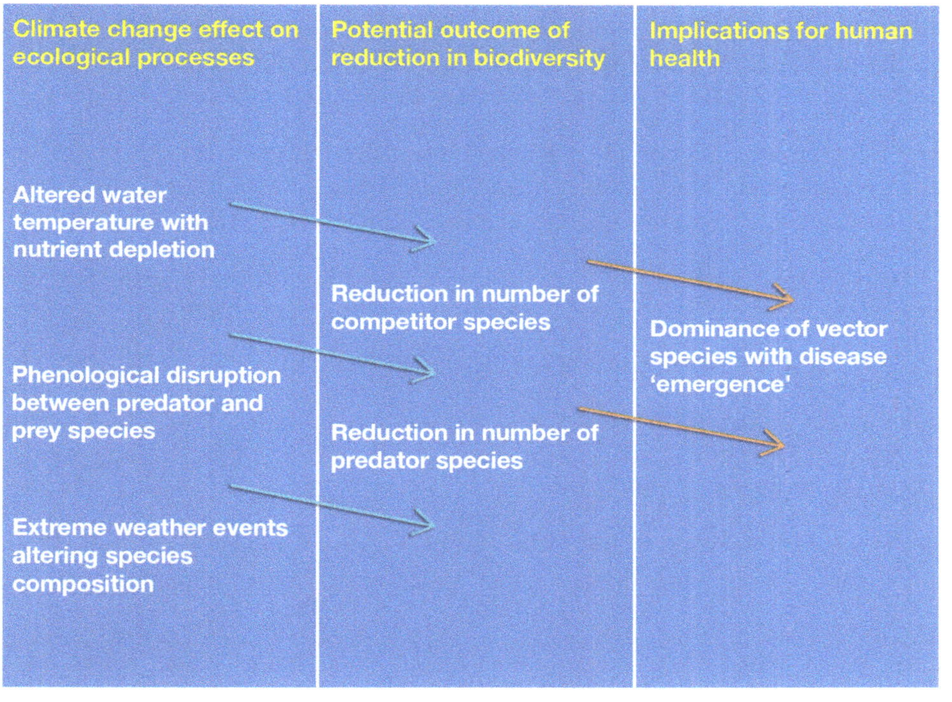

Figure 24.1 Potential relationships between climate change, biodiversity loss and the 'emergence' of vector-borne disease problems.

Source: Authors' work.

Acknowledgements

We thank an anonymous reviewer for helpful comments and Scott Carver for earlier discussions.

References

Carver, S., Spafford, H., Storey, A. & Weinstein, P. 2010. The roles of predators, competitors, and secondary salinisation in structuring mosquito (Diptera: Culicidae) assemblages in ephemeral water bodies of the wheatbelt of Western Australia. *Environmental Entomology* 39, 798–810.

Jardine, A., Corkeron, M. & Weinstein, P. 2011. Dryland salinity and vector-borne disease emergence in southwestern Australia. *Environmental Geochemistry and Health* 33, 363–70.

McMichael, A.J. 1993. *Planetary Overload. Global Environmental Change and the Health of the Human Species*. Cambridge University Press, Cambridge, UK.

McMichael, A.J., Woodruff, R.E., Whetton, P., Hennessy, K., Nicholls, N., Hales, S., et al. 2003. *Human Health and Climate Change in Oceania: A Risk Assessment*. Commonwealth Government, Canberra, Australia.

Millennium Ecosystem Assessment 2005. Synthesis Reports. Available at: www.maweb.org/en/Reports.aspx, accessed 30 January 2015.

Nimmo, J.R. 1928. An unusual epidemic. *Medical Journal of Australia* i, 549–50.

O'Reilly, C.M., Alin, S.R., Plisnier, P.-D., Cohen, A.S. & McKee, B.A. 2003. Climate change decreases aquatic ecosystem productivity of Lake Tanganyika, Africa. *Nature* 424, 766–8.

Ostfeld, R.S. & Keesing, F. 2000. The function of biodiversity in the ecology of vector-borne zoonotic disease. *Canadian Journal of Zoology* 78, 2061–78.

Russell, R.C. 2002. Ross River virus: ecology and distribution. *Annual Review of Entomology* 47, 1–31.

Saino, N., Ambrosini, R., Rubolini, D., von Hardenberg, J., Provenzale, A., Hüppop, K., et al. 2011. Climate warming, ecological mismatch at arrival and population decline in migratory birds. *Proceedings of the Royal Society B: Biological Sciences* 278, 835–42.

Tong, S., Bi, P., Parton, K., Hobbs, J. & McMichael, A.J. 1998. Climate variability and transmission of epidemic polyarthritis. *The Lancet* 351, 1100.

Weinstein, P. 1997. An ecological approach to public health intervention: Ross River virus in Australia. *Environmental Health Perspectives* 105, 364–6.

Weinstein, P. 2005. Human health is harmed by ecosystem degradation, but does intervention improve it? A research challenge from the Millennium Ecosystem Assessment. *EcoHealth* 2, 228–30.

Willig, M.R. & Walker, L.R. 1999. Disturbance in terrestrial ecosystems: salient themes, synthesis, and future directions. In: Walker, L.R. (ed.) *Ecosystems of Disturbed Ground*. Elsevier Science, Amsterdam, The Netherlands, 747–67.

25

DETECTION AND ATTRIBUTION OF CLIMATE CHANGE EFFECTS ON INFECTIOUS DISEASES

MELANIE BANNISTER-TYRRELL, DAVID HARLEY AND TONY MCMICHAEL

Abstract

Infectious agents are likely to be sensitive to climate change if their life cycle includes periods of exposure to ambient conditions. Several studies have attempted to attribute changes in patterns of infectious diseases to recent climate change, such as resurgent malaria in the East African Highlands and the northward expansion of tick-borne encephalitis and Lyme disease in Europe and Canada. However, debate continues over the relative importance of climate change compared to social, demographic and other factors. Methods for the detection and attribution of climate change impacts on human infectious diseases have not been clearly defined. There are several areas of contention in the literature on appropriate methods for the detection of climate change effects on infectious diseases, including the availability and appropriate use of climate data, identifying regions where changes are most likely to be observed and the biological importance of small temperature increases and threshold effects. Definitions and strategies for the detection and attribution of climate change impacts on human infectious diseases are discussed and compared to approaches to the detection and attribution of climate change impacts in other fields. 'Consistency analysis' is proposed as a feasible methodological approach to address research questions about the impact of recent climate change on infectious diseases.

Introduction

Infectious agents whose life cycle includes a life stage or extended periods exposed to ambient weather conditions (including time within vectors or hosts) are sensitive to climate variability. Anthropogenic (or human-induced) climate change will alter the patterns of many human infectious diseases, because the development rates, lifespan and reproductive capacity of climate-sensitive infectious agents, their vectors and hosts are influenced by higher temperatures and increased climate variability (Hoberg et al., 2008; Costello et al., 2009).

Most research on climate change and infectious disease has focused on vector-borne diseases (Kovats et al., 2001; Gage et al., 2008). For example, evidence has emerged of an influence of recent regional climate change on malaria occurrence in the East African Highlands (Pascual et al., 2006; Alonso et al., 2010; Chaves and Koenraadt, 2010). Earlier studies that did not find an association (Hay et al., 2002; Shanks et al., 2002) have been criticised (Patz et al., 2002; Pascual et al., 2006; Omumbo et al., 2011). Even so, the global impact of climate change on malaria, compared to interventions and economic development that have led to malaria control, remains unclear (Gething et al., 2010; Béguin et al., 2011).

There is similar debate regarding climate in relation to tick-borne diseases. Northward expansion of the tick vectors of tick-borne encephalitis (TBE) has been documented in Europe (Lindgren et al., 2000; Lindgren and Gustafson, 2001; Daniel et al., 2003; Danielová et al., 2006), while other authors argue that the spatial and temporal heterogeneity evident in the European-wide TBE resurgence is not consistent with the relatively uniform climate change that has occurred in this region (Sumilo et al., 2007; Randolph, 2010).

In relation to the detection and attribution of climate change impacts, other climate-sensitive diseases considered include cholera (Lipp et al., 2002; Rodo et al., 2002), dengue, other waterborne infections (Hunter, 2003), food-borne infections (Tirado et al., 2010) and soil-transmitted helminthiases (Weaver et al., 2010).

Methods for the detection and attribution of climate change impacts on human health are not as well developed as in fields such as ecology (Parmesan and Yohe, 2003), perhaps due to the greater complexity in disease systems where human behaviours and ethical and logistical issues of accessing health data and working within health systems, must also be considered. Contested methodological issues for detecting climate change influences on infectious diseases include the appropriate use of climate data, the geographical range over which changes in incidence are likely to be observed, the requisite length of time-series data and the biological importance of small temperature increases and threshold effects. We discuss here the difficulties in the detection and attribution of the impact of recent climate change on infectious diseases. This is part of a larger ongoing challenge for climate change-related research in various topic areas seeking to establish methods and criteria for assessing the climate attributability of observed changes in physical, biological and ecological systems.

Climate change is important for, and, ultimately, critical to, long-term human well-being and survival. While uncertainties exist about the detailed nature of climate impacts, impacts on infectious diseases are anticipated to pose significant, increasing, perceived and real threats. Our purpose in this chapter is to highlight the challenges in studying climate change impacts on infectious diseases. We suggest that new approaches will produce a less polarised and more productive discussion of climate change impacts on infectious diseases. Improved understanding of these impacts and further projected risks should increase the impetus for mitigation and facilitate the development of strategies for adaptation.

Detection

Climate change detection is the process of demonstrating that the climate has changed significantly, relative to natural climate variability, and that the change has persisted for several decades (Hegerl et al., 2006; Stott et al., 2010). In climate and health studies, detection is the process of demonstrating that significant changes in disease incidence or transmission risk (such as change in the distribution of vectors) are congruous with demonstrated climate change in space and time. Correlation must be supported with evidence for climate sensitivity of the agents, vectors and hosts of the disease (Kovats et al., 2001).

Climate change has heterogeneous impacts on infectious disease transmission, due to regional differences in the extent of warming, exposure to ambient conditions during the life cycle of infectious agents and the interaction between climate and other factors that affect incidence. The detection of climate change effects on infectious diseases is governed by the interaction between extrinsic and intrinsic biological factors[1] and the role of social conditions (Weiss and McMichael, 2004). Change in incidence will occur when environmental conditions reach or exceed the thermal and moisture tolerances of diseases. For example, rising temperatures have led to the altitudinal expansion of malaria in the East African Highlands (Pascual et al., 2006; Alonso et al., 2010), yet prolonged drought is

1 Extrinsic factors, including temperature, water availability, soil structure, pH and sunlight, determine the favourability of the environmental conditions that influence the development and reproductive rates of the agents, vectors and hosts of infectious diseases. Intrinsic factors include ecological regulation of the agent, vector and host populations; for example, the availability of food, water and breeding sites limit maximum population size.

associated with the contraction of the malaria transmission range in the Sahel (Mouchet et al., 1996). As incidence increases, intrinsic biological factors, including herd immunity, limit transmission. Conversely, range contractions may lead to reduced population immunity over time if endemic transmission ceases, which leaves populations vulnerable to infrequent epidemics (Bangs and Subianto, 1999). Table 25.1 presents a schematic to highlight how extrinsic climate influences and intrinsic saturation effects may interact to alter infectious disease transmission under a changing climate, using the example of herd immunity.

Table 25.1 Interaction between extrinsic climate influences and intrinsic herd immunity (saturation) effects.

	Potential effects of warming on infectious disease incidence	
Climate context[a]	Low herd immunity (epidemic transmission)	High herd immunity (endemic transmission)
Cool climate + warming	Transmission thresholds reached, virgin soil epidemics may occur	Minimal increased incidence, endemic transmission maintained
Warm climate + warming	Larger epidemics, increased duration of epidemic season endemic transmission	Minimal increased incidence, endemic transmission maintained
Hot climate + warming	Transmission thresholds exceeded. Partial or full range contraction may occur, with risk of infrequent epidemics	Partial or full range contraction of host or disease, with subsequent decrease in immunity, leaving population at risk of epidemics

[a] Cool, warm and hot climate defined with respect to the thermal tolerances of the disease agent, vector or host; for example, much of Europe may become a 'hot' climate for TBE (Randolph, 2004). Regions where high herd immunity prevents increased incidence may nonetheless experience an increased abundance of vector/host populations. This may make long-term control or eradication efforts substantially more difficult.

Source: Authors' work.

Climate-sensitive diseases with high incidence, due to short duration of immunity (such as malaria and cholera), are particularly likely to alter in incidence consequent upon climate change (Dobson, 2009). Similarly, incidence changes in infectious diseases that have short incubation periods and epidemic transmission will be more readily detectable than diseases with long incubation periods and/or endemic transmission, such as lymphatic filariasis (Gage et al., 2008).

In contrast, the provision of health services, sanitation and other public health strategies may reduce disease transmission, and these non-climate societal factors may mask the effect of climate change. In this case, climate change potentiates transmission, but no change in incidence is currently detectable. However, if a decline in the quality of health service provision occurs, then climate change impacts may become apparent over a relatively short period. Therefore, when discussing climate change influences on infectious diseases, we need to be aware of the difference between climate change influences and our ability to detect this influence, which may be masked by improvements in health service delivery. Analysis of malaria in 27 African countries demonstrates that climate change has heterogeneous observable impacts on malaria incidence against diverse economic backgrounds (Egbendewe-Mondzozo et al., 2011). The finding that TBE in endemic regions of Europe has not responded consistently to climate change (Sumilo et al., 2007) may nonetheless be an expected *observable* impact of climate change due to interactions between biological factors and social conditions.

Assuming climate change impacts on infectious diseases are most likely to be observed where extrinsic factors are a dominant influence on disease, the most likely types of changes to infectious diseases to be observed under climate change include:

- Range shifts: spatial changes in the incidence of infectious diseases are most likely to occur at the edge of currently known geographical ranges, where unstable epidemic transmission occurs and conditions may be marginal for transmission (Chaves and Koenraadt, 2010).
- Seasonal shifts: climate change may induce changes in the duration of the transmission season.
- Changes in transmission intensity: regions that currently experience epidemic transmission may shift to endemic transmission.

Scale Effects

To correlate regional anthropogenic warming with changes in infectious diseases, a minimum of 20 years of data is required, preferably 50 years (Hegerl et al., 2006). As the climate is currently unstable, attempts to detect a statistically significant warming trend in conjunction with changes in disease incidence need to be updated regularly (Stott et al., 2010).

The spatial scale of climate and disease data has also been shown to be critical for detecting climate change impacts on infectious diseases. Continental-scale maps and indices of malaria transmission risk are too coarse to capture transmission dynamics at the margins of current distributions, where local malaria transmission can be maintained by small numbers of vectors and climate change, weather anomalies and diurnal temperature variations have a marked effect on transmission intensity (Pascual and Bouma, 2009; Paaijmans et al., 2010). The application of malaria suitability indices (developed for use at large spatial scales; Hay et al., 2002) has been criticised (Patz et al., 2002;

Pascual et al., 2006). Similarly, the use of global climate gridded data sets at coarse resolution for studies on regional climate change and malaria trends has been criticised (Patz et al., 2002; Omumbo et al., 2011). Global gridded climate data sets provide spatially interpolated climate data that are reliable at continental and global scales but not at regional scales, particularly in regions with steep climate gradients and sparse local meteorological stations that provide input data to the global climate models (Patz et al., 2002; Omumbo et al., 2011).

Threshold Effects

Non-stationarity such as threshold effects in time-series data adds further complexity. Non-stationarity describes shifts in the dominant influence on the periodicity of epidemic infectious diseases over time (Cazelles et al., 2005). The absence of a significant correlation between climate change and disease transmission over the full length of a time series may mask significant effects in discrete intervals within the time series, particularly when the largest outbreaks coincide with conditions that deviate substantially from the climate average. Rodo et al. (2002) demonstrated a strong correlation between cholera incidence and climate conditions during El Niño Southern Oscillation (ENSO) events at three- to four-year cycles, but weak correlation at other times. There may be thresholds at which major influences on transmission change from factors such as vector control, which may co-occur with environmental conditions that are suitable for transmission, to environmental conditions being dominant influences that overwhelm attempts to adapt to increased transmission. Existing studies may need to be re-evaluated using statistical methods that can detect the climate thresholds at which discernible impacts on infectious diseases occur, such as transient climate-disease couplings (Rodo et al., 2002).

Climate Change: Weak but Persistent Signal

A further difficulty in detection studies is assessing the importance of small, 'non-significant' climate trends. Tests of statistical significance do not reveal the biological importance of small trends in average climate conditions. Zhou et al. (2004) showed that although statistically significant temperature increases occurred for only three sites of seven across the East African Highlands, climate variability increased significantly in five of seven sites, and that increased climate variability correlated with the increased frequency of malaria epidemics. Furthermore, Pascual et al. (2006) showed that a 0.5°C increase in monthly average temperatures increased *Anopheles* mosquito abundance by 30–40 per cent in a mosquito simulation model. Given that Bouma (2003) reports a non-significant

0.5°C rise in minimum December and January temperatures in Madagascar (months predictive of malaria incidence in his statistical model), climate warming may need to be reconsidered as a contributing factor to malaria resurgence in highland provinces of Madagascar. Further complexity is introduced by the effect of diurnal temperature ranges; if small temperature increases occur in regions with cool mean temperatures (<18°C), then the effect of diurnal temperature variation has been demonstrated to increase substantially the potential for malaria transmission (Paaijmans et al., 2009, 2010).

Sampling Effects

Compounding the difficulty of identifying significant climate trends, several factors can increase the risk of false positive (chance) findings in the search for climate change impacts on infectious diseases. As the number of observers increases, it becomes increasingly likely that agents, vectors or hosts may be found outside the presumed range; however, this may reflect either an observation at the extreme end of a stable distribution or an observation within the true range assumed novel due to inaccurate existing data. Population growth can produce similar risks of false positive findings through the increased density of agents, vectors or hosts at the edge of the known distribution. Many published studies are the result of opportunistic surveillance of diseases with good baseline data and for which changes have already been noted, rather than systematic analysis of any positive, negative or neutral impacts of climate change on the incidence and range of climate-sensitive diseases, as has been done in ecology (Parmesan and Yohe, 2003). Surveillance for range shifts may minimise the confounding effects of non-climate factors within the known range.

Attribution

Attribution is 'the process of establishing the most likely causes for a detected change with some level of confidence' (Stott et al., 2010). Significant correlation between changes in disease incidence and regional climate change (i.e. detection) is not sufficient to attribute a causal relationship. Kovats et al. (2001) suggest that attribution would require a 'trend in disease over many years which is significantly correlated with a change in climate, but not with any other potential driving mechanism'. A rigorous definition of attribution would require establishing an unbiased, causal relationship between observed changes in infectious diseases and climate change *and* establishing that the observed climate change is anthropogenic in origin. However, there are considerable difficulties in achieving this standard in epidemiology. Changes in infectious diseases are reported at regional scales at which anthropogenic climate change may be difficult to detect above the level of natural variability, and also factors other than anthropogenic greenhouse gas emissions may influence regional climate trends (Stott et al., 2010).

The scientific consensus on anthropogenic global change emerged through the collation of thousands of observations from individual sites; the attribution of warming trends to anthropogenic influences at any one site would not be possible. Similarly, attribution cannot be demonstrated formally for any single study, or possibly even any single disease. The causal effects of climate change on infectious disease may become unambiguously apparent by conducting a systematic analysis of trends across diverse diseases and geographic regions. Uncertainty in attribution for individual studies does not prohibit achieving an acceptable level of confidence in attribution based on cumulative synthesis (Parmesan and Yohe, 2003). No meta-analysis has been published of the magnitude of range shifts or other changes in multiple infectious diseases due to climate change. As with analyses of the impacts of climate change on species ecology (Parmesan and Yohe, 2003), the most systematic method for assessing whether climate change is impacting infectious diseases is to assess whether the changes observed for diverse climate-sensitive infectious diseases are consistent with the predicted effects of climate change. This represents a departure from previous debates in the literature, particularly for TBE (Randolph, 2010), that have focused on the unique, especially entomological, characteristics of particular diseases rather than assessing whether climate change has similar distributional effects on a number of infectious diseases.

Full attribution of changes in infectious diseases to climate change requires:

- meteorological evidence of climate change at regional scales
- spatiotemporally correlated change in infectious disease frequencies
- evidence that other factors cannot account for all of the observed change.

A simpler alternative for the detection and attribution of climate change impacts, called consistency analysis, has been proposed in ecology (Parmesan and Yohe, 2003), and we suggest could also be applied to infectious diseases. Consistency analyses involve demonstrating a significant relationship between regional climate change and changes to infectious diseases that are not fully explained by other factors. Consistency analyses are strengthened considerably when similar effects are observed for several diseases in multiple regions. Few individual studies can demonstrate all aspects of a consistency analysis, though the work of Alonso et al. (2010) is a notable exception. The finding that warming in the East African Highlands accounts for approximately 40 per cent of the observed increase in malaria cases is a substantial contribution to the field (Alonso et al., 2010). It should be noted that authors disputing a correlation between climate change and malaria in the East African Highlands have not quantified other possible contributing factors to malaria resurgence at a regional scale. On a global scale, the impact of economic development on reducing the global malaria burden has been estimated (Gething et al., 2010), but this finding cannot explain local increases in malaria incidence.

A qualitative assessment of consistencies in the types of changes in infectious diseases observed under recent climate change may be a good starting point for analysis. An example of a qualitative assessment measure is 'sign switching' (Parmesan and Yohe, 2003). Range expansion along the warming margins of the current distribution and range contraction along the cooling margins has been defined as a diagnostic 'fingerprint' of climate change impacts on species distribution (Parmesan and Yohe, 2003) and is applicable to infectious diseases. Several studies documenting altitudinal and latitudinal range shifts for several diseases and their vectors have been discussed previously in this chapter. Temporal sign switching may be evident for malaria in the East African Highlands; malaria incidence increased in the East African Highlands in the 1940s–50s and from the 1970s onwards, but decreased in the 1960s (Malakooti et al., 1998), which is broadly consistent with 20th-century temperature trends. Rigorous analysis is required to test whether temperature trends explain apparent sign-switching variation in malaria incidence after controlling for other factors such as malaria control and demographic change. A consistency analysis would require demonstrating regional climate change in each of these instances, and also assessing the overall coherence of the changes. Coherence would emerge if the overall pattern of change were consistent with predictions under climate change, such as both altitudinal and latitudinal shifts (i.e. coherent direction of change) are observed for several diseases.

The feasibility of quantitative consistency analysis of the recent impacts of climate change on infectious diseases is limited by the relatively small number of studies that have been published, and the risk of publication bias. Numerical estimates of mean range shifts, changes in duration of transmission season or net changes in incidence are not yet possible, though a method for this type of assessment has been presented for natural systems (Parmesan and Yohe, 2003).

Future Work

We suggest that it is now possible to document systematically consistent changes in infectious diseases in response to climate change across diverse agents, vectors and hosts using consistency analysis, and that this is a more appropriate and informative approach than the usual disease-specific research. Detecting a climate change signal in global changes in infectious diseases' incidence will require interdisciplinary collaboration with common understanding of priority regions for human health. Targeted surveillance efforts, including geographical information system mapping and molecular surveillance, should be integrated with archival distribution records to establish baseline geographic distributions and to monitor change (Hoberg et al., 2008; Weaver et al., 2010). Multi-disease, multi-site studies that document infectious disease shifts that are consistent, neutral or inconsistent with the predicted effects of climate change should be prioritised, and the effect of climate change needs to be quantified relative to the effect of other factors.

Although full attribution of changes in infectious diseases to recent climate change may not yet be possible for most diseases, it is timely to move beyond polarised debates about whether climate or other influences dominate (Brisbois and Ali, 2010). The approaches discussed here may offer a way forward to improved methods for the detection and attribution of recent climate change effects on infectious diseases, which will narrow uncertainty boundaries for projections of future transmission under climate change.

References

Alonso, D., Bouma, M.J. & Pascual, M. 2010. Epidemic malaria and warmer temperatures in recent decades in an East African highland. *Proceedings of the Royal Society B: Biological Sciences* 278, 1661–9.

Bangs, M.J. & Subianto, D.B. 1999. El Niño and associated outbreaks of severe malaria in highland populations in Irian Jaya, Indonesia: a review and epidemiological perspective. *The Southeast Asian Journal of Tropical Medicine and Public Health* 30, 608–19.

Béguin, A., Hales, S., Rocklöv, J., Åström, C., Louis, V.R. & Sauerborn, R. 2011. The opposing effects of climate change and socio-economic development on the global distribution of malaria. *Global Environmental Change* 21, 1209–14.

Bouma, M.J. 2003. Methodological problems and amendments to demonstrate effects of temperature on the epidemiology of malaria. A new perspective on the highland epidemics in Madagascar, 1972–1989. *Transactions of the Royal Society of Tropical Medicine and Hygiene* 97, 133–9.

Brisbois, B.W. & Ali, S.H. 2010. Climate change, vector-borne disease and interdisciplinary research: social science perspectives on an environment and health controversy. *EcoHealth* 7, 425–38.

Cazelles, B., Chavez, M., McMichael, A.J. & Hales, S. 2005. Nonstationary influence of El Niño on the synchronous dengue epidemics in Thailand. *PLoS Medicine* 2, e106.

Chaves, L.F. & Koenraadt, C.J.M. 2010. Climate change and highland malaria: fresh air for a hot debate. *The Quarterly Review of Biology* 85, 27–55.

Costello, A., Abbas, M., Allen, A., Ball, S., Bell, S., Bellamy, R., et al. 2009. Managing the health effects of climate change. *The Lancet* 373, 1693–733.

Daniel, M., Danielová, V., Kříž, B., Jirsa, A. & Nožička, J. 2003. Shift of the tick *Ixodes ricinus* and tick-borne encephalitis to higher altitudes in Central Europe. *European Journal of Clinical Microbiology and Infectious Diseases* 22, 327–8.

Danielová, V., Rudenko, N., Daniel, M., Holubová, J., Materna, J., Golovchenko, M., et al. 2006. Extension of *Ixodes ricinus* ticks and agents of tick-borne diseases to mountain areas in the Czech Republic. *International Journal of Medical Microbiology* 296, 48–53.

Dobson, A. 2009. Climate variability, global change, immunity, and the dynamics of infectious diseases. *Ecology* 90, 920–7.

Egbendewe-Mondzozo, A., Musumba, M., McCarl, B.A. & Wu, X. 2011. Climate change and vector-borne diseases: an economic impact analysis of malaria in Africa. *International Journal of Environmental Research and Public Health* 8, 913–30.

Gage, K.L., Burkot, T.R., Eisen, R.J. & Hayes, E.B. 2008. Climate and vectorborne diseases. *American Journal of Preventive Medicine* 35, 436–50.

Gething, P.W., Smith, D.L., Patil, A.P., Tatem, A.J., Snow, R.W. & Hay, S.I. 2010. Climate change and the global malaria recession. *Nature* 465, 342–5.

Hay, S.I., Cox, J., Rogers, D.J., Randolph, S.E., Stern, D.I., Shanks, G.D., et al. 2002. Climate change and the resurgence of malaria in the East African highlands. *Nature* 415, 905–9.

Hegerl, G.C., Karl, T.R., Allen, M., Bindoff, N.L., Gillett, N., Karoly, D., et al. 2006. Climate change detection and attribution: beyond mean temperature signals. *Journal of Climate* 19, 5058–77.

Hoberg, E.P., Polley, L., Jenkins, E.J., Kutz, S.J., Veitch, A.M. & Elkin, B.T. 2008. Integrated approaches and empirical models for investigation of parasitic diseases in northern wildlife. *Emerging Infectious Diseases* 14, 10–17.

Hunter, P.R. 2003. Climate change and waterborne and vector-borne disease. *Journal of Applied Microbiology* 94, 37–46.

Kovats, R.S., Campbell-Lendrum, D.H., McMichel, A.J., Woodward, A. & Cox, J.S.H. 2001. Early effects of climate change: do they include changes in vector-borne disease? *Philosophical Transactions of the Royal Society of London. Series B: Biological Sciences* 356, 1057–68.

Lindgren, E. & Gustafson, R. 2001. Tick-borne encephalitis in Sweden and climate change. *The Lancet* 358, 16–18.

Lindgren, E., Talleklint, L. & Polfeldt, T. 2000. Impact of climatic change on the northern latitude limit and population density of the disease-transmitting European tick *Ixodes ricinus*. *Environmental Health Perspectives* 108, 119–23.

Lipp, E.K., Huq, A. & Colwell, R.R. 2002. Effects of global climate on infectious disease: the cholera model. *Clinical Microbiological Reviews* 15, 757–70.

Malakooti, M.A., Biomndo, K. & Shanks, G.D. 1998. Reemergence of epidemic malaria in the highlands of western Kenya. *Emerging Infectious Diseases* 4, 671–6.

Mouchet, J., Faye, O., Julvez, J. & Manguin, S. 1996. Drought and malaria retreat in the Sahel, West Africa. *The Lancet* 348, 1735–6.

Omumbo, J., Lyon, B., Waweru, S., Connor, S. & Thomson, M. 2011. Raised temperatures over the Kericho tea estates: revisiting the climate in the East African highlands malaria debate. *Malaria Journal* 10, 12, doi: 10:12 doi:10.1186/1475-2875-10-12.

Paaijmans, K.P., Read, A.F. & Thomas, M.B. 2009. Understanding the link between malaria risk and climate. *Proceedings of the National Academy of Sciences (USA)* 106, 13844–9.

Paaijmans, K.P., Blanford, S., Bell, A.S., Blanford, J.I., Read, A.F. & Thomas, M.B. 2010. Influence of climate on malaria transmission depends on daily temperature variation. *Proceedings of the National Academy of Sciences (USA)* 107, 15135–9.

Parmesan, C. & Yohe, G. 2003. A globally coherent fingerprint of climate change impacts across natural systems. *Nature* 421, 37–42.

Pascual, M. & Bouma, M.J. 2009. Do rising temperatures matter. *Ecology* 90, 906–12.

Pascual, M., Ahumada, J.A., Chaves, L.F., Rodó, X. & Bouma, M. 2006. Malaria resurgence in the East African highlands: temperature trends revisited. *Proceedings of the National Academy of Sciences (USA)* 103, 5829–34.

Patz, J.A., Hulme, M., Rosenzweig, C., Mitchell, T.D., Goldberg, R.A., Githeko, A.K., et al. 2002. Climate change (communication arising): regional warming and malaria resurgence. *Nature* 420, 627–8.

Randolph, S.E. 2004. Evidence that climate change has caused 'emergence' of tick-borne diseases in Europe? *International Journal of Medical Microbiology Supplements* 293, 5–15.

Randolph, S.E. 2010. To what extent has climate change contributed to the recent epidemiology of tick-borne diseases? *Veterinary Parasitology* 167, 92–4.

Rodo, X., Pascual, M., Fuchs, G. & Faruque, A.S. 2002. ENSO and cholera: a nonstationary link related to climate change? *Proceedings of the National Academy of Sciences (USA)* 99, 12901–6.

Shanks, G.D., Hay, S.I., Stern, D.I., Biomndo, K. & Snow, R.W. 2002. Meteorologic influences on *Plasmodium falciparum* malaria in the Highland Tea Estates of Kericho, Western Kenya. *Emerging Infectious Diseases* 8, 1404–8.

Stott, P.A., Gillett, N.P., Hegerl, G.C., Karoly, D.J., Stone, D.A., Zhang, X., et al. 2010. Detection and attribution of climate change: a regional perspective. *Wiley Interdisciplinary Reviews: Climate Change* 1, 192–211.

Sumilo, D., Asokliene, L., Bormane, A., Vasilenko, V., Golovljova, I. & Randolph, S.E. 2007. Climate change cannot explain the upsurge of tick-borne encephalitis in the Baltics. *PLoS ONE* 2, e500.

Tirado, M.C., Clarke, R., Jaykus, L.A., McQuatters-Gollop, A. & Frank, J.M. 2010. Climate change and food safety: a review. *Food Research International* 43, 1745–65.

Weaver, H.J., Hawdon, J.M. & Hoberg, E.P. 2010. Soil-transmitted helminthiases: implications of climate change and human behavior. *Trends in Parasitology* 26, 574–81.

Weiss, R.A. & McMichael, A.J. 2004. Social and environmental risk factors in the emergence of infectious diseases. *Nature Medicine* 10, S70–S76.

Zhou, G., Minakawa, N., Githeko, A.K. & Yan, G. 2004. Association between climate variability and malaria epidemics in the East African highlands. *Proceedings of the National Academy of Sciences (USA)* 101, 2375–80.

26

PATTERNS OF ECOLOGICAL CHANGE AND EMERGING INFECTIOUS DISEASE IN THE AUSTRALASIAN REGION

RO MCFARLANE

Abstract

An unusually rapid and widespread increase in apparently new and changing infectious diseases has occurred globally over the past four decades. This has also been a time of accelerated global ecological change. Associations between the two phenomena are unclear: emerging infectious diseases (EIDs) are reported more frequently in wealthy countries, with greater capacity for resources for surveillance and detection than less affluent centres, even though the latter are often undergoing accelerated socioecological change. Here, a series of transdisciplinary studies is reviewed that test the hypothesis that specific ecological change accounts for a significant component of the rise in EIDs in the Australasian region. Amongst the range of mechanisms, factors such as wildlife adaptation to changing landscapes and selection for antimicrobial resistance appear to be of major significance. However, exploring multi-scale complex relationships is a challenge to epidemiology. The importance of framing the scale of relationships and limitations of available data are discussed. Despite obstacles, insight into approaches to mitigating disease risk at a landscape level is expanding.

Introduction – Global Patterns, Global Questions

The past four decades have seen an unusually rapid and widespread increase in apparently new and changing infectious diseases in humans, domesticated animals, wildlife and plants. Some 335 novel or re-emerging infectious diseases of humans have been described since the 1940s (Jones et al., 2008). The majority of these 'emerging infectious diseases' (EIDs) – defined as infectious diseases that are novel or expanding in pathogenicity and range (Morse, 1995) – have occurred since the 1970s. The increase in EIDs has coincided with an acceleration of anthropogenic ecological change, defined as a change in interactions among living organisms with each other and with their environments, driven by the increasing global human population. Links between the two phenomena have been postulated (McMichael, 2004).

The rise in EIDs has been linked broadly to changing ecosystems; climate and weather; economic development and land use; human demographics and behaviour; international travel and commerce; poverty and social inequality; breakdown in public health measures; lack of political will; intent to harm (such as bioterrorism); and the impacts of new technologies and industries (Smolinski et al., 2003). This multitude of potential influences on pathogen, vector and host(s) has also been discussed in terms of complex social–ecological systems (Wilcox and Colwell, 2005). The socioecological system perspective on disease causation reinforces a broader discussion of anthropogenic ecological change as systemic health risk (e.g. McMichael and Wilcox, 2009). Understanding the role of ecological change poses many challenges for epidemiology. Many of the speculated relationships are not easily tested. Available ecological information may describe a dynamic of interest at a scale other than that at which disease is understood, and multiple influences may act and interact across multiple scales. This chapter describes our approach to assembling a robust evidence base to understand the role of ecological change in EIDs of the Australasian region. By framing issues at appropriate scales and exploring relationships where data are available, we hope to add complexity and insight progressively.

Reviews of EIDs alert us to two major areas of ecological change resulting in new human–pathogen interactions. Approximately 20 per cent of global (human) EIDs are antimicrobial-resistant (AMR) pathogens and 75 per cent are zoonoses, most from wildlife, particularly wild mammals (Taylor et al., 2001; Jones et al., 2008). A modest overlap between these two groupings also exists. The small remainder includes environmental pathogens, opportunistic pathogens (such as those affecting immunocompromised individuals) and other less easily grouped diseases. These patterns potentially tell us much about our changing ecological impact.

Human influence on the selection of AMR is complex, but a direct relationship is clear. Prescriptions of antibiotics began in the 1930s and AMR was recognised shortly thereafter, steadily increasing until now, where multidrug-resistant organisms are common and widespread, including in many intensive livestock production systems (Levy and Marshall, 2004). Belatedly, research has turned to understanding the role of antibiotics and AMR in the natural systems in which they evolved. We are also only beginning to understand the lability and significance of environmental contamination with human and animal drug-resistant organisms (Finley et al., 2013). Similarly, there are many issues surrounding the rise in anti-fungal, malarial, parasitic and viral resistance, and in vectorcidal resistance following their widespread use.

The relationship between the rise in (wildlife) zoonoses and anthropogenic ecological change is less obvious. The traditional view of zoonotic and crowd diseases arising from ancient humanity's shift to densely populated agrarian settlements with domesticated animals (e.g. McNeill, 1976) sheds little light on the rise, now, of zoonotic pathogens of wild animals. There is a reported positive association between high mammal diversity, human density and zoonotic infectious diseases of wildlife origin (Jones et al., 2008; Morand et al., 2014), but it is difficult to undertake detailed global assessments. Data on EID emergence are usually more comprehensive in developed temperate regions, as are data on many other potential explanatory variables (such as the role of ecological and sociodemographic parameters).

Exploring the importance of ecological change as a driver of EIDs is complicated by many factors. Advances in diagnostic technology, surveillance, fundability of research and even digital search engines have had (incompletely quantified) influence on the number of EIDs reported. According to one study, reporting of EIDs peaked in the 1980s (once the underlying reporting bias for papers from less-developed countries (LDCs) was addressed). This was a decade associated with taxonomical reclassification and diagnosis of novel co-infections with HIV/AIDS (Jones et al., 2008).

The rise in numbers of EIDs is not necessarily accompanied by an increase in the burden of disease. HIV/AIDS is unique in its combined novelty, significance and the proliferation of novel co-infections recognised during and since the 1980s. Many other EIDs are of minor or only potential population health importance, or of importance primarily for their scientific novelty, a fact that undermines research on novel EIDs in countries struggling to address other major health impacts (Butler, 2012). Many of the most important human EIDs (e.g. multi-drug-resistant tuberculosis and malaria) are old scourges with new twists. HIV/AIDS also illustrates the lag period that may follow ecological changes, and the spatially and temporally dispersed social changes that may result in infectious disease emergence. For this disease, the events that led to ancestral virus spilling from non-human primates to humans appear to have occurred in the early 20th century (or perhaps even prior to this) (Sharp et al., 2001). Social and demographic changes in the late 20th century gave rise to a global pandemic.

Even as a signal of ecological change, human EIDs only tell part of the story. EIDs of plants and animals not involved in human disease transmission receive much less research and reporting effort, but are also a feature of recent decades. Wheat rust Ug99, white spot baculovirus syndrome of shrimp and porcine respiratory and reproductive syndrome are examples of EIDs that have arisen from, and caused collapse in, intensively produced human food production (Singh et al., 2011; Wang et al., 2006; Zhou et al., 2008). Intensive livestock production has proven to be a highly effective amplifier of zoonotic disease (Liverani et al., 2013). Infectious diseases of wildlife are also emerging in vulnerable species, degraded ecosystems and where least expected. The pandemic amphibian chytridiomycosis is responsible for multiple species extinctions even in pristine habitats; Tasmanian Devil Facial Tumour has decimated its marsupial carnivore host, a species not long ago regarded as a pest. Although there has been a vigorous literature on EIDs as a global phenomenon in a changing world, our understanding is biased to one host (humans) and to well-resourced developed countries.

Patterns of EIDs in the Australasian Region

To examine the hypothesis that ecological change accounts for a substantial component of the rise in zoonotic EIDs, a series of transdisciplinary studies based on the Australasian region were designed by the author under the doctoral supervision of Professors Tony McMichael and Adrian Sleigh and Dr Peter Black (McFarlane et al., 2011, 2012, 2013, 2014). These studies reflected Tony's support for research that explored the awkward, important issues, and for epidemiology that – in an inventive and insightful way – sought to address these challenges. The postulated drivers of EIDs examined in these studies have a history and forward trajectory, and cannot be considered in isolation from other processes. In this way, each study contributed detail to the complex systems perspective of socioecological change as a health risk that Tony's work brought to global research.

The EID literature for Australasia is dominated by reports published by the sparsely populated, developed country, Australia. The region also includes smaller, developed New Zealand and the developing Melanesian nations. This region adjoins that of the adjacent, densely populated, rapidly developing Southeast Asia and East Asia to its north, which have been the origin of numerous EIDs of global concern, including highly pathogenic avian influenza (H1N1) of poultry origin and SARS (severe acute respiratory syndrome) coronavirus and Nipah viruses of bat origin. These adjoining regions have important social and ecological influences on Australasia. In Australia, other bat-borne viruses and zoonotic arboviruses, including the southern expansion of Japanese Encephalitis Virus, are of concern (Mackenzie, 2001).

A systematic literature review of the databases Scopus, CABI and Web of Science for 1973–2010, using search terms 'emerging infectious disease(s)' and 'emerging communicable diseases(s)' of humans and animals by country (25) and region, identified a large number of articles (Australasia (n = 192), Southeast Asia (n = 257) and East Asia (n = 491)). China, Japan, Australia, Hong Kong and Taiwan were the subject of >100 papers each; South Korea, Indonesia, Thailand, Malaysia, Singapore, New Zealand and Vietnam were the subject of 16–99 papers; the remaining countries featured in <16 papers. Four diseases were the topic of large numbers of articles: SARS coronavirus (n = 125), highly pathogenic avian influenza (n = 49), amphibian chytridiomycosis (n = 20) and HIV/AIDS (n = 18). Across the regions, interest in zoonoses was high. However, ecological factors were rarely discussed as the primary focus of an EID article (n = 33).

A total of 104 emerging or re-emerging human diseases were reported in the reviewed literature (McFarlane et al., 2012; Morand et al., 2014). Zoonotic diseases (n = 70) accounted for 67 per cent of the total of these diseases, and 63 per cent of these were zoonoses of wildlife origin (n = 44). AMR (n = 14) and environmental pathogens (n = 9) accounted for 14 per cent and 9 per cent of EIDs, respectively. There were also 53 EIDs of livestock and 23 EIDs of wildlife reported. The collective Asian–Australasian region contains one-third of the human population and approximately one-third of globally reported human EIDs (Jones et al., 2008).

In Australia, the country with the largest EID literature in the region, 90 diseases (59 diseases of humans, of which 30 were zoonoses; 12 diseases of domestic animals; 18 diseases of terrestrial wildlife) meet the criteria for emerging or re-emerging diseases in the interval 1973–2010 (McFarlane et al., 2013). Of the human diseases, 51 per cent are zoonotic (66 per cent of these from wildlife), 15 per cent are classified as environmental pathogens and 10 per cent are AMR pathogens. Non-wildlife zoonoses (n = 10) include food-borne disease, AMR and canine pathogens. The majority of the remainder of human EIDs are re-emerging and/or re-identified viruses. A full list is available as online supplementary material (McFarlane et al., 2013).

The large volume of EID literature from Australia, including that of animal disease, reflects Australia's capacity to research and report EIDs. The small number of EIDs reported in the rest of Australasia – and in proportion to the population in Southeast Asia and East Asia – make intra- and interregional comparisons problematical. Reporting bias appears to be acting strongly against those countries to the east and north of Australia where fewer EIDs (and hence available data) have been reported and where socioecological change is occurring rapidly and extensively.

EIDs identified through the literature review were examined further with reference to ecological change. First, we examined the characteristics of the wildlife hosts of zoonotic EIDs identified from the multi-region literature review to gain insight into changing human–animal relationships. Second, we looked at the patterns of infectious disease emergence and ecological change within Australia's own tumultuous post-colonisation history. Third, we looked in detail at a particular Australian zoonosis, Hendra virus disease, thus providing the opportunity to study ecological drivers at both the broad and finer scales.

Biodiversity Change, Synanthropy and Zoonotic Disease in the Asian–Australasian Regions

In the first study, we found that the identified (mammalian) hosts of emerging zoonoses of wildlife origin across the Australasian–Asian regions were proportionate in terms of their taxonomic distribution to total mammals in the study region, as reported by the International Union for the Conservation of Nature (IUCN, 2012). However, wildlife hosts were 15 times more likely (OR = 15.02; 95 per cent CI 5.87, 38.41) to be associated ecologically with humans and human-modified environments (i.e. to be synanthropic) than to be restricted to intact natural habitat (McFarlane et al., 2012). These wildlife hosts were also more likely (relative to non-host species) to be species classified as being at little or no conservation risk. While some hosts were also species consumed as bushmeat, or were encountered at the leading edge of natural vegetation clearances, hosts were found overwhelmingly to be species that could exploit anthropogenic ecological change.

The relationship between synanthropy and EID hosts can be understood with reference to biodiversity change in the ecologically diverse Asian–Australasian regions. Approximately one-third of global terrestrial mammal species (n = 1,823) occur here: about one-quarter of these utilise human modified environments (the trait used to define synanthropic species in our study). The majority of hosts are not at conservation risk, and many are classified as pest and invasive species (IUCN, 2012). Almost half of the total 1,823 species are in a conservation risk category and threatened from extensive land clearing, hunting, the impact of invasive species or extreme weather events or climate (IUCN, 2012). Anthropogenic ecological change is taking a heavy toll on many species, but is selecting inadvertently for those that can live with people or exploit human environments. By this process, human exposure to synanthropic species, their numbers and their pathogens may be increased.

Synanthropy is a characteristic of a diverse range of species. For example, in Australia some 30 species of bats, 22 species of the largest marsupial order (kangaroos, possums, etc) and less than 10 species each of rodents, insectivorous marsupials, bandicoots, introduced hoofed mammals, carnivores, rabbits and hares make their homes in human-modified environments. Of these, some 20 species of bats and 0–5 species in the other orders find useful resources in urban environments.

The predominance of bats in urban environments is observed in (all) other regions globally – often greater in diversity than synanthropic rodents by an order of magnitude (IUCN, 2012). This is of particular interest because of the unforeseen emergence of numerous EIDs from bats in the past two decades. Nipah virus emerged in Malaysia in 1999 in a piggery where mangoes were co-produced, with the fruit crop providing a ready food source for local fruit bats (Johara et al., 2001). The principle host bat species commonly roosts and feeds in mainland orchards and coconut palm groves in preference to remnant native forest (IUCN, 2012). SARS coronavirus emerged from insectivorous horseshoe bats in southern China in 2003 after amplification in farmed civet cats, and possibly racoon dogs. These bats (and carnivores) are sold in local wet markets, but they are also synanthropic species. Horseshoe bats roost in the artificial caves created by roadworks, and multiple spillovers back and forth to domestic animals have been demonstrated prior to 2003 (Lau et al., 2010).

Elsewhere, synanthropic rodents and shrews have emerged as hosts of novel pathogens (e.g. hantaviruses), or with other novel hosts in new environments as hosts of re-emerging diseases (e.g. alveolar echinococcosis, leptospirosis, cutaneous leishmaniasis). Primate sources of 'monkey malaria' (Plasmodium knowlesi), Mi Tri and Zika viruses and the zoonotic reservoir of Chikungunya virus in Southeast Asia are macaques, particularly the highly synanthropic long-tailed macaques in the south and rhesus monkeys in the north (McFarlane et al., 2012).

Change in the diversity and number of synanthropic wildlife over time is difficult to assess, potentially limiting this as an explanation of how anthropogenic ecological change contributes to the rise in wildlife EIDs. However, global land transformation occurred very slowly from the first agricultural settlements some 10,000 years ago until its acceleration in the 20th century. The proportion of global (ice-free) land remaining in its natural state is now estimated to be 22 per cent (two-thirds of this in cold and dry regions with low productivity), having passed the 50 per cent mark (half natural, half human modified) some time in the first half of the 20th century (Ellis, 2011). Land transformation has continued to accelerate, and it is in the latter part of the 20th century that the pressure has been greatest on wild species to adapt to human environments.

Even so, ecological change has not occurred uniformly across the globe. Certainly, in Australia, there was no urban or Western-style agricultural land use, or associated synanthropic wildlife (with the exception of the dingo), before European colonisers displaced its predominantly hunter–gatherer Indigenous inhabitants over 225 years ago (McFarlane et al., 2013).

Recent Patterns of Development and Disease in Australia

The second study looked at the evidence for a relationship between ecological change and EIDs within (data-rich) Australia. In this country, the interval of post-hunter–gatherer land-use change is shorter and better documented than most other regions, and it is also an island continent. Since colonisation in 1788, Australia has lost approximately 50 per cent of its forest and woodland cover, with much of the rest degraded (Bradshaw, 2012). Its mammals, primarily highly endemic marsupials, experienced the highest extinction rate in the developed world. Agricultural and pastoral enterprises now account for 61 per cent of land use, and there is an extensive mining sector. The majority (87 per cent) of the population of 23 million is concentrated in urban centres that are located predominantly in the high-rainfall, biodiverse coastal regions.

Multiple emergences of indigenous zoonotic and vector-borne diseases have occurred after dramatic intervals of natural vegetation removal in the past, and in the recent decades that define EIDs, in Australia (see McFarlane et al., 2013, for full details, figures and references). Loss of natural habitat through land-use change affects zoonotic disease transmission by changing the density or abundance of disease-related organisms; the species composition of communities; the life cycle of vectors or pathogens; exposure pathways or by selection pressure on organisms that results in increased pathogen virulence (Myers and Patz, 2009). As land-use change intensifies and natural elements and processes are replaced by industrial food production and urban development – a major transition of the late 20th century in Australia, as elsewhere – do we see an increased rate of infectious disease emergence?

Our study found a positive temporally sequenced and biologically plausible association with land-use change (the majority with the extreme transitions) for approximately 22 per cent of Australian EIDs reported in the literature since 1970 (McFarlane et al., 2013). However, it is difficult to establish land-use change–EID causality beyond this or to quantify attribution for most diseases, and certainly not at a multi-disease level. Many processes are too complex or distally acting to demonstrate specificity, consistency or biological gradient, if indeed these metrics are relevant. For some diseases, the effect of land-use change may be incremental and reversible. For environmental pathogens such as *Burkholderia pseudomallei* (the cause of melioidosis) or *Mycobacterium ulcerans* (the cause of Buruli ulcer), the relationships between land-use change and disease emergence may be relatively straightforward. However, extreme stages of land-use change lead to state shifts in ecological communities that are irreversible. This makes many land-use change–EID effects one way and limits traditional analyses.

A striking example of ecological transformation relates to the increasing urbanisation of the four flying fox (fruit bat) species of the Australian mainland and the emergence of zoonotic Hendra virus, Australian bat lyssavirus (ABLV) and Menangle virus. All four bat species have been affected by natural vegetation clearing and have increased their reliance on vegetation in urban and peri-urban coastal areas. However, the relationships between habitat loss, urbanisation and disease emergence are incompletely understood, and are complicated further by the southern range extension (and contraction) of two species. Hendra, ABLV and Menangle viruses have been present in flying foxes prior to their emergence as human and animal disease and are endemic across their hosts' geographic ranges, an area collectively larger than that in which the diseases have been observed.

For Hendra virus disease, the relatively small number of geographically dispersed outbreaks since 1994 (most of the c.50 outbreaks have occurred since 2011) have challenged analysis of the ecological drivers of emergence. A temporal and spatial association between recent large-scale loss of habitat and Hendra emergence, most frequently in Queensland, can be demonstrated at a coarse scale (Bradshaw, 2012; McFarlane, 2013). However, temporally and geographically proximal, quantifiable environmental factors in local Hendra emergence have not been demonstrated beyond the proximity of horses to flying fox camps and seasonality at higher latitudes (McFarlane et al., 2011). The effect of urbanisation on virus dynamics has been modelled for Hendra virus and can explain periodic outbreaks of that disease (Plowright et al., 2011). Incorporating hypotheses from multiple disciplines including the ecological factors discussed here (and others, including viral factors, bat ecology, horse management) at the multiple scales relevant to each variable is now being undertaken to build the complex picture of why this disease has emerged (Plowright et al., 2015).

Future Risks and Research

Our understanding of ecological change and EIDs is scarcely beyond the conceptual mapping stage at this time. Meta-analyses risk simplifying risk factors, and data are often poor where ecological change is most dramatic. Other large-scale processes are also potentially important. Social factors within the Australasian–Asian region that have not been discussed here include the rising human population; the rapidly increasing wealth, resource and consumer demands of developing economies; the growth in intensive animal production systems (growth in pig, poultry and aquaculture production has been globally significant in East and Southeast Asia in recent decades; Thornton, 2010); patterns of human and livestock movement; changing diets; and improvements and failures in diagnostic, reporting and biosecurity measures.

Conceptual mapping of causal EID relationships is valuable by itself and gives insights into future risk. The rising human population, resource demand and the limited availability of new agricultural land is driving the intensification of land use. A dominant, simplified human ecosystem with large numbers of few species (dominated by humans, domestic animals, invasive and synanthropic wildlife) must affect the nature and patterns of zoonotic disease outbreaks. Livestock already make up a staggering 20 per cent of terrestrial animal biomass, 85 per cent of which is pig and poultry, increasingly within intensive production systems (Steinfeld et al., 2006; FAO, 2011). Zoonotic diseases are predicted to remain a substantial burden for urban and subsistence livestock keepers and intensive production units with inadequate biosecurity (Steinfeld et al., 2008; Grace et al., 2012).

It is difficult to predict the future importance of wildlife as hosts of EIDs. Ongoing loss of biodiverse equatorial forests is a potential source of future novel zoonotic risk, but we are currently close to the limit of remaining unconverted productive land outside these rainforest zones (Ellis, 2011). New opportunities for wildlife pathogen amplification may arise as new centres of intensive livestock production develop (e.g. in Africa) (Butler and McFarlane, 2011). Research continues to focus on the role of biodiversity to generate and/or regulate zoonotic disease emergence. However, this must take into account the clumped spatial distribution of biodiversity and the majority, simplified, human-dominated ecosystems in which this is embedded. Climate change may reshuffle vectors, wildlife, agriculture and people so that new opportunities for wildlife zoonoses emerge or reduce population immunity to existing risks (McMichael et al., 2006). It is also possible that the observed rise in EIDs of wildlife origin is a transient phenomenon marking the end stages of wildlife displacement and demise.

Widespread AMR, reduced investment in developing new antimicrobials and ever larger numbers of humans with impaired immune systems (due to poor nutrition and chronic diseases such as HIV/AIDS) are likely to ensure ongoing opportunities for AMR EIDs. Contamination of communities, water, soil and wildlife with large numbers of AMR organisms also impedes the control of emerging pathogens. Inadvertent selection of vectorcidal resistance and the creation of new niches for vectors or environmentally sourced microbes (such as urban wetlands or the translocation to air-conditioning systems of pond-dwelling Legionella and their symbiotic amoeba) are simple reminders of the extent to which we can drive disease emergence through change in human environments.

In a general sense, continued change in the environment and its micro- and macroorganisms will result in continued change in infectious disease. Although many disease mechanisms are relatively specific and difficult to use for generalised predictions, existing research is suggesting approaches to mitigating risk. For example, some cross-species movement and mutations of the influenza virus may be limited by avoiding the proximity of intensive pig and poultry farms, human population centres and wetlands of importance to (internationally) migrating wildfowl. Proper treatment of biological waste and its containment may also control the movement of antibiotic resistance by migratory waterfowl from contaminated wetlands (Cole et al., 2005). Risk of Hendra virus infection diminishes with reduced spatial overlap of horses with flying foxes (McFarlane et al., 2011). Even in the absence of a unified understanding of the role of ecological change in disease emergence, there is the opportunity to research, cost and communicate adaptive management strategies for safer microbial environments.

Conclusion

Concurrent, accelerated socioecological change may account for a significant component of the rise in EIDs observed globally and locally. Assessing these associations is impeded by an uneven research effort across countries of different wealth and history of ecological disruption. A series of transdisciplinary studies has explored the relationships between land use, biotic change and EIDs in the Australasian region. Zoonoses, particularly those of wild mammalian origin, are the largest group of EIDs. Organisms with antimicrobial resistance and those of environmental origin are also major causes of disease. Synanthropic wild mammals dominate as hosts of zoonotic EIDs in the Australasian–Asian regions. In the Australian context, we have explored temporally sequenced and biologically plausible relationships between land-use change and EIDs, particularly those of environmental and wildlife origins. However, patterns observed at a landscape scale may not be important at a smaller scale (and vice versa). By progressively exploring and mapping key relationships, we are building a better understanding of how change in complex systems drives infectious disease emergence, and how we can use this information to mitigate risk.

References

Bradshaw, C. 2012. Little left to lose: deforestation and forest degradation in Australia since European colonization. *Plant Ecology* 5, 109–20.

Butler, C.D. 2012. Infectious disease emergence and global change: thinking systemically in a shrinking world. *Infectious Diseases of Poverty* 1, 5 [17p].

Butler, C.D. & McFarlane, R. 2011. Beware of pigs near wings: piggeries, birds, bats and human health. *EcoHealth* 7, 46.

Cole, D., Drum, D.J.V., Stallknecht, D.E., White, D.G., Lee, M.D., Ayers, S., et al. 2005. Free living Canada Geese and antimicrobial resistance. *Emerging Infectious Diseases* 11, 935–8.

Ellis, E.C. 2011. Anthropogenic transformation of the terrestrial biosphere. *Philosophical Transactions of the Royal Society of London A* 369, 1010–35.

Food and Agriculture Organization (FAO) 2011. *World Livestock 2011 – Livestock in Food Security*. Food and Agriculture Organization of the United Nations, Rome, Italy.

Finley, R.L., Collignon, P., Larsson, D.G.J., McEwen, S.A., Li, X.-Z., Gaze, W.H., et al. 2013. The scourge of antibiotic resistance: the important role of the environment. *Clinical Infectious Diseases*, doi:10.1093/cid/cit355.

Grace, D., Mutua, F., Ochungo, P., Kruska, R., Jones, K., Brierley, L., et al. 2012. *Mapping of Poverty and Likely Zoonoses Hotspots*. Zoonoses Project 4 Report to Department for International Development. International Livestock Research Institute, London, UK.

International Union for the Conservation of Nature (IUCN) 2012. IUCN Red List of Threatened Species. Available at: www.iucnredlist.org, accessed 1 June 2012.

Johara, M.Y., Field, H., Rashdi, A.M., Morrissy, C.J., van der Heide, B., Rota, P., et al. 2001. Nipah virus infection in bats (Order *Chiroptera*) in peninsular Malaysia. *Emerging Infectious Diseases* 7, 439–41.

Jones, K.E., Patel, N.G., Levy, M.A., Storeygard, A., Balk, D., Gittleman, J.L., et al. 2008. Global trends in emerging infectious diseases. *Nature* 451, 990–4.

Lau, S.K.P., Li, K.S.M., Huang, Y., Shek, C.T., Tse, H., Wang, M., et al. 2010. Ecoepidemiology and complete genome comparison of different strains of Severe Acute Respiratory Syndrome-related *Rhinolophus* bat coronavirus in China reveal bats as a reservoir for acute, self-limiting infection that allows recombination events. *Journal of Virology* 84, 2808–19.

Levy, S.B. & Marshall, B. 2004. Antibacterial resistance worldwide: causes, challenges and responses. *Nature Medicine* 10, S122–9.

Liverani, M., Waage, J., Barnett, T., Pfeiffer, D.U., Rushton, J., Rudge, J.W., et al. 2013. Understanding and managing zoonotic risk in the new livestock industries. *Environmental Health Perspectives* 121, 873–7.

McFarlane, R., Becker, N. & Field, H. 2011. Investigation of the climatic and environmental context of Hendra virus spillover events 1994–2010. *PLoS One* 6, e28374.

McFarlane, R., Sleigh, A. & McMichael, A.J. 2012. Synanthropy of wild mammals as a determinant of emerging infectious diseases in the Asian and Australasian region. *EcoHealth* 9, 24–35.

McFarlane, R., Sleigh, A.S. & McMichael, A.J. 2013. Land use change and emerging infectious disease on an island continent. *International Journal Environmental Research and Public Health* 10, 2699–719.

McFarlane, R.A. 2014. *Linking Patterns of Ecological Change and Emerging Infectious Disease in the Australasian region*. PhD Thesis. The Australian National University, Canberra, ACT, Australia, 228.

Mackenzie, J. 2001. Emerging diseases in the Australasian region. In: Davis, J. & Lederberg, J. (eds) *Emerging Infectious Diseases From the Global to the Local Perspective*. National Academy Press, Washington, DC, USA, 65–7.

McMichael, A.J. 2004. Environmental and social influences on emerging infectious diseases: past, present and future. *Philosophical Transactions of the Royal Society of London Series B* 359, 1049–58.

McMichael, A.J. & Wilcox, B.A. 2009. Climate change, human health, and integrative research: a transformative imperative. *EcoHealth* 6, 163–5.

McMichael, A.J., Woodruff, R.E. & Hales, S. 2006. Climate change and human health: present and future risks. *The Lancet* 367, 859–69.

McNeill, W.H. 1976. *Plagues and Peoples*. Anchor Press, Garden City, New York, USA.

Morand, S., Jittapalapong, S., Suputtamongkol, Y., Abdullah, M.T. & Huan, T.B. 2014. Infectious diseases and their outbreaks in Asia-Pacific: biodiversity and its regulation loss matter. *PLOS One* 9, e90032.

Morse, S.S. 1995. Factors in the emergence of infectious diseases. *Emerging Infectious Diseases* 1, 7–14.

Myers, S. & Patz, J. 2009. Emerging threats to human health from global environmental change. *Annual Review of Environment and Resources* 34, 223–252.

Plowright, R., Foley, P., Field, H., Dobson, A., Foley, J., Foley, J.E., et al. 2011. Urban habituation, ecological connectivity and epidemic dampening: the emergence of Hendra virus from flying foxes (*Pteropus* spp.). *Proceedings of the Royal Society B* 278, 3703–12.

Plowright R.K., Eby, P., Hudson, P.J., Smith, I.L., Westcott, D., Bryden, W. L., et al. 2015. Ecological dynamics of emerging bat virus spillover. *Proceedings of the Royal Society B: Biological Sciences* 282, 20142124.

Sharp, P.M., Bailes, E., Chaudhuri, R.R., Rodenburg, C.M., Santiago, M.O. & Hahn, B.H. 2001. The origins of acquired immune deficiency syndrome viruses: where and when? *Philosophical Transactions of the Royal Society B Biological Sciences* 356, 867–76.

Singh, R.P., Hodson, D.P., Huerta-Espino, J., Jin, Y., Bhavani, S., Njau, P., et al. 2011. The emergence of Ug99 races of the stem rust fungus is a threat to world wheat production. *Annual Review of Phytopathology* 49(1):465-481.

Smolinski, M., Hamburg, M. & Lederberg, J. 2003. Microbial threats to health: emergence, detection and response. In: Institute of Medicine (ed.) *Shaping the Future for Health*. National Academies Press, Washington, DC, USA, 53–148.

Steinfeld, H., Gerber, P., Wassenaar, T., Castel, V., Rosales, M. & de Haan, C. 2006. *Livestock's Long Shadow*. Food and Agricutural Organization, Rome, Italy.

Steinfeld, H., Mooney, H., Neville, L., Gerber, P. & Reid, R. 2008. *Livestock in a Changing Landscape*. Policy Brief No. 6. UNESCO-SCOPE-UNEP, Paris, France. Available at: unesdoc.unesco.org/images/0015/001591/159194e.pdf, accessed 2 February 2015.

Taylor, L., Latham, S. & Woolhouse, M. 2001. Risk factors for human disease emergence. *Philosophical Transactions of the Royal Society B Biological Sciences* 356, 983–989.

Thornton, P. 2010. Livestock production: recent trends, future prospects. *Philosophical Transactions of the Royal Society B* 365, 2853–67.

Wang, M., Lin, X., Ma, G., & Bai, X. 2007. Emerging viral diseases of fish and shrimp. (Issues in Infectious Diseases Vol. 4). In: Lal, S.K. (ed.) *Emerging Viral Diseases of Southeast Asia*. S. Karger AG, Basel, Switzerland, 35–58.

Wilcox, B.A. & Colwell, R.R. 2005. Emerging and re-emerging infectious diseases: biocomplexity as an interdisciplinary paradigm. *Ecohealth* 2, 244–57.

Zhou, Y.J., Hao, X.-F., Tian, Z.-L., Tong, G.-Z., Yoo, D., An, T.-Q., et al. 2008. Highly virulent porcine reproductive and respiratory syndrome virus emerged in China. *Transboundary and Emerging Diseases*, 55, 152–64.

27

BIODIVERSITY KEEPS PEOPLE HEALTHY

PIM MARTENS AND CARIJN BEUMER

Abstract

Biodiversity and health mutually interact. Generally speaking, the greater the decline in biodiversity, the higher are the risks to human health – certainly over the long term (Corvalán et al., 2005). Guiding the health transition towards an era of sustainable health demands an integrated policy that embraces social, economic and ecological elements, recognising the complex relationships between them and looking further than a typically four-year period to the next government election.

Introduction: Biodiversity is Linked to Human Health

As stated by the World Health Organization (WHO) in its report, *Our Planet, Our Health, Our Future*, '[he]alth is our most basic human right and one of the most important indicators of sustainable development (WHO, 2011). Intuitively, we know that nature affects human health. However, people are generally less well acquainted with the fact that biodiversity – the rich variety of species – is in every way essential, indeed, indispensable, to the maintenance of human health and well-being (Corvalán et al., 2005). Without the complex web of interrelations and functional connections between different species in the natural environment, there would be few prospects for human health (Chivian, 2002). The way we are heading with our current trends in exploiting and degrading our environment may lead us towards tipping points that would reduce the ability of nature to provide the ecosystem services upon which all of us depend (CBD, 2010).

In order to sustain the ability of happy and healthy lives as humans, we need to foster an integrated way of thinking that directly connects the human sphere to the biosphere – our surrounding natural environment. This integrated ecosociological way of thinking is the basis for a sustainable development towards a thriving future of human-natural life (Capra, 1996; Laszlo, 1996, 2006; Beumer et al., 2008; Beumer and Martens, 2010).

Health is essential in achieving a sustainable development process. Sustainable development needs healthy people to address global issues effectively. Health can also be used as a measure to monitor progress in the process of sustainable development (UNCSD, 2012). As is stated in *The Future We Want* – the outcome report of the RIO+20 Conference of the United Nations Commission on Sustainable Development (UNCSD) – '[s]ustainable development will not be achieved in [the] presence of [a] high burden on communicable/non-communicable diseases' (UNCSD, 2012). Nevertheless, although the UNCSD recognises the importance of ecosystemic health to the sustenance and improvement of human health, it does not directly link biodiversity to this issue.

Fortunately, the recognition of the important connections between biodiversity and human health has increased during the past decade. A growing number of reports have been published on the topic of the complex relation between biodiversity and human health, and new opportunities emerge that may support biodiversity conservation in the light of human health and well-being. Many of these studies address ecosystemic health and human health inclusively in the context of sustainable development (WHO, 2011). The Convention on Biological Diversity (CBD) states in its strategic Aichi Biodiversity Targets that '[b]y 2020, ecosystems that provide essential services, including services related to water, and contribute to health, livelihoods and well-being, are restored and safeguarded' (CBD, 2011). Additionally, the CBD adopted 17 decisions referring to human well-being and health (WHO, 2011). The World Health Organization in its report, *Our Planet, Our Health, Our Future* (WHO, 2011), discusses some of the important connections between biodiversity and human health, and how ecosystem services – of which many are provided by a healthy biodiversity – are significant determinants of human well-being and health. Important insights reported in the documents of the Millennium Ecosystem Assessment (Corvalán et al., 2005; Duraiappah and Naeem, 2005) and in the reports of the Intergovernmental Panel on Climate Change (IPCC, 2007) increasingly guide local and global policymakers and institutions like WHO in reviewing their decisions in the light of the importance of ecosystems and biodiversity for human well-being and health.

The relationship between biodiversity and human health starts with the basics: are adequate supplies of healthy food, clean water and air of good quality available? A healthy ecosystem supplies these 'ecosystem services' free of charge (Costanza et al., 1997; TEEB, 2009). But, besides these primary services, there are many other, different ecosystem services that contribute to maintaining, boosting and improving human health (see Box 27.1). Even apart from these useful aspects, the richness of species has its own intrinsic value (Des Jardins, 2006).

Box 27.1 Examples of ecosystem services.

(Chivian, 2002; Huynen et al., 2004; Corvalán et al., 2005; TEEB, 2009)

Pollination

Insects, like bees and wasps, pollinate crops, providing us with a range of vegetables, fruit and grains for our food: the natural source of vitamins, fibre and many other nutrients indispensable to our bodily health.

Clean air

The leafy crown of forests and woods functions as a filter and chemical plant that regulates the atmosphere's composition. It cleans the air and contributes to the regulation of temperature, humidity and climate.

River basins

Forests regulate the flow of water to downstream areas, ensuring a fairly regular, predictable flow pattern. In this way, forests contribute to safety while also ensuring that water for drinking and/or irrigation does not immediately drain away.

Freshwater purification

Wetlands absorb and recycle nutrients from human settlement. As the water flows through the wetlands, the plants, microbes and sediments that are present cleanse it of harmful pollutants, such as nitrogen and phosphorus.

Management of potential infestations and disease-causing organisms

Many crops, insects, rodents, bacteria, moulds and other infestations compete with humans for food, influence the production of fibres and spread diseases. Some animals and microbes serve us by protecting us naturally against these infestations, which can cause diseases in plants, animals and humans.

Stabilising the countryside, protecting against erosion

Forests and grasslands provide a variety of natural ways to protect the soil against erosion, once again contributing to the safety of inhabited areas and crop security (the opportunity to use the soil for agriculture).

Carbon removal on the land and from the global climate

Land-based ecosystems are major carbon stores, both in plant tissues and the organic components of the soil. By absorbing carbon, such ecosystems help to restrain the increase of carbon dioxide in the atmosphere, thus contributing to limit climate change. The effects of climate change on human health are extremely complex and include such components as malaria, dengue fever and the West Nile virus, tick distribution, or the health effects of changing ecosystem services resulting from a changing natural environment.

Social and cultural services

Ecosystems supply crucial habitats for plants, animals and microbes, which have their own intrinsic value, as well as supplying services to humankind, such as food-crop pollination, physical and psychological health, sporting and leisure activities and other cultural, artistic and aesthetic services.

Genetic databank

The vast amount of genetic information stored in ecosystems – a great deal of which is still unknown to us – represents an opportunity to find solutions to an immense range of challenges, such as the alleviation of diseases. Nature can also represent a model for the discovery of ways to remedy health issues: during its long hibernation, for instance, the black bear (*Ursus americanus*) does not develop osteoporosis, while the polar bear's unusual energy metabolism may point the way to remedies for type 2 diabetes in humans.

Inspiration

Nature can inspire art and provide new technological discoveries, such as waterproof materials or energy generation from organic materials via photosynthesis.

These ecosystem services owe their existence to a dynamic, complex network of functions, relationships and interactions between the various species in their native habitats. In recent years, we have seen much research into the relationships between biodiversity and ecosystem stability and productivity, in terms of experimental research in the field, the formulation of concepts and theories through to quantitative field observations. This research has shown that greater biodiversity is linked to an increase in an ecosystem's stability: 'diversity = stability' (McCann, 2000; Rees, 2010; Ives and Carpenter, 2007; MacDougall et al., 2013). All the research conclusions lead unequivocally to the conclusion that biodiversity is an essential precondition for the maintenance and, indeed, the flourishing of human health and well-being.

The global loss of biodiversity may lead – directly or indirectly, in the short or long term – to a massive loss of health for humankind. The alarm bells are ringing throughout the world among ecologists, and also among eco-epidemiologists. Biodiversity has never vanished at such a rate as now: 1,000 times faster than the normal evolutionary rate at which species disappear (CBD, 2010). At the time of writing, the Red List maintained by the International Union for the Conservation of Nature (IUCN) contains 24,216 animal and plant species threatened with extinction, which is 1500 more than the year before. A total of 61,914 species were studied when the list was compiled (IUCN, 2012).

Ecosystems and Our Health

Many human activities that contribute to increasing prosperity are responsible for the loss of biodiversity, and thus for a reduction in our chance for a healthy life. This paradox illustrates the natural tension between the maintenance of biodiversity (and thus health) and prosperity. Not that the extinction of a given species by definition brings about a specific disease. But, a certain degree of biodiversity is necessary for a well-functioning ecosystem as a whole and for the services it supplies to humanity (Sala et al., 2000; Chapin et al., 2001). A great deal of research is still needed to discover the precise nature of the relationships between human health, biodiversity and ecosystems. Nevertheless, as seen above, a number of authors and institutions have already emphasised the link between nature and health (Chapin et al., 2001).

Agricultural and oceanic diversity, for example, are crucial in providing global food security. For instance, plants such as maize, rice and wheat are together responsible for 60 per cent of humankind's food supply. In the future, our food supply will also come to depend on the development of new crops derived from today's wild plants, since disease and pesticide resistance will ultimately render our present crops unfit for food production. The vitality of these crops – and with it, our food supply – relates directly to the variety of species (Fehr, 1984). So, we need natural diversity to maintain the health of our agricultural crops and our food (Fehr, 1984). On the other hand, the expansion of agriculture around the world – especially through monocultural methods – can contribute to the reduction of the resilience of ecosystems through the loss of often very rich forest biodiversity and by increasing contacts between humans, domestic animals and wildlife, with the increased risk of pathogen transfer as a result (WHO, 2011).

Maintaining healthy genetic diversity will be crucial in maintaining ecosystem and human health, including, for example, in the battle against growing antibiotic resistance (Jarlier et al., 2012). Much research money and attention is currently being spent on new genetically engineered food species and new ways of modifying pathogenic vectors and viruses in order to battle (infectious) diseases. There are serious health risks to humans and the global ecosystem involved with modifying living organisms with biotechnology (de Vendômois et al., 2012). What will the systemic impacts be, for example, of modifying malaria mosquitoes in a way that interferes with their malarial transmission capacity (Wang and Jacobs-Lorena, 2013)? Biodiversity decline or tempering with biodiversity in other ways can increase the spread of infectious diseases by reducing ecosystemic resilience and the capacity of ecosystems to buffer pests and diseases (Matt and Gebser, 2010). Genetically modified (GM) species introduced for food security or for human health reasons may, just as other invasive alien species have, become invasive over time and add to the decrease of biodiversity and ecosystem resilience (Jeschke et al., 2013). Many questions concerning the complex relationships between human health, ecosystemic properties and modified species are still unanswered.

Exotic life forms that penetrate our own ecosystem can cause health problems for humans, both directly and indirectly (IUCN, 2009). Exotic birds, insects and rodents can carry and transfer diseases, causing harm to the health of humans and native species. Exotic plants, such as certain algae, can overrun freshwater ecosystems, choking them and thus ultimately reducing biodiversity. It is often extremely difficult to combat exotic infestations, with heavy social and economic costs. Populations can simply explode from a lack of natural enemies in the new surroundings, and native species are driven away. The pesticides used to combat exotics lead to the pollution of soils and fresh water, with associated damage to valuable native insects, other species and human health (Pyšek and Richardson, 2010).

So, the relationship between environmental change, health and biodiversity is complicated. This also means that more biodiversity is not better by definition. Existing ecosystems are often in a dynamic but subtle equilibrium, which can be disrupted easily by changes that new species bring with them. For example, new species or species from another region, transported to or thriving in a new area under a changing climate, can cause very serious local or regional problems, creating hazards both to humans and to the environment.

A Paradigm Shift: From Symptom to System

Many of the health effects that can be caused by a loss of biodiversity can be mitigated by technological developments, improved hygiene and by eliminating the disease-causing agents using chemicals and pesticides, plus the continuous development of new medicines for improved treatments and disease management. These approaches provide options for attacking symptoms, and are of proven effectiveness. But, future investments aimed at alleviating the damage to health from the rapidly increasing loss of natural ecosystems will cost far more than investing today in a healthy global ecosystem. Mother Nature, after all, has known throughout the ages how to maintain equilibrium and stay healthy – and 'for free'. We have a lot to learn from her.

Greater biodiversity, in the main, also leads to the more efficient use of available natural resources, since there is more likelihood that species will be present that can respond to specific changes in a given habitat. The species that populate the world today are the result of a process of natural selection that has been continuing for three billion years, and which has conferred on them a significant degree of specialisation and great efficiency in the way they tackle a wide range of problems. We have a lot to learn from that, too.

The modern, narrow focus on 'treating the symptoms' can lead to serious health hazards, as we have seen in our use of antibiotics in the intensive cattle rearing industry (Jarlier et al., 2012). The more antibiotics we use to combat the symptoms of disease, the faster the bacteria develop resistance and the less we can use antibiotics to treat sick people. The way we currently use antibiotics shows how a reductionist focus on combating symptoms can lead us literally down a 'dead-end street'.

If we are to cope with disease in a sustainable way, we shall have to move towards an ecological approach: how can we take preventive measures to ensure that we improve our resistance to disease? How can we plan and manage our natural environment, our agriculture and the urban environment to help us do so?

The way we cope with disease and health will have to undergo a shift in paradigm to become based far more on such a 'systemic approach'. Of course, (new) diseases will always emerge and the symptoms will have to be alleviated. But, what we need to do now is shift our focus to a 'health ecology', in which we start to understand illness and health in terms of a global system of complex relationships between humans, animals and nature.

Whom we can learn much from, too, for our necessary transition towards a more ecosocio systemic approach to health are traditional Indigenous communities. Many communities with ancient traditional knowledge on crops, herbs and their specific uses are now being 'visited' by large food and pharmaceutical companies. Potential medicines and new food sources are abundant in areas rich in biodiversity. Often, these biodiversity hotspots are located near or in Indigenous community areas in developing countries. Access to regular health care is often poor, and the communities depend on their resources and traditional knowledge of ecosystems for subsistence. States and international property right regulations do not protect these Indigenous populations, their resources and their traditional ecological knowledge enough from the practices of commercial companies that enter the community areas for private gains by imposing patent claims on organisms that can be used as ingredients for medicines, foods (Mackey and Liang, 2012), pesticides (Orozco and Poonamallee, 2014) or cosmetics (Jolly et al., 2012). Often, communities become victims of biopiracy when bioprospecting is used by companies to gain exclusive intellectual property rights (IPRs) over resources and knowledge developed by others. Even after the adoption of the Nagoya Protocol – which aims to combat biopiracy and encourages equitable and joint benefit sharing of resources while sustainably managing biodiversity (UNEP-CBD, 2011) – global governance remains ineffective in protecting local communities from biopiracy (Mackey and Liang, 2012). Biopiracy does not only enhance ethical concerns about equity, environmental justice and the question of the right to 'own' living organisms (Jolly et al., 2012); it also directly affects the health and well-being of local communities: by violating people the right to breed, develop and even use their own developed knowledge, resources and ethnomedicine further without paying the prospecting companies (Laursen, 2012); by the depletion of the biodiversity resources the communities depend on for subsistence (Mackey and Liang, 2012); or by conflicts that arise (Jolly et al., 2012). Obviously, bioprospecting is not the way we can learn sustainably about biodiversity and its relation to our health from other communities and civilisations, and the way towards benefit sharing as proposed by the Nagoya Protocol of the CBD should be walked very cautiously, and questioned at every step: for, after all, who is to decide what benefits are going to be shared with whom (Orozco and Poonamallee, 2014)?

Trade-offs: Short-term Gains versus Long-term Losses?

Changes in the environment that are beneficial to our health can be viewed as trade-offs with the ecosystem's existing equilibrium. Often, though, their positive effect involves only a short-term benefit to our health. It turns out that the long-term costs (ecological, economic, social and health related) of this short-termism are far higher than estimates have suggested. One example is the extermination of vampire bats in Latin America. These bats can infect cattle with rabies. So, in the short term, the local food supply benefits, as does the local population's health. Over the long term, however, this action leads to an explosive growth in the mosquito population, which allows other diseases to flourish, such as malaria or dengue fever.

Another example is the drainage of the swamps in America's Great Lakes region, which eliminated the malaria mosquitoes, thus improving human health. But, the loss of these swamps – wetlands – from the drainage networks can lead to major problems with traditional livelihoods (the collapse of local fisheries, for instance). The long-term effect of technological fixes for the health issues caused by the local environment are sometimes pushed into the background, as was the case (and increasingly is, once again) with the use of dichlorodiphenyl-trichloroethane (DDT) to combat malaria.

In brief, the relationship between humankind, biodiversity and health is an ambiguous one. On the one hand, greater species' biodiversity can signify a larger reservoir of pathogens. On the other hand, there are many indications that increased diversity can reduce the spread to humans of a number of disease-causing agents. Think, for example, of preventing the spread of Lyme disease by maintaining a natural ecosystem. If sufficient numbers of large mammals such as deer can inhabit a sufficiently large area, then the ticks will prefer them to humans.

The Ecological Footprint of Health Care

Seen in a wider perspective – that of global human health – it appears that the changes throughout the world that we have witnessed in recent years are both a blessing and a curse. We have increased economic growth and achieved rapid development in both technology and medicine, which have improved the life expectancy and the health of many peoples. On the other hand, many aspects of globalisation are imperilling human health. Consider not only the reduction of biodiversity that we have been discussing but also the erosion of social conditions, the widening gap between rich and poor (both within and between countries) and the accelerated pace of consumption.

The health industry itself is having a major impact on the entire ecosocial system. Here, we can – again – cite the use of antibiotics and increased bacterial immunity; the mountainous waste of time-expired medicines and other medical waste (including nuclear waste) from hospitals and care homes; the exploitation and patenting of organisms from the rainforest to manufacture medicines; the pharmaceutical industry's chemical pollution; hormones released into the water from the use of birth control drugs, which affect the fertility and even the sex of the fish population.

The way we use our land for agriculture and cattle rearing, which involves the use of pesticides, also weakens the complex natural equilibrium in many ecosystems. The current paradigm that prefers quick cures and short-term prosperity to long-term prosperity magnifies the likelihood of serious ecological harm. The massive mortality among bee populations, for example, is being ascribed increasingly to the use of neonicotine, an insect nerve poison that has recently been banned from Europe (EEA, 2013) but is still being applied in many other parts of the world, like the USA, Asia and Africa.

Despite all these problems, there is also a good side to this story: many avenues are available to reduce the ecological footprint of the industries that aim to contribute to human health. If these avenues are followed by pharmaceutical and food-producing companies, then a systems approach is a prerequisite. Health interventions must be viewed in the wider context of complex relationships within the entire ecosocial system. Progress, both economic and technological, has brought us great benefits, but we must investigate and appraise the long-term consequences of health interventions.

The Health Transition

Health care in the Western world has progressed from a society in which infectious diseases were the greatest cause of mortality to one dominated by chronic diseases. This is called the 'health transition' (Huynen, 2008). In a globalising world, this trend will only be reinforced. The next logical step is to look at what the transition implies for our future health situation. To do this, we use three possible future scenarios (Martens, 2003; Huynen, 2008).

A sustainable world

A global, integrated, systems approach to humankind and nature will ensure a sustainable equilibrium for human health. Both a degree of economic growth and an improvement in sociocultural and ecological conditions (including countering the loss of biodiversity) will have a beneficial effect on health and prosperity, in the short term as well as (in fact, mainly) in the long term.

A market-oriented world

Medical technology provides quick fixes for health problems. Health risks from consumer lifestyles and biodiversity losses can be limited, time and again, thanks to new developments in technology and medicine: quick fixes. A precondition for this scenario is a constantly growing economy.

A fragmented, market-oriented world

The rise of infectious diseases, both known and new ones, has a significant, adverse impact on the health of the world's population. Combined with improved mobility, this will lead to microbiological resistance, problems with the provision of health care, increasing environmental problems and a further decrease in biodiversity, with declining stability of the biosphere.

While these future situations are fictional, they are based on exhaustive scenario studies (Gallopin et al., 1997; Glenn and Gordon, 1998; Hammond, 1998; WBCSD, 1998; IPCC, 2000; Corvalán et al., 2005; UNEP, 2007) and so they may be regarded as possible future phases in the health transition (Huynen, 2008). 'Incidents' like the outbreak and subsequent spread of new infectious disease like the coronavirus, antibiotic-resistant Enterohaemorrhagic *Escherichia coli* and other bacterial infections that are resistant to antibiotics show what can happen to our future health under certain 'business as usual' conditions. Our view is that it is imperative to make the transition to another, more sustainable and ecological approach to health. We regard that in the most desirable scenario, the possibility of continuing economic growth (the precondition in scenario 2) is nothing but a utopian dream (Martens, 2013). We need to refocus on other types of 'growth' and 'development' as essential for our future health and well-being. These are the 'development' of a global systemic ecological literacy (Mitchell and Mueller, 2009) and the 'growth' of a healthy, diverse and thriving ecosocial system (Beumer and Martens, 2010).

Conclusion: Sustainable Health is Ecosocio Health

In our view, the most desirable vision of the future couples economic development and globalisation with a growing social and ecological awareness. Here, sustainability is accorded high priority and economic growth remains within the parameters set by social and ecological goals. As a result, the risks to human health will decline, even as biodiversity increases.

We have shown that biodiversity and health mutually interact. Generally speaking, the greater the decline in biodiversity, the higher are the risks to human health – certainly over the long term. In a world where countries, ecosystems and economies are increasingly dependent on each other, a marginal degree of biodiversity makes a poor foundation for the health of all people, be they rich or poor.

So, in our view, policymakers cannot escape the need to conserve biodiversity. Guiding the health transition towards an era of sustainable health demands an integrated policy that embraces social, economic and ecological elements, recognising the complex relationships between them and looking further than a typically four-year period to the next election.

Poverty and inaccessible health care will tend to accelerate rather than resolve the inverse relationship between biodiversity and health. This chapter, in other words, is not simply a jeremiad against prosperity. Rather, it is a plea for a sustainable approach to development that pays attention to long-term effects and to the entire ecosocial system of Planet Earth, on which we all live.

References

Beumer, C. & Martens, P. 2010. Noah's ark or world wild web? Cultural perspectives in global scenario studies and their function for biodiversity conservation in a changing world. *Sustainability* 2, 3211–38.

Beumer, C., Huynen, M. & Martens, P. 2008. Finding paradise in a complex web: the inter-relation of biodiversity, ecosystems and human health. In: Westra, L. (ed.) *Reconciling Human Existence With Ecological Integrity*. Earthscan, London, UK.

Capra, F. 1996. *The Web of Life: A New Scientific Understanding of Living Systems*. Anchor Books, New York, USA.

Convention on Biological Diversity (CBD) 2010. *Global Biodiversity Outlook 3*. Convention on Biological Diversity, Montreal, Canada.

CBD 2011. *Strategic Plan for Biodiversity 2011–2020 and the Aichi Targets: Living in Harmony with Nature*. UN Convention on Biological Diversity, United Nations Environment Programme, Montreal, Canada.

Chapin, F.S., Sala, O. & Huber-Sannwald, E. (eds) 2001. *Global Biodiversity in a Changing Environment: Scenarios for the 21st Century*. Springer-Verlag, New York, USA.

Chivian, E. (ed.) 2002. Biodiversity: its importance to human health. Center for Health and the Global Environment & Harvard Medical School, Harvard, Massachusetts, USA.

Corvalán, C., Hales, S. & McMichael, A.J. (eds) 2005. *Millennium Ecosystem Assessment. Ecosystems and Human Well-Being: Health Synthesis*. World Health Organization, Geneva, Switzerland.

Costanza, R., D'Arge, R., De Groot, R., Farber, S., Grasso, M., Hannon, B., et al. 1997. The value of the world's ecosystem services and natural capital. *Nature* 387, 253–60.

de Vendômois, J.S., Cellier, D. & Séralini, G.-E. 2012. Debate on GMOs health risks after statistical findings in regulatory tests. *International Journal of Biological Sciences* 6, 590–8.

Des Jardins, J. 2006. *Environmental Ethics. An Introduction to Environmental Philosophy*. Thomson Wadsworth, Belmont, California, USA.

Duraiappah, A.K. & Naeem, S. 2005. *Ecosystems and Human Well-Being. Biodiversity Synthesis. Millennium Ecosystem Assessment*. World Resources Institute, Washington DC, USA.

European Environment Agency (EEA) 2013. Neonicotinoid pesticides are a huge risk – so ban is welcome, says EEA. European Environment Agency. Available at: www.eea.europa.eu/highlights/neonicotinoid-pesticides-are-a-huge, accessed 10 June 2013.

Fehr, W.H. 1984. *Genetic Contributions to Yield Gains of Five Major Crop Plants*. Crop Science Society of America, Madison, Wisconsin, USA.

Gallopin, G., Hammond, A., Raskin, P. & Swart, R. (eds.) 1997. Branch points: global scenarios and human choice. Stockholm Environment Institute (SEI), Stockholm, Sweden.

Glenn, J.C. & Gordon, T.J. 1998. *1998 State of the Future: Issues and Opportunities*. American Council for the United Nations University, Washington, DC, USA.

Hammond, A. 1998. *Which World? Scenarios for the 21st Century: Global Destinies, Regional Choices*. Earthscan, London, UK.

Huynen, M. 2008. *Future Health in a Globalising World*. Maastricht University Press, Maastricht, The Netherlands.

Huynen, M.M.T.E., Martens, P. & De Groot, R.S. 2004. Linkages between biodiversity loss and human health: a global indicator analysis. *International Journal of Environmental Health Research* 14, 13–30.

Intergovernmental Panel on Climate Change (IPCC) 2000. Special Report on Emissions Scenarios. Intergovernmental Panel on Climate Change, Geneva, Switzerland.

Intergovernmental Panel on Climate Change (IPCC) 2007. *Contribution of Working Group II to the Fourth Assessment Report of the Intergovernmental Panel on Climate Change*. Cambridge University Press, Cambridge, UK.

International Union for the Conservation of Nature (IUCN) 2009. *Life Support. Human Health and the Environment*. International Union for the Conservation of Nature, Gland, Switzerland.

International Union for the Conservation of Nature (IUCN) 2012. Summary statistics. International Union for the Conservation of Nature, Gland, Switzerland. Available at: www.iucnredlist.org/about/summary-statistics#Tables_1_2, accessed 10 June 2013.

Ives, A.R. & Carpenter, S.R. 2007. Stability and diversity of ecosystems. *Science* 317, 58–62.

Jarlier, V., Carlet, J., McGowan, J., Goossens, H., Voss, A., Harbarth, S., et al. 2012. Priority actions to fight antibiotic resistance: results of an international meeting. *Antimicrobial Resistance and Infection Control* 1, 1–3.

Jeschke, J.M., Keesing, F. & Ostfeld, R.S. 2013. Novel organisms: comparing invasive species, GMOs, and emerging pathogens. *AMBIO* 42, 541–8.

Jolly, J.M., Baglione, S.L. & Zimmerer, T. 2012. An empirical study of bioprospecting: ethical issues in conflict. *World Journal of Social Sciences* 2, 146–58.

Laszlo, E. 1996. *The Systems View of the World: A Holistic Vision for Our Time.* Hampton Press Inc, Cresskill, New Jersey, USA.

Laszlo, E. 2006. *Chaos Point: The World at the Crossroads.* Hampton Roads Publishing Company, Charlottesville, Virginia, USA.

Laursen, L. 2012. Monsanto to face biopiracy charges in India. *Nature Biotechnology* 30, doi:10.1038/nbt0112-11.

McCann, K.S. 2000. The diversity-stability debate. *Nature* 405, 228–33.

MacDougall, A.S., McCann, K.S., Gellner, G. & Turkington, R. 2013. Diversity loss with persistent human disturbance increases vulnerability to ecosystem collapse. *Nature* 494, 86–9.

Mackey, T.K. & Liang, B.A. 2012. Integrating biodiversity management and indigenous biopiracy protection to promote environmental justice and global health. *American Journal of Public Health* 102, 1091–5.

Martens, P., Huynen, M.M.T.E.. 2003. A future without health? Health dimension in global scenario studies. *Bulletin of the World Health Organization* 81, 896–901.

Martens, P. 2013. Grey, green or blue economy? It's sustainability, stupid! Available from: sustainable-learning.org/2013/03/grey-green-or-blue-economy-its-sustainability-stupid/, both accessed 1 July 2015.

Matt, F. & Gebser, R. 2010. Biodiversity decline can increase the spread of infectious diseases, mainly based on Keesing et al. 2010. The Economics of Ecosystems and Biodiversity (TEEB). Available at: www.TEEBweb.org./, accessed 3 February 2015.

Mitchell, D.B. & Mueller, M.P. 2009. A philosophical analysis of David Orr's theory of ecological literacy: biophilia, ecojustice and moral education in school learning communities. *Cultural Studies of Science Education* 6, 193–221.

Orozco, D. & Poonamallee, L. 2014. The role of ethics in the commercialization of Indigenous knowledge. *Journal of Business Ethics*, 119, 275–86.

Pyšek, P. & Richardson, V. 2010. Invasive species, environmental change and management, and health. *Annual Review of Environment and Resources* 35, 25–55.

Rees, W.E. 2010. Thinking 'resilience'. In: Heinberg, R. & Lerch, D. (eds) *The Post Carbon Reader: Managing the 21st Century's Sustainability Crises.* Watershed Media, Post Carbon Institute, Santa Rosa, California, USA, 1–12.

Sala, O.E., Chapin, F.S., Armesto, J.J., Berlow, E., Bloomfield, J., Dirzo, R., et al. 2000. Global biodiversity scenarios for the year 2100. *Science* 287, 1770–4.

The Economics of Ecosystems and Biodiversity (TEEB) 2009. *TEEB for Policy Makers – Summary: Responding to the Value of Nature*. United Nations Environment Programme, Bonn, Germany.

United Nations Conference on Sustainable Development (UNCSD) 2012. *The Future We Want: Outcome Document Adopted at RIO+20*. United Nations Conference on Sustainable Development, Rio de Janeiro, Brazil.

United Nations Environment Programme (UNEP) 2007. *Global Environmental Outlook 4. Environment for Development (GEO4)*. United Nations Environment Programme, Nairobi, Kenya.

UNEP-CBD 2011. Report of the Tenth Meeting of the Conference of the Parties to the Convention on Biological Diversity. United Nations Environment Programme – Convention on Biological Diversity, Nagoya, Japan.

Wang, S. & Jacobs-Lorena, M. 2013. Genetic approaches to interfere with malaria transmission by vector mosquitoes. *Trends in Biotechnology* 31, 185–93.

World Business Council for Sustainable Development (WBCSD) 1998. *Exploring Sustainable Development: Global Scenarios 2000–2050*. World Business Council for Sustainable Development, London, UK.

World Health Organization (WHO) 2011. *Our Planet, Our Health, Our Future. Human Health and the Rio Conventions: Biological Diversity, Climate Change and Desertification*. World Health Organization, Geneva, Switzerland.

28

A CASE STUDY OF URBAN TREES, PUBLIC HEALTH AND SOCIAL EQUITY

MICHAEL BENTLEY

Abstract

Research demonstrates positive associations between urban greenness and human health; yet, the underlying causal mechanisms are less well understood. Moreover, urban greenness is distributed inequitably. This chapter describes a case study that explores some of the ways in which the quality and quantity of urban trees (as an aspect of urban greenness) relate to public health and social equity in a southern Australian context. The research used a theoretically informed, ecological public health model derived from four foundational principles of ecological public health – conviviality, equity, sustainability and global responsibility – to reveal a set of ecohealth-promoting mechanisms linking urban greenness to public health and social equity. Ecohealth in urban areas is created and lived by its human and non-human inhabitants within the convivial settings of their everyday life. While social determinants shape the health of people, the socio-natural processes of urban environmental metabolism shape urban development and the quality and distribution of trees as an urban forest. As urban trees can affect health and well-being positively, their uneven distribution is inequitable. Further case studies are needed to understand how urban trees relate to environmental and social determinants of health in different urban contexts.

Introduction

> A marvellous thing about trees is that they solve their problems without moving. They are model citizens, decorative, quiet, calm and courageous. (Joignot, 2012, p. 28)

The dynamic process of global urbanisation, what Rayner and Lang (2012) call the 'urban transition', is resulting in the rapid growth of urban areas with more than one million people (Sadler et al., 2010). In these urban areas, the external environment comprises two distinct, juxtaposed spaces: 'grey space' and 'green space', which can be broken down further, as Figure 28.1 depicts.

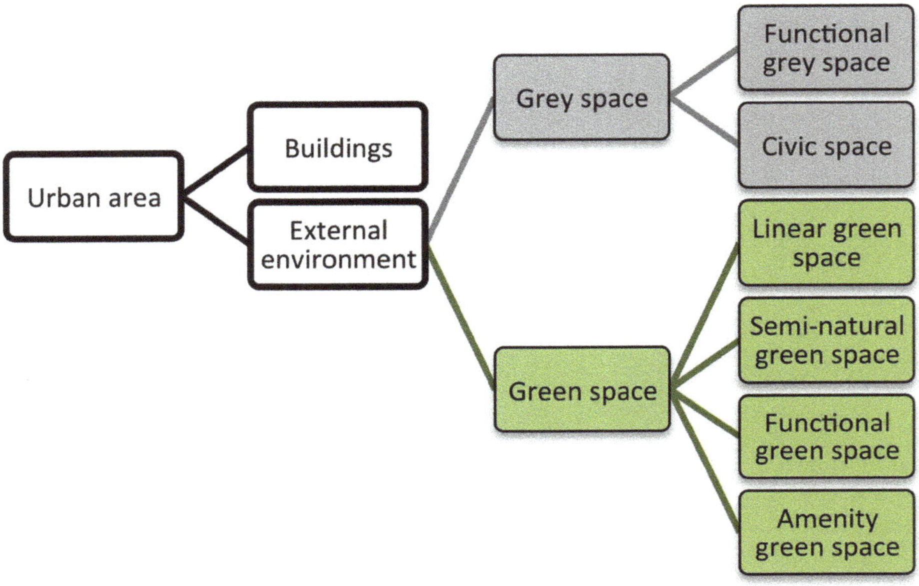

Figure 28.1 Grey and green space in urban areas.
Source: Adapted from Swanwick et al., 2003.

The increasingly dense urban built environment is placing pressure on the infrastructure of green spaces – the trees, parks and gardens. The health and well-being benefits of green space have been documented widely (Bell et al., 2008; Maas et al., 2009; Sadler et al., 2010). The green infrastructure is related to a healthy social ecosystem (Kuo, 2003), which is also important for urban biodiversity (Hostetler et al., 2011).

Trees are a significant element of green space and feature in all four classes (Figure 28.1). Urban trees are considered important for many reasons. Environmentally, there are benefits from having trees in urban areas. Urban trees contribute towards mitigating the heat island effect in cities (Coutts et al., 2013) and sequestering carbon (Nowak and Crane, 2002). Urban trees have substantial social (Kuo, 2003) and economic (Moore, 2009) value. Nevertheless, trees are distributed inequitably in cities (Landry and Chakraborty, 2009). The spatial distribution of urban trees in Australia has been shown to be related to income and education – areas of socio-economic disadvantage have fewer trees (Kirkpatrick et al., 2011), which raises concerns for social and environmental justice (Heynen and Perkins, 2005), and for public and community health (Nilsson and Sangster, 2008; Coutts et al., 2013).

Tony McMichael stressed the importance of the 'complex social and environmental systems that are the context for human health, [and] thinking more about population health in ecologic terms' (McMichael, 1999, p. 896). By way of this chapter, I add a mere leaf to McMichael's tree of knowledge by exploring some of the ways in which urban trees relate to public health and social equity. In so doing, I use a case study based on research conducted in suburban areas in Adelaide, South Australia (Bentley, 2012).

Research Methodology

The research (on which the case study draws) was situated in a critical realist paradigm and used critical methodological pluralism, a methodology which combines theory and methods to come up with an explanation of the phenomenon of interest (Danermark et al., 2002). The research question was: In what ways does urban greenness relate to public health and social equity in a southern Australian context? The case study explores the patterns produced by the underlying mechanisms linking urban trees to public health and social equity, and the context in which these patterns occur. Knowledge about the underlying mechanisms can be 'actively constructed from facts, events and experience' (Poland et al., 2008, p. 307), using various theoretical perspectives to understand and explain underlying structures. In other words, to understand the context and reveal the underlying mechanisms needs more than empirical data alone. The choice of methods in a critical realist enquiry is generally mixed methods and case studies. From a critical realist perspective, it is important that mixing methods 'must be governed not only by the research question but, more fundamentally, also by the ontological perspective from which you proceed' (Danermark et al., 2002, p. 153). That is, critical methodological pluralism 'is critical … in the sense that it opposes an unreflecting employment of methods' (Danermark et al., 2002, p. 176).

The methods in this research were a mix of intensive and extensive procedures. Critical realist research reframes qualitative and quantitative methods as intensive and extensive procedures to identify the 'generative mechanisms [of urban trees] and describe how they are manifested in real events and processes' (Danermark et al., 2002, p. 162). Intensive methods 'focus on generative mechanisms' and extensive methods look at the 'empirical patterns produced by a particular mechanism or structure of mechanisms' (Danermark et al., 2002, pp. 165–6).

I employed a variety of extensive methods (mapping, analysis of census and social health data, narrative reviews and summaries of relevant plans and policies, local newspaper media) and intensive methods (analysis of researchers' field notes and secondary analysis of interviews (n = 38) from the 'Location and Health' project (Baum et al., 2007), observational methods – field notes, photography and sound recordings) in the study.

The research found that while social determinants of health and health equity, such as income, education and housing, still shape the health of people, urban metabolism is the main driving mechanism behind the inequitable distribution of trees (as the canopy of the urban forest), and how the urban forest relates to public health and social equity.

The Adelaide Case Study

The case study looks at four suburbs of Adelaide, the capital city of South Australia. Adelaide's linear position between the Adelaide Hills and Gulf St Vincent defines and constrains its geography. Two of the suburbs are located in the northern metropolitan area – an area of relative most socio-economic disadvantage. The northern metropolitan area developed from pre-existing open woodland areas and experienced an urban sprawl, largely because of the post-war population boom that sought employment in the then new manufacturing industries. The decline in manufacturing has resulted in high levels of unemployment and social housing. The other two suburbs are in the eastern metropolitan area – an area of relative least socio-economic disadvantage. The eastern metropolitan area evolved from forested land and retained some remnant vegetation. The area contains some of the earliest colonial properties and most expensive housing. The northern case study suburbs are characterised by relatively high levels of rented housing and low levels of tertiary education (compared to the eastern case study suburbs). The eastern suburbs are relatively greener and have more than twice the household income of the northern suburbs (Table 28.1).

Table 28.1 Suburb characteristics.

	North		East	
	1	**2**	**1**	**2**
Housing tenure type (per cent)				
Fully owned	18	25	46	53
Rented	49	42	19	1[illegible]
SEIFA IRSD[a] score	745	788	1,097	1,123
SEIFA IRSD quintile[b]	5	5	1	1
Median household income (A$)	561	578	1,182	1,597
Median household size (persons)	2.4	2.4	2.4	2.7
Proportion of people with tertiary (bachelor degree or higher) education (per cent)	5	9	52	52
Proportion of houses with street/front yard tree cover (per cent)	24	50	78	88
Residential greenness rating (per cent)	53	63	76	8[illegible]

Notes:

[a] SEIFA = socio-economic indexes for areas; IRSD = index of relative socio-economic disadvantage.

[b] 1 = area of relative least disadvantage; 5 = area of relative most disadvantage.

Source: Table summarised from data used in the case study of urban greenness, public health and social equity (Bentley, 2012).

Compared with the least relatively disadvantaged areas, the most relatively disadvantaged areas have worse self-rated health and higher rates of mental health problems, health risk factors (smoking, physical inactivity and obesity), chronic health conditions and premature mortality from avoidable, treatable and preventable causes (Public Health Information Development Unit, 2010, p. 96).

Adelaide's geographical position also makes it a unique urban biological entity (Tait, 2005). The presence of trees is a significant contributor to objective and subjective measures of greenness (Tait et al., 2005). Urban greenness is distributed inequitably in Adelaide. The distribution of vegetation is uneven across metropolitan Adelaide, with the south-eastern suburbs rating highly compared with the remaining suburbs in the north, west and south. Importantly, the 'lack of greenness could not be totally attributed to the current level of land use factors' (Goodwins and Noyce, 1993, p. 3). This pattern persists to the current day (see the contrasting levels of tree cover in Figure 28.2).

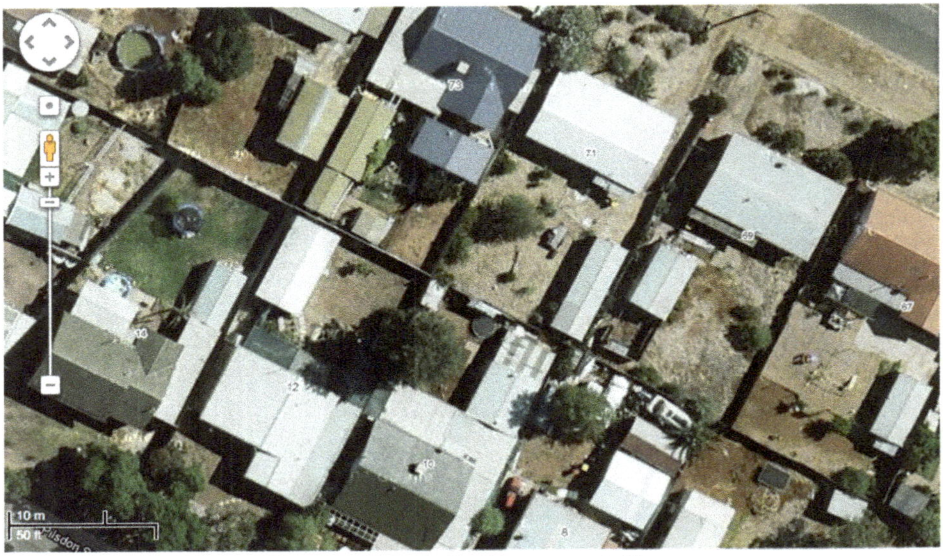

NORTH 1 Proportion of houses with street/front tree cover: 24%
Median tree cover score: 2.0 (n=7)[a]

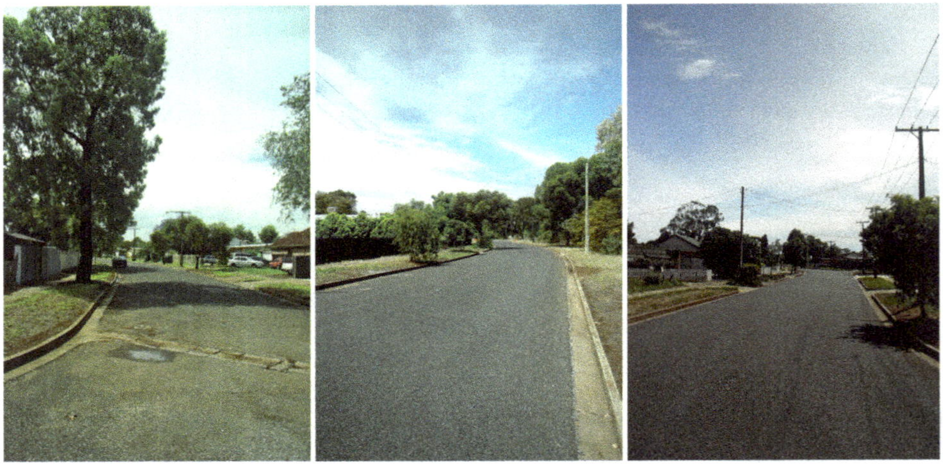

Figure 28.2 Characteristics of urban trees in northern and eastern Adelaide suburbs.

Source: Google, DigitalGlobe (overhead images above are at the same 10 m scale) and author's photographs.[b]

Notes:

[a] Tree cover score is derived from 3 × 3 grids overlayed on street-level photographs and measuring the number of squares with tree cover. For instance, in the left hand North 1 photo above, tree cover makes up 3.0 squares out of the nine squares. All photographs were taken on consecutive days in early summer at street intersections (automatic exposure with ISO 100 and 18 mm lens settings).

[b] Note that, for conciseness, one northern and one eastern suburb are featured in this figure.

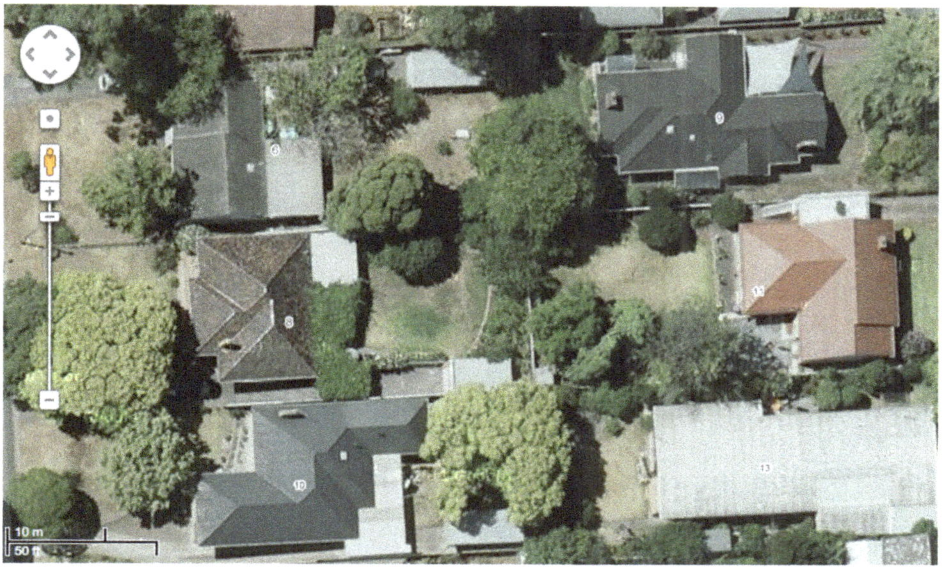

EAST 2 Proportion of houses with street/front tree cover: 88%
Median tree cover score: 3.8 (n=10)

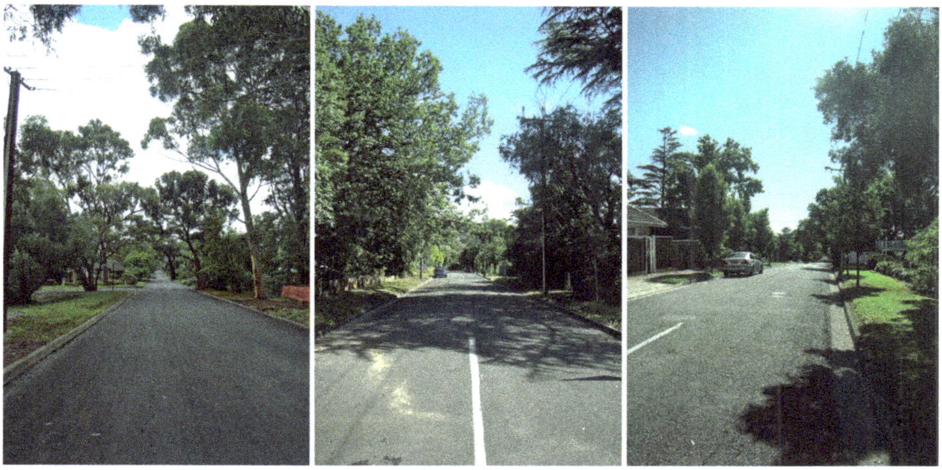

This case study will not be generalisable to rural areas or to urban areas in poorer countries. However, in relation to generalisability, case studies 'are generalizable to theoretical propositions and not to populations or universes' (Yin, 2009, p. 15). A benefit of using a critical realist approach is that explanation, which is based on theory and methods, can provide theoretical generalisability (Yin, 2009) to similar contexts.

Theoretical Perspective

> Place-sensitive approaches will enable scholars of well-being to better appreciate the significance of local interconnections that frame the lives of local populations and their experience of (and relationships with) environments and socio-cultural values attached to these locations. (Panelli and Tipa, 2007, p. 456)

This case study is place based. However, places (neighbourhoods, local areas, etc) are also part of an open ecosystem. Thus, the case study takes an ecological public health perspective, which acknowledges humans as part of the ecosystem, not separate from it (Rayner and Lang, 2012). There are broader public health concerns that affect the health of humans and the ecosystem (e.g. water, pollution, climate change). There are social aspects that affect well-being (e.g. amenity, access to green space) differentially. Moreover, social equity is related to environmental equity in urban areas (Falk et al., 1993), which also has consequences for the well-being of the non-human inhabitants (e.g. loss of habitat, reduced biodiversity).

The ecological public health thinking behind the case study is based on a theoretically derived model of ecological public health, which describes the relationships between different convivial communities interacting with each other in equitable ways (Bentley, 2014). Theories of more-than-human agency (the activities of non-human actors) inform ways of living together (conviviality) in urban areas. Political ecology links the equity concerns about environmental and social justice. At the core of this ecological public health thinking is the concept of conviviality. According to the Oxford dictionary, the origin of 'conviviality' lies in the Latin *convivialis*, which can be taken literally to mean 'live with'. In an ecological sense, this can connote the relations of the entities of an environment to each other and their surroundings. Conviviality necessitates a shift in thinking separately about health and ecology. Living with the non-human inhabitants of urban areas opens up new ways of thinking about health ecology and the equitable distribution of convivial areas. Conviviality has been conceptualised as 'a political project that is concerned with a more broadly conceived accommodation of difference, better attuned to the comings and goings of the multiplicity of more-than-human inhabitants that make themselves at home in the city' (Hinchliffe and Whatmore, 2006, p. 125).

In an ecological sense, nature is part of the urban fabric. In Australia, a general pattern is for people to separate the natural environment from their built environment (Head and Muir, 2005). The private space of the backyard (or back garden) is best for people and the natural environment (the 'bush' in Australia) is best for wildlife. Nevertheless, in between these spaces, people and wildlife encounter each other in the green infrastructure of neighbourhoods, streets, local parks and bushland areas in different ways. Urban trees play an active role, for example, in providing shade, ameliorating the local climate and acting as a wildlife corridor. This is not to say that trees 'possess the particular and extraordinary capabilities of humans … [but] they do possess very significant forms of active agency, which have usually been assumed to exist only in the human realm' (Jones and Cloke, 2008, p. 81). It is the role and distribution of trees that I now focus on.

The Urban Metabolism of Trees

Trees are part of the connections and interactions between people and things. Local government councils plant street trees and maintain public parks and gardens. Homeowners (and many home renters) create, alter and maintain private gardens (some spilling out on to the public footpaths).

The concept of urban metabolism has been used in socioecological frameworks for health to illustrate how physical and social resources are transformed or metabolised by urban systems and processes, resulting in outcomes that influence liveability, environmental quality and waste (Kearns et al., 2007; Schandl et al., 2012).

In this chapter, I propose that urban trees and urban forests are central to the processes of urban metabolism: they contribute to mitigating air pollution, harvesting stormwater, ameliorating heat island effects and providing psychosocial or mental support to humans who interact with them. They contribute to an aesthetic quality that is related to a healthy social ecosystem (Kuo, 2003). Key to their ongoing existence and care are political processes that may or may not protect them; for example, pressures on urban development, road clearances, dangers from falling limbs to pedestrians and drivers, risk of same-species disease transmission. Political contestations around urban forests lead to their uneven distribution, with the socio-natural transformations of urban forests changing urban areas in ways that may be health promoting or damaging. From an equity perspective, these political processes produce unjust outcomes.

Urban forests are socially produced (Heynen and Perkins, 2005). For example, with the exception of some significant trees in the eastern metropolitan area that pre-date European settlement, most of Adelaide's urban forest has evolved since 1,836. All 38 native tree species remain, and 60 introduced species have been added to the mix (Tait, 2005). Yet, the distribution remains uneven and, as urban trees affect health and well-being positively (Nilsson and Sangster, 2008), it is also inequitable.

The socio-natural processes of urban environmental metabolism have been shown to be a strong mechanism in explaining the uneven distribution of the urban forest:

> Urban trees necessarily exist within the urban built environment, and thus should be expected to change (to be cut or die and not be replanted, to be planted, etc) in relation to urban consumption patterns. These consumption patterns are necessarily related to class and other power relations. (Heynen, 2006, p. 513)

The spatial distribution of urban trees in Australia is related to income and education – areas of socio-economic disadvantage have fewer trees (Kirkpatrick et al., 2011). Housing tenure may explain some of this inequitable distribution. People who are renting dwellings are less likely to have trees in their front gardens (Kirkpatrick et al., 2011). There was a strong relationship between median household income and trees in front yards or street frontage in the case study suburbs (the correlation coefficient of median household income and trees in front yards or street frontage is 0.92, with a coefficient of determination of 0.84). There was also a strong relationship between the proportion of dwellings being rented and trees in front yards or street frontage in the case study suburbs (the correlation coefficient of rented dwellings and trees in front yards or street frontage is –0.98, with a coefficient of determination of 0.95).

Kirkpatrick et al. also found an association between rates of unemployment and the density of street/front garden trees and concluded:

> It would be possible to plan to double the number of street trees in Australian cities in present circumstances, but that significant increases in garden tree numbers would depend on increasing the income and higher education attainment of lower socio-economic groups. (Kirkpatrick et al., 2011, p. 244)

The social equity statistics in the Adelaide case study support this conclusion. The different proportions of higher education attainment in the northern (less than 10 per cent) and eastern (over 50 per cent) suburbs are stark. The median household income in eastern suburbs is more than twice that of the northern suburbs (Table 28.1).

Heynen (2006) draws on the concept of the consumption fund of the urban built environment – 'the circuit of capital that contains most urban ecological resources, such as urban forests, that are vital to the health of urban systems in general' (Heynen and Perkins, 2005, p. 105) – to show how political processes contribute to urban forest metabolism.[1] In Heynen's study, 'median household income was shown to significantly contribute to local metabolization in urban forest canopy cover and residential forest canopy cover' (Heynen, 2006, p. 513). There was a similar finding in the Adelaide case study. Furthermore, in the Adelaide case study, activism to save urban trees was strongest in more affluent areas, which supported the hypothesis that community groups could contribute to an uneven canopy cover (Conway et al., 2011).

In the Adelaide case study, the agency of trees was acknowledged in interviews with residents from the areas of relatively higher income and relatively less disadvantage, where the urban forest was denser:

> We have the beautiful gentle breezes at night on a hot day. It's generally cooler where we are because of the shade of the trees, so it's very pleasant from that perspective visually as well. (Female, 49 years old, East 1)

The agency of trees has some explanatory power in informing ways of living together (conviviality) in urban areas and casting biodiversity in a new light. Large urban trees play an important role in providing vital habitat resources for the city's non-human inhabitants (Stagoll et al., 2012). But, the respondent above also saw a downside of trees and yet, at the same time, acknowledged the need to live together with them.

> [The trees have] always been an issue because they block our drains and they're staining our pavers ... But the nice thing is and the important thing is I love the trees, I just wish they weren't gum trees. ... getting a house somewhere where there's no trees would be awful because you wouldn't get the lovely birds in the morning, so it's a compromise, so we've had to learn to live with them. (Female, 49 years old, East 1)

These comments reflect the dichotomous positions on trees in suburban areas. For instance, people like the bird life that trees attract, but not the risk of falling limbs (Head and Muir, 2005). Local media reports from the eastern suburbs highlight these risk concerns.

> **Sheltering under trees may not be such a hot idea**: Looking for shade under a tree may not be the greatest idea, with the SES reporting a growing number of falling branches during the current heatwave. SES deputy chief officer Matt Maywald says trees can drop their branches without warning during hot weather. 'Commonly eucalypts are affected, but the problem is not limited to this variety of tree, so people should not be complacent,' Mr Maywald said. ... The SES is advising people to

1 Heynen uses 'metabolism' rather the more neutral 'change', as the socio-natural transformations of urban areas are the result of neoliberal political processes.

> avoid standing or parking under trees with large, overhanging branches and to ensure their children do not climb or play around at-risk trees. (*Eastern Courier*, 13 November 2009)
>
> **Tree policy goes out on a limb**: Falling tree limbs that cause property damage, injury and even death are looming as a 'significant risk' for councils, prompting an independent inquiry into tree management by the Local Government Association (LGA). The LGA says the recent drought, combined with the overall ageing of Adelaide's street trees, has led to a significant increase in falling branches recently. (*Eastern Courier*, 27 April 2010)

Trees also featured prominently in local news stories from the eastern suburbs, in the context of the prolonged drought that affected much of south-eastern Australia from 2003 to 2010.

> **Summer's new autumn for Adelaide streetscapes**: Still in summer, yet some parts of the city already look like mid-autumn. Adelaide's deciduous trees, such as plane trees, are dropping leaves weeks earlier than usual, apparently caused by the scorching summer and ongoing drought. University of Adelaide tree expert Dr Jennifer Watling said the trees were suffering from heat and water stress. (*Eastern Courier*, 25 February 2009)
>
> **1800 eastern trees axed**: More than 1800 dead, dying or dangerous trees have been axed across the drought-ravaged eastern suburbs this past year, sparking calls for more stormwater harvesting. ... Treenet Director David Lawry — whose organization researches the state of local trees and gives feedback to councils and communities — said people had 'no right to blame' climate change for killing trees in the east, considering Adelaide was losing 160 gigalitres of stormwater each year instead of harvesting it. (*Eastern Courier*, 8 September 2009)

What was also notable in the case study was the uneven distribution of watered private gardens across the case study suburbs. Most of the northern blocks are reasonably sized. Many yards are not watered. There are few trees in the backyards. Most of the eastern blocks are also reasonably sized. Yet, most yards have some watered areas. All the yards have one or more trees (Figure 28.2). This pattern follows the income distribution. That is, the high-income suburbs have more watered areas. The price of water in Adelaide has a fixed (water-supply charge) and a variable (water-use charge) component.

On the whole, there is an unequal distribution of the urban forest across the case study suburbs that is related to household income and housing tenure, two of the social determinants of health. Moreover, the processes of urban metabolism influence the quality and quantity of urban trees and their relationship to social equity and mental health. There is a body of experimental evidence to support the restorative effects of urban greenness on mental health and well-being (Tzoulas et al., 2007). The 'Location and Health' project (Baum et al., 2007) found statistically significant differences in mental health (derived from the SF-12 standardised self-reported health measure) between the northern suburbs and the eastern suburbs. The results were lowest in the north and highest in the east. In the eastern areas of relative least socio-economic disadvantage, the case study reveals some support for the project of conviviality. There is a stronger focus on environment and biodiversity in local government plans that cover the eastern suburbs. Local government plans that cover the northern suburbs focus more on social and economic development.

Discussion and Conclusion

The Ottawa Charter for Health Promotion acknowledges that the 'inextricable links between people and their environment constitutes the basis for a socio-ecological approach to health' (World Health Organization, 1986, p. ii). There is congruence in the standpoints of health promotion and urban ecology. The Ottawa Charter states: 'Health is created and lived by people within the settings of their everyday life; where they learn, work, play and love' (World Health Organization, 1986, p. iii). Relatedly, the new field of reconciliation ecology calls for 'inventing, establishing and maintaining new habitats to conserve species diversity in places where people live, work and play' (Rosenzweig, 2003, p. 7).

Further work is needed on the contribution of urban trees to public health and social equity. The geographical context is important – efforts at reconciliation ecology are strongest where access to natural corridors is closer (Loss et al., 2009). There are still gaps in knowledge about the biodiversity values of green space and ecological connectivity in urban green space (Bell et al., 2008). Moreover, as urban areas are part of an ecosystem, concerns that manifest locally may have their roots or causes in other parts of the system, climate change for instance (Wilbanks and Kates, 1999). The sustainability of the urban forest requires an understanding of the local and global thresholds that can trigger irrevocable changes in urban living. Climate change and water are two concerns likely to affect the quality of Adelaide's urban trees.

In my research, I set out to investigate the question: In what ways does urban greenness relate to public health and social equity in a southern Australian context? Through an ecological public health lens, I revealed a set of ecohealth-generating mechanisms that manifest in the South Australian context under contingent conditions. That is to say, the answer to the research question is tentative – each of these mechanisms could be explored in different contexts. Others have called for 'a truly integrative framework for analysing all aspects of urban systems covering environment and health' (Schandl et al., 2012, p. 381).

This case study is a modest response to that call. The cities where the majority of the world's population now live provide a setting for human and more-than-human health. To understand the links between environment and health in urban areas, there needs to be a shift to biosensitive cities – 'in tune with, sensitive to, and respectful of, the processes of life' (Schandl et al., 2012, p. 382). Furthermore, an ecological public health perspective on biosensitive cities would '[refuse] the old settlements between society and nature, between humans and the rest ... [and] is serious about the heterogeneous company and messy business of *living together*' (Hinchliffe and Whatmore, 2006, p. 134) (italics in original). An ecological public health should be convivial, equitable, sustainable and ethical (Bentley, 2014). However, the inequitable distribution of trees as part of urban green space raises social and environmental justice concerns. It remains to assess the extent to which conviviality can inform social and environmental justice, how political ecology informs sustainable urban environments and how the local informs the global (Bentley, 2014). Further case studies are needed to understand how urban trees relate to environmental and social determinants of health in different urban contexts.

References

Baum, F., Ziersch, A., Zhang, G., Putland, C., Palmer, C., MacDougall, C., et al. 2007. *People and Places: Urban Location, Social Capital and Health*. Flinders University, Adelaide, Australia.

Bell, S., Hamilton, V., Montarzino, A., Rothnie, H., Travlou, P. & Alves, S. 2008. *Greenspace and Quality of Life: A Critical Literature Review*. Greenspace Scotland, Stirling, Scotland, UK.

Bentley, M. 2012. Urban Greenness, Public Health and Social Equity: A South Australian Study. DrPH dissertation, Flinders University, Adelaide, SA, Australia.

Bentley, M. 2014. An ecological public health approach to understanding the relationships between sustainable urban environments, public health and social equity. *Health Promotion International* 29, 528–37.

Conway, T.M., Shakeel, T. & Atallah, J. 2011. Community groups and urban forestry activity: drivers of uneven canopy cover? *Landscape and Urban Planning* 101, 321–9.

Coutts, A.M., Tapper, N.J., Beringer, J., Loughnan, M. & Demuzere, M. 2013. Watering our cities: the capacity for water sensitive urban design to support urban cooling and improve human thermal comfort in the Australian context. *Progress in Physical Geography* 37, 2–28.

Danermark, B., Ekström, M., Jacobsen, L. & Karlsson, J.C. 2002. *Explaining Society: Critical Realism in the Social Sciences*. Routledge, London UK and New York, USA.

Falk, J., Hampton, G., Hodgkinson, A., Parker, K. & Rorris, A. 1993. Social Equity and the Urban Environment: Report to the Commonwealth Environment Protection Agency. University of Wollongong, Wollongong, NSW, Australia.

Goodwins, D. & Noyce, T. 1993. *A 'Greenness' Rating for the Suburbs of Metropolitan Adelaide*. Government of South Australia, Adelaide, SA, Australia.

Head, L. & Muir, P. 2005. Living with trees – perspectives from the suburbs. In: Calver, M., Bigler-Cole, H., Bolton, G., Dargavel, J., Gaynor, A., Horwitz, P., Mills, J., Horwitz, P. & Wardell-Johnson, G. (eds) *Proceedings of the 6th National Conference of the Australian Forest History Society*. Millpress, Rotterdam, The Netherlands, 84–95.

Heynen, N. 2006. Green urban political ecologies: toward a better understanding of inner-city environmental change. *Environment and Planning A* 38, 499–516.

Heynen, N. & Perkins, H.A. 2005. Scalar dialectics in green: urban private property and the contradictions of the neoliberalization of nature. *Capitalism Nature Socialism* 16, 99–113.

Hinchliffe, S. & Whatmore, S. 2006. Living cities: towards a politics of conviviality. *Science as Culture* 15, 123–38.

Hostetler, M., Allen, M. & Meurk, C. 2011. Conserving urban biodiversity? Creating green infrastructure is only the first step. *Landscape and Urban Planning* 100, 369–71.

Joignot, F. 2012. Trees give us more than we recognise. *The Guardian Weekly* 186, 28–9.

Jones, O. & Cloke, P. 2008. Non-human agencies: trees in place and time. In: Knappett, C. & Malafouris, L. (eds) *Material Agency: Towards a Non-anthropocentric Approach*. Springer, New York, USA, 79–96.

Kearns, A., Beaty, M. & Barnett, G. 2007. A socio-ecological perspective on health in urban environments. *NSW Public Health Bulletin* 18, 48–50.

Kirkpatrick, J.B., Daniels, G.D. & Davison, A. 2011. Temporal and spatial variation in garden and street trees in six eastern Australian cities. *Landscape and Urban Planning* 101, 244–52.

Kuo, F. 2003. The role of arboriculture in a healthy social ecology. *Journal of Arboriculture* 29, 148–55.

Landry, S.M. & Chakraborty, J. 2009. Street trees and equity: evaluating the spatial distribution of an urban amenity. *Environment and Planning A* 41, 2651–70.

Loss, S.R., Ruiz, M.O. & Brawn, J.D. 2009. Relationships between avian diversity, neighborhood age, income, and environmental characteristics of an urban landscape. *Biological Conservation* 142, 2578–85.

Maas, J., Verheij, R.A., de Vries, S., Spreeuwenberg, P., Schellevis, P.F.G. & Groenewegen, P.P. 2009. Morbidity is related to a green living environment. *Journal of Epidemiology and Community Health* 63, 967–73.

McMichael, A.J. 1999. Prisoners of the proximate. Loosening the constraints on epidemiology in an age of change. *American Journal of Epidemiology* 149, 887–97.

Moore, G.M. 2009. Urban trees: worth more than they cost. 10th National Street Tree Symposium. Available at: www.treenet.org/symposium/proceedings-archive/symposium-2009/?vid=3, accessed 18 February 2015.

Nilsson, K. & Sangster, M. 2008. Forests, trees and human health and well-being. *Forest and Landscape*. Cost Action E39, Copenhagen, Denmark.

Nowak, D. & Crane, D. 2002. Carbon storage and sequestration by urban trees in the USA. *Environmental Pollution* 116, 381–9.

Panelli, R. & Tipa, G. 2007. Placing well-being: a Maori case study of cultural and environmental specificity. *EcoHealth* 4, 445–60.

Poland, B., Frohlich, K.L. & Cargo, M. 2008. Context as a fundamental dimension of health promotion program evaluation. In: Potvin, L. & McQueen, D. (eds) *Health Promotion Evaluation Practices in the Americas*. Springer, New York, USA, 299–317.

Public Health Information Development Unit 2010 (cited in Bentley, 2012, p. 96). www.adelaide.edu.au/phidu/, accessed 2 July 2015.

Rayner, G. & Lang, T. 2012. *Ecological Public Health Reshaping the Conditions for Good Health*. Routledge/Earthscan, Abingdon, UK.

Rosenzweig, M. 2003. *Win-win Ecology: How Earth's Species Can Survive in the Midst of Human Enterprise*. Oxford University Press, New York, USA.

Sadler, J., Bates, A., Hale, J. & James, P. 2010. Bringing cities alive: the importance of urban greenspaces for people and diversity. In: Gaston, K. (ed.) *Urban Ecology*. Cambridge University Press, Cambridge, UK, 230–60.

Schandl, H., Boyden, S., Capon, A. & Hosking, K. 2012. 'Biosensitive' cities – a conceptual framework for integrative understanding of the health of people and planetary ecosystems. *Current Opinion in Environmental Sustainability* 8, 378–84.

Stagoll, K., Lindenmayer, D.B., Knight, E., Fischer, J. & Manning, A.D. 2012. Large trees are keystone structures in urban parks. *Conservation Letters* 5, 115–22.

Swanwick, C., Dunnett, N. & Woolley, H. 2003. Nature, role and value of green space in towns and cities: an overview. *Built Environment* 29, 94–106.

Tait, C. 2005. Trees and urban green areas. In: Daniels, C. & Tait, C. (eds) *Adelaide. Nature of a City: The Ecology of a Dynamic City from 1836 to 2036*. Biocity: Centre for Urban Habitats, Adelaide, SA, Australia, 101.

Tait, C.J., Daniels, C.B. & Hill, R.S. 2005. Changes in species assemblages within the Adelaide metropolitan area, 1836–2002. *Ecological Applications* 15, 346–59.

Tzoulas, K., Korpela, K., Venn, S., Yli-Pelkonen, V., Kaźmierczak, A., Niemela, J., et al. 2007. Promoting ecosystem and human health in urban areas using Green Infrastructure: a literature review. *Landscape and Urban Planning* 81, 167–78.

Wilbanks, T. & Kates, R. 1999. Global change in local places: how scale matters. *Climatic Change* 43, 601–28.

World Health Organization 1986. Ottawa Charter for Health Promotion. *Health Promotion* 1, i–iv.

Yin, R. 2009. *Case Study Research: Design and Methods*. Sage, Thousand Oaks, California, USA.

29

REFLECTIONS ON THE VIRULENCE OF INFECTIONS

Heirlooms and Temporary Exhibits

ROBIN A. WEISS

Abstract

Infection has played a crucial role in human evolution – from the ancient acquisition of vital organelles such as mitochondria to the 'fossil' viral elements that constitute so much of our genome – but we usually focus on pathogens. When a virus infects a new host species, large changes may occur in pathogen-host ecology and virulence. Some viruses with RNA genomes (e.g. influenza viruses, henipaviruses and severe acute respiratory syndrome (SARS) coronavirus) can leap across relatively large host taxa, causing epidemics in the naïve population. This phenomenon is exemplified by changes in the mode of transmission and virulence of influenza A viruses when they move from waterfowl to chickens, and from chickens to mammals. Increasing virulence is also evident with retroviruses such as human immunodeficiency viruses (HIV) and the leukaemia virus of koalas. Viruses with DNA genomes (e.g. poxviruses, herpesviruses and papilloma viruses) usually have a greater fidelity to their host, but may devastate a closely related host species provided they gain access to it, as when the New World myxomatosis virus was introduced into European rabbits in Australia. Other virulent pox- and herpes virus infections occur when a host species or populations separated by geography and time regain contact through globalisation or through artificial introduction as captive or invasive species. The epidemics among humans indigenous to the Americas and the Pacific islands following the arrival of Europeans serve as a model for the likely fate of Neanderthals and Denisovans when modern humans reached them out of Africa.

Introduction

> No scientist is admired for failing to solve problems that lie beyond their competence. If politics is the art of the possible, research is surely the art of the soluble. Good scientists study the problems they think they can solve. (Medawar, 1967)

Medawar exhorts us to dismiss insoluble questions – when the intellectual and practical means to answer them are not yet available – as idle speculation. All too often, however, we take refuge in asking small questions that are too easily soluble and which will never lead to Kuhnian paradigm shifts (Kuhn, 1962). An exception was Tony McMichael, who had the art of asking penetrating questions before others had formulated them, but for which at least partial answers could be provided. I first met Tony when he was at the London School of Hygiene and Tropical Medicine and I had moved to University College London, 400 metres up Gower Street. Tony had that freshness and clarity of mind that crossed easily between social sciences and medical sciences, and despite our different backgrounds, we established an easy rapport. I was privileged to speak at the launch of Tony's book, *Human Frontiers, Environments and Disease* (McMichael, 2001).

In 2001, the Royal Society invited me to deliver the Leeuwenhoek Lecture and I rashly chose to speak on the origin of human infectious diseases at the London School. The Australian President of the Royal Society, Bob May, looked bemused as I donned a yellow biohazard suit while he introduced me. I asked the audience to imagine that I had recently received a heart transplant from a pig, in order to illustrate the potential infection hazards of xenotransplantation (Weiss, 1998). My purpose was to explain that novel infectious diseases did not always emerge from 'backward' parts of the world. Consider the transmissible spongiform encephalopathies: while kuru, a form of Creutzfeldt–Jakob disease (CJD), did emerge from certain ritual cannibalistic practices in Papua New Guinea, advances in medical technology such as human pituitary transplants gave rise to iatrogenic CJD, and 'advances' in food technology such as mechanised extraction of neural tissue from beef carcasses led to mad cow disease and to variant CJD in humans (Schwartz, 2003).

The editor of *Nature Medicine* attended my Leeuwenhoek Lecture and later invited me to contribute an article to an issue devoted to emerging infectious diseases. She wished me to address broad aspects of the emergence of infections rather than remain in my comfort zone of the cellular and molecular biology of HIV/AIDS. Feeling ill-equipped to write a review covering this degree of breadth, I realised that there was one person above any other who could co-author the article, and I was delighted that Tony (by then back in Canberra) agreed to do so. It is reprinted in this volume (Weiss and McMichael, 2004).

In homage to Tony, I shall raise some questions on the origins, spread and virulence of infectious diseases in the hope that the time is ripe to consider how to solve them. We have the exciting prospect of bringing together social aspects of infectious diseases with their molecular biology (Pulliam, 2008; Wood et al., 2012), and neither discipline should ignore the other.

The Human Body as an Ecosystem

What constitutes an infection? The vast majority of microbes that live in and on the human body are not classified as infections, merely as fellow travellers, and we depend on some of them for good health, the beneficial strains of *Escherichia coli* for instance. As a 'metagenome', our human body contains a minority of human cells (Table 29.1). The human microbiome comprises immensely diverse species, representing about 3 kg of our body mass. The bacterial biofilms in our mouths alone contain upwards of 1,000 species. Moreover, the invasion of the human body goes deeper: some 8 per cent of our chromosomal DNA sequences represent fossil retrovirus genomes. Most, but not all, are defunct. The placental fetal–maternal interface depends on the expression of ancient retroviral envelope glycoproteins to form the syncytiotrophoblast (Weiss and Stoye, 2013). There are DNA traces of RNA viruses such as bornavirus in our chromosomes, too (Feschotte and Gilbert, 2012). If we include retrotransposons among the virus-like fragments that have invaded the human genome, then we carry more DNA derived from infective processes than the genes encoding human proteins (Weiss and Stoye, 2013).

Table 29.1 The human metagenome.

10^{13} human cells	1 sp.
10^{11} eukaryotes	~10^2 spp.
10^{15} bacteria	~10^4 spp.
10^{17} viruses	~10^3 spp.

Source: Author's work (multiple sources).

The numbers listed represent a very rough estimate because the tally and load of organisms in the healthy human body is still incomplete. The eukaryotes include fungi, protozoa and helminths. Less than 1 per cent of the species (spp.) are known pathogens.

Eukaryotic (nucleated) cells themselves represent a successful evolutionary outcome of invasion by different microbes. Mitochondria (and photosynthetic plastids in plants) derive from once independent microbes. Then, eukaryotic cells learned to form multicellular organisms in which cells and tissues could evolve different functions. Nick Lane believes that the emergence of eukaryotic cells is a rarer event than the evolution of microbial life (Lane, 2010), which might explain why we have not yet come across signals of intelligent life on other planets.

On the other hand, pathogens can emerge from normal tissues that have never previously followed an infectious lifestyle. Prions causing transmissible spongiform encephalopathies are encoded by a normal gene but acquire self-propagating epigenetic 'chain reactions' that lead to disease when a misfolded protein triggers similar misfolding in neighbouring molecules (Schwartz, 2003). Genetic predisposition to prion disease is evident where a single amino-acid residue in the protein sequence renders it more liable to misfolding. The cancer that threatens the survival of the endangered Tasmanian devil is derived from an escaped somatic cell originating from one animal (Murchison et al., 2012). A similar but more ancient transmissible pathogen of dogs, canine transmissible venereal tumour, is a somatic cell clone that probably originated ~11,000 years ago and which has spread worldwide (Murgia et al., 2006). As a sexually transmitted infection, it is hardly surprising that it is most prevalent among lower socio-economic canine communities such as pie dogs in India.

What is a Pathogen?

Among the plethora of micro-organisms cohabiting with us, a few are pathogenic. And many of these are conditional pathogens, behaving as harmless companions most of the time but exerting a disease profile when the host is out of condition owing to other factors. Several epidemic and endemic diseases are caused by conditional pathogens. Paradoxically, some infectious diseases have increased in incidence as the prevalence of the pathogen diminishes. Once common infections of infancy have become rarer, and the age of first infection is therefore delayed. The mid-20th-century epidemic of poliomyelitis is an example. When almost all of us acquired poliovirus infection early in infancy when maternal antibodies were present, the virus seldom spread from its natural home in the gut to damage the central nervous system. But, clean, middle-class children acquiring delayed infection when they went to swimming pools were more susceptible to paralysis. Similarly, the gamma-herpes virus, Epstein–Barr virus (EBV), engenders little more than a sore throat in infancy, but can cause infectious mononucleosis when acquired at a higher dose by teenagers. These examples are reminiscent of the 'hygiene hypothesis', whereby early exposure to infectious agents and to antigens may, by influencing the direction of maturation of the immune system, be protective against later infectious and autoimmune diseases.

Some of the chronic diseases of adults may also have an infectious component in their aetiology. Until Barry Marshall famously swallowed *Helicobacter pylori*, epidemiologists did not regard gastric ulcers and stomach cancer as infectious diseases. As molecular methods of microbial detection become more sophisticated, other common microbes may prove to be pathogens for diseases prevalent in the ageing population.

The Power of Molecular Phylogenetics

Until recently, the origin of viruses and other parasites was based on data from historical and ecological surmises. With the development of powerful forensic DNA sequencing technology, we can apply more stringent methods to investigate origins. Analysis of simian immunodeficiency virus (SIV) genomes reveals that four distinct transfer events to humans took place because each of the four HIV-1 groups has SIV relatives in chimpanzees, which are genetically closer than the human HIV-1 groups are to each other (Figure 29.1). Only one virus lineage, HIV-1 group M, has become pandemic and has diverged into the diverse clades (subtypes A–K) and the recombinant strains we see today (Ndung'u and Weiss, 2012). Thanks to molecular phylogenetics applied to urine samples from painstaking field studies, the geographic origin of group M could be located to a small area in south-east Cameroon, because that was where chimpanzees with SIV of similar sequence were found.

Molecular sequencing proved that the HIV strains infecting children in Benghazi in Libya pre-dated the arrival of the Bulgarian nurses who came to care for them, and who were accused under the Ghadaffi regime of deliberately spreading AIDS (de Oliveira et al., 2012). The same technique demonstrated conclusively that the *Vibrio cholerae* strain causing the cholera outbreak in Haiti following the 2010 earthquake really was introduced, albeit unwittingly, by UN emergency forces from Nepal (Frerichs et al., 2012). Ironically, 40 years earlier, Haitian UN peacekeeping forces returning from the Katangan war in the Congo were probably the vector that introduced HIV subtype B to the West (Pepin, 2011). If John Snow, born 200 years ago, came back today, I think he would delight in applying molecular epidemiology to tracking transmissible diseases.

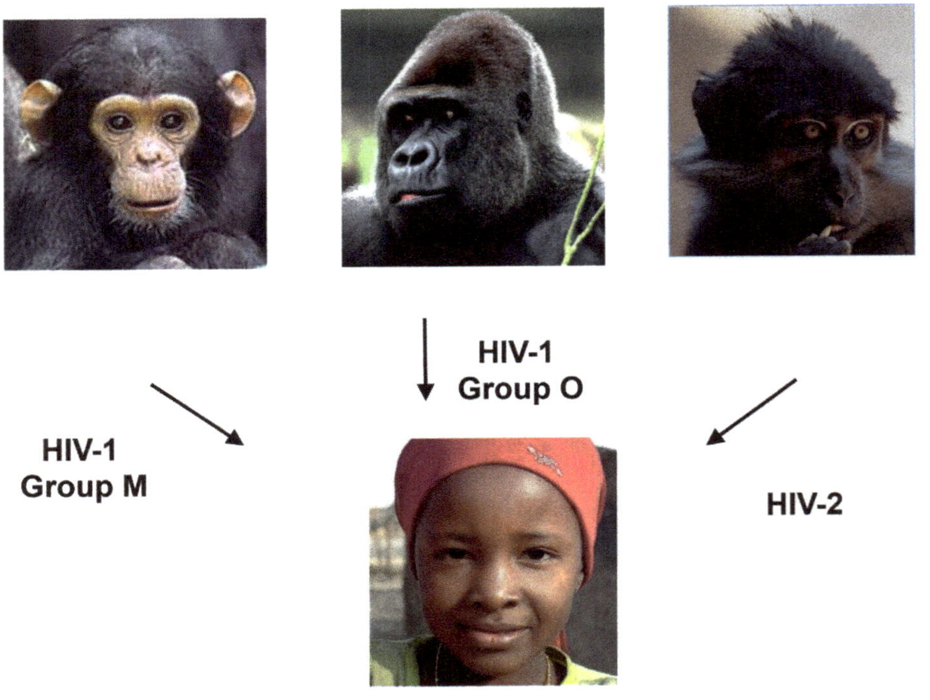

Figure 29.1 Multiple cross-species origins of human immunodeficiency viruses (HIV).

The pandemic strain of HIV-1 group M came from a specific population of chimpanzees (*Pan troglodytes troglodytes*) in Cameroon about 90 years ago and has infected approximately 65 million humans to date. HIV-1 group O came either from gorillas (*Gorilla gorilla*) or chimpanzees and has infected about 10,000 humans, while two other SIVcpz transfers have spread to only a handful of humans each. HIV-2 has been introduced from sooty mangabey monkeys (*Cercocebus atys*) to humans in West Africa on at least six separate occasions. It has spread to Europe and India, but its prevalence is waning, for poorly understood reasons. See Ndung'u and Weiss, 2012.

Source: Author's work.

Molecular sequencing of complementary DNA from the RNA of influenza A virus genomes showed that during the recent epidemic of swine-origin H1N1, the virus was imported several times into the UK (Baillie et al., 2012). Temporal and geographical movements of viruses can be tracked through phylogenies, and deep sequencing can reveal the evolution of virus populations within one infected individual. Sequencing and rescue of the influenza virus from archival specimens from the 1918/19 pandemic helped to pinpoint its origin as an avian virus, and may explain why it was highly pathogenic (Taubenberger et al., 2001).

With increasing refinement of DNA amplification and sequencing from ancient specimens, it is becoming possible to determine origins previously based on historical studies; for instance, whether the virulent form of syphilis that appeared in 1493 really came from Hispaniola (Harper et al., 2008). The Justinian

Plague in 541 CE and the Black Death in Europe in 1347/8 were discussed by McMichael (McMichael, 2010), and it has been confirmed that the latter was caused by *Yersinia pestis*, perhaps by two distinct clades (Haensch et al., 2010). It may soon become possible to elucidate which particular pathogens lay behind more ancient plagues through the molecular analysis of archaeological specimens.

A caveat is that as DNA sequencing techniques become ever more sensitive, allowing single cell and microbe amplification, the greater the danger becomes of contamination by extraneous DNA fragments. For example, much publicity was given in 2009 to a virus related to the xenotropic murine retrovirus putatively detected in blood samples from people suffering from chronic fatigue syndrome, but the whole edifice crumbled on more detailed and objective analysis (Weiss, 2010). Thus, candidates for viruses possibly contributing to other chronic diseases like multiple sclerosis need to be examined with genuine curiosity mixed with healthy scepticism.

Family Heirlooms and New Acquisitions

The title of this section is a metaphor first coined by Tony McMichael (McMichael, 2001). *Family heirlooms* are the human infectious agents that have co-evolved with us ever since we and the other great apes diverged from each other. The gamma-herpesviruses, EBV and Kaposi's sarcoma-associated virus, KSHV, are maternal heirlooms; they are typically transmitted from mother or grandmother to offspring via saliva, but can also be transmitted sexually or by sexual kissing later in life. Our closest extant relative, the chimpanzee, carries a virus closely related to EBV, while other apes and monkeys harbour more distant relatives of EBV in parallel with the evolutionary distance of the host (see Figure 29.2).

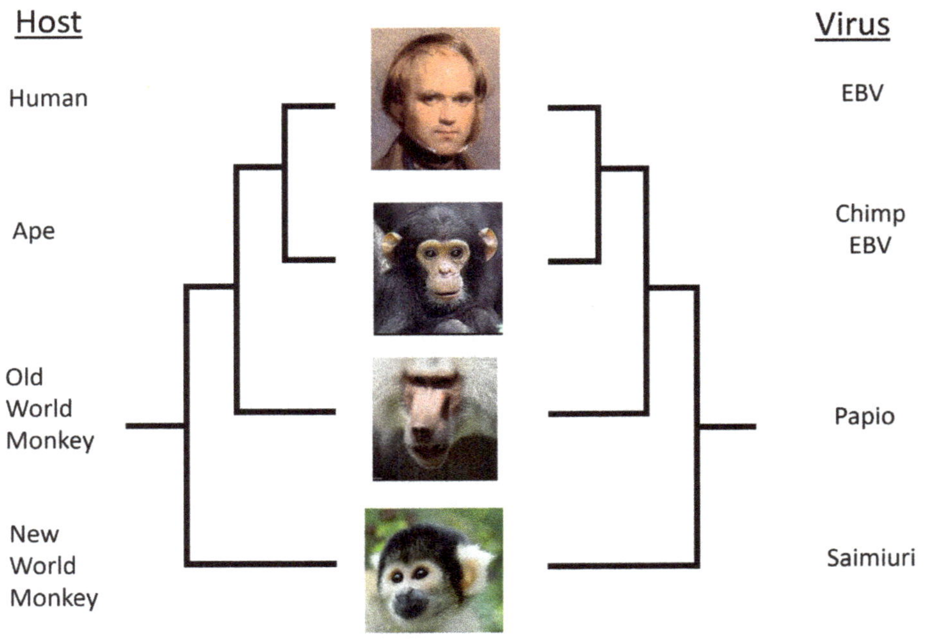

Figure 29.2 Co-speciation of lymphocryptic herpesvirus (EBV) genomes and their hosts. The estimated time back to the most recent common ancestor is broadly the same for virus and host.

Source: Author's work.

I used to assume that each of the eight known human herpesviruses came down to us adhering strictly to host lineage, but now it appears that there has been more horizontal exchange of family heirlooms within families than we formerly imagined, including the EBV lineage (Ehlers et al., 2010). Such horizontal transfers may lead to large changes in virulence, as argued below. There remain puzzles: humans harbour two distinct herpes simplex viruses, HSV-1 and HSV-2. Phylogenetic analysis of HSV genomes indicates that HSV-2 is much closer to chimpanzee herpesvirus than to HSV-1 (Luebcke et al., 2006). This observation raises the question whether humans have always had the two types on board (separated in their anatomical silos) ever since the viruses diverged about eight million years ago, or whether HSV-1 has been acquired horizontally (Luebcke et al., 2006; Weiss, 2009).

New acquisitions are the infections that we have picked up in 'recent' times, such as measles about 10,000 years ago and HIV less than 100 years ago (McMichael, 2001; Weiss and McMichael, 2004). Tony McMichael documented different episodes in the emergence of pandemic infections and the changing patterns of human migration, ecology and behaviour that promoted their emergence (McMichael, 2001). Many prehistoric and historic disease agents came from domesticated livestock, or from animals which themselves found a suitable habitat in becoming our companions, such as dogs and rats. In contrast, recent outbreaks of novel virus infections tend to originate in wildlife (McFarlane et al., 2012). The SARS coronavirus, Hendra and Nipah paramyxoviruses, and Ebola and Marburg filoviruses came from exotic species such as primates (Ebola) and civet cats (SARS), although the paramyxoviruses came from bats via horses (Hendra) and pigs (Nipah). But, all these animals are temporary amplifying vessels for viruses that have their long-term reservoir in bats (Wood et al., 2012). Extending McMichael's metaphor, we can regard outbreaks that naturally peter out as *temporary exhibits*.

The challenge is to ascertain which novel outbreaks are likely to become long-term acquisitions or disappear like Ebola. SARS engendered enormous fear and economic damage, although less than 1,000 persons worldwide died as a result of SARS infection (McLean et al., 2005). In contrast, the World Health Organization's (WHO) figure for annual human mortality from rabies is 55,000, and this figure may well represent a substantial underestimate of actual deaths. Yet, each human is a dead-end host for rabies, so there is no fear of a rabies pandemic.

Although WHO claimed that intelligent surveillance controlled the SARS epidemic, it probably played a minor role (McLean et al., 2005). What saved the SARS outbreak from becoming a major pandemic was more mundane biology. In contrast to influenza, people infected with the SARS coronavirus only become infectious to others after they develop serious symptoms and retire to bed. Moreover, only a minority of those with SARS were what became known as super-spreaders. As with Ebola virus, those at greatest risk for acquiring secondary infection were carers – family members and nurses. In other words, SARS transmission was inefficient and the overall reproductive rate of the virus was low, $R0 = <1$.

It might have gone otherwise for SARS. A novel, highly pathogenic coronavirus (Van Boheemen et al., 2012) arising in Saudi Arabia in mid-2012 had killed 6/13 infected people in the Middle East and Europe by February 2013, and we do not yet know what the outcome will be. HIV initially struggled to take off (Pepin, 2011), and as mentioned, only one of the ten transfers from apes and monkeys has become pandemic. This is not because the environmental or social conditions differed for each transfer. Rather, subtle differences in the properties of the virus strains themselves determined how efficiently they could adapt to their new host. Despite Colin Butler's timely warning (Butler, 2012) that overemphasis on novel emerging pathogens diverts attention from other important health problems and determinants, the example of HIV/AIDS shows that to ignore them altogether would be foolhardy.

Our burgeoning understanding of the molecular biology of species-specific host restriction factors (Duggal and Emerman, 2012) that a virus has to overcome to establish itself in a new species may help in forecasting which new outbreaks pose the greatest threat to become pandemic. Moreover, analysis of the amplification and reduction of genetic sequences within the viral genome can reveal past patterns of adaptation in the Red Queen evolutionary race between virus and host (Elde et al., 2012).

The Concept of Virulence

I regard disease caused by viruses as collateral damage to viral replication. True, there are a few pathological symptoms that may be induced specifically to aid onward transmission, such as the behavioural changes induced by rabies virus. In most cases, however, disease is only indirectly related to transmission dynamics. For instance, the paralysis induced in a small proportion of those infected by poliovirus is related to high viral load, but the neurological effects are not themselves relevant to polio transmission. Some symptoms of illness are a sign of a healthy reaction to the infection, such as the fever and aches induced by interferon. But an overstimulation of such an innate immune reaction, often referred to as a 'cytokine storm', may in itself be fatal. Severity tends to be associated with novel infections where there is no immunological memory and no previous selection in the host for survival.

Virulence is neither positively nor negatively related with the efficiency of epidemic spread. There is a tendency for initially highly virulent infections to become attenuated over time, as Girolamo Fracostoro observed for syphilis in the 16th century and Frank Fenner witnessed for myxomatosis (Fenner and Ratcliffe, 1965). In contrast, the virulence of untreated HIV-1 infection over the past 25 years appears to be increasing (Herbeck et al., 2012). Virulence in the individual has little impact on the population when it occurs at the extremities of lifespan – in infancy and in old age. However, viruses newly introduced into a host population (like the 1918–19 influenza pandemic and HIV) are virulent at all ages – which has greater consequences for society (Weiss and McMichael, 2004).

Cross-species Virulence

The virulence of infection in a new host species is difficult to predict. Most zoonoses are barely detectable, being ill-adapted to the new host, yet some are devastating. I shall reflect on a few virus examples.

Influenza and other avian viruses

In public health terms, we rightly fear the emergence of a highly pathogenic virus that is also highly transmissible. That is why there has been so much concern about the highly pathogenic H5N1 influenza virus that kills chickens and humans alike. Luckily, the H5N1 virus has not yet adapted to efficient human-to-human transmission and remains a zoonotic infection. While the public health experts were looking eastwards in trepidation, the H1N1 influenza virus quietly escaped from pigs in Mexico and spread rapidly across the globe. The mortality of this virus is low and is restricted mainly to a rare human genotype (Everitt et al., 2012). However, a reassortant virus between H5N1 and H1N1 might be quite a different matter.

Why do chickens and humans alike suffer from influenza virus infection when the natural hosts, waterfowl, do not usually become ill? There is no clear answer, but it behoves us to consider the ecology of the infection in different hosts. In ducks and geese, influenza is an enteric, waterborne infection, whereas in both chickens and humans, it is respiratory. Thus, the mode of transmission differs, as well as virulence. The transfer from duck to chicken may well involve a more drastic change for the virus than that of chicken to mammal. However, we understand the avian to mammalian switch better at the molecular level because the stereochemistry of the sialic acid receptors differs for influenza virus in these two classes of host.

It strikes me that the social dynamics of different species of birds is being largely ignored in discussions of avian reservoirs of potential human infection. Migratory birds have an enormous geographic range. We do not know whether it was a stowaway mosquito or an imported bird that brought West Nile virus to New York in 1999, but we do know that it took only two years to reach the US West Coast. Apart from migration, there is 'epideictic' behaviour, whereby some avian species live for part of their life cycle in extraordinarily crowded habitats while they may be highly dispersed and sparsely distributed at other times (Wynne-Edwards, 1962). Large avian colonies, such as seabird nesting sites or the mass roosts of starlings in cities like London, resemble the dense human habitation that facilitates the spread of epidemic infections, whereas dispersed birds (such as the jungle fowl progenitors of the domestic chicken) are more like hunter-gatherer humans whose viruses need to establish persistent infections to be passed vertically through generations. It would be interesting to investigate whether the species exhibiting crowd behaviour are more effective reservoirs for the emergence of viruses. Likewise, many species of bats live in huge colonies when not on the wing, and they are the reservoirs of many types of RNA virus (lyssa-, filo- and henipaviruses) that do them little harm but are highly pathogenic for terrestrial mammals (Wood et al., 2012).

Poxviruses

Poxviruses typically establish short-lived, acute infections. If the host survives, it becomes immune to reinfection, and a relatively large population of naïve subjects is needed for maintenance of the virus. Some like smallpox virus are highly pathogenic, and this may be a marker of its relatively recent introduction into humans, about 2,000 years ago (McMichael, 2001). Myxoma virus is an endemic, low pathogenic virus in American lagomorphs such as the jackrabbit (*Sylvilagus* spp.), but it became a mass killer when introduced by accident or deliberately into European rabbits. This is the most famous example of high virulence upon cross-species transfer (Fenner and Ratcliffe, 1965). But, high virulence in cross-species infection is not inevitable. Cowpox is not virulent in humans, but as Edward Jenner demonstrated, it confers acquired immunity to smallpox (Weiss and Esparza, 2015). This lack of virulence may be due to the large evolutionary distance between bovines and humans. More closely related species show a similar pattern to myxomatosis in rabbits. For instance, the dieback of indigenous red squirrels in the UK since the introduction of American grey squirrels 100 years ago appears to be due less to competition for habitat than to a grey squirrel poxvirus (Sainsbury et al., 2008).

Retroviruses

Some retroviruses represent the extreme family heirloom in being transmitted as chromosomally integrated DNA genomes in the host. As already mentioned, ~8 per cent of human DNA is derived from retrovirus infection. In this way, the virus gets a free ride through the generations, but intact genomes can re-emerge as infectious agents (Weiss and Stoye, 2013). The host carrying the endogenous virus often evolves resistance to reinfection at the cellular level, so that viral load remains low, but such viruses can infect foreign species and hence are called xenotropic. An example is an endogenous gamma-retrovirus transmitted through the germ line of Asian species of mice. In the 1970s, it spread to gibbons held in captivity in Southeast Asia, and it has also spread to koalas in Australia. It causes acute leukaemia in both the new hosts. Interestingly, it is becoming newly endogenous in koalas in colonising their germ line (Tarlinton et al., 2006) (see Figure 29.3).

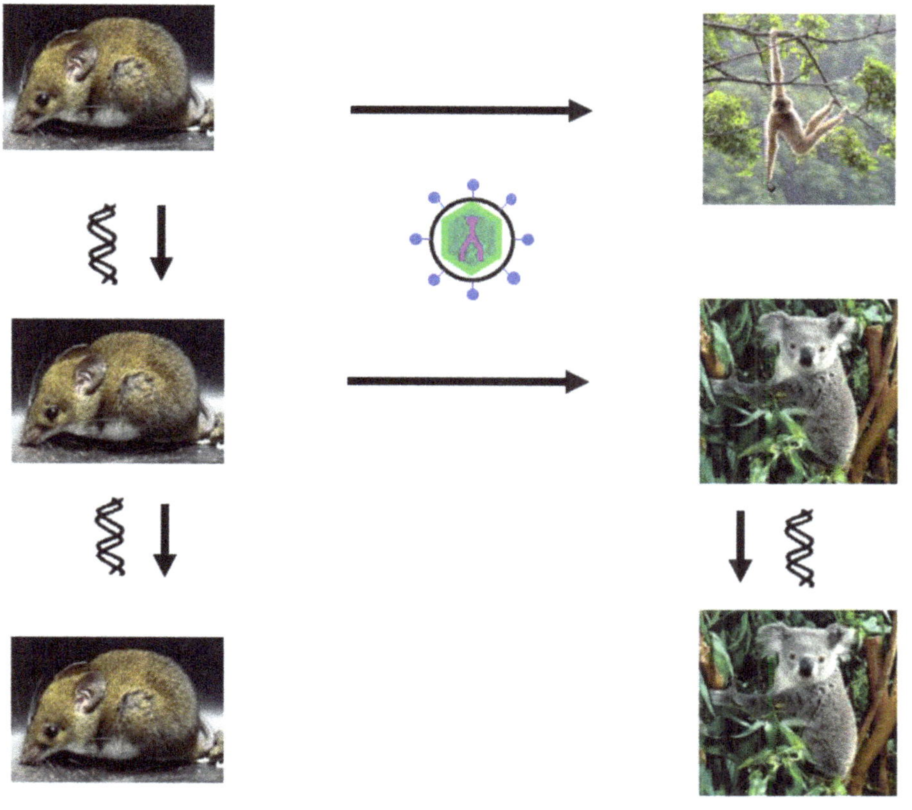

Figure 29.3 Gamma-retrovirus genomes can be transmitted either vertically as Mendelian traits or horizontally as infectious virus particles.

The evolutionary dynamics of such contrasting modes of transmission are drastically different. Two Asian species of mouse, the Ricefield mouse (*Mus caroli*) and the Fawn-coloured mouse (*Mus cerviclor*), carry closely related Mendelian retroviruses that are more distantly related to the leukaemia viruses of house mice (*Mus musculus*). The similarity in genomes of the two murine retroviruses indicates that this genome reservoir has been present in Southeast Asian mice for tens of thousands of years before these species diverged. During the 20th century, this virus gave rise to two distinct infectious epidemics causing leukaemia, one in gibbon apes and another in koalas. The koala retrovirus is in the process of becoming endogenous in the koala genome. It may be significant that the lar gibbons first known to be infected were captive animals held at ground level, where they would have had more contact with mice than in the canopy of the rainforest. How the Asian mice gained contact with koalas in Australia is not known, but it may have been through the importation of rice and other goods by ship.

Source: Author's work.

Herpesviruses

Herpesviruses are heirloom viruses that set up long-term persistent infections ideally suited to maintenance in small, isolated host populations like hunter-gatherers. The virus can be activated decades after initial infection and transmitted to the next generation. Although human herpesviruses such as herpes simplex, cytomegalovirus and EBV cause disease in some individuals, infection is not commonly fatal. Like poxviruses, however, herpesviruses can be lethal to related but distinct host species. This has long been known for human exposure to herpes B virus of macaques. More recently, this phenomenon has come to light in elephants held in zoos. An alpha-herpesvirus of African elephants is lethal to Indian elephants, while causing nothing more serious than a cold sore in its own host. Conversely, the Indian counterpart is highly pathogenic to African elephants (Richman et al., 1999).

Conclusion

I have argued that the virulence of cross-species virus infections can be devastating. RNA viruses often cross into quite unrelated hosts. Modern-day examples of novel viral diseases in humans tend to come from wildlife, and particularly from species that associate with humans (McFarlane et al., 2012; and discussed by Ro McFarlane, this volume). One factor of this wildlife origin may be that humans have already had ample time to acquire infections from livestock, such as measles from rinderpest of cattle.

Cross-species infections by DNA viruses are more likely to originate in species closely related taxonomically to their new host, and also often show a marked increase in virulence. The separation of species or populations halts selection for attenuation for the other species' virus, so that when related species meet again, their herpesviruses and poxviruses may present a disastrous situation in the new host. If Indian elephants unwittingly acted as bioterrorists to their African counterparts (and possibly to Hannibal's 'third' species and mammoths, too?), and if myxomatosis was so lethal to European rabbits, we could surmise that when modern humans met Neanderthals and Denisovans, they almost certainly introduced them to lethal viruses (Weiss, 2009). Our hominid cousins would have been just as susceptible to human diseases they had not previously encountered as the Indigenous Americans and Pacific Islanders were to Old World viruses exported by European colonisation.

Of course, the transfer might also have gone in the opposite direction. We do not know what infections modern humans acquired from Neanderthals and Denisovans, but we certainly had contact because we acquired some of their genes (Meyer et al., 2010). Today, ecotourism can threaten endangered great apes if they acquire infections such as common colds and measles from humans. Such 'anthoposes' may account for more ancient animal infections; it seems as if bovine tuberculosis may have come from humans (Brosch et al., 2002).

Overall, in this dynamic world where climatic change, human expansion and habitat destruction continue, we should expect to witness further surprising episodes of novel infections with curious origins and threatening virulence.

References

Baillie, G.J., Galiano, M., Agapow, P.-M., Myers, R., Chiam, R., Gall, A., et al. 2012. Evolutionary dynamics of local pandemic H1N1/2009 influenza virus lineages revealed by whole-genome analysis. *Journal of Virology* 86, 11–8.

Brosch, R., Gordon, S.V., Marmiesse, M., Brodin, P., Buchrieser, C., Eiglmeier, K., et al. 2002. A new evolutionary scenario for the *Mycobacterium tuberculosis* complex. *Proceedings of the National Academy of Sciences (USA)* 99, 3684–9.

Butler, C.D. 2012. Infectious disease emergence and global change: thinking systemically in a shrinking world. *Infectious Diseases of Poverty* 1, 5.

de Oliveira, T., Pybus, O.G., Rambaut, A., Salemi, M., Cassol, S., Ciccozzi, M., et al. 2012. Molecular epidemiology: HIV-1 and HCV sequences from Libyan outbreak. *Nature* 444, 836–7.

Duggal, N.K. & Emerman, M. 2012. Evolutionary conflicts between viruses and restriction factors shape immunity. *Nature Reviews Immunology* 12, 687–95.

Ehlers, B., Spiess, K., Leendertz, F., Peeters, M., Boesch, C., Gatherer, D., et al. 2010. Lymphocryptovirus phylogeny and the origins of Epstein–Barr virus. *Journal of General Virology* 91, 630–42.

Elde, N.C., Child, S.J., Eickbush, M.T., Kitzman, J.O., Rogers, K.S., Shendure, J., et al. 2012. Poxviruses deploy genomic accordions to adapt rapidly against host antiviral defenses. *Cell* 150, 831–41.

Everitt, A.R., Clare, S., Pertel, T., John, S.P., Wash, R.S., Smith, S.E., et al. 2012. IFITM3 restricts the morbidity and mortality associated with influenza. *Nature* 484, 519–23.

Fenner, F. & Ratcliffe, F.N. 1965. *Myxomatosis*. Cambridge University Press, Cambridge, UK.

Feschotte, C. & Gilbert, C. 2012. Endogenous viruses: insights into viral evolution and impact on host biology. *Nature Reviews Genetics* 13, 283–96.

Frerichs, R.R., Keim, P.S., Barrais, R. & Piarroux, R. 2012. Nepalese origin of the cholera epidemic in Haiti. *Clinical Microbiology and Infection* 18, E158–63.

Haensch, S., Bianucci, R., Signoli, M., Rajerison, M., Schultz, M., Kacki, S., et al. 2010. Distinct clones of *Yersinia pestis* caused the Black Death. *PloS Pathogens* 6, e1001134.

Harper, K.N., Ocampo, P.S., Steiner, B.M., George, R.W., Silverman, M.S., Bolotin, S., et al. 2008. On the origin of the treponematoses: a phylogenetic approach. *PloS Neglected Tropical Diseases* 2, e148.

Herbeck, J.T., Müller, V., Maust, B.S., Ledergerber, B., Torti, C., Di Giambenedetto, S., et al. 2012. Is the virulence of HIV changing? A meta-analysis of trends in prognostic markers of HIV disease progression and transmission. *AIDS* 26, 193–205.

Kuhn, T. S. 1962. The *Structure of Scientific Revolutions*. University of Chicago Press, Chicago, USA.

Lane, N. 2010. *Life Ascending*. Profile Books, London, UK.

Luebcke, E., Dubovi, E., Black, D., Ohsawa, K. & Eberle, R. 2006. Isolation and characterization of a chimpanzee alphaherpesvirus. *Journal of General Virology* 87, 11–9.

McFarlane, R., Sleigh, A. & McMichael, A.J. 2012. Synanthropy of wild mammals as a determinant of emerging infectious diseases in the Asian and Australasian region. *EcoHealth* 9, 24–35.

McLean, A.R., May, R.M., Pattison, J. & Weiss, R.A. (eds) 2005. *SARS: A Case Study in Emerging Infections*. Oxford University Press, Oxford, UK.

McMichael, A.J. 2001. *Human Frontiers, Environments and Disease: Past Patterns, Uncertain Futures*. Cambridge University Press, Cambridge, UK.

McMichael, A.J. 2010. Paleoclimate and bubonic plague: a forewarning of future risk? *BMC Biology* 8, 108.

Medawar P.B. 1967 *The Art of the Soluble*. Methuen & Co, London, UK.

Meyer, M., Kircher, M., Gansauge, M.-T., Li, H., Racimo, F., Mallick, S., et al. 2010. A high-coverage genome sequence from an archaic Denisovan individual. *Science* 338, 222–6.

Murchison, E.P., Schulz-Trieglaff, O.B., Ning, Z., Alexandrov, L.B., Bauer, M.J., Fu, B., et al. 2012. Genome sequencing and analysis of the Tasmanian devil and its transmissible cancer. *Cell* 148, 780–91.

Murgia, C., Pritchard, J.K., Kim, S.Y., Fassati, A. & Weiss, R.A. 2006. Clonal origin and evolution of a transmissible cancer. *Cell* 126, 477–87.

Ndung'u, T. & Weiss, R.A. 2012. On HIV diversity. *AIDS* 26, 1255–60.

Pepin, J. 2011. *The Origins of AIDS*. Cambridge University Press, Cambridge, UK.

Pulliam, J.R.C. 2008. Virus host jumps: moving towards a predictive framework. *EcoHealth* 5, 80–91.

Richman, L.K., Montali, R.J., Garber, R.L., Kennedy, M.A., Lehnhardt, J., Hildebrandt, T., et al. 1999. Novel endotheliotropic herpesviruses fatal for Asian and African elephants. *Science* 283, 1171–6.

Sainsbury, A.W., Deaville, R., Lawson, B., Cooley, W.A., Farelly, S.J., Stack, M.J., et al. 2008. Poxviral disease in red squirrels *Sciurus vulgaris* in the UK: spatial and temporal trends of an emerging threat. *EcoHealth* 5, 305–16.

Schwartz, M. 2003. *How the Cows Turned Mad*. University of California Press, Berkeley, California, USA.

Tarlinton, R.E., Meers, J. & Young, P.R. 2006. Retroviral invasion of the koala genome. *Nature* 442, 79–81.

Taubenberger, J.K., Reid, A.H., Janczewski, T.A. & Fanning, T.G. 2001. Integrating historical, clinical and molecular genetic data in order to explain the origin and virulence of the 1918 Spanish influenza virus. *Philosophical Transactions of the Royal Society of London Series B Biological Sciences* 356, 1829–39.

Van Boheemen, S., de Graaf, M., Lauber, C., Bestebroer, T.M., Raj, V.S., Zaki, A.M., et al. 2012. Genomic characterization of a newly discovered coronavirus associated with acute respiratory distress syndrome in humans. *mBio* 3, e00473-12.

Weiss, R.A. 1998. Transgenic pigs and virus adaptation. *Nature* 391, 327–8.

Weiss, R.A. 2009. Apes, lice and prehistory. *Journal of Biology* 8, 20, doi:10.1186/jbiol114.

Weiss, R.A. 2010. A cautionary tale of virus and disease. *BMC Biology* 8, 124.

Weiss, R.A. & McMichael, A.J. 2004. Social and environmental risk factors in the emergence of infectious diseases. *Nature Medicine* 10, S70–S76.

Weiss, R.A. & Stoye, J.P. 2013. Our viral inheritance. *Science* 340, 820–1.

Weiss RA & Esparza J, 2015. The prevention and eradication of smallpox. *Philosophical Transactions of the Royal Society of London Series B*. 370: 20140378. doi.org/10.1098/rstb.2014.0378.

Wood, J.L.N., Leach, M., Waldman, L., MacGregor, H., Fooks, A.R., Jones, K.E., et al. 2012. A framework for the study of zoonotic disease emergence and its drivers: spillover of bat pathogens as a case study. *Philosophical Transactions of the Royal Society of London Series B Biological Sciences* 367, 2881–92.

Wynne-Edwards, V.C. 1962. *Animal Dispersion in Relation to Social Behaviour*. Oliver & Boyd, London, UK.

PART 7

TRANSFORMATION

REPRINT 1

The Sustainability Transition: A New Challenge

ANTHONY J. MCMICHAEL, KIRK R. SMITH
AND CARLOS F. CORVALÁN

McMichael, A.J., Smith, K.R. & Corvalan, C.F. 2000.
The sustainability transition: a new challenge. *Bulletin of the World Health Organization* 78(9), 1067.

Pages: 531 to 534

Editorial

The sustainability transition: a new challenge

Anthony J. McMichael,[1] Kirk R. Smith,[2] & Carlos F. Corvalan[3]

As several of the papers in this special issue show, environmental health hazards are currently most prevalent in developing countries at the household level. Among the commonest hazards are indoor air pollution, arsenic and infectious agents in drinking-water, and local environmental exposure to lead. Finding ways to reduce these risks more quickly remains an important item on the global agenda because of the significant burden of disease they impose.

At the United Nations Conference on the Human Environment in 1972, much of the concern was about chemical contaminants, the depletion of natural resources, and urbanization. This reflected problems resulting from rapid industrialization in the West and the Soviet bloc countries, as well as uncontrolled agricultural and industrial expansion in the newly independent developing countries. Earlier there had been serious episodes of air pollution, such as the London fog of 1952, organic mercury poisoning in Minamata, Japan (disclosed in 1956), accumulations of heavy metals (especially lead and cadmium), pesticide toxicity, and exposures to environmental ionizing radiation. Similar toxicological hazards persist today. Since 1972, we have had the major accidents of Bhopal, Seveso and Chernobyl, and it is highly probable that there will be more.

Meanwhile, a further set of large-scale environmental problems has emerged and moved towards centre-stage. They add up to the conviction that we are living beyond the Earth's means, and that the continued increase in human numbers and economic activity poses a serious problem for the world as a whole. In September 1999 the United Nations Environment Programme (UNEP) issued its *Global environment outlook 2000*, whose final chapter begins as follows.

> "The beginning of a new millennium finds the planet Earth poised between two conflicting trends. A wasteful and invasive consumer society, coupled with continued population growth, is threatening to destroy the resources on which human life is based. At the same time, society is locked in a struggle against time to reverse these trends and introduce sustainable practices that will ensure the welfare of future generations." (*1*)

The report urges all national governments to recognize the urgent need for concerted and radical action in order to make the transition to a sustainable system.

Some of the health implications of living in a destabilized global ecosystem are reviewed in this issue. They include the impact of climate change on vector-borne diseases (Githeko et al., pp. 1136–1147), the health effects of El Niño (Kovats, pp. 1127–1135), and the challenge of protecting health in a time of rapid change (Woodward et al., pp. 1148–1155).

The sustainability transition involves ensuring that the natural ecological, geophysical and chemical systems that support life on Earth can continue to function. The aim here is for those alive today to meet their own needs without making it impossible for future generations to meet theirs. To do this we have to bequeath to them a biosphere that is intact. This in turn calls for an economic structure within which we consume only as much as the natural environment can produce, and make only as much waste as it can absorb.

The three determinants of human disruption of the environment are population size, levels of material production and consumption, and types of technology (*2*). During the 20th century, carbon dioxide emissions increased almost fourfold. Climatologists think that for the concentration of carbon dioxide to be tolerable for most ecosystems, emissions need to be reduced to about two thirds of their current level. Much of the technology needed to reduce carbon dioxide emissions without forfeiting our material standards of living already exists. The real challenge is political: to adopt the technologies and the practices that will ensure sustainability.

Overall, then, the threat to the environment and to human health comes not so much from increasing human numbers as from increasing use of environmentally damaging technologies (*3*). Major problems would arise in an unmanaged "development" transition that generalized to all countries the patterns of production and consumption typical of today's rich countries. By attempting to run the planet at full-speed-ahead, with current technologies and an expanding consumer demand, we are putting too much pressure on Earth's biophysical systems.

The sustainability transition cannot be expected to occur on its own or as the inevitable outcome of current trends. It will only occur if we make it happen, and do so in the near future. This is a task for the international community, as it feels its way towards more effective forms of global decision-making. One of the strongest sources of motivation for making the transition will be a clear understanding of the risks to human health posed by our overloading of the biosphere. The closing years of the 20th century put us clearly on notice that we must work together to get onto a path of ecologically sustainable social and economic development. The level of health attained by the world's population will be the ultimate criterion of how well we succeed. ■

[1] Professor of Epidemiology, Department of Epidemiology and Population Health, London School of Hygiene and Tropical Medicine, Keppel Street, London WC1E 7HT (email: tony.mcmichael@lshtm.ac.uk). Correspondence should be addressed to this author.

[2] Professor, Environmental Health Sciences, University of California, Berkeley, CA 94720-7360, USA

[3] Scientist, Protection of the Human Environment, World Health Organization, Geneva, Switzerland.

Ref. No. **00-0907**

1. **United Nations Environment Programme.** *Global environment outlook 2000.* London, Earthscan, 1999.
2. **Ehrlich PR, Holdren JP.** Impact of population growth. *Science*, 1971, **171**: 1212–1217.
3. **McMichael AJ, Powles JWP.** Human numbers, environment, sustainability and health. *British Medical Journal*, 1999, **319**: 977–980.

END OF REPRINT 1

The Sustainability Transition: A New Challenge

ANTHONY J. MCMICHAEL, KIRK R. SMITH
AND CARLOS F. CORVALÁN

30

MANAGING DECLINE

Global Change Requires Local Action

TREVOR HANCOCK

Abstract

Ecosystem decline and collapse is not just a plausible alternative future but an unfolding present-day reality. It will be accompanied by the decline and collapse of societies and communities that depend on those ecosystems, and will have a dramatic impact on population health. Decline can be thought of as a form of long, slow crisis or a slowly unfolding disaster, and may be the prelude to collapse. After briefly reviewing the declining condition of some key elements of the global ecosystem, I conclude that we need a game plan to guide us through the ecological decline that we are already experiencing, and through the social changes this will require. I call this 'managing decline'; it begins with a willingness to acknowledge and accept the reality of ecological decline, and may need to include setting up 'decline management' units, rather as we have set up disaster management units, to help us manage the transition through decline and avoid collapse. As with so many important innovations, managing decline will begin at the local level. Indeed, this is beginning to happen, best exemplified by the synergy between *healthy* and *sustainable* cities and, more recently, the emergence of the Transition Towns movement.

Context: Declines in All That Sustains Life

As a health futurist with a particular interest in alternative futures and preferable futures, I have long recognised that 'decline and collapse' is a plausible alternative future that we face (Bezold and Hancock, 1993, 1994). Indeed, we face the real option of both the decline and collapse of ecosystems and the accompanying decline and collapse of the societies and communities that are embedded in and depend on those ecosystems. Yet, it is in many ways the future whose name we dare not speak – or at least, that we prefer not to explore. In workshops, it is, of course, seen as an undesirable future, although not improbable – and nobody likes to examine the undesirable.

But, the reality is that decline and collapse is not just a plausible alternative future but an unfolding present-day reality. In the 20 years since Tony McMichael wrote *Planetary Overload* (McMichael, 1993) the state of our planetary ecosystems and the sustainability of our natural resources have declined significantly.

Average annual global CO_2 emissions increased from 22.6 billion tonnes (Bt) in 1992 to 33.9 Bt in 2011, an increase of 50 per cent (Olivier *et al.*, 2012), with CO_2 levels at Mauna Loa, Hawaii hitting 400 ppm in May 2013 for the first time in about three million years (Gillis, 2013), while the average annual global temperature has increased from 14.15°C in 1992 to 14.53°C in 2012 (December–November),[1] and the Arctic summer sea ice minimum in 2012 was the lowest ever recorded and has declined '49 percent below the long-term average (1979–2000)' (NOAA, 2012).

The Global Living Planet Index (LPI – a measure of the state of the world's biological diversity based on vertebrate population trends from around the world) has declined from 0.82 in 1992[2] to 0.72 in 2007. Even more seriously, the Tropical LPI has declined from 0.55 in 1992 to 0.40, while the Temperate LPI has actually increased from 1.22 to 1.29 (Zoological Society of London, 2010), suggesting the temperate (and mostly high-income) countries have preserved and even enhanced the condition of their living species at the expense of the tropical ecosystems located largely in middle- and low-income countries, which have been exploited largely to maintain the way of life of the high-income countries.

The Global Ecological Footprint in 1990 was 2.7 hectares (ha) per person, and was the same in 2008, but since the population had increased from 5.3 billion to 6.7 billion, this actually represents a 26 per cent increase in the total footprint. This is reflected in the fact that the footprint/biocapacity ratio increased from 1.18 in 1990 to 1.52 in 2008, which is an increment of 2.5 times the demand for nature's renewable resources since 1961 (Global Footprint Network, 2012). Thus, we went from using just over one planet's worth of biocapacity to using more than one and a half planet's worth. Clearly, this is unsustainable, and yet most standard projections of population and economic growth show that demand on the Earth's biocapacity will continue to expand as the new population and economic engines of China, India, Brazil, Indonesia, Russia, Nigeria and many

1 Calculated from 'Global Land–Ocean Temperature Index in 0.01 degrees Celsius (base period: 1951–1980)' raw data available from NASA's Goddard Institute for Space Studies at data.giss.nasa.gov/gistemp/tabledata_v3/GLB.Ts+dSST.txt, accessed 28 December 2012.

2 Baseline for all measures of 1.0 in 1970.

other countries continue to grow. If the whole world had the same consumption patterns as the USA (8.0 ha per person in 2007) or of high-income countries as a whole (6.1 ha per person), we would need, respectively, more than three or more than two Planet Earths to meet our global demand.

In 1968, an international think tank of industrialists, scientists and politicians – called The Club of Rome – asked a group at the Massachusetts Institute of Technology, USA, to model the effects of major global trends on the health of the planet. The MIT group built a world computer model to investigate five major trends of global concern – accelerating industrialisation, rapid population growth, widespread malnutrition, depletion of non-renewable resources and a deteriorating environment. The results were published in their 1972 book, *The Limits to Growth* (Meadows et al., 1972). The first of their three general conclusions was:

> If the present growth trends in world population, industrialization, pollution, food production, and resource depletion continue unchanged, the limits to growth on this planet will be reached sometime within the next 100 years. The most probable result will be a sudden and uncontrollable decline in both population and industrial capacity. (Meadows et al., 1972)

Although the authors were widely attacked for their conclusions, in their 20-year review, they found the trends relatively unchanged. They stated that they would rewrite their first basic conclusion as follows:

> Human use of many essential resources and generation of many kinds of pollutants have already surpassed rates that are physically sustainable. Without significant reductions in material and energy flows, there will be in the coming decades an uncontrolled decline in per capita food output, energy use, and industrial production. (Meadows et al., 1992)

Almost 20 years after that, Turner looked back at the original Club of Rome scenarios and the actual record since then and concluded that:

> Thirty years of historical data compare favourably with key features of a business as usual scenario called the 'standard run' scenario which results in collapse of the global system midway through the 21st century. (Turner, 2008)

In short, as the UN's Millennium Ecosystem Assessment noted:

> Human activity is putting such a strain on the natural functions of Earth that the ability of the planet's ecosystems to sustain future generations

> can no longer be taken for granted ... Nearly two-thirds of the services provided by nature to humankind are found to be in decline worldwide. (Millennium Ecosystem Assessment, 2005)

Clearly, ecological decline is well under way, and given the inertia and time lag built into Earth's natural systems, it will continue for many years to come, even were we to start doing everything right today – and there seems little prospect of that, given the inertia and time lag that is also built into our social systems. Given that bleak reality, it seems logical that we should begin to treat ecological decline as a present-day reality, not an improbable or undesirable future, and act accordingly.

But, ecological decline is not in some way separate from us. We, as biological beings, as a species, and the societies and communities we have created as a social animal, are ultimately dependent on the so-called 'ecosystem goods and services' that the Earth 'provides' for us.[3] These include such basic necessities as the production of oxygen, water and food, the great cycles of water, nitrogen and carbon, the recycling of 'wastes', and so on. So, when ecosystems decline or collapse, so too do the communities and societies that are embedded in and dependent on them (Diamond, 2005). Thus, we face the very real possibility, indeed, the probability, that at least some communities and societies around the world, if not the entire edifice of our modern technological society, will decline or collapse in the coming decades.

Faced with such a prospect, we need a game plan to guide us through the ecological decline that we are already experiencing, which will only get worse, and through the social changes this will require. I call this 'managing decline'.

Managing Decline

'Decline' is a complex concept that can be thought of in several ways:

- It is a slow process and, as such, may be thought of as a form of long, slow crisis or a slowly unfolding disaster.
- It is, or may be, the prelude to collapse, which might also be just an accelerated form of decline, or could be sudden and unexpected, a sort of phase shift.
- Ecological and social decline and collapse are likely to be interwoven.

3 In stating this, I am not taking an anthropocentric view. I do not believe that the Earth's ecosystems were put there for our benefit, but that, like all species, we depend on the natural processes that 'produce' a set of 'goods and services' essential for life, goods and services that we have to share with all other species because they are part of the web of life that we, too, are part of.

The first step in managing decline is to recognise reality, not turn away from it. An analogy is that we do not think denial is a healthy response to a serious and life-threatening disease. One has to face it and deal with it, both in terms of managing the disease and managing the impact of the disease on one's life. Well, as a society and as a planetary civilisation, we have to face the reality of ecosystem and resource decline, try to manage it, and try to manage the impact of the decline on our community, society and global well-being.

'Managing decline' has several dimensions:

- Understanding the types of ecological decline we face, their scale and likely timelines, and their implications for society.
- Finding ways to handle the social disruptions that will result (at different times and in different places around the world) with the least harm to people; a form of long, slow disaster management plan.
- Finding ways to slow and reverse the ecological decline, which means slowing and then reversing the impact of humans on the Earth's ecosystems, which, in turn, means a radical shift in the way our societies work.
- Finding ways to identify the potential 'tipping points' where either or both of ecological and societal decline can slide off swiftly into collapse and chaos, so that emergency action can be taken to try to avert the situation.

If we are going to come to these understandings and find our way forward, we need intellectual, social, political and organisational mechanisms to help us do so. What I propose is really no different to something we have become quite accustomed to; namely, setting up disaster management organisations. However, I am unaware of any organisation or institution that has a mandate at present to address decline, rather than an acute disaster.

The first challenge is perhaps largely an intellectual one – to understand the dimensions of ecological decline and its implications for societal decline, to begin to 'map' this and to try to understand what might be the early warning signs of impending collapse. As such, universities would seem to be the place to start, or perhaps a dedicated think tank. This would necessarily have to occur in more than one place, because ecosystem and societal characteristics vary from region to region, even from country to country. But, it would also be necessary for there to be a global organisation, perhaps at the United Nations (UN), or through a global non-governmental organisation (NGO), or a university with a global reach and mandate. These groups or units would also need to be effective in communicating their work to the general public and political and other societal leaders, because action requires awareness.

The next stage, although perhaps occurring simultaneously, would be to start to set up 'decline management' units and programmes, rather as we have set up disaster or emergency management units. These would have to be government organisations, and indeed might be added to existing emergency management units. Again, they would need to be established at both a global and a regional level, and within individual countries. And, as is the case with existing disaster management programmes, public communication would be an important role for them, too.

Of course, all this is predicated on there being a willingness to acknowledge and accept the reality of ecological decline in the first place, and its implications for our communities and societies. Sadly, but perhaps predictably, as the crisis worsens, there seems to be even less willingness today to face the facts than what was seen a generation ago. So, regrettably, as has been the case only too often in the past, we will likely need to experience disaster – sometimes several times – before we develop the political and public will to respond. But, given the scale of the decline and collapse that we face, the question is whether, by then, it will be too late.

Global Change, Local Action

I first became involved in thinking about healthy cities in the early 1980s at the city of Toronto, and by the early 1990s, about the time that Tony McMichael published *Planetary Overload* (McMichael, 1993) I was involved in the development of the emerging global movement for healthy cities and communities. My focus was on linking the concept to that of *sustainable* cities (Hancock, 1994, 1996, 1997, 2000). It seemed to me then, and still does, that health and sustainability are two sides of the same coin, and that there is much to be gained on both sides from a closer collaboration; indeed, a synthesis.

Moreover, my involvement with Healthy Cities since the movement first started in Europe and Canada more than 25 years ago has confirmed for me that if there is any hope, it will be found at the local level. Following the Second International Conference on Health Promotion in Adelaide, Australia, which was focused on healthy public policy, Kickbusch, Draper and O'Neill remarked that the local level

> is where the practice of healthy public policy is developing most rapidly and where its effects are most visible. There are clear reasons for this: many of the problems that have environmental or service dimensions are most obvious at the local level. So are the changes needed. Politicians at this level are more closely in touch with their electors and respond more clearly to their concerns. Governmental structures, even in large cities,

> interact more easily with each other and find ways to coordinate their planning and action more readily than at the national level. (Kickbusch et al., 1990)

In that same publication, I suggested characteristics that might make healthy public policy both more easy and more difficult to undertake at the local level. Local-level characteristics that make healthy public policy easier include:

- a degree of local intimacy among key actors in the smaller social networks and the more human scale of the community;
- policymakers (politicians and staff) live close to where they work and their decisions affect themselves, their friends, neighbours and family;
- smaller bureaucracies may make response times faster and feedback easier;
- closer links between the community and policymakers;
- the possibility of linking community advocacy and community action directly to policy change and to policymakers.

On the other hand, some of the issues that make healthy public policy more difficult at the local level include:

- a number of 'mega issues', especially economic issues, may be nationally or even internationally determined;
- local government may lack the jurisdiction or power to alter policy;
- central government may be opposed to local initiatives and autonomy;
- central government may dump on local governments, decentralising the burden or responsibility for policy, but not the power and resources to implement it;
- local politicians may claim they are powerless to act, thus shifting blame upwards;
- local jurisdictions (especially the smaller ones) may lack adequate resources and expertise (Hancock, 1990).

Nonetheless, in spite of these potential difficulties and obstacles, it remains the case now, as it was then, that there has been relatively little development of healthy public policy at provincial and national levels. On the other hand, there has been considerable experience in the development and application of healthy public policy at the local level. In recent years, we have seen such leadership in the development of, for instance, municipal by-laws to control smoking, the development of biking paths and an increased emphasis on walkability, the creation of food policy councils and other approaches to creating food security at the local level, and so on. The same is true with respect to the creation of sustainability policy, where many of the major advances have come at the municipal level, from action on climate change and energy efficiency to recycling, from bans on cosmetic pesticide use to the restoration of natural areas.

There is, moreover, another interesting difference about local governments when compared with provincial/state or federal/national governments, and that is in how they measure progress – and what that says about their values and their focus. While higher levels of government are focused – indeed, fixated – on the gross domestic product (GDP) (which was never intended to measure social progress anyway), I have never known a municipal government measure its progress in that way; rather, they focus on quality of life. For example, the Federation of Canadian Municipalities has been developing and supporting a Quality of Life Reporting System for some 20 years.[4] What this tells us is that municipal governments value people rather than just the economy, and are focused on the environmental, social, economic and other conditions that enable people to have a high quality of life; higher orders of government could learn a lot from municipal governments!

So, I believe that it is to the local level that we should now look for the first steps towards managing decline.

Indeed, this is precisely what is happening with the emergence in the past few years of the Transition Towns movement, which began in the small town of Totnes, Devon, in the UK, in 2005. Described as being focused on 'small-scale local responses to the global challenges of climate change, economic hardship and shrinking supplies of cheap energy',[5] this grass-roots movement has expanded to encompass over 1000 initiatives worldwide, in 34 countries, with 13 national hubs. Taking the view that we cannot continue to 'operate on the assumption that our high levels of energy consumption, our high carbon emissions and our massive environmental impact can go on indefinitely', and that we need to make the transition to a lower energy future, the Transition Towns movement believes that 'the best place to start transitioning away from this unviable way of living is right within our own communities, and the best time is right now'.

Moreover, and importantly, their work is not focused simply on avoiding the worst that could happen.

Transition Towns are 'actively and cooperatively creating happier, fairer and stronger [and, I would add, healthier] communities, places that work for the people living in them and are far better suited to dealing with the shocks that'll accompany our economic and energy challenges and a climate in chaos'.

4 See www.fcm.ca/home/programs/quality-of-life-reporting-system.htm.

5 All quotes about Transition Towns are taken from their website, www.transitionnetwork.org/support/what-transition-initiative, accessed 13 January 2013.

Conclusion

The focus on models of change to cope with declines in all that supports living systems needs to be located at the local level. Transition Towns are taking the first steps in managing decline, and are doing so in a positive and locally based manner that engages people. From the global perspective, optimism is hard to muster. However, locally based, realistic approaches such as Transition Towns provide the hope that we can, indeed, manage decline and transition to a more positive future.

References

Bezold, C. & Hancock, T. 1993. Introduction and overview of health futures (Appendix 5). In: Taket, A. (ed.) *Health Futures in Support of Health For All WHO/HST, 93.4*. World Health Organization, Geneva, Switzerland, 69–89.

Bezold, C. & Hancock, T. 1994. Possible futures, preferable futures. *Healthcare Forum Journal* 37, 23–9.

Diamond, J. 2005. *Collapse: How Societies Choose to Fail or Succeed*. Viking Press, New York, USA.

Gillis, J. 2013. Heat-trapping gas passes milestone, raising fears. *New York Times* (10 May). Available at: www.nytimes.com/2013/05/11/science/earth/carbon-dioxide-level-passes-long-feared-milestone.html?pagewanted=all&_r=0, accessed 5 February 2015.

Global Footprint Network 2012. The National Footprint Accounts, 2011 edition. Available at: www.footprintnetwork.org/en/index.php/GFN/page/footprint_data_and_results, accessed 24 June 2013. Data tables from the 2010 Edition (2007 data) are available at: www.footprintnetwork.org/images/uploads/NFA_2010_Results.xls, accessed 24 June 2013.

Hancock, T. 1990. Developing healthy public policies at the local level. In: Evers, A., Farrant, W. & Trojan, A. (eds) *Healthy Public Policy at the Local Level*. Westview Press, Boulder, Colorado, USA, 7–11.

Hancock, T. 1994. A healthy and sustainable community: the view from 2020. In: Chu, C. & Simpson, R. (eds) *Ecological Public Health: From Vision to Practice*. Griffith University, Brisbane, Australia, and Centre for Health Promotion, Toronto, Canada, 245–53.

Hancock, T. 1996. Planning and creating healthy and sustainable cities: the challenge for the 21st century. In: Price, C. & Tsouros, A. (eds) *Our Cities, Our Future: Policies and Action for Health and Sustainable Development*. WHO Healthy Cities Project Office, Copenhagen, Denmark, 65–88.

Hancock, T. 1997. Healthy, sustainable communities: concept, fledgling practice and implications for governance. In: Roseland, M. (ed.) *Eco-City Dimensions: Healthy Communities, Healthy Planet*. New Society Press, Gabriola Island, British Columbia, Canada, 42–50.

Hancock, T. 2000. Healthy communities must be sustainable communities too. *Public Health Reports* 115, 151–6.

Kickbusch, I., Draper, R. & O'Neill, M. 1990. Healthy public policy: a strategy to implement the Health for All philosophy at various governmental levels. In: Evers, A., Farrant, W. & Trojan, A. (eds) *Healthy Public Policy at the Local Level*. Westview Press, Boulder, Colorado, USA.

McMichael, A.J. 1993. *Planetary Overload. Global Environmental Change and the Health of the Human Species*. Cambridge University Press, Cambridge, UK.

Meadows, D., Meadows, D., Randers, J. & Behrens, W. III 1972. *The Limits to Growth*. Universe Books, New York, USA.

Meadows, D.H., Meadows, D.L. & Randers, J. 1992. *Beyond the Limits: Global Collapse or a Sustainable Future*. Chelsea Green Publishing Co, White River Junction, Vermont, USA.

Millennium Ecosystem Assessment 2005. Living beyond our means: natural assets and human wellbeing (statement from the Board). Available at: www.maweb.org/documents/document.429.aspx.pdf, accessed 8 August 2011.

NOAA 2012. Arctic Report Card – Data visualizations and graphics from the NOAA climate.gov team. Available at: www.climatewatch.noaa.gov/article/2012/2012-arctic-report-card, accessed 31 December 2012.

Olivier, J.G.J., Janssens-Maenhout, G. & Peters, J.A.H.W. 2012. Trends in Global CO2 emissions. PBL Netherlands Environmental Assessment Agency, The Hague, the Netherlands; Joint Research Centre, Ispra, Italy. Available at: edgar.jrc.ec.europa.eu/CO2REPORT2012.pdf, accessed 31 December 2012.

Turner, G. 2008. *A Comparison of the Limits to Growth with Thirty Years of Reality*. CSIRO, Canberra, ACT, Australia.

Zoological Society of London 2010. Data tables from the 2010 Living Planet Report. Available at: static.zsl.org/files/lpr2010-index-values-1610.xls, accessed 1 July 2015.

31

ELEMENTAL EPIDEMIOLOGY

The Complex Association Between Mineral Extraction and Health

MARTIN MCKEE

Abstract

While much attention has, rightly, been devoted by the public health community to the unsustainability of our addiction to activities that involve burning the Earth's finite supplies of hydrocarbons, this is not the only way in which we are threatening the health of the world's population by depleting resources. The quest to control supplies of minerals, many of them present in small quantities, is having profound consequences for health. This chapter examines these consequences, including environmental contamination, conflicts and violence as warlords seek control of mineral-rich land, and the working conditions of those who mine these materials. These examples illustrate the importance of taking the broadest possible perspective on the determinants of health in a complex, interlinked world.

Introduction

It has been suggested that the reason why humans have never been contacted by inhabitants from other planets is because, long before sentient beings reach the stage when they can travel across space, they have already destroyed their own planets. For several decades, Tony McMichael was warning us that we risked repeating this mistake (McMichael, 1993, 2001). Blending insights from epidemiology, climate science and behavioural sciences, he rendered visible what would otherwise have remained invisible (such as how seemingly unconnected events such as landslides and forest fires in geographically dispersed lands were linked through man-made climate change), confronting us with difficult, but essential, questions of whether we were asking our planet to bear a load that was unsustainable (McMichael, 2001, 2012). In particular, he held us to account for the stewardship of our carbon resources and, especially, our propensity to take complex hydrocarbons needed for many of the materials that made modern life so easy and simply burn them. In this chapter, I examine a related issue. How well have we performed in our stewardship of some of the Earth's other resources?

An (Uneven) Abundance of Riches

The atomic composition of the universe is the result of a complex set of nuclear reactions, going back to the Big Bang, when much of the hydrogen and helium were created. However, the speed of this process left little time for the next largest elements to be formed, so that lithium, beryllium and boron remained relatively uncommon, even today, and there was no time to form carbon, with the next largest nuclei.

The process then moved to the stars. Alpha particles (helium nuclei) combined to form ever larger elements, explaining why those elements with even numbers of protons were more common than those with odd numbers, as well as why iron was so common (iron-56 is the largest stable nucleus that can be created by combining alpha particles, and so is the end of the line for this process). Other elements came about as a result of neutron capture and, to a lesser degree, fission of those nuclei that were unstable.

These processes gave rise to the overall composition of Earth, formed from the condensation of interstellar material. Initially, the slowly solidifying lump of molten rock was believed to be fairly homogeneous, but this changed over time as iron and those metals, such as nickel, that most easily formed alloys with it sank, while those elements that formed oxides remained on the crust. Flowing water dissolved and released many of these oxides, depending on the prevailing conditions of temperature and pressure arising from the constant volcanic activity (Fleischer, 1954). The consequence of this and other processes, such as those linked to tectonic movements (McDonald, 2005), meant that many elements were concentrated in particular places; for example, because they were leached out of rock formations or because they were left behind when other elements were leached out.

It is only because of these processes that it has been possible for humans to extract them from the Earth's surface. The concentration of elements in certain places made it possible to mine them commercially, especially as some related elements, such as silver, gold and platinum, were concentrated in the same places. Yet, not all elements were concentrated to the same extent. One group that largely escaped these processes is a set of 17 elements, all but two heavy elements, with atomic numbers between 57 and 71, making them relatively uncommon in the universe. However, they are also relatively dispersed on Earth, giving rise to their description as 'rare earths'. They are found in significant amounts in some places, such as the small Swedish mining town of Ytterby, which gave its name to no fewer than four elements, yttrium, erbium, terbium and ytterbium. Elsewhere, however, they are found only in very low concentrations.

The extraction of all but the most common and concentrated elements, such as iron or aluminium, can involve enormous effort. Thus, it can take one tonne of ore to extract one gram of gold. The ores with the highest yields of many elements are already depleted. Save some new discoveries in unexpected places, we are already exploiting ores with yields far below what would have been considered viable even a few decades ago. However, the extraction of these elements from ores where they have lain undisturbed for millennia begins a process of human-led dispersal, whereby they are distributed throughout the environment, in rubbish dumps or as litter, across the planet. In effect, we are speeding up the phenomenon known as entropy, whereby, over time, the universe will reach a cold, homogeneous, and dead state. While there will still be vast quantities of these elements in ocean water and sediment reserves, it will no longer be economically viable to extract them in useable quantities.

This is becoming increasingly problematic as we find new uses for many elements that were previously little more than chemical curiosities. Tantalum, for example, is an essential component of mobile phones. Neodymium and lanthanum are necessary for the production of hybrid cars. Iridium is used to make crucibles in which large, high-quality single crystals used in the electronics industry are grown. Neodymium, dysprosium and samarium are used in high-strength magnets. Promethium is used in nuclear batteries, and scandium is used in aerospace components. A number of others, such as yttrium, holmium and erbium, are used in specialist lasers. There is, however, a finite amount of these elements on Earth, unless at some stage in the future we discover how to create controlled, large-scale nuclear fusion, at best a distant prospect.

The growing demand for these elements has important implications for those countries that, by an accident of geology, have deposits of these substances. Some will find themselves in an economically extremely powerful position. Others, especially if their governments are too weak to safeguard their resources, may become victims of conflict, as warlords seek to control the resources. All these scenarios have consequences for human health.

Taking Control of Earth

Those who control a finite resource have power over those who need it. It is possible to view much of human history as a struggle for control over scarce resources, whether it was the expansion of the Roman Empire as it sought to maintain its supplies of maize from North Africa, the Spanish conquest of South America in pursuit of silver, or the colonisation of Asia by European powers in search of spices. More recently, few believe those politicians who deny that at least some of the causes of conflict in the Middle East lie in the quest for control of oil.

At the beginning of the 20th century, the struggle is no longer for control of spices but of those minerals that are increasingly in demand. One country, China, now dominates the global debate of access to many of these resources. In particular, it has developed a near monopoly on the production of the rare earths. It has used the power that comes with this monopoly position.

Since 2005, China has reduced the amount of rare earths it exports, from just under 60,000 tonnes per year to just over 30,000 tonnes in 2011. This led to a steep increase in world prices. However, it also stimulated a number of responses in other countries, including a referral to the World Trade Organization on the basis that its export quotas were illegal, the relocation of companies that used them in manufacturing (especially Japanese companies) to China and the opening up of production in other parts of the world, such as the USA and Australia, where it had previously been economically non-viable. As a consequence, prices have fallen back somewhat. However, while the widespread dispersion of rare earths means that there are alternative sources, China's actions serve as a warning. European powers once colonised large parts of the world to ensure control of natural resources. Nowadays, the process is different. Wealthy countries are not seeking to govern other countries. Instead, sovereign wealth funds and similar entities are taking advantage of international settlement procedures that enable them to enforce property rights to buy up large tracts of land. So far, this has been mainly for agricultural production, but, increasingly, it is likely that it will be to secure control over strategic stocks of minerals. The likely price rises may place in peril the affordability of many of the new technologies on which the world depends for clean energy, with negative implications for our planet.

A related issue is the health consequences of extraction. In China, activity centres on the mines at Bayan Obo in the north of Inner Mongolia (Bontron, 2012). The ores are brought 120 km south to the town of Batou, where two-thirds of Chinese production is processed. Because these elements are in such low concentrations, they can be extracted and purified only with great difficulty. The processes used involve strong acids (now deemed by the International

Agency for Research on Cancer as a Group 1 carcinogen; International Agency for Research on Cancer, 2012) and give rise to large amounts of waste that is corrosive and contains many toxic chemicals. The waste is also radioactive as a result of the thorium that is extracted at the same time. The inevitable result is that the land around Batou, which once supported agricultural production, is now unusable. Moreover, the air is heavily polluted with sulphuric acid mists and pollutants from the coal-fired electricity generators used to power the local industry.

Despite growing awareness of the hazards, and in some cases extensive programmes to clean up polluted areas in countries such as China and Malaysia, similar stories can still be told in many other parts of the world. For example, the extraction of gold, silver and platinum involves the extensive use of cyanide, which too often has leaked into watercourses, destroying wildlife.

Conflict Commodities

The song, 'Oh my darling Clementine', serves as a reminder that the 1848–55 California gold rush was accompanied by many individual tragedies, although the fate of the indigenous inhabitants of the land on which the gold was found has often received less attention. Today, there are many similar land grabs going on, some for gold, but more often for other substances. Perhaps the best known are 'blood diamonds', made famous by a movie of the same name and now subject to a raft of international measures, of varying degrees of success, to control the trade. Blood diamonds played a key role in the civil war in Sierra Leone, leading to the death and maiming of thousands of people, illustrated horrifically by the pictures of young children with both hands severed by machetes. However, there are many others.

The one that has given rise to most deaths is the quest to control coltan reserves in the Democratic Republic of Congo (DRC). Coltan is an abbreviation for columbite-tantalite, a compound containing the element tantalum, and the DRC is an increasingly important producer. When refined, it forms a heat-resistant powder that can hold a very high electric charge, leading to its widespread use in capacitors and energy storage cells in a wide range of portable electronic devices such as mobile phones and laptops. Unfortunately, the coltan that is mined in the DRC contributes little to the welfare of its people. Warlords from Rwanda, Uganda and Burundi have deployed militia forces in the DRC to achieve control of the trade in coltan and other natural resources. The resulting conflict has been characterised by widespread atrocities, while the money they have raised has contributed to instability and rapidly growing inequality in the neighbouring countries in which they are based (Montague, 2002).

'Oil and Democracy Do Not Mix'

This oft-cited quotation is from an op-ed in the *New York Times* in which Ottaway (2005) notes that only two of the world's top ten oil producers are fully democratic, with three more only partially so. However, this is not just an assertion. Ross (2001) conducted a pooled time-series using cross-national data from 113 countries between 1971 and 1997 and showed that oil exports were associated strongly with authoritarian rule but, crucially, that export of other types of minerals had a similar antidemocratic effect, while the other types of commodity exports studied (food and non-food agricultural products) did not. In subsequent analyses, he found some support for three possible explanations: a 'rentier effect', whereby resource-rich governments used patronage to dampen democratic pressures; a 'repression effect', whereby they used their resources to strengthen their internal security and thus repress popular movements; and a 'modernisation effect', whereby growth, driven by the export of oil and minerals, failed to bring about the social changes that produced democratic governments.

This interpretation is important because of the contribution of democratic governance to health, increasing the responsiveness of governments to the needs of their people, including their health needs, and encouraging representation of their poorest citizens (Mulligan et al., 2004). Greater democracy is associated with lower infant mortality (Lena and London, 1993; Navia and Zweifel, 2003). Children in Africa, born to the same mother before and after political changes, have different health outcomes; infant mortality falls when multi-party elections lead to a change of leader, but not where the incumbent wins or when the change of leadership is undemocratic (Kudamatsu, 2006). In these ways, dependence on extractive industries can act through political processes to undermine health.

Mines and Health

Miners face increased risks of injuries and a large number of illnesses through physical exposures, including those from dust, such as silicosis, and those from toxic chemicals, such as mercury poisoning (Eisler, 2003). However, mineral miners are also at high risk of tuberculosis (TB) (Packard, 1987; Rees and Murray, 2007). Miners in sub-Saharan Africa have a higher incidence of TB than in any other working population in the world (Government of South Africa, 2007), reflecting both the intensity of exposure to infection in confined spaces, both in the mines and in accommodation blocks (Leon et al., 1995), and the effects of silica dust exposure, which increases the risk of pulmonary TB (Hnizdo and Murray, 1998; Churchyard et al., 2000; Rees and Murray, 2007). Miners are also at high risk of HIV infection because of the extent of sex work associated with mining facilities (Campbell, 1997). Miners in this region have three–four times the prevalence of HIV compared with non-miners, while partners of migrant miners have also been found to have a significantly greater prevalence of HIV (Lurie et al., 2003). However, mines are not only a risk to those who work in and around them. They act as incubators of infectious diseases, which then spread into the general population as miners circulate between the mines and their often distant homes (Basu et al., 2011). Thus, the intensity of mining is associated significantly with overall rates of TB in the countries of Africa (Stuckler et al., 2011).

Conclusion

Tony McMichael changed the way we thought about the determinants of human health, looking far upstream for the answers to exploring some of the greatest challenges facing humanity. This necessitated a breadth of vision, as well as an ability to make connections across complex chains of causation. Fundamentally, he was concerned about how we interacted with our environment and the ecosystems in which we were embedded, and the scarce resources we inherited. In a small way, this chapter seeks to reinforce and, indeed, to bolster this tradition.

References

Basu, S., Stuckler, D. & McKee, M. 2011. Addressing institutional amplifiers in the dynamics and control of tuberculosis epidemics. *American Journal of Tropical Medicine and Hygiene* 84, 30–7.

Bontron, C. 2012. En Chine, les terres rares tuent des villages. *Le Monde*. Available at: www.lemonde.fr/asie-pacifique/article/2012/07/19/en-chine-les-terres-rares-tuent-des-villages_1735857_3216.html, accessed 5 February 2015.

Campbell, C. 1997. Migrancy, masculine identities and AIDS: the psychosocial context of HIV transmission on the South African gold mines. *Social Science & Medicine* 45, 273–81.

Churchyard, G.J., Kleinschmidt, I., Corbett, E.L., Murray, J., Smit, J. & De Cock, K.M. 2000. Factors associated with an increased case-fatality rate in HIV-infected and non-infected South African gold miners with pulmonary tuberculosis. *The International Journal of Tuberculosis and Lung Disease* 4, 705–12.

Eisler, R. 2003. Health risks of gold miners: a synoptic review. *Environmental Geochemistry and Health* 25, 325–45.

Fleischer, M. 1954. The abundance and distribution of the chemical elements in the earth's crust. *Journal of Chemical Education* 31, 446–51.

Government of South Africa 2007. *Tuberculosis Strategic Plan for South Africa, 2007–2011*. Ministry of Health, South Africa.

Hnizdo, E. & Murray, J. 1998. Risk of pulmonary tuberculosis relative to silicosis and exposure to silica dust in South African gold miners. *Journal of Occupational and Environmental Medicine* 55, 496–502.

International Agency for Research on Cancer. 2012. *Occupational Exposures to Mists and Vapours from Strong Inorganic Acids; and Other Industrial Chemicals*. IARC, Lyon, France.

Kudamatsu, M. 2006. Has democratization reduced infant mortality in sub-Saharan Africa? Evidence from micro data. ISER Discussion Paper No. 685. Institute of Social and Economic Research, Osaka, Japan.

Lena, H.F. & London, B. 1993. The political and economic determinants of health outcomes: a cross-national analysis. *International Journal of Health Services* 23, 585–602.

Leon, R., Davies, A., Salomon, M. & Davies, J. 1995. *Commission of Enquiry into Safety and Health in the Mining Industry*. Government Printers, Pretoria, South Africa.

Lurie, M.N., Williams, B.G., Zuma, K., Mkaya-Mwamburi, D., Garnet, G.P., Sturm, A., et al. 2003. The impact of migration on HIV-1 transmission in South Africa: a study of migrant and nonmigrant men and their partners. *Sexually Transmitted Diseases* 30, 149–56.

McDonald, I. 2005. *Mineral Deposits and Earth Evolution*. Geological Society, London, UK.

McMichael, A.J. 1993. *Planetary Overload: Global Environmental Change and the Health of the Human Species*. Cambridge University Press, Cambridge, UK.

McMichael, A.J. 2001. *Human Frontiers, Environments and Disease: Past Patterns, Uncertain Futures*. Cambridge University Press, Cambridge, UK.

McMichael, A.J. 2012. Insights from past millennia into climatic impacts on human health and survival. *Proceedings of the National Academy of Sciences (USA)* 109, 4730–7.

Montague, D. 2002. Stolen goods: coltan and conflict in the Democratic Republic of Congo. *SAIS Review* XXII, 103–18.

Mulligan, C., Gil, R. & Sala-i-Martin, X. 2004. Do democracies have different public policies than nondemocracies? *Journal of Economic Perspectives* 18, 51–74.

Navia, P. & Zweifel, T.D. 2003. Democracy, dictatorship and infant mortality revisited. *Journal of Democracy* 14, 90–104.

Ottaway, M. 2005. Tyranny's full tank. *New York Times*. Available at: www.nytimes.com/2005/03/31/opinion/31ottaway.html, accessed 5 February 2015.

Packard, R. 1987. *White Plague, Black Labor: Tuberculosis and the Political Economy of Health and Disease in South Africa*. University of California Press, Berkeley, California, USA.

Rees, D. & Murray, J. 2007. Silica, silicosis and tuberculosis. *The International Journal of Tuberculosis and Lung Disease* 11, 474–84.

Ross, M.L. 2001. Does oil hinder democracy? *World Politics* 53, 325–61.

Stuckler, D., Basu, S., McKee, M. & Lurie, M. 2011. Mining and risk of tuberculosis in sub-Saharan Africa. *American Journal of Public Health* 101, 524–30.

32

FREEING POLICY FROM THE PROXIMATE

Expanding the Scope of Public Health Practice to Match Epidemiological Insights

DEVIN C. BOWLES

Abstract

Human health depends on the health of eco-planetary systems, many of which are under increasing anthropogenic pressure. In recent years, epidemiology has expanded its range of enquiry temporally and spatially, confirming many of these dependencies. Using climate change as a case study, I demonstrate that the capacity for public health action to mitigate the health effects of global ecological degradation has not kept pace.

There are several impediments to action. Diffuse responsibility impedes focusing efforts for change. Relatively slow mechanisms linking planetary-scale degradation with health impacts create an intergenerational conflict of interests. The momentum of both socio-economic and physical systems, such as the climate system, delays the feedback of consequences and hinders action. Over-determination of ecological pressure, in which multiple stressors could each individually degrade ecosystems, compounds the problem of diffuse responsibility and complicates resource allocation. The complexity of ecological degradation and constraints on effective solutions facilitate individual and societal self-deception, and thus corruption.

Despite these barriers, upstream intervention may be the only way to prevent the myriad ill effects of global environmental problems on human health. Epidemiologists should expand the scope of their power to impact the factors leading to global-scale ecological disruption. Several strategies are discussed.

Introduction

Ecological systems necessary for human health are under increasing threat from diverse anthropogenic pressures. Threats of concern include biodiversity loss, disruptions to the nitrogen cycle and climate change, which has been labelled as the century's greatest health threat (Costello et al., 2009). As A. J. McMichael elucidates, a subset of epidemiologists is responding by expanding the spatial and temporal scope of their enquiry beyond proximate health risk factors to include population-level influences on health (McMichael, 1999). While only a minority of epidemiologists are directly involved, the discipline's overall understanding of the environmental and social systems that imbed health is increasing. Pathways from ecological disruption to ill health remain only partially described, but include undernutrition, poverty, limited access to ecosystem services, conflict over resources and decreased genetic diversity on which to base medical innovation. Negative consequences may be borne by all people, perhaps especially by those who contribute least to ecological disruption. While the spatial-temporal scope of epidemiological enquiry has expanded in line with humanity's pressure on the environment, the capacity for public health action lags.

Using climate change as a case study, I discuss barriers and enablers that affect public health issues mediated by global-scale environmental change. I suggest strategies by which epidemiology could help to meet the challenges posed by environmental degradation, including shifting the research and policy focus further upstream, altering the discipline's role in informing policy, in informing policy to better influence policy levers, and rethinking communication among professionals and with the public. Such strategies would contribute to a healthier planet, and, thereby, to healthier populations.

Ecological Stress and Human Health

There is an apparent paradox between the pattern of increasing health globally and the likelihood that health outcomes will stagnate or decline in future. However, both history and ecology are replete with examples of increased health and fertility being followed by substantial population contractions, in part from premature death, when the population surpasses the resource base (Diamond, 2005; Zhang et al., 2007, 2011). The disciplines of history and ecology are clear on these points, but their lessons have been missed by many people. Epidemiology and public health are in a unique position to highlight the current dangers precisely because of their recent successes.

Humanity continues to increase pressure on the ecological systems that support human health. The Holocene, the period of environmental stability in which civilisation arose and prospered, has given way to the Anthropocene, the current period in which humans are the major force shaping Earth's ecology (Crutzen, 2002; Steffen et al., 2011). Nine interrelated ecological limits have been identified that could tip the planet from the stability characterising the Holocene and decrease its capacity to sustain humanity (Rockström et al., 2009).

Three safety thresholds have already been crossed, and this now could disrupt the worldwide ecological balance. Biodiversity loss may be occurring at a rate broadly comparable with the five previous mass extinctions, including that of the dinosaurs. If current losses continue, a sixth mass extinction event, in which the planet loses at least three-quarters of its species in a geologically short period, would occur (Barnosky et al., 2011). Agriculture and fertiliser production have substantially disrupted the nitrogen cycle, removing 35 million tonnes of N2 from the atmosphere annually for human use. Much of it flows into waterways, where it can disrupt ecology and lead to anoxic areas (Rockström et al., 2009). The concentrations of greenhouse gases are outside of humanity's safe operating space (Rockström et al., 2009), with deleterious effects on human health already evident (Epstein and Ferber, 2011; McMichael, 2012). While abundant human health requires functioning and robust ecosystems, anthropogenic pressure continues to expand.

Impediments to Epidemiological Intervention

A growing body of research exists on the 'knowledge-to-action gap' in health care, including the conversion of primary research into tools such as practice guidelines and the uptake of such tools by practitioners (Graham et al., 2006). Two-way interactions between research and practice are essential to facilitate practice that is based on the best available evidence and a research agenda influenced by practitioners to maximise utility and uptake (Graham et al., 2006). However, despite efforts to close the gap between research and practice, there remains a significant lag – estimated at up to 17 years – between knowledge production and mainstream practice in many areas of health care (Balas and Boren, 2000); furthermore, patients do not receive appropriate care at over two in five of their encounters with the American and Australian health systems (McGlynn et al., 2003; Runciman et al., 2012). This suggests that, true to the Greek roots of the word, epidemiology is better at the *study* of health than in the *practice* of improving it.

The knowledge-to-action literature focuses largely on medical and paramedical practice, with less attention paid to other determinants of health, including ecological determinants (Graham et al., 2006). The task of bridging the knowledge-to-action gap for ecological health determinants possesses all of the challenges that it does for medical practice, and important additional challenges. Five characteristics make widespread ecological harm difficult to reverse. As discussed below, they also impede effective amelioration by epidemiologists: diffuse responsibility, intergenerational conflicting interests, momentum, over-determination and corruption.

Diffuse responsibility

Responsibility for socio-economic drivers of ecological degradation is diffuse and spread over multiple levels of organisation. In the same way as responsibility for emerging medical epidemics such as diabetes and heart disease is dispersed across a wide range of actors, from individuals to organisations, regulators and politicians, so too does responsibility for ecological damage. As is the case for medical researchers attempting to use their findings to help reduce the prevalence of chronic disease, so must the epidemiologist attempting to preserve ecological health often contend with multiple sources of responsibility for degradation. Carbon dioxide, next to methane, is the main anthropogenic greenhouse gas and has numerous sources, including oil, coal and natural gas. These are consumed in myriad industries and across millions of sites daily.

Deforestation reduces the natural absorption of carbon dioxide, increasing its atmospheric concentration and further driving climate change. People who drive cars, use electricity generated at a coal-fired plant or who eat meat raised on feed farmed from the sites of clear-cut forests are also contributing to carbon dioxide emissions and thus bear some level of responsibility for current trends. At a higher level of organisation, those who structure incentives and subsidise energy in ways that encourage fossil fuel use are promoting consumption as a means of self-actualisation. They lobby governments against effective action on international treaties and deliberately disseminate misinformation about climate change. It is these entities that bear an even greater responsibility for contributing to climate change (Pearse, 2007; Hamilton, 2010). This trend may be exacerbated by the reliance on gross domestic product (GDP) as a measure of economic success, despite the fact that it was not designed to measure well-being (Kubiszewski et al., 2013). Diffuse responsibility impedes intervention because of the behaviour of so many people at different levels that would require change, and because unilateral strategies that target a single level or single aspects of the bigger issue (i.e. the types of strategies that are sufficiently straightforward as to be feasible) generally fail to establish sufficiently broad and sustainable change.

Diffuse responsibility also leads to the tragedy of the commons, in which people overexploit common resources when benefits are individual but when costs are shared (Diamond, 2005). Put another way, the act of pollution is often facilitated because polluters do not bear the cost of negative externalities (Balmford et al., 2002). Theoretically at least, the tragedy of the commons could be averted if players would agree to a regulatory regime that aligned individual interests with common interests. To date, however, countries have failed to create an international regulatory system capable of averting climate change (Gardiner, 2006).

Problems associated with the tragedy of the commons are exacerbated by multiple levels of responsibility, each of which can claim that climate change is best solved by other levels. For example, an oil executive could argue that he or she is only satisfying consumer demand, while the driver of a fuel-inefficient vehicle can blame the manufacturer for his or her carbon dioxide emissions. The diffusion of responsibility complicates intervention by creating a situation of conflicting interests and ethical tension. Many of the worst effects of climate change, including on food production and reduced labour productivity, are in equatorial countries that have benefitted the least due to greenhouse gas emissions. Climate change will impact the health primarily of those who cannot afford to buffer themselves from it, by paying more for food when agricultural output falls (Cribb, 2010), or by buying an air conditioner to cope with heat stress. The ethical tension arises from the fact that the poor do not bear primary responsibility for climate change, which is the product of wealthy and middle-class lifestyles, yet they are suffering the harms from a changing climate.

Intergenerational conflicting interests

There is also a strong temporal conflict of interests (Gardiner, 2006). Carbon dioxide can persist in the atmosphere for centuries, where total concentrations depend on previous emissions. Changes to the climate from increased carbon dioxide can take years to unfold. Many of the effects of climate change similarly take time to manifest, including sea level rise from thermal expansion and melting glaciers. Those living a century hence will have to contend with a climate impacted by present-day emissions, even if humanity has stopped its carbon dioxide production completely by then (Friedlingstein et al., 2011). The current generation, thus, will not face the worst impacts of the climate it creates (Gardiner, 2006). This leads to a situation allied to the tragedy of the commons described above, except that intergenerational regulatory frameworks are impossible. Unborn generations are incapable of making or enforcing agreements with the present generation. Rational pursuit of narrowly defined, 'economically rational' self-interest is claimed by some to mean the current generation would emit without regard to future generations (Gardiner, 2006).

The effects of many other forms of environmental destruction also take time to manifest, creating similar dynamics. Relevant phenomena that could disrupt civilisation include the accumulation of other persistent pollutants, resource depletion and disruption to elemental cycles such as nitrogen and phosphorus (Rockström et al., 2009).

Momentum

The term 'momentum' is often used to describe the lag between anthropogenic perturbations on the climate systems and the full effects of these perturbations. A similar lag exists in many socio-economic and political systems. Physical infrastructure associated with greenhouse gas emissions lasts for years, or decades. Incentives to utilise these 'investments' fully mean that they are unlikely to be decommissioned until it is considered economical to do so (i.e. by the measures of mainstream economics), regardless of their contribution to climate change. Coal-fuelled power plants built today may still be operational in 2050. The commitment for Los Angeles to become coal-free by 2025 offers some hope that this lag can be shortened, at least in some instances.

Elements of infrastructure are often interlinked with each other and with cultural norms, perpetuating existing infrastructure–cultural connections and hindering qualitative/substantive change. For example, high levels of automobile ownership, which represent substantial citizen investment, create a disincentive for governments to moderate road funding. Limited budgets mean that roads are built at the expense of other transportation infrastructure, increasing the incentive of citizens to continue to invest in cars. Cultural and emotional attachment to automobiles further impedes the rapid alteration of transport networks. Dependence on automobile infrastructure influences other aspects of development planning, increasing urban sprawl and dwelling size, and placing further pressure on the planet through ever-increasing contributions to climate change, resource depletion and air pollution.

Over-determination

Over-determination is a situation in which there are multiple causes which, individually, would result in a given outcome. Over-determined outcomes are thus difficult to change. When applied to ecological degradation, it requires distinct strategies to combat separate problems to preserve individual ecosystems or species. This complicates environmental resource allocation, especially in a context of limited government budgets. Over-determination compounds the problem of diffuse responsibility because one ecosystem can be under threat from multiple sources, each of which can blame others for any degradation that occurs. Over-determination impedes effective action while increasing the action required.

Ecosystems important to human health are under multiple threats. Ocean acidification, caused by the absorption of increasing levels of atmospheric carbon dioxide, is the twin of climate change. It interferes with the chemistry used by many marine organisms, including corals, to make their shells, and could eventually make shell production impossible. Ocean acidification, overfishing and pollution each pose existential threats to coral reefs (Bradbury, 2012). Bradbury argues that, together, they have created a situation in which 'there is no hope of saving the global coral reef ecosystem', though small pockets of functioning reef ecosystems may remain (Bradbury, 2012). Rising ocean temperatures that cause coral bleaching place additional stress on reef ecosystems. Reef ecosystems are an important food source for humanity and the primary source of protein for many in developing countries.

Other ecosystems important to human well-being are also under multiple threats. The Amazonian rainforest is shrinking from logging and land-use change, while altered precipitation patterns associated with climate change could lead to drought and enhance forest fire risk (Davidson et al., 2012). Even at the global level, humanity continues to promote several largely separate anthropogenic risks to the planet (Rockström et al., 2009).

Corruption

Diffuse responsibility, conflicts among intergenerational interests, momentum and over-determination all impede humanity's response to broad-scale environmental problems. Humanity lacks the conceptual tools to address effectively the ethical and practical issues that climate change raises (Gardiner, 2006). The complexity of problems and the practical constraints on effective solutions facilitate self-deception, at both the individual and the organisational level. Consequently, there is ample room for vested interests to manipulate the debate through a number of psychosocial mechanisms: pandering, hypocrisy, complacency, distraction, selective attention, unreasonable doubt and delusion. These mechanisms are also open to individuals for self-deception. The enhanced manipulation of others and self-deception leads to moral corruption by facilitating unethical behaviour (Gardiner, 2006, pp. 407–8). This is magnified in situations when action to preserve the environment is pitched against individual interests due to the tragedy of the commons.

Upstream Intervention

The challenges of mitigating climate change and other global environmental problems are immense, yet upstream intervention may be the only way to prevent the resultant deterioration of human health. Climate change, like other large-scale ecological insults, will harm health through myriad pathways (Epstein and Ferber, 2011). According to one framework, primary effects will be those of the climate acting directly on human health, such as through increased rates of heatstroke (Butler and Harley, 2010). Secondary effects will operate via the web of life, such as changing ranges of mosquito-borne diseases. Tertiary effects are those which manifest through socio-economic and political pathways (Butler and Harley, 2010).

Climate change will change the distribution of many resources and likely diminish many renewable resources globally in the long term. This will combine with other factors to amplify food insecurity and malnourishment among many of the world's poor in the coming decades (Cribb, 2010).

Climate change is associated with conflict historically (Zhang et al., 2007, 2011), and increased resource conflict from climate change is predicted by the academy (Mazo, 2010; Hendrix and Salehyan, 2012; Bowles et al., 2014) and by the world's militaries (Sullivan et al., 2007; Morisetti, 2012). Climate change may also increase the risk of genocide. While individual causal pathways between climate change and ill health might be interrupted, their diversity and sheer number precludes comprehensive downstream health intervention. Upstream intervention that limits the rate and extent of climate change is required if all, or even most, of the health consequences of greenhouse gas emissions are to be averted.

Power and Epidemiology

Power relations are rarely examined in the medical knowledge-to-action gap literature (Graham et al., 2006). Yet, power relations are acknowledged as being of fundamental importance in the social sciences (Foucault, 1980; Comaroff and Comaroff, 1991), and become especially salient when actors are pursuing different and sometimes opposing goals. Maintaining and improving health is a primary goal of most actors within the health system. The goals of those with the greatest influence over ecological well-being, including multinational petroleum, mining, manufacturing and logging corporations, governments, advertisers and real estate developers, are more diverse, and health is often not among their priorities. Currently, epidemiologists can exert little power over these actors to ensure that their activities are consistent with current, let alone future, public health priorities. More insidiously, these actors cannot necessarily be relied on to influence the research agenda helpfully, to maximise its utility in achieving ecological or human health. Some may use their influence to bias the research agenda away from such questions in order to protect their own short-term interests. To facilitate planetary and human health, epidemiologists must increase their influence over domains not traditionally associated with health.

Overcoming Barriers

Humanity is disrupting rapidly a number of global ecological processes necessary for the flourishing of, and even maintenance of, human health. The challenge is of a greater scale than any previously faced by epidemiologists. Impediments to preserving health through ecological protection are substantial and fundamentally different from previous challenges to public health. Old solutions will not suffice.

For new ecological protection measures to overcome barriers and achieve widespread, sustainable change, one or more of the enablers in Table 32.1 may be required.

Table 32.1 Environmental protection enablers.

Enabler	Climate change examples
Substantial ongoing funding to establish national or international programmes	• Direct national funding of clean energy infrastructure • Funding of public transportation systems
Regulatory measures that require or facilitate change in practice	• Government-mandated emission standards for cars or power plants • Government-funded industry bailouts linked to improved environmental practices • Carbon taxes
Market forces that encourage organisations to change practice	• Boycotts of environmentally unfriendly products • Clean energy becoming less expensive than fossil fuel-based energy • Carbon trading schemes
Integration of successful local strategies into existing national or international networks or programmes	• A 'health in all policies' approach to governing that recognises the links between ecological and human health • Integration of local energy-efficient building design principles into all future government-funded buildings

Source: Author's work.

Most countries could afford to engage in substantial and accelerated change in their energy infrastructure (enabler 1), but this has so far been politically unfeasible. They could realistically set up a system of incentives and disincentives, such as implementing carbon taxes and ending oil subsidies (enabler 2), which would nudge energy companies towards more sustainable energy production. Enhancing the influence of epidemiological theory and research in the policy debate that determines such action is therefore necessary, and, indeed, critically important. The participation of developing countries is essential, given their rapidly growing ecological footprints, as is the involvement of developed countries. While such countries want to avoid economic disadvantage, their populations could experience many health co-benefits from a number of mitigation strategies. For instance, green cities planned to facilitate decreased car use would lead to reduced incidence of obesity and cardiovascular disease.

However, it is not just at the policy level where epidemiology has a role. In the context of climate change, substantial increases in access to government policy levers are unlikely without a widespread understanding of the threat that climate change and other ecological health determinants play. Epidemiologically informed education of the general population is therefore critical. This should begin at school, but cannot wait until the next generation attains the vote, and should target adults as well. Such education could serve to alter the salience of distal consequences, and help to increase consumer demand for clean energy. This approach offers particular opportunities for epidemiology because health – consistently rated as a high voting priority in community surveys (Research Australia, 2012) – has not yet been linked strongly to climate change in the public discourse. The public may, therefore, be more responsive to messages that climate change will impact health, and consequently will be more likely to support mitigation and adaptation measures than after exposure to environmental or national security messages (Myers et al., 2012). However, given the five impediments discussed above, no large-scale shift in the market towards clean infrastructure (enabler 3) is likely until its cost approaches that of traditional energy. Government taxes and subsidies, if structured correctly, could force this equality of pricing.

Finally, since the amelioration of climate change requires 'silver buckshot', ecological and epidemiological thinking needs to occur in unfamiliar realms, unaccustomed to such considerations (enabler 4). The concept of 'health in all policies' (Ståhl et al., 2006; Puska, 2007) might be extended to include ecological health, on which human health depends. Incentive creation will be required, both in government and private enterprises unused to thinking in such terms. Another necessary condition for success will be enhancing ecological and epidemiological wisdom in these areas. Two parallel strategies are useful: increasing the number of experts and embedding epidemiology and ecology in the core curriculum of the education system, including at universities.

In the 1800s, public health practitioners revolutionised health care by expanding the accepted purview of health specialists to include social and economic determinants of health. Today's global environmental threats to health are qualitatively different in ways that preclude previous solutions. However, an expansion of discipline and its tools similar to that experienced in the 19th century is required. Recently, as Tony McMichael both chronicled and exemplified, epidemiologists have been enhancing their understanding of the importance of ecological stability for human health. It is unsurprising that he had already begun to expand epidemiological action to have some influence over the ecological determinants of health, having provided advice to the Australian Prime Minister and the Chief Scientist. Clearly, much remains to be done. Continuation of his work is vital to the future health of the planet and its inhabitants.

References

Balas, E.A. & Boren, S.A. 2000. Managing clinical knowledge for health care improvement. *Yearbook of Medical Informatics* 2000, 65–70.

Balmford, A., Bruner, A., Cooper, P., Costanza, R., Farber, S., Green, R.E., et al. 2002. Economic reasons for conserving wild nature. *Science* 297, 950–3.

Barnosky, A.D., Matzke, N., Tomiya, S., Wogan, G.O.U., Swartz, B., Quental, T.B., et al. 2011. Has the Earth's sixth mass extinction already arrived? *Nature* 471, 51–7.

Bowles, D.C., Braidwood, M. & Butler, C.D. 2014. Unholy Trinity: climate change, conflict and ill health. In: Butler, C.D. (ed.) Climate Change and Global Health, CABI, Wallingford, UK, 144–52.

Bradbury, R. 2012. A world without coral reefs. *New York Times*. New York, USA. www.nytimes.com/2012/07/14/opinion/a-world-without-coral-reefs.html?_r=0, accessed 5 July 2015.

Butler, C.D. & Harley, D. 2010. Primary, secondary and tertiary effects of eco-climatic change: the medical response. *Postgraduate Medical Journal* 86, 230–4.

Comaroff, J. & Comaroff, J.L. 1991. *Of Revelation and Revolution*. Vol. 1: Christianity, Colonialism, and Consciousness in South Africa. University of Chicago Press, Chicago, Illinois, USA.

Costello, A., Abbas, M., Allen, A., Ball, S., Bell, S., Bellamy, R., et al. 2009. Managing the health effects of climate change: Lancet and University College London Institute for Global Health Commission. *The Lancet* 373, 1693–1733.

Cribb, J. 2010. *The Coming Famine: The Global Food Crisis and What We Can Do to Avoid It*. University of California Press, Berkeley, California, USA.

Crutzen, P.J. 2002. Geology of mankind. *Nature* 415, 23.

Davidson, E.A., de Araujo, A.C., Artaxo, P., Balch, J.K., Brown, I.F., Bustamante, M.M.C., et al. 2012. The Amazon basin in transition. *Nature* 481, 321–8.

Diamond, J. 2005. Collapse: How Societies Choose to Fail or Succeed. Viking, New York, USA.

Epstein, P.R. & Ferber, D. 2011. *Changing Planet, Changing Health: How the Climate Crisis Threatens Our Health and What We Can Do About It*. University of California Press, Berkeley, California, USA.

Foucault, M. 1980. *The History of Sexuality: An Introduction*. Vintage Books, New York, USA.

Friedlingstein, P., Solomon, S., Plattner, G., Knutti, R., Ciais, P. & Raupach, M. 2011. Long-term climate implications of twenty-first century options for carbon dioxide emission mitigation. *Nature Climate Change* 1, 457–61.

Gardiner, S.M. 2006. A perfect moral storm: climate change, intergenerational ethics and the problem of moral corruption. *Environmental Values* 15, 397–413.

Graham, I.D., Logan, J., Harrison, M.B., Straus, S.E., Tetroe, J., Caswell, W., et al. 2006. Lost in knowledge translation: time for a map? *Journal of Continuing Education in the Health Professions* 26, 13–24.

Hamilton, C. 2010. *Requiem for a Species: Why We Resist the Truth about Climate Change*. Allen & Unwin, Sydney, New South Wales, Australia.

Hendrix, C.S. & Salehyan, I. 2012. Climate change, rainfall, and social conflict in Africa. *Journal of Peace Research* 49, 35–50.

Kubiszewski, I., Costanza, R., Dorji, L., Thoennes, P. & Tshering, K. 2013. An initial estimate of the value of ecosystem services in Bhutan. *Ecosystem Services* 3, e11–e22.

McGlynn, E.A., Asch, S.M., Adams, J., Keesey, J., Hicks, J., DeCristofaro, A., et al. 2003. The quality of health care delivered to adults in the United States. *New England Journal of Medicine* 348, 2635–45.

McMichael, A.J. 1999. Prisoners of the proximate: loosening the constraints on epidemiology in an age of change. *American Journal of Epidemiology* 149, 887–97.

McMichael, A.J. 2012. Insights from past millennia into climatic impacts on human health and survival. *Proceedings of the National Academy of Sciences (USA)*. 109, 4730–7.

Mazo, J. 2010. *Climate Conflict: How Global Warming Threatens Security and What to Do About It*. Routledge, the International Institute for Strategic Studies, London, UK.

Morisetti, N. 2012. Climate change and resource security. *BMJ* 344, e1352.

Myers, T.A., Nisbet, M.C., Maibach, E.W. & Leiserowitz, A.A. 2012. A public health frame arouses hopeful emotions about climate change. *Climatic Change*, 113, 1105-12,

Pearse, G. 2007. *High & Dry: John Howard, Climate Change and the Selling of Australia's Future*. Viking/Penguin, Camberwell, VIC, Australia.

Puska, P. 2007. Health in all policies. *The European Journal of Public Health* 17, 328.

Research Australia 2012. What do Australians think about health & medical research? 2012 opinion poll – views of over 1000 Australians. Research Australia, Sydney, NSW, Australia.

Rockström, J., Steffen, W., Noone, K., Persson, A., Chapin, F.S., Lambin, E.F., et al. 2009. A safe operating space for humanity. *Nature* 461, 472–5.

Runciman, W.B., Hunt, T.D., Hannaford, N.A., Hibbert, P.D., Westbrook, J.I., Colera, E.W., et al. 2012. CareTrack: assessing the appropriateness of health care delivery in Australia. *Medical Journal of Australia* 197, 100–5.

Ståhl, T., Wismar, M., Ollila, E., Lahtinen, E. & Leppo, K. 2006. *Health in all Policies. Prospects and Potentials*. Finnish Ministry of Social Affairs and Health, Helsinki, Finland.

Steffen, W., Grinevald, J., Crutzen, P. & McNeill, J. 2011. The Anthropocene: conceptual and historical perspectives. *Philosophical Transactions of the Royal Society A: Mathematical, Physical and Engineering Sciences* 369, 842–67.

Sullivan, G.R., Bowman, F., Ferrell, L.P.J., Gaffney, P.G.I., Kern, P.J., Lopez, T.J., et al. 2007. *National Security and the Threat of Climate Change*. The Center for Naval Analysis (CAN) Corporation, Alexandria, Virginia, USA.

Zhang, D.D., Brecke, P., Lee, H.F., He, Y.-Q. & Zhang, J. 2007. Global climate change, war, and population decline in recent human history. *Proceedings of the National Academy of Sciences (USA)* 104, 19214–9.

Zhang, D.D., Lee, H.F., Wang, C., Li, B., Pei, Q., Zhang, J., et al. 2011. The causality analysis of climate change and large-scale human crisis. *Proceedings of the National Academy of Sciences (USA)* 108, 17296–301.

33

YOU'VE GOT TO BE CAREFUL IF YOU DON'T KNOW WHERE YOU'RE GOING BECAUSE YOU MIGHT NOT GET THERE (YOGI BERRA)

KRISTIE L. EBI

Abstract

The future is uncertain, not just in terms of the magnitude and pattern of climate change but also how socio-economic development will unfold and what that pathway could mean for the vulnerability and resilience of future populations to the health risks of climate change. Scenarios are standard tools for exploring how these health risks might change under different development assumptions (and how climate change could itself affect development), including the timing and effectiveness of adaptation and mitigation policies. Scenarios typically include qualitative and quantitative descriptions of atmospheric composition, climate change and associated physical impacts, and socio-economic development pathways. Although existing scenarios contain factors relevant for exploring health risks in a changing climate, additional variables are needed to project social, economic, demographic and ecological dynamics likely to affect future health burdens, as well as to describe how governance and institutions might change to increase resilience to current and future health risks. New scenarios are needed to explore health-related questions about the future. Professor McMichael's extensive publications on global environmental change focus on questions of how climate change could affect the future sustainability of life on Earth, including how history can illuminate factors determining population health vulnerability.

Introduction

Climate change will continue to alter weather patterns over coming decades, including more frequent and intense extreme weather and climate events; increases in the average and local variability of temperature, precipitation and other weather variables; and rises in sea level (e.g. IPCC, 2007, 2012). Projections of the magnitude and pattern of these changes offer an opportunity for public health (and other sectors) to modify current policies and measures proactively and develop new means to manage known and anticipated risks effectively and efficiently.

While projections of how the climate could change are necessary, they are insufficient to project health impacts and manage risk. Climate is one of many drivers of climate-sensitive health outcomes. Other drivers also will change over coming decades, including increases in population (albeit not uniformly around the world), the social determinants of health will change from global to local scales, new technologies will be identified and the policy environment for adaptation and mitigation will evolve at the international and national level. Understanding how these other drivers might change will be important for understanding the magnitude and extent of possible impacts. This information is critical for effective risk management, including identifying opportunities for modifying current and planned policies and measures to increase resilience over future decades.

Scenarios are standard tools to understand the magnitude and extent of changes in climate and associated risks, the degree to which mitigation and adaptation policies can reduce risks, the interactions among and trade-offs between climate change impacts, and adaptation and mitigation policies, and the relationship between climate change and development. Scenarios typically include qualitative and quantitative descriptions of socio-economic development pathways, atmospheric composition, and climate change and associated physical impacts.

One focus of Professor McMichael's extensive publications is on questions of how global environmental change could affect the future sustainability of life on Earth, including insights into thinking about development pathways (c.f. McMichael, 2001, 2008, 2012; McMichael and Lindgren, 2011).

Approaches to and History of Scenario Development

There are two basic approaches for developing scenarios (Ebi and Gamble, 2005). One is to envision a particular future at a particular date and then work backwards to determine the policies, measures and technology developments that are needed to achieve that future. This was the approach used for the Millennium Development Goals (MDGs) (UN Millennium Project, 2005). Specific activities (e.g. national programmes, funding) were recommended to achieve each goal, with the activities updated regularly based on monitoring and evaluation of the efforts to achieve national targets. For example, one goal is to reduce by two-thirds, between 1990 and 2015, the under-five mortality rate. In 2010, it was reported that the number of children in developing countries who died before they reached the age of 5 dropped, between 1990 and 2008, from 100 to 72 deaths per 1000 live births (www.un.org/millenniumgoals/pdf/MDG_FS_4_EN.pdf). However, of the 67 countries defined as having high child mortality rates, only 10 are currently on track to meet the MDG target. Activities were proposed or initiated to accelerate the reduction in child mortality to reach the goal in a timely manner.

Another approach, commonly used in the global change research community, is to describe internally consistent pathways from the near to the far future that can be used to explore the possible impacts of climate change under different development pathways, including the possible costs, benefits and harms of adaptation and mitigation policies. Over the past decade, projections of climate change and scenario-based analyses of impacts, adaptation and mitigation have been based primarily on the Intergovernmental Panel on Climate Change (IPCC) Special Report on Emission Scenarios (SRES) (Nakicenovic et al., 2000), developed to represent the range of driving forces and emissions in the scenario literature, including reflecting current understanding about underlying uncertainties. The SRES scenarios were developed by first creating internally consistent storylines of possible future worlds (Nakicenovic et al., 2000).

The four main storylines (labelled A1, A2, B1 and B2) describe the relationships between the driving forces of greenhouse gases and sulphur emissions, and their evolution, with each storyline representing different demographic, social, economic, technological and environmental development pathways. The axes of the scenarios are worlds with a more global versus a more regional focus, and worlds with a more economic versus a more social/environmental focus (see Table 33.1). For each storyline, several scenarios were developed using different models to examine the range of possible outcomes associated with similar assumptions about driving forces. Forty scenarios were quantified for the SRES report, six of which were selected as illustrative scenarios (one for each of the storylines, plus additional high and low emissions variants of the A1 storyline). By design, the SRES scenarios assumed no specifically targeted climate mitigation and adaptation policies and measures.

Table 33.1 The Intergovernmental Panel on Climate Change emission scenarios from the special report on emission scenarios.

Driving forces	Economics	Environmentalism
Globalisation	A1 (market forces; economic and technological convergence)	B1 (sustainable development; economic and technological convergence)
Regionalisation	A2 (market forces; slower economic growth)	B2 (sustainable development; slower economic growth)

Source: Nakicenovic et al., 2000.

Quantification of the storylines resulted in estimated emissions of greenhouse gases and sulphur that were used as input to climate models for projecting how patterns of weather variables, such as temperature and precipitation, could vary with climate change. These projections have been used to estimate possible impacts associated with each scenario (IPCC, 2007).

The Millennium Ecosystem Assessment (MEA) was a large assessment of the current status, present trends and longer-term challenges to the world's ecosystems, including climate change and other sources of stress (MEA, 2005). The MEA sought to assess changes in ecosystems in terms of the services they provided to people. It also examined the effects of ecosystem change on human well-being and identified and assessed methods to mitigate and respond to ecosystem change. Scenarios to 2050, with more limited projections to 2100, were developed in an iterative process, including consultations with potential scenario users and experts (Carpenter et al., 2005).

Two basic dimensions of uncertainty in long-term ecosystem stresses were identified: globalisation (continuation and acceleration of present global integration trends) versus reversal of these trends (increasing separation and isolation of nations and regions); and whether responses to increasing ecosystem stresses were predominantly reactive (waiting until evidence of deterioration and loss of services were clear) or predominantly proactive (taking protective measures in advance of their clear need). The extreme values of each of these dimensions yielded four scenarios (see Table 33.2).

Table 33.2 The Millennium Ecosystem Assessment scenarios.

Ecosystem management	World development	
	Global	Regional
Reactive	Global orchestration	Order from strength
Proactive	Techno-garden	Adapting mosaic

Source: Carpenter et al., 2005.

One chapter in the MEA described the implications for human well-being of the four scenarios based on qualitative analysis of the storylines, quantitative model results and an assessment of the assumptions underpinning the scenarios (Butler et al., 2005). The extensive work on describing the components of human well-being (basic material needs for a good life; health; good social relations; security; and freedom of choice and action) will be helpful in underpinning the development of new scenarios for use by the health sector to explore the possible impacts of and adaptation and mitigation response options to manage the risks of global environmental change.

The Global Environmental Outlook 4 (GEO-4) conceptual framework is based on the drivers–pressures–state–impacts–responses framework that reflects the key components of the complex chain of cause and effect relationships that characterise the interactions between society and environment at all spatial scales (Agard et al., 2007). Environmental changes are induced by drivers and caused by pressures, which also affect each other. Responses include measures by society for mitigating and adapting to environmental changes.

Through the GEO-4 scenario exercise, stakeholders explored the interplay between environmental issues in atmosphere, land, water and biodiversity. The scenarios were based on assumptions related to institutional and socio-political effectiveness, demographics, economic demand, trade and markets, scientific and technological innovation, value systems, and social and individual choices, and highlighted areas of uncertainty in the coming decades. The main scenarios are:

- Markets first: the private sector, with active government support, pursues maximum economic growth as the best path to improve the environment and human well-being.
- Policy first: the government sector, with active private- and civic-sector support, implements strong policies intended to improve the environment and human well-being, while still emphasising economic development.
- Security first: the government sector and the private sector vie for control in efforts to improve, or at least maintain, human well-being for mainly the rich and powerful in society.

Sustainability first: the civic, government and private sectors work collaboratively to improve the environment and human well-being for all, with a strong emphasis on equity.

Limitations of Current Scenarios

As the brief summaries of different scenarios indicate, some drivers of global change included in these scenarios are highly relevant to future health burdens, as well as to the effectiveness of future public health and health-care organisations and institutions whose mission is to manage adverse health outcomes. Drivers include population growth, general socio-economic development and the relative emphasis on developing new technologies and investing in research. Factors such as the extent to which countries collaborate suggest regional and international priorities for addressing adverse health outcomes in countries, particularly low-income countries, requiring external funding to manage risks.

Although important for developing narratives on how public health and health care might evolve over the coming decades, additional variables are needed to project social, economic, demographic and ecological dynamics that could affect future health burdens, as well as to describe how governance and institutions might change to increase resilience to current and future health risks (Ebi and Gamble, 2005). For example, the effectiveness of vector control programmes, drug and pesticide resistance, land-use change, travel and a range of other variables not captured by the SRES and other scenarios will affect possible alterations in the geographic range of malaria due to climate change.

Projections and descriptions are needed, from the local to the global scale, to provide decision makers with policy-relevant insights into how the future might unfold. Health researchers and practitioners have been slow to provide input on the variables needed, resulting in scenarios without the richness needed to inform policy- and decision makers on the health risks of global change and the options for managing those risks effectively, including estimates of the health co-benefits and co-harms of mitigation and adaptation policies.

Scenarios also could be enriched with descriptions of the possible impacts of climate change on the frequency, duration, spatial extent and timing of extreme weather and climate events. The IPCC *Special Report on Managing the Risks of Extreme Events and Disasters to Advance Climate Change Adaptation* (IPCC, 2012) concluded that recent projections suggested the frequencies of heatwaves and of heavy precipitation are likely to increase in the 21st century over many regions.

There is evidence that droughts will intensify over the coming century in southern Europe and the Mediterranean region, central Europe, central North America, Central America and Mexico, north-east Brazil and southern Africa, but confidence is limited because of issues regarding how to classify and measure a drought, the lack of observational data and the inability of models to include all the factors that influence droughts (IPCC, 2012). In addition, it is very likely that average sea level rise will contribute to upward trends in extreme coastal high-water levels. Further, the projected precipitation and temperature changes imply changes in floods, although, overall, there is low confidence at the global scale regarding climate-driven changes in the magnitude or frequency of river-related flooding, due to limited evidence and because the causes of regional changes are complex.

The effectiveness of particular policies and measures depend on local circumstances, including geography, development pathways, social and cultural contexts, financial and human resources and other factors. Developing scenarios to illustrate the possible risks of extreme weather and climate events would be helpful to ensure that disaster risk management and adaptation activities take into consideration how factors determining risk could evolve over time.

Health Transitions

One approach to thinking about future public health and health-care pathways is from the perspective of past health transitions (Ebi, 2008). Over the past century, the populations in higher-income countries experienced socio-economic, demographic and epidemiologic transitions from high to low fertility and mortality rates, as well as from high infectious to high chronic disease morbidity and mortality (Omran, 1998; Martens, 2002). Incorporating health transitions into scenarios could provide more nuanced descriptions of possible future population health. Typically, three stages are used to describe these health transitions: the age of famine and infectious diseases, the age of receding pandemics and the age of chronic diseases (Omran, 1998).

- The age of famine is characterised by high fertility and low life expectancy, with infectious diseases the primary causes of death, inadequate food and safe water supplies, limited access to health care and education, insufficient social and economic capital and slow technology development. Many of the least-developed countries are in this stage.
- The age of receding pandemics is characterised by somewhat lower mortality rates and increased life expectancy, primarily from increased access to safe water and adequate nutrition, leading to a reduction in the prevalence of infectious diseases (Omran, 1998). Higher-income countries entered this stage

in the middle of the 19th century. Countries with economies in transition and some low-income countries are in this stage.

- The age of chronic diseases is characterised by improvements in health care and the social determinants of health (Martens, 2002). Chronic diseases are the dominant causes of death, with continued improvements in social circumstances and economic growth, further increases in life expectancy and low fertility rates. High- and middle-income countries are in this stage.

Although many developed countries passed through these phases sequentially, health transitions in developing countries are more complex because recent and current socio-economic and political conditions differ from those prevailing when high-income countries were developing (Ebi, 2008). Many currently developing countries are simultaneously in an age of receding pandemics and an age of chronic disease, with high burdens of infectious and chronic diseases (Martens, 2002). Public health and health care are struggling to cope with this double burden, trying to reduce disease epidemics while also trying to reduce the health consequences of lifestyle choices, high levels of environmental exposures and other factors contributing to chronic disease burdens.

Possibilities for the next stages in the health transition include an age of emerging infectious diseases, an age of medical technology and/or an age of sustained health and an age of reduced life expectancy (Olshansky and Ault, 1986; Olshansky et al., 1998; Martens, 2002).

- An age of emerging infectious diseases could result from the re-emergence of currently controlled infectious diseases and the simultaneous emergence of new infectious diseases. This transition would be characterised by increasing infectious disease rates in high- and low-income countries, with falling life expectancies and economic productivity. Factors facilitating this transition would include travel and trade, microbiological resistance, human behaviour, breakdowns in health systems and increased pressure on the environment (Barrett et al., 1998). A number of worldwide events and trends suggest this transition is possible.
- Increased economic growth, investments in social and medical services and improvements in technology could lead to an age of medical technology and/or sustained health, with associated reductions in lifestyle-related diseases and the elimination of most infectious diseases (Martens, 2002). Life expectancy would increase, with implications not only for medical care and other services but also for sectors from water to energy consumption.
- Another possible pathway for future population health is a decrease in life expectancy and economic productivity owing to an increased burden of lifestyle-related diseases in high- and low-income countries. Trends supporting this health transition include projections for the burden of

obesity and other lifestyle-related diseases in most countries (Mokdad et al., 1999, 2001).

Global issues not considered in many of these pathways could affect health transitions in complex and non-linear ways (Ebi, 2008). Population health and economic growth are affected increasingly by conditions that transcend national borders and political jurisdictions, such as macroeconomic policies associated with international financial institutions, global trade agreements, water shortage and pollution that crosses borders (Labonte and Spiegel, 2003). Further, climate change could affect a transition through potentially devastating impacts on ecosystems, agricultural productivity and water availability (Butler and Harley, 2010). More work is needed to consider how these and other trends could influence socio-economic development, to further our understanding of the range of possible futures in which global change will be operating.

Discussion

Scenarios are valuable tools for exploring the range of possible interactions between human and natural systems and climate and other global environmental changes. However, developing scenarios is complex because of the multiple and interacting drivers of climate-sensitive health outcomes, with interactions among the drivers.

Ebi and Gamble (2005) recommended that scenario building should first determine why the scenario was being built, such as risk management, to inform policy or for communication purposes. The purpose will influence the baseline variables to be included, the geographic and temporal scale of the scenario and the focus on vulnerability versus impact. The purpose also will determine the kind of scenario needed to achieve the aim, and the appropriate methods and tools for generating the scenario.

Scenarios developed to date have not focused sufficiently on health issues. Modifications of scenarios are needed that specifically identify and address health-related questions about the future. Considerations in health scenario development include:

- Identifying key determinants of population health and how they may evolve into the future. This includes consideration of how to incorporate development pathways.
- Incorporating adaptation, mitigation and adaptive capacity.
- Incorporating thresholds and non-linear events, such as extreme weather and climate events.

- Identifying events or processes that could change projected trends, leading to alternative futures.
- Identifying and characterising critical uncertainties.
- Involving stakeholders in scenario development.

Conclusion

While the future is inherently uncertain, scenarios are important tools for providing insights into how the future could unfold and what those changes might mean for avoiding, preparing for, responding to and recovering from climate change impacts. Such insights are critical for informing strategies, policies and measures to increase population health resilience now and in the future.

References

Agard, J., Alcamo, J., Ash, N., Arthurton, R., Barker, S., Barr, J., et al. 2007. *Global Environment Outlook: Environment for Development (GEO-4)*. United Nations Environment Programme (UNEP), Nairobi, Kenya.

Barrett, R., Kuzawaa, C., McDade, T. & Armelagos, G. 1998. Emerging and re-emerging infectious diseases: the third epidemiologic transition. *Annual Review of Anthropology* 27, 247–71.

Butler, C.D. & Harley, D. 2010. Primary, secondary and tertiary effects of the eco-climate crisis: the medical response. *Postgraduate Medical Journal* 86, 230–4.

Butler, C.D., Oluoch-Kosura, W., Corvalán, C., Fobil, J., Koren, H., Pingali, P., et al. 2005. Human well-being across the scenarios. In: Carpenter, S.R., Pingali, P.L., Bennett, E.M. & Zurek, M.B. (eds) *Ecosystems and Human Well-Being: Scenarios Vol 2*. Island Press, Washington, DC, USA, 409–29.

Carpenter, S.R., Pingali, P.L., Bennett, E.M. & Zurek, M.B. (eds) 2005. *Ecosystems and Human Well-Being: Scenarios Vol 2*. Island Press, Washington, DC, USA.

Ebi, K.L. 2008. Healthy people 2100: modeling population health impacts of climate change. *Climatic Change* 88, 5–19.

Ebi, K.L. & Gamble, J.L. 2005. Summary of a workshop on health scenarios development: strategies for the future. *Environmental Health Perspectives* 113, 335–8.

Intergovernmental Panel on Climate Change (IPCC) 2007. *Climate Change 2007: Synthesis Report. Contribution of Working Groups I, II and III to the Fourth Assessment Report of the Intergovernmental Panel on Climate Change* [Core Writing Team, Pachauri, R.K. & Reisinger, A. (eds)]. IPCC, Geneva, Switzerland.

IPCC (ed.) 2012. *Managing the Risks of Extreme Events and Disasters to Advance Climate Change Adaptation. A Special Report of Working Groups I and II of the IPCC* [Field, C.B., Barros, V., Stocker, T.F., Qin, D., Dokken, D.J., Ebi, K.L., Mastrandrea, M.D., Mach, K.J., Plattner, G.-K., Allen, S.K., Tignor, M. & Midgley, P.M. (eds)]. Cambridge University Press, Cambridge, UK.

Labonte, R. & Spiegel, J. 2003. Setting global health research priorities. *BMJ* 326, 722–3.

McMichael, A.J. 2001. Human Frontiers, Environments and Disease: Past Patterns, Uncertain Futures. Cambridge University Press, Cambridge, UK.

McMichael, A.J. 2008. Public health, the environment and the 21st century: a wider field of vision (Editorial). *European Journal of Public Health* 18, 101.

McMichael, A.J. 2012. Insights from past millennia into climatic impacts on human health and survival. *Proceedings of the National Academy of Sciences (USA)* 109, 4730–7.

McMichael, A.J. & Lindgren, E. 2011. Climate change: present and future risks to health, and necessary responses. *Journal of Internal Medicine* 270, 401–13.

Martens, P. 2002. Health transitions in a globalizing world: towards more disease or sustained health? *Futures* 34, 635–48.

Millennium Ecosystem Assessment (MEA) 2005. *Ecosystems and Human Well-being. Synthesis.* Island Press, Washington, DC, USA.

Mokdad, A.H., Serdula, M.K., Dietz, W.H., Bowman, B.A., Marks, J.S. & Koplan, J.P. 1999. The spread of the obesity epidemic in the United States, 1991–1998. *Journal of the American Medical Association* 282, 1519–22.

Mokdad, A.H., Bowman, B.A., Ford, E.S., Vinicor, F., Marks, J.S. & Koplan, J.P. 2001. The continuing epidemics of obesity and diabetes in the United States. *Journal of the American Medical Association* 286, 1195–200.

Nakicenovic, N., Alcamo, J., Davis, G., de Vries, B., Fenhann, J., Gaffin, S., et al. 2000. *IPCC Special Report on Emissions Scenarios (SRES).* Cambridge University Press, Cambridge, UK.

Olshansky, S.J. & Ault, A.B. 1986. The fourth stage of the epidemiologic transition: the age of delayed degenerative diseases. *Milbank Quarterly* 64, 355–91.

Olshansky, S.J., Carnes, B.A., Rogers, R.G. & Smith, L. 1998. Emerging infectious diseases: the fifth stage of the epidemiologic transition? *World Health Statistics Quarterly* 51, 207–17.

Omran, A.-R. 1998. The epidemiological transition theory revisited thirty years later. *World Health Statistics Quarterly* 51, 99–119.

UN Millennium Project 2005. *Investing in Development: A Practical Plan to Achieve the Millennium Development Goals*. Earthscan London, UK.

34

CLIMATE CHANGE, VIOLENCE, AND THE AFTERLIFE

KIRK R. SMITH

Abstract

Climate change poses challenges to decision making because actions today have their most severe consequences many decades in the future. Using perspectives from the moral philosopher, Samuel Scheffler, and the social historian, Steven Pinker, I explore how a shift of human values needed to make difficult and expensive decisions today to protect the future may actually fit existing trends and values in society if the implications of the work of McMichael and others to document climate impacts comes to be fully accepted. Scheffler's 'afterlife conjecture' is that believable threats to even an indefinite human future actually affect today's values profoundly; that we in a sense care more for the future than the present. Some future climate scenarios would place humanity in a world very much altered from today, i.e. threaten Scheffler's afterlife and thus today's values. Pinker, in contrast, documents the worldwide reduction in violence over human history that is still spreading. Climate change will harm many groups not able to protect themselves – arguably violence by one group on another that could be ameliorated by extending Pinker's long-term societal tendency for violence reduction forward in time as well as historically. The insights of philosophers and historians may be essential to learn how to change values in time to avoid the worst impacts from climate change.

Introduction

The first two volumes of the McMichael trilogy served to pioneer and then frame modern understanding of the impacts of global change on human health (McMichael, 1993, 2001). The third puts it into a broad historical context (McMichael, in press). The challenge facing us now is to find ways to place these understandings within the continuum of human experience, extending also into the future. Without doing so, expecting society to alter behaviour today to reduce climate change a century away seems futile, given numerous, more immediate demands. Scholarly contributions from two entirely different fields, however, together offer a path to start thinking about establishing this continuum. They come from the moral philosopher, Samuel Scheffler, on the 'afterlife' (Scheffler, 2012) and the psychologist and social historian, Steven Pinker, on the history of violence (Pinker, 2011).

Scheffler's Afterlife

Scheffler has articulated compelling arguments that, in contrast to common understanding, people actually value the future far more than they realise; indeed, in some fundamental ways, this valuation of the future not only exceeds that of the present but also even their own lives. He defines the 'collective afterlife' as the continuation of society through unnamed and non-specific populations, who will carry forward the human experience well past our own lives, and even past the lives of our children and grandchildren.

He uses thought experiments postulating worlds with no 'afterlife'; for example, through a chemical or disease that causes humanity to become infertile, as depicted by P.D. James in her novel, *The Children of Men* (James, 1992). In this scenario, no one dies prematurely, yet, Scheffler argues, people still suffer, because they perceive the absence of an afterlife, i.e. the break in the continuation of human society after their own deaths and those of everyone they know. By asking us to consider how the things we would value in daily life would change in such circumstances, he forces us to recognise that much of what seems of value today is actually premised on the unstated assumed existence of an afterlife.

Indeed, as Scheffler points out, it is hard to imagine what would actually be of value in such a circumstance. Would anyone work on a cure for cancer, for example? Or a solution for climate change? Such tasks are undertaken routinely now by people who know their own lives are as limited as are those of all they know and love. This does not deter them from taking on goals with pay-offs far in the future. Even valuing such simple pleasures as a good book, a good meal and a good holiday may actually be premised on subconscious expectation that humanity will persist following their death. Scheffler states:

- 'The fact that we and everyone we love will cease to exist matters less to us than would the non-existence of future people whom we do not know and who, indeed, have no determinate identities.'

- 'Or to put it more positively, the coming into existence of people we do not know and love matters more to us than our own survival and the survival of the people we do know and love.'
- 'The fact that, in certain respects, we care less about our own survival than about the survival of humanity shows something important and insufficiently appreciated about the limits of our egoism.'

Climate change does not threaten human survival in the way that absolute infertility would, but climate scenarios exist that portray major disruptions in the continuum of human experience. Scenarios, for example, in which large areas of Earth are no longer inhabitable, except in cities built like space colonies. These are currently considered low probability events by climate scientists; although not that low, being, for example, far more likely than events that many people dread and which are also less severe, such as nuclear reactor accidents. Neither are climate catastrophes far off in an indefinite future, such as the burn-out of the Sun. Some scenarios start to become severe well within the lifetimes of babies born this decade, i.e. by 2100.

What is Rational?

Scheffler's 'afterlife conjecture' calls into question the large discount rates used by standard economic and political thinking that assume implicitly that solving today's short-term problems will be enough to protect the future. Today's activities have long-term consequences, however, and the conjecture can be stated as:

- What combination of severity and probability of future climates might risk crossing the afterlife threshold, calling into questions actions that still optimise present values today?

That is, might any such combination threaten our reasonable expectation of the continuation of human existence as we know it? If so, this would fundamentally threaten all that we value in this generation, and may force us to reverse the usual discounting rules.

The Nobel economist, Amartya Sen, famously once described the 'rational economic man', who operates to maximise present value as if he were alone in space in time, as 'close to being a social moron' (Sen, 1977). Others have also criticised *Homo economicus* as a conceit that peppers economic textbooks but rarely, if ever, occurs in life. From the future, actions to maximise short-term well-being ('optimise present value') cannot be considered rational if they impose sufficient impacts on the future to cross the Scheffler afterlife threshold, thus also destroying many of the values we place in the present.

The History of Violence: A Positive Story

For me, Steven Pinker's book presents a detailed and convincing narrative and statistical analysis of trends of violence over human history. He argues that violence in essentially all its forms (*inter alia*, war, crime, torture, terrorism, genocide, slavery, racism, riots, violent sports, animal cruelty, religious fanaticism and intolerance, suppression of minorities, homosexuals and women, duelling, infanticide, burning witches, human sacrifice) has declined dramatically in the world, particularly in the last 200 years. Even the official creed of the US Marine Corps has shifted in recent years from protect god and country and leave no man behind to 'protect all persons at all times, even the enemy'. Not that all forms of violence have been eradicated or that no reversals are possible, but the toll is orders of magnitude less than before, and trends still look good.

War and other institutionalised violence, for example, has decreased globally in the era after World War II, when true global institutions, greatly improved communications and expanded trade has spearheaded the longest peace among great powers in human history. Pinker argues that we are now engaged in the halting process of extending worldwide the right to be violence free.

Is Climate Change a Form of Violence?

Today's world is not the final frontier, however. The next stage of anti-violence evolution may need to be launched across temporal boundaries into the future. Our science tells us clearly that damage to others, including from climate change, can be propagated across time by our own present actions, even some actions that seem rational or apparently harmless in the short term. Science also informs us that the inadvertent target of most such climate impacts is the most vulnerable; the very groups which rationally should be the focus of contemporary efforts to enlarge the frontier of rights and empathy during anti-violence evolution. In other words, the bulk of climate-threatening actions most endanger the future well-being of the groups society is just beginning to include within the global anti-violence boundary.

Violence, as usually defined, is harmful action taken by one identifiable person or group directly against another identifiable person or group. It is usually framed in the context of trauma in which direct causality and aetiology are not much in question, to use health terminology. This is true whether machetes or nuclear weapons are used, both of which have killed hundreds of thousands in recent memory, although the former much more than the latter – or whether perpetuated by rogue nation states or abusive husbands.

The impacts of climate change, however, although partly acting through trauma, do not have the same immediate direct linkage. Causality and aetiology are still in question for some impacts today, and even as the connections become more statistically clear with increasing global warming, there will not be the direct clarity of cause and effect as when people wield swords against one another.

Nevertheless, people can be harmed by actions taken by others, even if far distant in time and place. This is another form of violence, even if mediated by Earth's climate system. Violence, however, also carries a moral connotation, being made up of clear acts of commission, not merely of negligence, i.e. omission. Climate change has not yet crossed the boundary into clear acts of commission in the minds of most of the world – the visceral recognition that our emissions today are killing people tomorrow. It is more in the realm of a sin of omission today; climate change occurs because we are negligent in doing something about it. Nevertheless, perception is moving in the direction of considering our actions today as a form of commission, as the climate science shows more and more clearly how what we now do affects others, even those whose names cannot ever be known.

Violence to the Afterlife

Issues of intergenerational equity have long been part of the debate about climate change and other long-term environmental issues, such as nuclear waste (Smith, 1977). The works of Scheffler and Pinker, however, provide important extensions of that perspective from completely different realms – moral philosophy and social history. They give new ways to frame the evidence marshalled in the McMichael trilogy as leading to the needed changes in thinking about climate mitigation and the human future. On one side, understanding the negative changes that could come from the severe climate change that could occur well within the lifetime of children born today pushes us to contemplate what it would mean to cross what might be termed the 'Scheffler Afterlife Threshold'. This would be the point at which threats to the future from climate change might so alter our belief in the nature of what human life and society will become that it threatens how we value ourselves and our own lives today, one of Scheffler's main points about the afterlife. On the other side, strengthening our belief in the connection between current actions and future impacts shifts the moral argument away from omission towards commission, i.e. makes our actions more like conscious violent acts against others. Thus, mitigation of climate change then could be seen as an extension of the long march of violence reduction in human history to our own future.

References

James, P.D. 1992. *Children of Men*. Alfred A. Knopf Inc, New York, USA.

McMichael, A.J. 1993. *Planetary Overload: Global Environmental Change and the Health of the Human Species*. Cambridge University Press, Cambridge, UK.

McMichael, A.J. 2001. *Human Frontiers, Environments and Disease: Past Patterns, Uncertain Futures*. Cambridge University Press, Cambridge, UK.

McMichael, A.J. in press. *When Climates Change. Famines, Fevers and Fates of Populations*, Oxford University Press, Oxford, UK.

Pinker, S. 2011. *The Better Angels of our Nature*. Viking, New York, USA.

Scheffler, S. 2013. *Death and the Afterlife*. Oxford University Press, Oxford, UK, New York, NY, USA. Also see: tannerlectures.berkeley.edu/2011-2012, accessed 12 February 2015.

Sen, A. 1977. Rational fools. *Philosophy and Public Affairs* 6, 317–44.

Smith, K.R. 1977. *The Interaction of Time and Technology*. PhD dissertation, University of California, Berkeley, California, USA.

35

ON THE NEED TO TRANSFORM GOVERNANCE TO REGULATE CORPORATIONS FOR THE SURVIVAL OF *HOMO SAPIENS*

PETER TAIT

Abstract

Widespread concerns about the state of health in the modern world, and in parallel about the increasingly damaged state of the environment, lead many to conclude that humanity's future is bleak. Many piecemeal solutions are attempted. However, using a primary health-care lens and looking for common causes that permit strategic action for finding solutions. I argue that the ultimate cause of our concerns is poorly regulated corporate behaviour within a capitalist, market-oriented politico-economic system. To rectify this governance failure, we need to reassert democratic control over governments. A programme is required to reform government and transform societal and corporate governance to make them democratically responsive to the needs of society and the environment.

Focusing on Social Determinants of Health

Dire warnings of the deleterious human effects on ecosystems and their consequences have been made for decades (McMichael, 1993; Rockström et al., 2009; McMichael and Butler, 2011). The primary health-care approach and social determinants of health theory show that health is promoted, or not, by how we arrange society (World Health Organization, 1986; Marmot and Wilkinson, 2006; Commission on Social Determinants of Health, 2008).

Extending this approach to seek common origins of and linkages between humanity's health, social and environmental problems permits a strategic approach to address the causes of the causes. Indeed, humanity's ability to survive requires working this far upstream.

The Need for Regulated Markets and Limiting Corporate Influence

Our current social arrangements have arisen from the co-evolution of several intersecting political, economic and technological strands (Fotopoulos, 1997; Christian, 2004; Attali, 2009). The present capitalist, liberal democratic socio-economic system focuses on increasing material prosperity through growing production and consumption. Economic and social relationships are transacted within an unregulated market. Profit for shareholders trumps all other considerations, including consumer and environmental well-being (Hastings, 2012).

Large corporations have become the dominant players in the current economic and political system. Corporations use their wealth and power to influence governments to maintain the economic system that furthers their interests (Denniss and Richardson, 2013). Meaningful citizen involvement in governance is undermined (Korten, 1996). The outputs of this system are increasing wealth disparity, unhealthy people, an exploding human population and environmental and ecological destruction. By overloading the natural world on which society relies, corporations are facilitating catastrophic declines in all that sustains life (McMichael, 1993; Commission on Social Determinants of Health, 2008; Harvey, 2011).

Corporations versus Democratic Processes

The determining cause of the current social and environmental situation is poorly regulated corporate behaviour. Corporate influence undermines government capacity to do this effectively (Korten, 1996). Denniss and Richardson (2013) provide examples of how, in recent Australian history, actions by banking, mining and gambling corporations have undermined government ability to rule in the interests of the whole of society. They note 'Big business exerts influence through campaign contributions, influence over university funding, sponsorship of think tanks and in other ways that create an agenda for low tax for the rich, low entitlements for the poor and poor services for the middle class. In articulating why he wrote his book, Sachs (2011) argued that democracy itself was being threatened by the power and corruption of big business' (p. 2).

Denniss and Richardson (2013, p. 6) concluded: 'Reforms such as the mining tax, the carbon tax and gambling reform … have been vetoed by the affected industries and, with such a veto in place, the government has found it virtually impossible to implement their reforms in their original guise'.

The societal influence of corporations happens at a more insidious level. Corporate ideology has colonised global society, not as geographical annexation of land and resources, but by retelling the narrative of Western society, redefining democracy, societal relations between people, between society and the environment, the nature of business, the economy and the role of government (Deetz, 1992). This narrative serves corporate ends for growth and concentrating wealth, and it warps the narrative necessary for a healthy, biosensitive (Boyden, 2010) society.

Government's role is to regulate society and corporations, via effective legislation and enforcement mechanisms and by influencing social norms. Consequently, I argue that a primary focus on corporate behaviour and regulating that behaviour will permit a biosensitive society to emerge.

The mechanism to change how governments act to reduce the power of the corporate sector is to increase the power of the citizen. This will require a democratising transformation of governance. In order to transform democracy, we need to explore what it is. Current liberal democracy lacks meaningful citizen involvement. It is electoral oligarchy (Burnheim, 1985). Elections are open to manipulation by vested interests. The only 'actual operating democracy' that we have record of is classical Athens, which provides a template on which to model a reformed democracy (Burnheim, 1985; Fishkin, 1991; Fotopoulos, 1997).

A set of common elements and principles pertain to 'real' democracy. The key is a method for making decisions by those who have to live with the consequences of those decisions. This is also a core primary health-care principle. A second set of elements recognises that decisions need to be made deliberatively, that is as an informed group considering its 'enlightened self-interest'.

The most vexatious issue in societies with large populations is that decision making requires some form of representation. As noted, representation by election is harmful. The cleanest method for representation is by statistical sampling from among those eligible. Elections are replaced by a lottery. Eligibility for standing requires criteria, which can be provided by a methodology such as Ulrichian boundary critique (Ulrich, 2005). Representation must embody the principle of 'every vote has the same value'. It must avoid vested interests gaining influence over decisions.

Finally, democratic institutional frameworks should be arranged to distribute political, economic and social power equally, and to constrain human ability to damage the natural world (Fotopoulos, 1997). The programme for rejuvenating democracy will require simultaneous reform of government and transformation of governance at the community level. Meadow's model for systemic change gives us a way for prioritising where we might apply levers for change (Meadows, 1999). Additionally, this model lends support to the view that a focus on governance reform is important.

Processes of Change

Societal change only occurs in response to action by, to paraphrase Margaret Mead, small numbers of concerned citizens. Citizens act through non-governmental organisations (NGOs), and together these make up civil society. Coalitions of NGOs create the social movements necessary to pressure government and the corporate sector to reform.

Changing the dominant paradigm has the highest-level impact. However, we know that changing attitudes and beliefs is the most difficult. Instead, changing people's behaviour leads to changes in beliefs as they seek to rationalise new behaviour (Nisbett and Wilson, 1977). So, a focus on changing government and institutional system-level behaviour is likely to be more effective in the short term. Governance and institutional reform will be synergistic.

Simultaneously, at the community level, a transformative process to strengthen democracy within communities, workplaces, municipalities and grass-roots organisations, and to build momentum for more widespread societal transformation, is required. The Transition Towns movement is an example of this in practice (Hopkins, 2009). Corporations themselves require transformation internally to democratise their governance and operations.

It is beyond the scope of this essay to discuss the spatial, geographic and temporal scales of transformation. Suffice it to say that modern democracy will have to accommodate the globalisation of our society and our economy, as well as recognise the standing of other species, the ecosystem and future generations.

Democratic Society, Better Health

Demonstrating empirically how a more democratic society regulating corporate behaviour achieves improved environmental, public and individual health is difficult. Three lines of evidence exist. First, the primary health-care model holds individual and community empowerment central to achieving better health (World Health Organization, 1986a). Democratic governance is the method for that empowerment to emerge. Second is evidence for the reverse occurring, as decreasing democracy and increasing inequality in the current socio-economic system drives societal unrest, poor health and environment damage (Commission on Social Determinants of Health, 2008; Rockström et al., 2009; Wilkinson and Pickett, 2009; McMichael and Butler, 2011). Third, the principles underlying diverse polycentric institutions that produce more effective natural resource management (Ostrom, 2009) approximate those of democracy outlined above, supporting the notion that more democratic institutions can produce better outcomes.

Conclusion

Framing the current human health situation on the one hand and the environmental/ecological situation on the other as consequent to poorly regulated corporate behaviour, and thus as a governance problem, provides a systemic, strategic focus for solutions. Citizens, NGOs and all aspects of civil society can become active in movements to transform government democratically. Individually, we need to continue to strongly promote democratic governance arrangements into the processes of our social, work and home lives. Focusing thus takes the foundational work of Tony McMichael, alerting us to the consequences of rampant corporations, forward towards action for healthier and ecologically sustainable human societies and a healthier, humanity-sustaining environment.

References

Attali, J. 2009. *A Brief History of the Future*. Allen & Unwin, Crows Nest, NSW, Australia.

Boyden, S. 2010. *Our Place in Nature: Past Present and Future*. Nature and Society Forum Inc, Canberra, ACT, Australia.

Burnheim, J. 1985. *Is Democracy Possible?: The Alternative to Electoral Politics*. University of California Press, Oakland, California, USA.

Christian, D. 2004. *Maps of Time: An Introduction to Big History*. University of California Press, Berkeley, California, USA, Los Angeles, California, USA, and London, UK.

Commission on Social Determinants of Health 2008. *Closing the Gap in a Generation: Health Equity Through Action on the Social Determinants of Health: Final Report of the Commission on Social Determinants of Health*. World Health Organization, Geneva, Switzerland.

Deetz, S.A. 1992. *Democracy in Age Corp Co: Developments in Communication and the Politics of Everyday Life*. SUNY Press, Albany, New York, USA.

Denniss, R. & Richardson, D. 2013. Corporate power in Australia, Policy Brief No. 45. The Australia Institute, Canberra, ACT, Australia.

Fishkin, J.S. 1991. *Democracy and Deliberation: New Directions for Democratic Reform*. Yale University Press, New Haven, Connecticut, USA, and London, UK.

Fotopoulos, T. 1997. *Towards an Inclusive Democracy: The Crisis of the Growth Economy and the Need for a New Liberatory Project*. Cassell, London and New York, USA.

Harvey, D. 2011. *The Enigma of Capitalism and the Crises of Capitalism*. Oxford University Press, Oxford, UK.

Hastings, G. 2012. Why corporate power is a public health priority. *BMJ* 345, e5124.

Hopkins, R. 2009. *The Transition Handbook*. Finch Publishing, Sydney, NSW, Australia.

Korten, D.C. 1996. *When Corporations Rule the World*. Kumarian Press, Berrett-Koehler Publishers, West Hartford, Connecticut, San Francisco, California, USA.

McMichael, A.J. 1993. *Planetary Overload: Global Environmental Change and the Health of the Human Species*. Cambridge University Press, Cambridge, UK.

McMichael, A.J. & Butler, C.D. 2011. Promoting global population health while constraining the environmental footprint. *Annual Review of Public Health* 32, 179–97.

Marmot, M.G. & Wilkinson, R.G. (eds) 2006. *Social Determinants of Health*. Oxford University Press, Oxford, UK.

Meadows, D. 1999. *Leverage Points*. The Sustainability Institute, Hartland, Vermont, USA.

Nisbett, R.E. & Wilson, T.D. 1977. Telling more than we can know: verbal reports on mental processes. *Psychological Review* 84, 231–59.

Ostrom, E. 2009. Beyond markets and states: polycentric governance of complex economic systems. *The American Economic Review* 100, 641–72.

Rockström, J., Steffen, W., Noone, K., Persson, Å., Chapin, F. III, Lambin, E., et al. 2009. Planetary boundaries:exploring the safe operating space for humanity. Ecology and Society 14, art 32 www.ecologyandsociety.org/vol14/iss2/art32, accessed 16 February 2015.

Sachs, J.D. 2011. *The Price of Civilization: Reawakening American Virtue and Prosperity*. Random House Publishing Group, New York, USA (cited by Denniss and Richardson, 2013).

Ulrich, W. 2005. A Brief Introduction to Critical Systems Heuristics (CSH). ECOSENSUS project, Open University, Milton Keynes, UK. Available at: www.google.com.au/url?sa=t&rct=j&q=&esrc=s&source=web&cd=1&ved=0CC8QFjAA&url=http%3A%2F%2Fprojects.kmi.open.ac.uk%2Fecosensus%2Fpublications%2Fulrich_csh_intro.pdf&ei=nYVOU4-RNcWrkgXPsoDQDA&usg=AFQjCNEwcSksuF-MpexqngW1RbAFtfsVJA&sig2=ZB0g2kj3kjSyZcAV-xe4Ng&bvm=bv.64764171,d.dGI, accessed 16 April 2014.

Wilkinson, R.G. & Pickett, K. 2009. *The Spirit Level: Why More Equal Societies Almost Always Do Better*. Allen Lane, London, UK.

World Health Organization 1986. *Ottawa Charter for Health Promotion*. World Health Organization, Geneva, Switzerland.

36

HUMAN HABITAT AND HEALTH

Interdisciplinary and Integrative Perspectives

ANTHONY G. CAPON

Abstract

Since 2008, for the first time in human history, more people live in cities than in the countryside. By mid-21st century, the United Nations estimates are for two to three billion additional people being housed in cities – more than one million extra every week. While cities can be desirable places, living there can pose risks to human health. Beyond cities, ecosystems are the planet's life-supporting systems on which human health and survival is dependent. Because cities concentrate people and economic activity, they also concentrate resource consumption and waste production. Thus, cities can affect the health of ecosystems. Consequently, cities should be planned, designed, developed and managed to protect not only the health of people but also ecosystems.

The International Council for Science (ICSU) recently launched a 10-year global interdisciplinary science programme on health and well-being in the changing urban environment. The programme will bring scientists together with counterparts in government, industry and communities to tackle critical urban policy and planning questions. The ambition of the programme is to build new knowledge and develop capacity for decision making in cities, and about them, and thereby protect and promote human health in sustainable ways. Tony McMichael's influence on my thinking in this regard is described.

Introduction

> ... the prime role of societies is to create enduring conditions that promote the population's wellbeing and health. (A.J. McMichael, quoted in Shetty, 2006)

Homo sapiens is undergoing a radical transformation of its ecology (McMichael, 2000). Since 2008, cities have been the dominant habitat for the human species. The majority of the world's people now live in cities and, for the foreseeable future, most population growth will be in urban areas (Figure 36.1). By the middle of the 21st century, two to three billion more people will need to be housed in the cities of the world – more than one million additional people every week. Most of this urban population growth will be in small and medium-sized cities in low- and middle-income countries. This urban transition provides an unparalleled opportunity to improve health outcomes for people and planetary systems through improved urban planning, design, development and management.

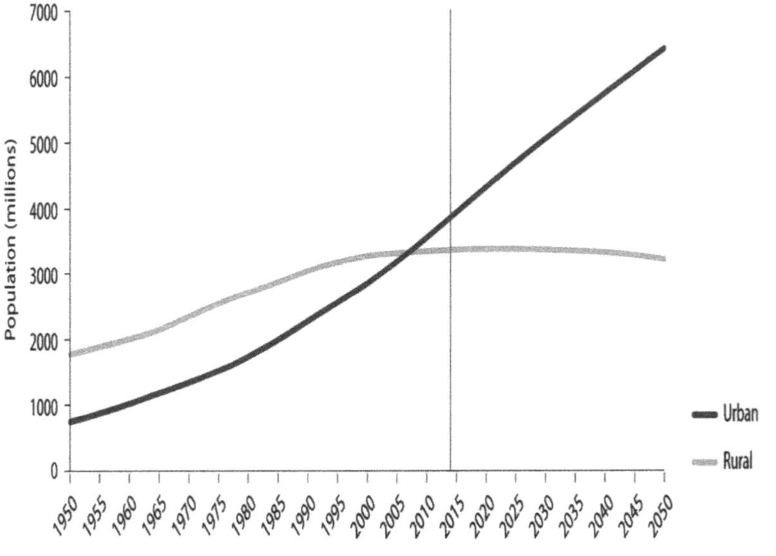

Figure 36.1 The urban and rural population of the world in millions, 1950–2050.

Source: United Nations Department of Economic and Social Affairs, Population Division, *World Urbanization Prospects: The 2014 Revision*, © 2014. Reprinted with the permission of the United Nations.

Cities can be great places to live. People are attracted to cities for work, education and social and cultural reasons, and access to food, health care and other services. However, cities can also be unhealthy places to live. Contaminated water, lack of sanitation, inadequate housing and overcrowding are health issues in many low-income cities. The way people live in cities affects their health via exposure to pollution, levels of physical activity, food choices, safety and social connection and participation (Capon and Blakely, 2007). These are determinants of common, contemporary health problems such as heart disease, chronic respiratory disease, obesity, diabetes, cancers, injury and depression.

The way people live in cities also affects the health of the environment through loss of biodiversity, changes to ecosystems, carbon emissions, climate change and environmental pollution. These environmental changes have feedback impacts on human health. While city dwellers, on average, often enjoy better health than those who live in the countryside, this masks health inequities within cities. Urban health inequities are detrimental to all city dwellers. Infectious disease outbreaks, social unrest, crime and violence are some ways that urban health inequities affect everyone (WHO and UN-HABITAT, 2005).

Population growth is increasing competition for planet Earth's finite resources. With rising incomes, per capita consumption is increasing in many parts of the world. This combination of increasing population and per capita consumption is increasing greatly the demands on planetary systems. To reduce potential conflict, it is essential that resources be shared more equitably. The availability of cheap liquid fuels during the 20th century enabled the development of energy-intensive cities, and many cities became reliant on the motor car for transport (Newman and Kenworthy, 1999). This era of cheap liquid fuels is now over. In order for cities to thrive in the future, they must adapt to rising liquid fuel prices and transition to be less energy-intensive places to live.

Because cities usually develop in places that are good for growing food, urban population growth consumes surrounding fertile agricultural land unless appropriate planning controls are in place. In almost every country, the proportion of people aged over 60 years is growing because of increased life expectancy and reduced fertility rates. This demographic transition presents challenges and opportunities in cities. From a health perspective, cities are confronting global epidemics of chronic diseases (i.e. heart disease, diabetes, chronic lung disease, cancers and depression) (Yach et al., 2005). As these epidemics mature, we should think of the built environment as a potential 'treatment' for chronic disease, as well as a place for 'prevention' of disease.

Personal Reflections: A Case Study in Collegial Influence

My interest in relationships between urban environments and human health was first sparked in 1991, when I was appointed Director of Public Health and Medical Officer of Health (MOH) in western Sydney, Australia.[1] MOH is a statutory appointment under the *NSW Public Health Act 1991*, with responsibility for protecting the health of a geographically defined population,

1 Participation in a 1993 British Council course on healthy cities led by John Ashton imbued me with a long-standing passion for improving urban health in sustainable ways.

in this case about one million people living along, and to the north of, the main western metropolitan railway line, from Auburn through Parramatta, Blacktown and Penrith to Hawkesbury and the Blue Mountains. This is a socioculturally diverse part of Sydney that includes several large relatively socio-economically disadvantaged communities. The landscape ranges from remnant Cumberland forest, through Hawkesbury River floodplain to the UNESCO world heritage listed parklands. While average health status in western Sydney is comparable to the rest of Australia, an aggregate analysis masks considerable health inequities across subregions.

Our research demonstrated that the pattern of urban development in western Sydney (similar to most of the outer metropolitan regions of Australia's large cities) was presenting risks to health for the people who lived there – from air pollution (Jalaludin et al., 2000) and food insecurity (Webb et al., 1998) to injury (Close et al., 1993) and newly emerging infectious diseases (Bell et al., 1996), among others. As interest in urban health developed, I reached out to Howard Frumkin,[2] who shared concern about the impacts of urban sprawl on public health in similar contexts in North America (Frumkin, 2002).

In 2002, I approached Tony McMichael. I knew of McMichael's work because *Planetary Overload* (McMichael, 1993) was, by then, considered a public health classic. His thoughtful commentary about urbanisation and health (McMichael, 2000) had already inspired me to think in more integrative ways about urban health problems in western Sydney. Our first encounter, in the Director's office at the National Centre for Epidemiology and Population Health (NCEPH),[3] The Australian National University (ANU), remains imprinted on my memory. As we discussed the health challenges facing the residents of outer metropolitan Australia, and I made a case for enhanced academic attention to these challenges, McMichael was clear that he would be delighted to help in any way he could. He expressed concern for the people affected and a readiness to contribute from an academic perspective. Since that first meeting, McMichael was a consistently wise and generous mentor to me. While he was a singular scholar, unlike many academics he was also committed strongly to the application of new knowledge in policy and practice (knowledge translation). He was well known as a tireless advocate for the urgent need for action on climate change in Australia and internationally.

2 At that time, Howard Frumkin was professor of environmental and occupational health at Emory University, Atlanta, USA. Subsequently, he directed the National Center for Environmental Health and Agency for Toxic Substances and Disease Registry at the Centers for Disease Control and Prevention, and is now Dean of the School of Public Health at the University of Washington in Seattle. Howard is another environmental health scholar who has been inspired by McMichael's contributions.

3 Having co-supervised field placements in western Sydney for a number of Master of Applied Epidemiology (MAE) trainees during Bob Douglas's tenure as founding NCEPH director during the 1990s, I was well acquainted with the centre and always ready to collaborate with their scholars.

At the same time, I contacted the CSIRO urban systems programme and arranged to meet with their Canberra-based team, led by Allen Kearns. This was a turning point for me, and I resolved to learn more about systems thinking[4] and its applications in population health research and intervention (Proust et al., 2012). In Australia, 2004 was declared the Year of the Built Environment. In recognition of the mounting evidence of detrimental health impacts of urban development, the Western Sydney Area Health Service Chief Executive Officer, Stephen Boyages, allowed me to spend the year advocating for policy responses across the three levels of government in Australia, in partnership with the land development and transport sectors. The House of Representatives Standing Committee on Environment and Heritage established an enquiry into the sustainability of Australian cities and, in this context, I spent much of that year exchanging with a diverse range of stakeholders – from members of parliament through planners, infrastructure builders and funders, to land developers and private bus operators (a mix of academics, civil society and business people). I even spent a memorable day in a truck traversing Sydney to experience first-hand the challenges of urban transport from the perspective of a delivery truck driver – essential qualitative research because the urban transport challenge is as much about the movement of resources as it is about the movement of people.

In 2006, McMichael chaired an Australian Academy of Science (AAS) Fenner Conference on the Environment[5] on the theme of 'Urbanism, Environment and Health'. Bruce Armstrong, from the University of Sydney (where I had an honorary academic appointment), had suggested an AAS Fenner Conference as one option for getting concerns about urban health and sustainability debated by the Australian public policy community. The inspiration for the conference was the seminal work of Stephen Boyden[6] on the ecology of cities and their people (Boyden et al., 1981). The conference brought researchers together with policymakers, practitioners and concerned citizens to examine the relationships between 'urbanism' – ways of living in urban areas – and the health of people and ecosystems. The outputs of the conference included two collections of papers on Australian urban health and sustainability challenges authored and edited to attract a policy audience (Capon and Dixon, 2007; Dixon and Capon, 2007).

4 Potential applications of systems thinking in population health research and practice definitely warrant more attention by the international public health community (Foresight: see www.gov.uk/government/publications/reducing-obesity-future-choices, accessed July 5, 2015).

5 AAS Fenner Conferences on the Environment are supported by a generous endowment from the late Frank and Bobby Fenner.

6 McMichael introduced me to Stephen Boyden. Apart from stimulating my interest in human ecology and health, Stephen inspired me to join the Frank Fenner Foundation (then known as the Nature and Society Forum) with its vision of *Healthy People on a Healthy Planet*. Some time later, McMichael told me that for a while he kept a copy of Stephen's book, *The Biology of Civilisation: Human Culture as a Force in Nature*, in his tennis bag in anticipation of moments when there would be room for inspiration.

The fifth Oxford Health Alliance Global Summit was held in Sydney in 2008, on the theme of 'Building a healthy future: Chronic disease and our environment'. The summit picked up this developing urban health agenda, and McMichael, a keynote speaker at the conference, was influential in the framing of the resultant Sydney Declaration (The NCD Alliance, 2013). In 2009, ANU led a successful bid for funding from the CSIRO Climate Adaptation Flagship to establish a multi-institutional research programme on 'Urbanism, Climate Adaptation and Health', which spanned thermal impacts, vector-borne disease, food security, air pollution, urban transport and urban form and housing.

Around this time, I was invited to join the planning group for the first International Council for Science (ICSU) global interdisciplinary programme on 'science for health and well-being' (SHWB).[7] McMichael had advised an earlier scoping group that had settled on the topic of 'Health and Well-being in the Changing Urban Environment – a Systems Analysis Approach' as the focus for the new 10-year programme. Inspired by the experience of the AAS Fenner Conference, I relished the opportunity to contribute to this ICSU process, which has since provided outstanding opportunities for collaboration with leading international scholars in the broad field of urban health and sustainability (Bai et al., 2012). The Chinese Academy of Sciences' Institute of Urban Environment in Xiamen was recently named as the host for the International Programme Office for this new programme, now sponsored jointly by the Inter-Academy Medical Panel and United Nations University (UNU).

Ways of Understanding

Evolutionary perspectives

There is value in understanding contemporary health problems from an evolutionary perspective. Most humans are now living in very different ways to those of our hunter-gatherer ancestors (Box 36.1). The evolutionary health principle postulates that if an animal's environment changes in a significant way, then it is likely that the animal will be less well adapted to the new conditions and will consequently show signs of physiological or behavioural maladjustment (Boyden, 2004). From an evolutionary perspective, chronic disease can be seen to arise from human maladaptation to the current ready availability of fossil fuel energy, contemporary food systems, patterns of urban settlement and ways of living.

---

7 As president of the International Union of Nutritional Sciences during 2001–05, Mark Wahlqvist was one of the agitants for an ICSU SHWB initiative.

Box 36.1 From city dweller to urban hunter-gatherer

For thousands of generations, our ancestors were hunter-gatherers. It was only about 10,000 years ago that humans began to take up farming as a way of life (Boyden, 2004). From an evolutionary perspective, the human body is well suited to the hunter-gatherer way of life – procuring plants and animals from the wild, by gathering and hunting – because it provides a natural diet and plenty of exercise. Nowadays, most people are living in ways that are very different from the way hunter-gatherers lived. Modern lifestyles can be very sedentary and modern diets can be far from natural. The way we live in cities contributes to many of our contemporary health problems. In order to design healthy cities, perhaps our ambition should be to plan and develop cities in ways that would enable people to live more like hunter-gatherers. What would such cities be like? *Urban hunter-gatherers* would get plenty of exercise in daily life – walking to school, up and down stairs in buildings, to the shops, to work. Bursts of intense physical activity – *hunting* – would occur when people ran fast (e.g. running late for the train) or when they cycled at speed. The *urban hunter-gatherer* could *gather* healthy food at local shops and markets, or from a community or street garden. While this may seem an unusual vision for the future of our cities, it may provide useful insights for the design of active and healthy cities.

Change in cities and their environs has been conceptualised as an evolutionary process with four distinctive stages – poverty, industrial, consumption and eco-city (Bai and Imura, 2000). Cities do not fit neatly into a single stage, rather they usually exhibit characteristics of more than one stage at any one time. The principal health concerns are different for each stage (Table 36.1), although this is also not clear-cut – chronic diseases are an increasing burden in low-income cities. The value of this typology is in identifying typical transitions in the evolution of cities, including the aspirational stage of healthy eco-city. The challenge becomes how cities might avoid the pitfalls of stages 2 and 3 by moving directly from stage 1 to eco-city.

Table 36.1 Stages of urban evolution and characteristic environmental conditions and health issues.

Stage	Characteristic environmental conditions	Characteristic health issues
1. Poverty	Contaminated water, lack of sanitation, inadequate housing	Infectious diseases, malnutrition, injury
2. Industrial	Air pollution and land contamination by chemicals and solid waste	Chronic respiratory disease, injury, heart disease, cancers
3. Consumption	High levels of consumption of water, energy and other resources	Chronic diseases (obesity, diabetes, heart disease, cancers), injury, depression
4. Healthy eco-city	Conditions of life in balance with nature	Maximum health potential

Source: Adapted from Capon, 2007.

Adaptive approaches

Climate change affects health in many ways – most of them adverse – and will do so increasingly over coming decades (McMichael et al., 2006). The threats include more frequent, and more intense, heatwaves, hurricanes and other extreme weather events. Coastal cities are particularly vulnerable to beach erosion and inundation. There are also indirect health impacts from changes to physical and biological processes, such as enhanced health risks from urban air pollution. In addition, there are flow-on health impacts from social, demographic and economic disruptions, such as declining rural incomes from agricultural production, with consequent urban migration. The health impacts of climate change are greater in low-income communities – those least responsible for climate change are affected the most.

Responses to climate change – so-called mitigation and adaptation actions – also affect health. These health impacts are mostly beneficial and have been called 'health co-benefits' (Haines et al., 2009). A co-benefit is an additional benefit arising from an action that is undertaken for a different principal purpose. Putative co-benefits from action on climate change (i.e. additional benefits beyond greenhouse gas reductions) include reduced air pollution, increased levels of physical activity, a healthier diet, improved energy security through a more diverse energy supply and less dependency on oil, a reduction in traffic congestion and new employment opportunities. Co-benefits are sometimes referred to as a 'no-regrets approach' because, even in the absence of a need to act on climate change, there are already strong arguments for many of the proposed actions. A figure in the foreword to this book shows a diagrammatic representation of the concept of co-benefits for health (Boyden, 2014). Human activities have direct human health impacts – via pathways including nutrition and level of physical activity – and indirect human health impacts – via the health of planetary systems (e.g. the climate system). It follows that there can be co-benefits for health from actions to address climate change. (For clarity, the arrows are presented as unidirectional. However, there are relationships in both directions.)

An understanding of health co-benefits could have profound implications for decisions about the future of cities. In the interest of our future health, the findings of research on health co-benefits should be accounted for in the design of cities. However, although the take-home message is a positive one – low-carbon ways of living are healthy ways of living – urban policymakers should be alert for potential unintended negative impacts, such as exacerbation of social inequity.

Eco-social perspectives on health

McMichael greatly influenced the way I think about human health futures. His arguments for integrative perspectives on the health of people, the places where they live and work and the health of broader planetary systems are compelling. Currently, I am transitioning the UNU International Institute for Global Health (UNU-IIGH) from its initial focus on health services research to eco-social perspectives on human health. Eco-social perspectives mean recognition of the ecological, economic and social foundations of human health. Fundamentally, future human health, well-being and survival depend on the health of planetary systems (McMichael, 1999, 2013).

The World We Want

As the world's people come together to shape a post-2015 development agenda, it is timely to consider the way human health and well-being should be framed in this agenda. The current proposal is for a new set of development goals that integrate poverty reduction with sustainable development. For this to be meaningful, all people – from across all nations and societal sectors – will have a part to play in achieving such sustainable development goals (SDGs). One challenge is representing urban health futures in this agenda. Cities are for people (Gehl, 2010). Health is relevant not only to urban planning and development; health should also be considered a key outcome of the ongoing management of cities. While the form and size of cities are highly variable – reflecting different histories, geographies, cultures, technologies, economies – human health needs are universal (Boyden, 2004). The increasingly urban habitat of the human species is a determinant of habits, including health behaviours and health. An essential prerequisite for achieving 'the world we want' is to embrace the eco-social perspectives on human health and well-being advanced by McMichael.

References

Bai, X. & Imura, H.A. 2000. Comparative study of urban environment in East Asia: stage model of urban environmental evolution. *International Review for Environmental Strategies* 1, 135–58.

Bai, X., Nath, I., Capon, A.G., Hasan, N. & Jaron, D. 2012. Health and wellbeing in the changing urban environment: complex challenges, scientific responses, and the way forward. *Current Opinion in Environmental Sustainability* 4, 465–72.

Bell, J.C., Jorm, L.R., Williamson, M., Shaw, N.H., Kazandjian, D.L.J., Chiew, R., et al. 1996. Legionellosis linked with a hotel car park – how many were infected? *Epidemiology and Infection* 116, 185–92.

Boyden, S. 2004. *The Biology of Civilisation: Understanding Human Culture as a Force in Nature*. UNSW Press, Sydney, Australia.

Boyden, S. 2014. The story of life and the future of civilisation. Available at: www.natsoc.org.au/biosensitivefutures, accessed 11 May 2014.

Boyden, S., Millar, S., Newcombe, K. & O'Neill, B. 1981. *The Ecology of a City and its People*. Australian National University Press, Canberra, ACT, Australia.

Capon, A.G. 2007. The way we live in cities. *Medical Journal of Australia* 187, 658–61.

Capon, A.G. & Blakely, E.J. 2007. Checklist for healthy and sustainable communities. *NSW Public Health Bulletin* 18, 51–4.

Capon, A.G. & Dixon, J. 2007. Creating healthy, just and eco-sensitive cities. *NSW Public Health Bulletin* 18, 37–40.

Close, G., Capon, A.G. & Wolfenden, K. 1993. What's new in injury surveillance. *NSW Public Health Bulletin* 4, 63–4.

Dixon, J. & Capon, A.G. 2007. Healthy, just and eco-sensitive cities: moving forward. *NSW Public Health Bulletin* 18, 209–12.

Frumkin, H. 2002. Urban sprawl and public health. *Public Health Reports* 171, 201–17.

Gehl, J. 2010. *Cities for People*. Island Press, Washington, DC, USA.

Haines, A., McMichael, A.J., Smith, K.R., Roberts, I., Woodcock, J., Markandya, A., et al. 2009. Public health effects of strategies to reduce greenhouse-gas emissions: overview and implications for policy makers. *The Lancet* 374, 2104–14.

Jalaludin, B.B., Chey, T., O'Toole, B.I., Smith, W.T., Capon, A.G. & Leeder, S.R. 2000. Acute effects of low levels of ambient ozone on peak expiratory flow rate in a cohort of Australian children. *International Journal of Epidemiology* 29, 549–57.

McMichael, A.J. 1993. *Planetary Overload. Global Environmental Change and the Health of the Human Species*. Cambridge University Press, Cambridge, UK.

McMichael, A.J. 1999. Prisoners of the proximate. Loosening the constraints on epidemiology in an age of change. *American Journal of Epidemiology* 149, 887–97.

McMichael, A.J. 2000. The urban environment and health in a world of increasing globalization: issues for developing countries. *Bulletin of the World Health Organisation* 78, 1117–26

McMichael, A.J. 2013. Population health in the Anthropocene: gains, losses and emerging trends. *The Anthropocene Review*, 1, 44–56.

McMichael, A.J., Woodruff, R.E. & Hales, S. 2006. Climate change and human health: present and future risks. *The Lancet* 367, 859–69.

NCD Alliance, The. 2013. *Healthy Planet, Healthy People: The NCD Alliance Vision for Health in the Post-2015 Development Agenda*. The NCD Alliance. ncdalliance.org/visionfor2015, accessed 20 March 2015.

Newman, P. & Kenworthy, J. 1999. *Sustainability and Cities: Overcoming Automobile Dependence*. Island Press, Washington, DC, USA.

Proust, K., Newell, B., Brown, H., Capon, A.G., Browne, C., Burton, A., et al. 2012. Human health and climate change: leverage points for adaptation in urban environments. *International Journal of Environmental Research and Public Health* 9, 2134–58.

Shetty, P. 2006. Tony McMichael: a visionary of the environment-health interface. *The Lancet* 368, 21.

United Nations Department of Economic and Social Affairs Population Division 2012. World urbanization prospects: the 2003 revision. United Nations, New York, USA. Available at: www.un.org/esa/population/publications/wup2003/WUP2003Report.pdf, accessed 31 March 2015.

Webb, K.L., Pelletier, D., Maretzki, A.N. & Wilkins, J. 1998. Local food policy coalitions: evaluation issues as seen by academics, project organizers, and funders. *Agriculture and Human Values* 15, 65–75.

WHO & UN-HABITAT 2005. *Hidden Cities: Unmasking and Overcoming Health Inequities in Urban Settings*. The WHO Centre for Health Development, Kobe, Japan.

Yach, D., Leeder, S.R., Bell, J. & Kistnasamy, B. 2005. Global chronic diseases. *Science* 305, 317.

37

TRANSFORMING HUMAN SOCIETY FROM ANTHROPOCENTRISM TO ECOCENTRISM

Can We Make It Happen in Time?

BOB DOUGLAS

Abstract

The publication of Tony McMichael's *Planetary Overload* in 1993 crystallised the emerging nature of the human predicament and the urgent need for a shift in the behaviour of our species. McMichael wrote, 'It is just now becoming conceivable that within several generations the human species may face threats to its survival because of its disruption of Earth's life supporting ecosystems.' Since then, human actions have resulted in the crossing of a number of critical system boundaries on which continuing human life on the planet depends. The survival of our species now demands transformative change in the way we relate to and care for the ecosystems on which survival and well-being depend. Global understanding of these matters has improved, while planetary overload has steadily worsened. We are going backwards, heading into eco-catastrophe, and we have succumbed to the psychological defence of denial. A change in the human mindset and in governance of the human economy will be needed to rescue us. We must now invest renewed efforts into the education of our young on the issue of ecocentrism and sustainability.

Introduction

Through more than 30 years of close professional association, Tony McMichael inspired a generation of epidemiologists and environmentalists. I argue in this paper that through his work, and others of his extraordinary ilk, we now know enough about what is threatening human futures to embark on a social engineering effort to change the human mindset in close collaboration with the up and coming generation, and especially schoolchildren.

In 1968, the ecologist Paul Ehrlich[1] published *The Population Bomb* (Ehrlich, 1968), in which he expressed grave doubts about the world's ability to feed itself in view of the massive growth in the human population that was under way. It was Ehrlich and Holdren (1971) who popularised the I = PAT equation, which proposed that the impact (I) of a population on the world's environment was a function of population size (P), its affluence (A) and its technological sophistication (T).

Then, in 1972, The Club of Rome published *The Limits to Growth* (Meadows et al., 1972), which suggested that continued human population growth and resource use could lead to the collapse of human civilisation during the 21st century. Like Tony McMichael, I was appalled at the conclusions of both Paul Ehrlich and The Club of Rome when I read them in the early 1970s. But, unlike Tony, I failed at the time to understand the environmental nature of the evolving crisis. I do claim credit, however, for recruiting Tony to the Foundation Chair of Occupational and Environmental Health at the University of Adelaide, and it was from that position that he published his seminal work, *Planetary Overload* (McMichael, 1993).

He said there: 'Our burgeoning numbers, technology and consumption are overloading Earth's capacity to absorb, replenish and repair. These global environmental problems pose health risks, not just from localised pollution but from damaged life-support systems … We cannot live apart from nature, remote from a great web of life … The risk arises from the disruption of natural systems because we are exceeding the biosphere's carrying capacity – that is, we are overloading the planet's metabolic capacity.'

Planetary Overload makes it clear that humans cannot live apart from an intact natural web of life. Since its publication, McMichael also drove home the point, and mobilised the evidence, that climate change was a huge threat to human health and well-being (McMichael et al., 1996). This is a message thoroughly crafted for the ears of his anthropocentric hearers. For we live in an age of blatant anthropocentricism. Humans generally believe that we are at the apex of the evolutionary pyramid and that Earth has been created for us to exploit. But, as Tony pointed out in the introduction to *Planetary Overload*, 'Humans are newcomers to our planet with no special immunity against the usual fate of biological species on Earth; namely extinctions.'

1 Ehrlich later regretted that his wife, Anne, was not listed as co-author.

Boundaries of Sustainability

In 2009, a group of senior Earth system and environmental scientists proposed a framework of planetary boundaries that were selected to define a safe operating space for humanity. The group asserted that, once human activity had passed certain thresholds or tipping points, which they called planetary boundaries, there was a risk of irreversible and abrupt planetary change. They pointed to nine Earth system processes which had boundaries that they considered to mark the safe zone for the planet. They argued that, because of human activities, three of these dangerous boundaries, especially climate change, biodiversity loss and biogeochemical flows, might have already been crossed, while others were in imminent danger of being crossed (Rockström et al., 2009). This work was updated in 2015 (Steffen et al., 2015).

Anthropocentrism is the Problem

I suggest that our anthropocentric mindset is the central problem, which we must address urgently. To do so will require a revolution in global thinking. We need somehow to build into the new mindset an understanding and response to the verities, which Tony spelled out in his book and which can be summarised by the term 'ecocentrism'. Humanity is currently hurtling down the anthropocentric highway towards a brick wall of total impossibility. Already, the signs that we are moving beyond the constraints imposed by physics, chemistry and biology are screaming at us on the billboards on the sides of the highway, but we ignore them. We are approaching a fork in the road, with a little sign that points down a bumpy track labelled 'ecocentric survival', but much of the traffic is travelling too fast to even notice the sign or the fork in the road.

We need to engineer a transition from the current, nearly universal human mindset, which sees humans as the superior species in total control of our planet, to a new operating paradigm where we recognise our utter dependence on healthy ecosystems and make their nurture central to our culture. Ecocentrism places welfare at the heart of the human social, psychological and economic enterprise. It understands the world as a collaborating system of networks, ecologies and relationships. It recognises that human systems are a subset of nature's systems and will survive only if they survive. A communal mindset shift of this kind will have profound consequences and will lead to changes in the way we live, govern ourselves and structure the global economy.

Mindset Shifts

I am talking here of a very large social engineering project. We must recognise that this shift in the communal mindset will need to have a number of dimensions – cognitive, ethical and spiritual – and it must also be practical in its operation and applications. Mindset change of this kind is unlikely to follow from promotion of fear and doom saying. It is more likely if people see in the new vision of an ecocentric future, the promise of a better and more fulfilling life. And, it is more likely where there is grass-roots involvement and people have a sense of empowerment about the changes that they will help to bring about. Mindset change will not come from a pulpit or a classroom teacher, but from one-on-one engagement among people of all ages who respect each other.

Malcolm Gladwell (2000) has drawn attention to the fact that shifts in the communal mindset and behaviour can occur quite rapidly when less than 20 per cent of the population decides, for whatever reason, to make the shift. Communal mindset changes occur frequently, and sometimes quite quickly. Cataclysmic events, like the attack on Pearl Harbour and the Great Depression (Gilding, 2011), can rapidly induce a shift in communal thinking. The Arab Spring is a recent example of a profound communal shift in mindset and action that followed the suicide by immolation of a street vendor in Tunisia (Anon., 2012).

Of course, we cannot predict the nature, timing or magnitude of unpleasant and cataclysmic events that could help to precipitate the shift. But, it is now very likely that such events will not be too far in the future. What we can do now is prepare the ground in modern society with new narratives about the benefits of a different mindset.

The Transform Australia Manifesto[2] outlines a vision for Australia where the well-being of both humans and the health of the planet are synonymous; where we accept that nature is our provider and we are its stewards; where we acknowledge that our economy, ecology and ecosystems are interdependent; and where a sustainable future for our descendants is therefore possible. Transform Australia is not a coherent organisation but a network of individuals who have come together in various conferences and small groups in the past three years to discuss the conditions needed for a viable future.

2 On Facebook see: www.facebook.com/pages/Transform-Australia/192700014096588, accessed 10 April 2015.

Collaboration, Partnering and Compassion

An essential feature of a new ecocentric mindset will be a new emphasis on collaboration and partnering and a de-emphasis on competition as a driver of our culture. The Transform Australia group has drawn heavily on the writings of Riane Eisler, whose book, *The Real Wealth of Nations* (Eisler, 2007), points to many examples in history, economics, sociology and biology that demonstrate the social, psychological and economic benefits of collaboration, both among humans and between humans and the planet. Our current economic model is driven by competition and barely values partnership, sharing and collaboration. It also fails utterly to value properly our environmental assets. Eisler identifies convincing Scandinavian and corporate examples where human well-being and economics have prospered as a result of economically valuing partnerism and collaboration. She and David Korten (Korten, 2010) have also drawn attention to the evidence from neurobiology of the stimulation of brain pleasure centres by collaborative and altruistic behaviour.

Another development relevant to this desirable mindset shift is an International Charter for Compassion (Armstrong, 2011), which has come together under the leadership of Karen Armstrong, a leading theological writer, who, in 2008, brought together representatives from Christianity, Buddhism, Hinduism, Confucianism, Judaism and Islam. The charter builds on the fact that the golden rule – doing to others what you would like them to do to you – is a common thread across these six great religions. The charter argues that humans urgently need to make compassion a clear, luminous and dynamic force in our polarised human world, and that it should be rooted in a principled determination to transcend selfishness. Compassion, it says, can break down political, dogmatic, ideological and religious boundaries. It will be born out of our interdependence and will be an enriching component of human relationships in a more fulfilled humanity. The charter concludes that compassion is indispensable to the creation of a just economy and peaceful global community. It complements Riane Eisler's view of partnerism and should be included in the essential re-engineering of human economics and governance.

The Economy

Tony McMichael had a great deal to say about economics in *Planetary Overload*. Much of what he said there continues to be true today. Ecological economics has evolved somewhat in the 21 years since his book appeared, but it is still far from mainstream. Our Australian economy, depending for its health on consumption-led growth in the gross domestic product (GDP), is insanely unfit for purpose.

Nobody doubts the benefits that have flowed to global society from economic growth in the past, but consumption-driven economic growth is no longer a viable option for countries like ours (Quaker Institute for the Future, 2012). Nor can we continue to ignore the obscene inequity between and within human populations, which is increasing under the operation of the current economic model (Wilkinson and Pickett, 2009). Designing a new steady state economy that values our ecosystems, shares wealth more equitably and promotes partnerism and compassion at the expense of competition and domination is theoretically feasible. But, implementing such a change will require new approaches to human governance that respect the relationship between human communities and their ecosystems, strengthen the nature of community and operate on newly enunciated democratic principles of subsidiarity. None of this will occur while anthropocentricism dominates our individual thinking and our collective mindset.

Governance

In *Planetary Overload*, on page 335, Tony wrote, 'The embryonic conventions emerging from the 1992 Earth Summit may yet foreshadow a new global environmental consciousness. Without such an international commitment it is hard to see how we humans, living in an increasingly overloaded world can make the necessary transition in awareness, values and collective rational action.' Quite so! Rio+20 (Rio plus 20 conference, 2012) demonstrated convincingly that this hope is as yet completely unrealised. We are still behaving as though individual human and national interests are all that count. The penny has not yet dropped that human survival depends on the health of the planet and that, until we bring our formidable intellects to this challenge, we will be wasting precious time on trivia. In the 2012 Australian Capital Territory (ACT) election, there was clear division between contending parties about their attitudes to the environment, but so anthropocentric is our collective mindset that neither side dared to draw attention to the obvious difference. Three of four Greens lost their seats, although it had been their initiative that had placed the ACT in a remarkably strong position with respect to carbon emissions targets. Similarly, Greens are being marginalised nationally, and the recent US presidential election stayed well away from issues like climate change. It is not yet clear what form future ecocentric governance will take. But, it is definitely clear that Australian democracy in its present form will not do the job. It is too susceptible to the interests of those who fund political campaigns and to the influence of advertising and the media. In these circumstances, public and environmental good takes second place to those of special interests.

A New Human Narrative

In the closing paragraph of *Planetary Overload*, Tony wrote as follows. 'Human history can be viewed as a succession of cultural and technological developments, enabling us to sidestep the natural ecological constraints on basic human biology.' And, finally, he wrote, 'we now depend on that same cultural ingenuity to find – soon – a path towards an ecologically sustainable, health supporting way of life.'

The vision for a new approach needs to be underpinned by a new cultural narrative that spells out the attractiveness of an ecocentric lifestyle. Developing the impetus for the new narrative requires fresh minds and new talents that will take us beyond a tired, self-centered, consumptive approach and will help us to rediscover the vitality of being an integral part of an evolving universe.

Empowering Youth

A transformation in mindset will not come about from the top down. But, I think it could follow from a determined empowerment of young people. They are less invested in and constrained than older generations by the operation of the current system and can build a new vision of a future for humanity that is both fulfilling and exciting, one to which they can actively contribute.

In Canberra, SEE-Change (www.see-change.org.au), a grass-roots, non-governmental organisation, worked with the ACT Education Department and Catholic and Independent schools and colleges on a project aimed at engaging all of the 67,000 ACT school and college students on what we have described as '2020 Vision' (www.see-change.org.au/?q=node/369). New national curriculum guidelines now obligate schools across the nation to introduce a sustainability theme across subjects for all age groups. Canberra's Centenary year was celebrated in 2013. We invited schools to use this occasion to look forward rather than backward. Curriculum materials have been developed to focus on how Canberra could change in the lead-up to 2020, when our legislators are committed to achieve a 40 per cent reduction in carbon emissions, relative to 1990 levels, and an energy system that is 90 per cent based on renewable sources. We worked with educators and other community groups towards a Youth Parliament on Sustainability, held in November 2013, when elected representatives from 26 schools and colleges and from grades 4 to 12, met to debate recommendations from green papers prepared by senior students about Canberra in 2020. They agreed on 24 recommendations and elected a Cabinet that will now meet with the Planning Committee of the ACT Legislative Assembly to discuss their views.

The Parliamentary White Paper that the Youth Parliament endorsed came about as a result of children across the education system, during 2013, considering the issues that now confront Canberra and our human world and applying their talents to planning for the world that they will inherit.

Can It All Happen in Time?

The concerns raised by McMichael in *Planetary Overload* were prophetic and are rapidly coming to pass. At a Canberra conference held recently, entitled 'The Future of Homo Sapiens' (Adams, 2012), Phillip Adams, in his keynote address, quoted the cellist Pablo Cassals, 'The situation is hopeless, we must take the next step.' I do not share the deep pessimism of many of the speakers at that symposium. Rather, I agree with Paul Gilding (2011) that 'humans are slow but not stupid', but that it will probably take a major disruption, which could come from a variety of sources, to move us towards the radical ecocentrism that will be required to avoid early extinction. In the meantime, I am heartened by evidence I see among young people's networks of their determination to find a better way forward. We need urgently to enable their building of the narrative that will shift the human mindset towards ecocentrism.

References

Adams, P. 2012. The Future of Homo Sapiens. Available at: manningclark.org.au/sites/default/files/mch_abstract_book-1.pdf, accessed 16 April 2014.

Anon. 2012. Street vendor Mohamed Bouazizi sets himself on fire – catalyst for Tunisian revolution/Arab Spring. Available at: slicethelife.com/2012/12/17/street-vendor-mohamed-bouazizi-sets-himself-on-fire-catalyst-for-tunisian-revolution-arab-spring, accessed 13 February 2014.

Armstrong, K. 2011. *Twelve Steps to a Compassionate Life*. Random House, New York, USA.

Ehrlich, P.R. 1968. *The Population Bomb*. Sierra Club, San Francisco, California, USA.

Ehrlich, P.R. & Holdren, J.P. 1971. Impact of population growth. *Science* 171, 1212–7.

Eisler, R. 2007. *The Real Wealth of Nations: Creating a Caring Economics*. Berrett-Koehler Publishers, San Francisco, California, USA.

Gilding, P. 2011. *The Great Disruption: Why the Climate Crisis Will Bring on the End of Shopping and the Birth of a New World*. Bloomsbury Press, London, UK.

Gladwell, M. 2000. *The Tipping Point: How Little Things Can Make a Big Difference*. Bloomsbury, London, UK.

Korten, D. 2010. *Agenda for a New Economy; From Phantom Wealth to Real Wealth*. Berrett-Koehler Publishers, San Francisco, California, USA.

McMichael, A.J. 1993. *Planetary Overload. Global Environmental Change and the Health of the Human Species*. Cambridge University Press, Cambridge, UK.

McMichael, A.J., Haines, A., Slooff, R. & Kovats, S. (eds) 1996. *Climate Change and Human Health*. World Health Organization, Geneva, Switzerland.

Meadows, D., Meadows, D., Randers., J. & Behrens, W. III. 1972. *The Limits to Growth*. Universe Books, New York, USA.

Quaker Institute for the Future 2012. Beyond the Growth Dilemma; Toward an Ecologically Integrated Economy. Available at: www.quakerinstitute.org/wp-content/uploads/2012/10/BGD-web.pdf, accessed 16 April 2014.

Rio plus 20 conference. 2012. Available at: www.uncsd2012.org/content/documents/814UNCSD%20REPORT%20final%20revs.pdf, accessed 16 April 2014.

Rockström, J., Steffen, W., Noone, K., Persson, Å., Chapin, F.S., Lambin, E.F., et al. 2009. A safe operating space for humanity. *Nature* 461, 472–5.

Steffen, W., Richardson, K., Rockström, J., Cornell, S.E., Fetzer, I., Bennett, E.M., et al 2015. Planetary boundaries: Guiding human development on a changing planet. *Science* 347, 736.

Wilkinson, R.G. & Pickett, K. 2009. *The Spirit Level: Why More Equal Societies Almost Always Do Better*. Penguin, London, UK.

38

ECOLOGICAL PUBLIC HEALTH

Leaders, Movements and Ideas to Shift the Boundaries Between the Normal and the Desirable

GEOF RAYNER AND TIM LANG

Abstract

Tony McMichael's 1999 essay, 'Prisoners of the Proximate: Loosening the Constraints on Epidemiology in an Age of Change', published by the *American Journal of Epidemiology*, is the authors' starting place for understanding current thinking and challenges in public health. Rayner and Lang argue that McMichael's essay presents the case for ecological reasoning to be applied in epidemiology. In so doing, it opens the door for an appreciation of complexity as a developing theme in the sciences and arts and for the interdisciplinary enhancement of public health thinking, several lines of which are considered. The chapter then outlines the main traditions and models of public health among which a newer approach, ecological public health, sits. The authors explore the conventional models of public health and why they believe an ecological perspective on health has particular advantages. Their core argument is that human and ecosystems health is interdependent and that climate change, land, water, air, microbial activity, all show that, in the 21st century, just as humans can no longer live by disregarding the health of ecosystems, nor can they continue with the fantasy, expressed through neoliberal thought, that individual desires, behaviours, consumption and ultimately patterns of health can be disconnected from the health of everyone and everything else. The cause of public health, they conclude, requires not only movements but also leaders.

Introduction

> Knowing is not enough; we must apply. Willing is not enough; we must do. (Johann Wolfgang von Goethe)[1]

In his essay, 'Prisoners of the Proximate', Tony McMichael gives an overview of the history and changing shape of epidemiology, concluding with an appeal for modern epidemiology to embrace an ecological public health conception (McMichael, 1999). We agree with that analysis and have argued the case from different starting points elsewhere (Rayner and Lang, 2012). In this chapter, we explore a key feature of ecological public health thinking – the centrality given to addressing complexity. The argument is that ecological thinking helps public health by accepting the normality of complex interactions while also explaining the necessity of multiple rather than single interventions or actions. Ecological thinking ought to be normal within public health, but it is not. To understand why not partly requires an historical look at the public health project. Other models of public health appeared to provide the answer, offering quicker fixes, narrower foci. In that sense, ecological public health does not make life easier for proponents!

The present chapter sets out to put the return of interest in complexity into historical context, arguing that it is the modern manifestation of a long-established approach to knowledge. This chapter then outlines the other main traditions and models of public health among which ecological public health sits. These emerged in the 19th and 20th centuries, as ill health became a dire result of industrialisation. We explore the advantages the models offer and why we believe an ecological perspective on health has particular advantages, yet why it makes public intervention apparently harder. Our core argument is that today ecological thinking becomes central, simply because the interconnection of human and ecosystems health is now self-evident. Climate change, land, water, air, microbial activity, all show that humans cannot live in an ecosystems-free bubble, even if they think they can. And yet the 20th century nurtured a fantasy that human health could somehow be disconnected. This is both poor science and poor politics and policy. It translates and corrals public health into a fantastic pursuit of private or personalised health.

---

1 www.iep.utm.edu/goethe, accessed 10 April 2015.

Complexity

Could anyone dispute that we live in an age of complexity? The notion is not, however, new. In the 16th century, William Shakespeare held his largely illiterate audience spellbound by his dramatic interweaving of historical narrative and psychology. Among the many claims for the sophistication of Shakespeare's literary work, it has been argued that his last great play, *The Tempest*, anticipated Darwinian evolutionary ideas (Love, 2010). Two centuries later, Johann Wolfgang von Goethe, remembered more today as a playwright than as a biologist (and a passionate advocate of Shakespeare), presented an evolutionary view of natural biology, arguing that art, poetry and science were interlinked and complementary. While his biological formulations differed considerably from Darwin, his admirer, the anatomist, Hermann von Helmholtz, claimed that Goethe's biological writings led to an accelerated acceptance of Darwinian science (Richards, 2006). Goethe's near contemporary, the French biologist, Jean-Baptiste Lamarck, a decorated soldier, may himself have lacked his counterpart's artistic pretensions (although he worked with botanic artists), but his influence was equally, or perhaps more, profound. He proposed that all organisms evolved from simple to complex forms due to their ability to pass on acquired changes to their offspring. Lamarck not only brought the word 'biology' into formal use, but set the dimensions of European evolutionary thought in the early 1800s (Corsi, 2005).

Nevertheless, it was only through the English naturalist, Charles Darwin (or more correctly, through Darwinism, since this attribution includes the co-discoverer of natural selection, Alfred Russel Wallace), that due scientific rigour was applied to the problem of how species changed and differentiated. Darwin revered Goethe and learned much from Lamarck, but the conceptual threads of his reasoning drew from a far broader intellectual cloth (Herbert, 2005). For Darwin, as for Goethe, nature was a thing of wonder. His concluding metaphor in *On the Origin of the Species* was a poetic description of an 'entangled bank' of nature where numerous organisms interacted 'in so complex a manner' (Darwin, 1859).

In contrast, the modern beginnings of the story of public health did not start with biology, even less, evolutionary biology, and although biomedical understandings of health and disease played a role, and were later to play the starring role, other perspectives and frameworks of action initially mattered more. The figure of Edwin Chadwick, journalist, researcher, lawyer, civil servant, close observer of Paris's revolutionary health scene, and philosopher's apprentice (to Jeremy Bentham), despite more recent criticisms (Hamlin, 1998), sets the scene for a quintessentially modern view of public health. Chadwick saw public health as a task of administration and environmental change more than of ministration to bodies, and further proposed that, technically, improvement was more an issue of improved sanitary engineering than of medical knowledge.

This is not to say that advances in biology and biomedical thinking at the population level played no part. Edward Jenner, the countryside General Practitioner, certainly exemplified that by modernising the ancient practice of immunisation. John Snow, too, is today celebrated as the founder of epidemiology (and voted by the readers of a medical magazine in 2003 as the 'greatest doctor' of all time). But their impact can be considerably overplayed. The worth of vaccination was hotly disputed until early in the 20th century (Williamson, 2007). And Snow's celebrity reputation was only established decades after his death (Vandenbroucke et al., 1991).

One reason why Thomas McKeown's critique of the role of medicine in improving public health has continued to scandalise supporters of the medical model of public health is not just because he considered biomedical interventions to have a more limited impact (until the 20th century) than claimed, but because he thought that the primary factors for improving population health lay only at the boundaries of formal public health action, and because he advocated the view that economic advancement and nutrition were key to public health improvement, a fundamentally Malthusian argument (McKeown, 1971). Such views later opened him to the charge that he paved the way for policy groups who argued that economic growth was the primary (not just a significant) pathway to improved public health (Szreter, 1988, 2002). On the contrary, we see such techno-economic perspectives in public health as only one specific mode of advance.

In fact, few celebrated figures in the history of ecological thought, apart from Wallace, had much or anything to say about human health, despite the pressing health circumstances they doubtless would have observed. Wallace, while wholly on the side of 'sanitary science', was highly critical of public health interventions of his day, like Jenner's vaccination (Weber, 2007). Their presence in this chapter's celebration of ecological public health is not specious. These thinkers and writers provide scientific and imaginative underpinnings for what must surely be a mainstream approach to public health today. Our argument here is that public health thinking does not need to be embarrassed by this rich intellectual history. On the contrary, it offers the perfect and broad canvass of ideas from which to critique the fetishisation of evidence-based interventions or a reductionist biomedicine. Public health thinking is, and always must be, a ferment of ideas, not just evidence. Furthermore, even a brief discussion of the origins of modern biology and ecological thought allows us, in a very different era, to understand that neither the consideration of complexity nor ecology is especially new, that art, science and creativity might, indeed must, coexist, and that, as Goethe exemplified, a more participatory comprehension of nature must substitute for one based on technological dominance and subservience. As bacteria teach us, they might initially be vanquished, only to defeat our powerful drugs later.

Ecology Addresses Complexity

Darwin may be associated with creating the foundations of modern ecology but he nowhere used the word, his own term of choice was 'the economy of nature', a term with roots in Linnaeus's botany and used by political economists and others of his day. By the turn of the 20th century, the new term had come to substitute. Coined by Darwin's German follower, Ernst Haeckel, its broadening acceptability may be due, in part, to the loss of focus on nature among economists and towards consumer notions of utility and desire (Schabas, 2005). Consumerism and the 'dismal science' of economics have systematically marginalised nature, other than as resources to be mined (often literally). Haeckel may be a mostly forgotten (even vilified) figure today – with detractors and defenders (Richards, 2007) – but his specification of ecology as an integrative science of species and environments remains relevant, even if the use of the term is confused by its association with the consumer products industry.

Complexity, for Darwin, is what occurs when species interrelate in their environmental setting, and he uses the term constantly. No 'balance of nature' was implied – as is the appeal today of much nature conservancy in a tradition of thought extending back to the ancient Greeks (Kricher, 2009) – but rather an unending process of dynamic interplay. A Darwinian understanding underlies all modern biology, and much of what is also called ecological thought, but it was another half-century after his death before the principles of natural selection were synthesised with the newly discovered science of genetics (after the rediscovery of Mendel's ideas in 1900) and the model – if not the detail – became complete. Complexity, unlike ecology, is no neologism. It draws from the Latin *complexus*, meaning to entwine, encircle or to be 'twisted together'.

Despite its extensive use by Darwin, its entry into scientific vocabulary is actually recent. Philosopher of science, Nicholas Rescher, notes that the term is absent from standard philosophical dictionaries and encyclopaedias, and even absent from most systems of metaphysical thought (Leibnitz, C. S. Peirce and A. N. Whitehead are seen as the 'honourable exceptions'; Rescher, 1998). Among complexity theorists, it is, of course, central, although in substance shifts according to topic or disciplinary field. Nevertheless, there are unifying properties. Complexity, says information scientist, John Holland, is 'emergent', always in a state of coming into being (Holland, 1998). It has been seen as the 'start position' from which evolution began (Lauterbur, 2005). Even if the fundamental laws governing the universe turn out to be simple (or rather, uncomplex), argues Nobel-winning physicist, Murray Gell-Mann, given that chance and indeterminacy exist (as introduced by quantum mechanics), complexity is always expansive (Gell-Mann, 1995).

For members of the multidisciplinary Santa Fe Institute (Gell-Mann, Holland and colleagues), complexity theory has offered a unifying systems-based perspective extending across life and non-life. It is constrained by start positions, dynamic relationships between parts, conditions of scale and systemic feedback. It forms a complement and corrective to the reductionist perspective that studies parts in isolation. In this picture, complexity is both an assessment about the changing fabric of reality (emergent, hyperbolic, etc), as well as a perspective on that reality. The principle of complexity offers a new conceptual basis not just for biology, physics and chemistry, but has implications that extend across all disciplines and areas of life, including health, public policy, cultural theory and more (Philippe and Mansi, 1998; Taylor, 2001; Tsoukas and Hatch, 2001; Geyer, 2003; Mitleton-Kelly, 2003; Pearce and Merletti, 2006; Rickles et al., 2007; Sandro et al., 2009; Geyer and Rihani, 2010).

Complexity may seem central to ecological thought, but the word 'ecology', since Haeckel invented it, has come to span dozens of specialist fields and overlapping and even antagonistic assumptions and methodologies. In considering natural ecology, for example, species interactions underlying complexity can be both antagonistic, involving predation, herbivory and parasitic, or mutualistic, such as involving the pollination of flowers by insects (Montoya et al., 2006). Some biologists stress the calculable properties of interrelationships, where, for example, the 'level' of complexity is presented as the number of entities and interconnections in a given system, as well as the effect of the entities on the system. In this manner, Edward O. Wilson has described complexity as 'the search for algorithms used in nature' (Wilson, 1998, p. 95). At this point, it might be useful to remember Goethe's complaint about mathematicians that they declared 'everything as worthless, inexact, and insufficient which cannot be submitted under their calculation' (Simms, 2005). The big question of how far the rules of biological complexity applied to human behaviour intrigued Darwin. Certainly since Darwin himself, there have been both influential thinkers and movements that have offered a more direct equation. There has also been an equally forceful movement claiming that while humans undoubtedly have biological roots, they now have autonomy from those roots.

Beginning with the Darwin-influenced philosopher, Charles S. Peirce (as mentioned by Rescher, above), it has been suggested that while all organisms require some minimal level of signalling of their presence to other organisms, human communication operates through far higher-level principles. Recent evolutionary anthropology has suggested that human cooperative and reflective modes of behaviour were first established through group foraging, with positive feedback loops between organic reconstruction, cognitive development and behavioural modernisation, the result being a continuous development of the human learning niche and the building of cultural inheritance (Sterelny, 2012). Society today operates far beyond the level of the group. The technologies, social processes and institutions that make up the world can only be conceived in their full extent through abstractions, constructs and models; systems that operate beyond the capacities of any single individual to understand. Human society has therefore become complex, not simply due to biological evolution or its extensions into culture (like the notion of memes), the laws of physics or, in some recent economic formulations, the evolution of the economic market, but because human society – through its art – makes it so (Dissanayake, 2009). More than through science perhaps, it is the richness and creativity of art and culture, as presented by Shakespeare or by Goethe, which is perhaps the most visible and engaging aspect of human complexity.

This, too, is an ecological perspective, but one that draws on an extension of the principle of Darwinian complexity into the cultural realm, as found, for example, in philosopher John Dewey's opposition to the Cartesian dualism found in much contemporary Western philosophical thought (Popp, 2007). Dewey once remarked: '[w]e have no word by which to name mind-body in a unified wholeness of operation' (Dewey et al., 2008, p. 27). Following Dewey, the modern task is not just to free analysis from biological reductionism, but its economic, psychological or sociological counterparts as well. Engaging with human complexity entails the recognition that human existence is constructed through multiple levels and interactions: material, biological, social and cultural. Thus, while culture grants people meaning and values, a fact that may account for humankind's recent and rapid evolutionary progress, compared to other species, at the same time, people are biological agents and recipients existing in a permeable relationship with others. It is because human society operates through multiple planes of complexity that even the most apparently private matters of health at all times reveal a parallel public health counterpart.

The systemic and complexity-based view of ecology first presented by Darwin and Wallace was later complemented by the concept of the ecosystem, introduced by Arthur Tansley early in the 20th century (Tansley, 1935). This concept reconfirmed that systemic thinking was essential, and that while ecosystems existed in variations of scale and density, no ecosystem could be understood in linear or reductionist terms alone. More recently, it has been proposed that quite minor, apparently confined perturbations in ecosystems and subsystems might lead to dramatic regime shifts, a feature that undermines classical approaches in mathematical ecology (Norberg and Cumming, 2008).

Ecological and complexity-based thought in the mid-20th century expanded through an heterogeneous mix of disciplines and thinkers. The British-American economist, Kenneth Boulding, presented the case for an integrated systems-based perspective reaching across the sciences, necessary, he thought, because of a trend towards the disintegration of scientific communication. Although thinking 'a general theory of practically everything' implausible, he presented the case for interdisciplinary systems theory. In effect, this was a multilayered conception of complexity expressed through a hierarchy of eight frameworks conveying varying principles, ranging from the clockworks of physics and astronomy, the control mechanism of cybernetics, the self-maintaining structure of cells and on to purposive behaviour and self-awareness of social animals (Boulding, 1956). His lasting contribution was perhaps the revival of an older specification of the economy with the recognition of natural limits, now known as ecological economics.

René Dubos, the French-American biologist, discovered gramicidin in 1939, the world's first commercially produced antibiotic. If he is chiefly remembered today as an ecological theorist rather than scientist, it was his ecological perspective on biotechnology and nutrition futures – now proved essentially correct – that warranted his reputation. Dubos observed that if society was not cautious about the use of antibiotics, bacteria would evolve according to the Darwinian principles operative in the rest of nature to get round them. In similar terms, he warned of the shift in diets, with consequences for trends in chronic disease. All human development involved evolutionary dynamics, he argued, but the critical factor in shaping disease response was 'the environmental conditions that undisciplined technology creates' (Dubos, 1968, p. 219). In other words, the poor use of powerful medicines and the marketing of processed foods provided the new aberrant – while seen as normal – conditions for disease to flourish. If only his ecological warnings had been taken seriously. Today, the situation of antimicrobial resistance is alarming (Spellberg et al., 2008; WHO, 2011).

Jay Forrester, known today as a management theorist, developed his perspective from the study of electronics systems. He argued that common intuitive judgements about cause and effect relationships failed to acknowledge the existence of feedback, either in production systems or, for that matter, in urban environments. The tendency was to consider issues in linear terms. Although people looked for links between cause and effect, Forrester argued that causes might not be proximate in time and space to witness the full resultant effects. What Forrester called 'system dynamics' established an approach to complexity that encompassed counter-intuitive behaviour, growth limits, non-linearity, tipping points and feedback – the latter term drawn from his electronic experience. In the hands of Donella Meadows and colleagues, Forrester's systems dynamics formed the basis of The Club of Rome study in the 1970s, repeated some years later, which modelled environmental stress against population growth, in the style of a vastly expanded Malthusian logic (Meadows et al., 1972, 1993).

Outwardly, Forrester's enterprise appeared utterly technocratic, but in essence the conclusion of his research was that there was no purely technical solution to the challenge of creating a sustainable society. Of these three, only Dubos offered a centrally public health focus, but the thinking of all three converged around points of system complexity, developing mismatch, a critique of technological consumerism and the promotion of sustainable patterns of living. These themes remain critical for the public health project today.

Models of Public Health: Different Approaches

Much of modern ecological thought, although not all of it, as we have shown, flows back to the Darwinian intellectual struggle to understand the interrelationships of living forms and the dynamics of change. Darwin memorably offered the 'entangled bank' as a simile for the interplay of visible and invisible life forms that collectively manifested themselves as an English hedgerow and roadside bank. His focus was on flora and fauna, rather than societal or cultural levels of existence. In our book, *Ecological Public Health*, we have suggested that while ecological thinking offers brilliant hope for analysing complexity, it has tended to be segmented into competing areas of discourse: the natural world and the social world. Indeed, many people in the public health world think ecological thinking is synonymous with the social-ecological model, often associated with the psychologist, Urie Bronfenbrenner (Bronfenbrenner, 1979). This is regrettable, as good public health requires analysis and the infrastructure for both. Instead, we propose a heuristic for re-integrating those two levels of analysis (Rayner and Lang, 2012). Reality may be viewed through four coexisting dimensions: (i) the material or physical; (ii) the biological and physiological; (iii) the cognitive or cultural; and (iv) the social dynamics of human interaction. Viewing problems through this multidimensional lens helps describe complexity while providing structure and pointers for actions. It offers a way of applying ecological public health in the modern world.

There are four definable and conventional models with which this ecological public health model competes (Lang and Rayner, 2012; Rayner and Lang, 2012). These models are: the sanitary-environmental and biomedical models, the rising social-behavioural model and the less discussed techno-economic model.

Sanitary-environmental model

The sanitary-environmental model is what most originally thought public health action to be. It focuses on the health of populations in their physical circumstances. It might equally be called the classical model of public health, for some of the measures with which it is associated are ancient, such as the laying of water pipes, sanitary engineering and the like. The Romans were its original masters.

In the 19th century, the challenge was to clean and clear up urbanisation and industrialisation's dirt and detritus – seen as the determinants of epidemic disease – and to rid society of nuisances to eye, ear and nose. Its advocates were known as sanitarians or hygienists. Its professionals were public health inspectors, engineers, town planners, building standards regulators, even street designers. In the richer parts of the world, these measures are now taken for granted, being embedded in law and convention. Infrastructure is governed by tight rules and highly organised arrangements for managing human, biological and material flows and waste.

Looking outside those societies that first industrialised, a different picture emerges. While such environments represent the modern equivalent of early 19th-century European cities, they operate on a much larger scale. Here, the model should thrive, as in Europe before it, but the model relies on the institutionalisation of material processes of change and an enabling political system. It required not only apprehensiveness about the consequences of inaction but also imagination and foresight – the appreciation that sewage did not need to swill in the streets or that deaths due to infectious disease could, and indeed should, be averted. Critically, it also required ample reserves of economic and political capital, perhaps only feasible during times of economic growth or political democratisation.

Biomedical model

This model comes in two, sometimes ill-at-ease, versions, one with a population orientation, the other an individual orientation. Population-based biomedical interventions first came into prominence in the early 1800s with vaccination, and much later through the establishment of public health laboratories. In its modern form, promoted by the English physician, Edward Jenner (1749–1823), vaccination was claimed as more scientific, more effective and with fewer side effects. (It had been in use in China over centuries.) Vaccination was probably the first example of the internationalisation of a biomedical public health measure. Today, vaccination has a powerful track record. In 1980, the World Health Assembly announced the eradication of smallpox.

In contrast, a more personalised version of the biomedical model now shapes our understanding of how the living body works and fails to work. From the 1880s, medicine began to cast aside ineffective treatments. It was only after the close of that century that, with the increasing use of aseptic techniques, post-surgical survival rates began to climb. After World War II, progress has been exceptional, but comes with a warning, and at great cost. In the 1960s, social epidemiologists like Thomas McKeown provided controversial reminders that improving nutrition was a more salient factor for health than medicine.

The case example is the USA. In the 1950s, the USA spent 4.4 per cent of gross domestic product (GDP) on healthcare, a low figure because, as William Schwartz of the Brookings Institution says, in those days 'doctors really couldn't do much' (Schwartz, 1998). The USA subsequently invested massively on devices and technologies ranging from the iron lung to computerised imaging (Rothman, 1997). In 2009, 17.4 per cent of US GDP was spent on health care, double high-income country averages. By 2040, it could rise to 30 per cent (Fogel, 2008). Despite these immense costs, unaffordable for all but the richest countries, US health-care arrangements remain socially fractured by access and outcome inequalities – and attempts to reform this situation deeply contentious; it is also deeply inefficient overall, the USA ranking only 37th out of 191 in international performance rankings (OECD Health Data, 2011). Many treatments improved vastly over time, but no amount of spending could halt the mounting scale of US diabetes or obesity, a result of its 'society design' more than any other factor. A fresh equation has seemingly taken root, that medicine, to quote political scientist, Aaron Wildavsky, equals health (Wildavsky, 1976).

Social-behavioural model

This model seems new, but is not. Rulers have attempted to influence the behaviour of their people for health reasons for centuries. King James of England and Scotland published a diatribe against tobacco in 1604 (Stuart, 1604). The model is older yet, when religious precepts that explicitly or implicitly include health, such as towards washing, or choice or preparation of foods, are included. The social-behavioural model is now the main rival to the biomedical model. It addresses the behavioural circumstances of health. Thus, since the 1950s, smoking, food and nutrition, and physical activity, increasingly are seen as major factors in chronic disease prevention, clinical areas where the biomedical model struggles.

Here, public health is engaged with rules and guides to behaviour. Early 20th-century social science focused on the undirected modernisation of behavioural rules over matters like eating, defecating, nasal blowing, spitting, etc, via the analysis of social-psychological mechanisms like embarrassment and shame.

If the royal court once decided such rules, increasingly the state, commerce and civil society assumed this role, and in a more intentionally directive manner (hence, 'nanny statism').

In the 19th century, newly mass-manufactured products were marketed with health messages, catering to an increasingly segmented consumer marketplace, like products for women. Personal health habits were changed by messages such as the value of regular bathing of bodies, cleanliness of the home and about women's domestic responsibilities and work. These were salutary. Today, the marketing firepower of transnational corporations is massive. In work done for the World Health Organization, we have shown that Coca Cola can spend more annually on its marketing of soft drinks than the entire biannual budget of the World Health Organization (Lang et al., 2006).

Ranged against the power of commerce, what leverage do public health advocates possess? What methods do they use? Is it psychology, marketing – reborn as social marketing (with pitiful budgets)? Or is it law? The Canadian public health writer, Nancy Milio, expressed it well in the mid-1970s. It could only be a 'minimal aim', she said, to make healthy choices easier: the unhealthy choices must also be blocked. And for the most widespread impact, the focus should be on 'national-level policy-making' which would in turn change 'the range of options for the largest number of people' (Milio, 1976). Oddly, the recent analytic focus on behaviour reunites public health and economics (the latter as 'behavioural economics'), which begets the latest fad, 'nudge', with the hidden ideological charm being that the state should do something (warn people, edit choices), but not much (Thaler and Sunstein, 2008; Rayner and Lang, 2011).

Techno-economic model

The techno-economic model is central in the public health literature but undesignated as a type, and deeply controversial to some historians, who have seen it as an attack on public health measures. It depends on two concepts: economic growth and knowledge growth.

Economic growth leads to a higher standard of living, which then leads to better nutrition. This was a view promoted by the social epidemiologist, Thomas McKeown, and, following him, by the Nobel Prize winning economist, Robert Fogel (who has named his version 'technophysio evolution') (McKeown, 1976; Fogel, 2004). Both hark back to political economists, Adam Smith and Thomas Malthus, on the economy of nature (as noted, for which the term 'ecology' later substituted), the former who indexed human prosperity to its rate of population growth and the latter who linked patterns of disease to population growth and agricultural productivity. Society's breakout from the 'Malthusian trap' is based heavily on knowledge. The conversion of knowledge into raised agricultural productivity and energy-heavy living and work technologies reduces physical stress on bodies and creates opportunities for easier, potentially richer lives.

There is no automatic link between economic growth and health. This may be so up to a basic level and depending on other factors, such as effective institutions, limited corruption, the rule of law and reasonable levels of democracy. The case for a link between improving standard of living and patterns of health is historically strong, but in the 21st century, diminishing returns seem to have set in. The USA was once among the healthiest societies in the world but, with mounting social inequality, an inferior, poorly accessible health-care system and a thin social safety net, health trends are moving in the opposite direction (Komlos and Baur, 2004). A cornucopia of food or consumer goods – the basis of modern US culture and trend now spreading worldwide – hardly provides the automatic key to improving health and well-being.

Ecological Public Health

Our last model draws us back to our introductory themes of ecology and complexity. Ecology, as noted, is a term that denotes interrelations of species and of nature, but its meaning extends far beyond this, permeating across fields of enquiry and social movements. Early in the 20th century, the term 'ecology' was drawn into sociology, largely from botany, as a means of examining human behaviour and social forms in environmental contexts (Park and Burgess, 1925). It already was obvious in the century before that ecological thought did not have to be 'environmental', and that environmentalism was not the sole domain of ecologists, even if they were interested (and most, beginning with Darwin himself, were not). It was neither an environmentalist nor ecologist (noting that neither term then existed) but the economist, J. S. Mill, who first recommended a 'stationary state' economy to preserve the natural environment, and conversely it was the naturalist, Alfred Russel Wallace, who proposed that pollution and inequality were merely the opposite sides of unregulated capitalism. Their joint proposals for saving and democratising nature and human health involved the common ownership of land and cooperative production. Such influences might be seen as liberal or socialist in conception, but the revival of ecological thought in the current period also has taken its cue from Thomas Malthus, often seen solely as a reactionary figure in history. For example, in the mid-1960s, parasitologist, Leo Kartman, presented an ecological account of challenges to public health, drawing on Malthus's views on the natural limits to human development (Kartman, 1967). John Hanlon, US Assistant Surgeon General, drew on Kartman's and René Dubos's critique of technological change, thus marking the first advocacy of an ecological public health approach by an important public health official (Hanlon, 1969). Here was an ecological perspective in two dimensions: natural and human ecology, each with a feedback to the other, but it was also true that the historical line from Darwinian-inspired ecology to Hanlon's use of the term was anything other than straight.

Alongside an explicit formulation of public health as being desirably 'ecological', this was mirrored by the emergence of ecological thought within disease epidemiology. McMichael termed this process one of 'methodological consolidation', an intellectual journey which began in the 1600s with the description and classification of death and disease, was bolstered by sanitarian theory in the 19th century, permutated into theories of specific cause and then onwards to broader causal models, to arrive at (in developed countries) a new public health context of rapidly declining infectious diseases and proportionally increasing chronic disease, an outcome, in the context of other intellectual developments we have noted, that spurred 'a more ecologic view of how the social and environmental conditions of life influence population health' (McMichael, 1999).

The implication was that epidemiology had become social epidemiology, which had then become ecological epidemiology. McMichael brought together a new stress on the environment, an appreciation of complexity, and other novel conceptual extensions, such as a life-course perspective. If his view of the new was a reassertion of the old, what was also seemingly apparent was that the determinants of health were increasingly delocalised, that understanding health amelioration required understanding of feedback effects – perhaps the first demonstration of which was made by M'Gonigle and Kirby (M'Gonigle and Kirby, 1936) in the 1930s. He understood that behavioural and cultural factors in health, if long present, were taking on new forms, and that the signs of biological feedback, as Dubos warned in the 1960s, were beginning to present.

More than half a century on, and perhaps taking a cue from the magisterial Ottawa Charter (WHO, 1986), major bodies like the US Institute of Medicine support an ecological perspective on public health (Institute of Medicine (US) Committee on Health and Behavior: Research Practice and Policy, 2001; Institute of Medicine, 2002). The need to develop these ideas is urged on by hard evidence of major changes reshaping the conditions on which human health depends: rapid, massive population growth; climate change; resource scarcity and price volatility; soil, sea and freshwater damage; biodiversity loss. In the past, specifically environmental threats to human health were mostly localised, although infectious diseases rarely recognised borders. Today, that biological dynamic continues, witnessed by the ceaseless tendency for bacteria, as Dubos saw, to reduce the effectiveness of antibiotics. Another strand of change has a more material basis in the link between industry, energy use and toxicity, with a double impact, on the human species and on the rest of nature. A third strand is cultural and societal, shaped by changing mass behaviour and aspirations. In sum, although ecological public health has been articulated as a perspective, it has never been formulated systematically. Our argument is that this is precisely what is now needed to help reshape how societies live, to inform policy and to integrate the long-term into short-term political choices.

Why Do This?

Why not stick to the simpler, conventional public health models? The short answer is that they no longer capture what evidence demands of a policy framework – a mix of overview and capacity to inform detailed actions. So often, public health is caught in 'policy cacophony', confronting multiple explanations when the political system demands only one, preferably with immediate beneficial effects (Lang and Rayner, 2007). Modern ecological public health thinking is able to face complex and dynamic biological, material, social and cultural dimensions of the human, living and physical world. It works better than the other models considered, in a number of ways:

- It draws on these conventional models and plays to their strengths.
- It is the one model of the five that is fully integrative.
- Drawing on complexity science and system dynamics, modern ecological thinking introduces questions of non-linearity, variations in scale, evolutionary mismatch and biological feedback, and other emergent qualities of nature and human behaviour.
- Aiming to build knowledge for action, it eschews the narrow, backward-facing, 'evidence-based' perspective.
- It engages multi-actor engagement: action is required by all.
- It is explicitly interdisciplinary, rejecting tiered and unequal multidisciplinary 'compartmentalism'– the critique derived from philosopher, John Dewey.
- It is interdimensional, incorporating the material, biological, social and cultural dimensions of life.
- It promotes the role of social movements in shifting and integrating public perspectives on health and politics.

How Ecological Public Health Helps Grapple With Reality

Tony McMichael usefully described both the growing sophistication of epidemiology and the intransigence of proximal thinking. Of course, the opposition to effective public health measures, let alone ecological public health, goes much further. Why is the failure to advocate this ecological perspective on public health so important now? Because the world of policy is awash with huge problems, so big that political processes are in danger of seeming unable (or is it unprepared?) to address them. These issues include the obvious ones: non-communicable diseases, climate change, the fragility of ecosystem services (including biodiversity), but they also include feedback into animal, plant and human biology, of which antimicrobial resistance is merely one form. These are vast and complex issues, which invite either silence or symbolic action only from policymakers. They are right; to tackle them requires not only vast expenditure and effort but also, as Dubos asserted half a century ago, the rethinking of economics linked to a certain technological and consumerist path. Given the short-termism of politics, it is much easier to park such issues than deal with them. Another reason is that the economy has primacy, an explanation that not only explained the historical delay in addressing pollution but today explains why nutrition-based diseases, such as obesity or diabetes, are addressed primarily on the basis of behavioural dimensions and not outcomes of business strategy and supply chains.

What progressive Victorians got right, in an age when mass political action was gaining sophistication, was the power of social movements and attempts to modify state structures newly sensitive to them. Of course, one should not sentimentalise such times. While the sanitarians achieved much in many important arenas of the health 'battle', other problems such as energy and pollution, and above all social inequality, were barely touched. Many actions in the name of health were also perceived, and some intended as repressive and socially judgemental. The veneer of reform in the name of health could sometimes barely disguise social contempt.

Today, if everything is so complex, as we and others argue, how it is possible to intervene in causation? We wonder, in fact, if the challenge today is really more difficult than 100 years ago. The scale, perhaps. As societies become more complex, the mechanisms for changing them or for scaling-up areas where progressive change has been won need to evolve to match. That is why models and conceptions of public health need to be updated; they must be appropriate for the times. Today, in an era when the warning signs of ecological damage are now so clear and so strongly evidenced, it is essential that this case is represented strongly in, and injected into, public health policies. The simple and central message that must be spread into policymaking processes is that human health and ecosystems health must be seen from within one unifying framework (Hancock, 2011). Longer time horizons must be set. Western energy-guzzling societies, for example, will not shift from being high carbon emitters overnight; but Germany is showing the way with regard to its power sources, aiming for 45 per cent of energy to be sourced from renewable sources by 2030 (Schiermeier, 2013), and the UK ambitiously set a target in its Climate Change Act 2008 to reduce its CO_2 emissions by 80 per cent by 2050 (Her Majesty's Government, 2008). Equally, societies that have seen supermarkets overflowing with food as symbols of success – banishing the Malthusian nightmare of excess population and underproduction of food – will not easily begin to shift their patterns of distorted eating and resulting diet-related ill health (notably obesity). Twenty-first-century ecological public health thinking must lengthen its time frames.

Another effect of subscribing to ecological public health thinking concerns the role of expertise. Medical models have consistently celebrated the specialist: the public health physician as detective, soothsayer and problem solver, all in one. Ecological public health, by contrast, necessarily draws on multiple disciplines and modes of action. This requires existing disciplines to have something not usually associated with public health – humility and preparedness to take difficult arguments seriously. If only more people had taken seriously the early warnings about overuse and the capacity of antimicrobial resistance to undermine the effectiveness of antibiotics, for instance. These miracle 'cures' were latched onto with joy by those who saw biology and nature as forces to be tamed, rather than worked within. Retrospectively, we can see, too, that the use of antibiotics coincided with a more consumer era for medicine. Where strict controls should have existed (as with pollution), their use instead was defined by choice. In this respect, ecological public health thinking easily can appear to spoil proffered advances. It cautions against potentially rebounding technical fixes and emphasises the need to think longer term about the possible consequences of intervention. More positively, it suggests the advantages of multiple, rather than single, lines of action. If ecological public health requires multidimensional analysis, actions are more likely to be effective if they are pursued across multiple dimensions of policy and action. To put it simply, combinations of intervention are more likely to have lasting effects, even if they are more difficult to parse into an evidence-based system of scrutiny over their impact.

Looking Ahead: What Difference Does This Make?

Most obviously, ecological public health provides a rationale for reinvigorating the public health task. It redefines what is meant by the health of the public in the 21st century. It redefines progress (Jackson, 2009). It proposes a rebalancing of emphasis on material wealth as the sole driver of life improvement by layering in more factors, more levels by which people's lives can be kept well. The evidence is strong that, beyond a certain basic level, wealth does not deliver endless health improvement. Indeed, inequalities may be more important than other prime factors (Wilkinson and Pickett, 2009). The ecological public health perspective goes further. It asks us to consider what is meant by progress itself. Is health the absence of disease? No, it is about well-being, and not just human but ecosystems health, too. And in an era where humanity has to face the consequences of two centuries of mining the Earth and the concentration of wealth into the hands of a minority of populations and countries, this is vital. In an era of climate change, biodiversity loss, water stress, soil erosion on unprecedented scales, the need to build conditions for human existence that support and nurture ecosystems health is urgent.

Practical tasks need to be undertaken if the public health movement and professions adopt an ecological public health perspective.

First, ecological public health itself needs to be championed within public health discourse. Reshaping the conditions for good health requires people to do things. That requires, in turn, a combination of leadership and collective action. This requires articulate social movements who 'get' the notions and advantages of ecological public health. That requires education, courses, entry into curricula, teaching and learning. Tony McMichael and colleagues have been too rare as they have charted powerful and inspiring lines of thinking. More programmes of research and development are needed across professional and scientific divides. This function – reaching beyond one's intellectual base camp or primary specialism – is essential for 21st-century public health. In our own book, we used the unfashionable word 'leadership'. Collegiate thinkers and teamworkers hesitate over leadership for its top-down authoritarian overtones, but what else is there? Champion? Coordinate? Initiate? Cooperate? Pathfinders? Scouts? Pilots? Auditors? Are we speaking of the qualities of individuals or teams, institutions or cultures? Our key point is that within organisations, within laboratories, within research teams, within institutions, within policymaking processes, within movements for ecological public health – anywhere that claims to be interested in health improvement – there must be people in groups who build knowledge, take on the opposing forces, encourage and facilitate better integration of human society with our environments. Better match between humans and ecosystems requires change agents. To put it starkly, the world will not change course without change agency.

One of the many reasons we have celebrated Tony McMichael is for his persistent, consistent capacity to supply cogent arguments that question narrow orthodoxy. For us, this is epitomised in his essay on the proximate and distal, a brilliant criticism of conservative thinking, with which we began this chapter. This imaginative leadership of ideas is critical because it has to challenge fragmentary, compartmentalised, departmentalised and uncritical thought. No one's eminence is beyond questioning, if done rationally and by tackling the evidence and the ideas, not the personalities. Who follows and adopts and runs with ideas? Our view is that public health is more than a collection of individuals, however inspired. Individuals matter, but just as science requires a 'community of inquirers', to recall C. S. Peirce's view on progress in science, so too the effective advocacy of ideas requires groups, organisations and movements (Rayner and Lang, 2012).

Although this chapter is written in affectionate homage to a great researcher, thinker and communicator, we end by stressing the word 'public' in ecological public health. Since the 1970s, the world's decision makers and power elite have subscribed broadly to and pursued a neoliberal framework for policy. How their ideas triumphed has been well chronicled elsewhere (Cockett, 1994). Their domination followed the societal perspective of Keynes and the Western architects of post-World War II political economy. Today, the neoliberal domination of political economic thought is, in turn, under stress. Advances in the developing and developed worlds have been threatened. The ruthless accumulation of money and power has been exposed (Tett, 2009). The rewriting of trade rules and conceptual as well as economic boundaries has been highlighted by social movements decrying unfairness. And yet, the primacy of individualism and market forces continues, as though these are concrete realities. In our view, public health is what the term says: the juxtaposition of two words 'health' and 'public'. Public health is about the health of the public. That means more than a vociferous minority of affluent individuals. It refers to collective health; we cannot be healthy if others are not. This requires conditions to be altered, knowing that variations in health will still exist, only the level has been ratcheted up. This societal, nay public, approach to health means societies are judged by how they look after and allow all, not just some, people to live with dignity and decency. Ecological public health is thus the project that has to combine those pursuits with ensuring that the ecosystems on which humanity depends themselves thrive. The 40-year neoliberal project is, to some extent, a block on ecological public health progress. But the intellectual and practical task is much more deeply rooted.

References

Boulding, K.E. 1956. General systems theory – the skeleton of science. *Management Science* 2, 197–208.

Bronfenbrenner, U. 1979. *The Ecology of Human Development*. Harvard University Press, Cambridge, Massachusetts, USA.

Cockett, R. 1994. *Thinking the Unthinkable: Think-Tanks and the Economic Counter-Revolution, 1931–1983*. HarperCollins, London, UK.

Corsi, P. 2005. Before Darwin: transformist concepts in European natural history. *Journal of the History of Biology* 38, 67–83.

Darwin, C. 1859. *On the Origin of Species by Natural Selection*. John Murray, London, UK.

Dewey, J., Boydston, J.A. & McDermott, J.J. 2008. *John Dewey: The Later Works, 1925–1953: 1935–1937*. Southern Illinois University Press, Carbondale, Illinois, USA.

Dissanayake, E. 2009. The artification hypothesis and its relevance to cognitive science, evolutionary aesthetics, and neuroaesthetics. *Cognitive Semiotics* 5, 148–73.

Dubos, R. 1968. *So Human an Animal: How We Are Shaped by Surroundings and Events*. Charles Scribner's Sons, New York, USA.

Fogel, R.W. 2004. Technophysio evolution and the measurement of economic growth. *Journal of Evolutionary Economics* 14, 217–21.

Fogel, R.W. 2008. *Forecasting the Cost of U.S. Health Care in 2040*. NBER Working Paper No. 14361. National Bureau of Economic Research, Washington, DC, USA.

Gell-Mann, M. 1995. *The Quark and the Jaguar: Adventures in the Simple and the Complex*. Henry Holt, New York, USA.

Geyer, R.R. 2003. Globalization, Europeanization, complexity, and the future of Scandinavian exceptionalism. *Governance* 16, 559–76.

Geyer, R.R. & Rihani, S. 2010. *Complexity and Public Policy: A New Approach to 21st Century Politics, Policy & Society*. Routledge, London, UK.

Hamlin, C. 1998. *Public Health and Social Justice in the Age of Chadwick: Britain 1800–1854*. Cambridge University Press, Cambridge, UK.

Hancock, T. 2011. It's the environment, stupid! Declining ecosystem health is THE threat to health in the 21st century (Commentary). *Health Promotion International* 26, 168–72.

Hanlon, J. 1969. An ecologic view of public health. *American Journal of Public Health* 59, 4–11.

Her Majesty's Government 2008. Climate Change Act. Available at: www.legislation.gov.uk/ukpga/2008/27/contents, accessed 10 February 2015.

Herbert, S. 2005. *Charles Darwin, Geologist*. Cornell University Press, New York, USA.

Holland, J.H. 1998. *Emergence: From Chaos to Order*. Oxford University Press, Oxford, UK.

Institute of Medicine 2002. *The Future of the Public's Health in the 21st Century*. National Academies Press, Washington, DC, USA.

Institute of Medicine (US) Committee on Health and Behavior: Research Practice and Policy 2001. *The Interplay of Biological, Behavioral, and Societal Influences*. National Academies Press, Washington, DC, USA.

Jackson, T. 2009. *Prosperity without Growth: Economics for a Finite Planet*. Earthscan, London, UK.

Kartman, L. 1967. Human ecology and public health. *American Journal of Public Health* 57, 737–50.

Komlos, J. & Baur, M. 2004. From the tallest to (one of) the fattest: the enigmatic fate of the American population in the 20th century. *Economics & Human Biology* 2, 57–74.

Kricher, J. 2009. *Balance of Nature: Ecology's Enduring Myth*. Princeton University Press, Princeton, New Jersey, USA.

Lang, T. & Rayner, G. 2007. Overcoming policy cacophany on obesity: an ecological public health framework for politicians. *Obesity Reviews* 8, 165–81.

Lang, T. & Rayner, G. 2012. Ecological public health: the 21st century's big idea? *BMJ* 345, e5466.

Lang, T., Rayner, G. & Kaelin, E. 2006. *The Food Industry, Diet, Physical Activity and Health: A Review of Reported Commitments and Practice of 25 of the World's Largest Food Companies. Report to the World Health Organisation.* City University Centre for Food Policy, London, UK.

Lauterbur, P.C. 2005. Demystifying biology: did life begin as a complex system? *Complexity* 11, 30–5.

Love, G.A. 2010. Shakespeare's Origin of Species and Darwin's Tempest. *Configurations* 18, 121–40.

McKeown, T. 1971. Medical issues in historical demography. In: Clarke, E. (ed.) *Modern Methods in the History of Medicine*. Athlone Press, London, UK, 57–74.

McKeown, T. 1976. *The Modern Rise of Population*. Edward Arnold, London, UK.

McMichael, A.J. 1999. Prisoners of the Proximate: Loosening the Constraints on Epidemiology in an Age of Change. *American Journal of Epidemiology* 149, 887–97.

Meadows, D.H., Meadows, D.L., Randers., J. & Behrens, W.III. 1972. *The Limits to Growth: A Report for the Club of Rome's Project on the Predicament of Mankind*. Universe Books, New York, USA.

Meadows, D.H., Meadows, D.L. & Randers, J. 1993. *Beyond the Limits: Confronting Global Collapse, Envisioning a Sustainable Future*. Chelsea Green Publishing, Post Mill, Vermont, USA.

M'Gonigle, G.C.M. & Kirby, J. 1936. *Poverty and Public Health. Left Book Club ed*. Victor Gollancz, London, UK.

Milio, N. 1976. A framework for prevention: changing health-damaging to health-generating life patterns. *American Journal of Public Health* 66, 435–9.

Mitleton-Kelly, E. (ed.) 2003. *Complex Systems and Evolutionary Perspectives on Organisations: The Application of Complexity Theory to Organisations*. Emerald Group Publishing, Bingley, UK.

Montoya, J., Pimm, S.L. & Solé, R.V. 2006. Ecological networks and their fragility. *Nature* 442, 259–64.

Norberg, J. & Cumming, G.S. 2008. *Complexity Theory for a Sustainable Future*. Columbia University Press, New York, USA.

OECD Health Data 2011. *How Does the United States Compare*. Organisation for Economic Co-operation and Development, Paris, France.

Park, R.E. & Burgess, E.W. (eds) 1925. *The City*. University of Chicago Press, Chicago, Illinois, USA.

Pearce, N. & Merletti, F. 2006. Complexity, simplicity, and epidemiology. *International Journal of Epidemiology* 35, 515–9.

Philippe, P. & Mansi, O. 1998. Nonlinearity in the epidemiology of complex health and disease processes. *Theoretical Medicine and Bioethics* 19, 591–607.

Popp, J.A. 2007. *Evolution's First Philosopher: John Dewey and the Continuity of Nature*. State University of New York, Albany, New York, USA

Rayner, G. & Lang, T. 2011. Is nudge an effective public health strategy to tackle obesity? No. *BMJ* 342, d2168.

Rayner, G. & Lang, T. 2012. *Ecological Public Health: Reshaping the Conditions for Good Health*. Routledge/Earthscan, Abingdon, UK.

Rescher, N. 1998. *Complexity: A Philosophical Overview*. Transaction Publishers, New Brunswick, New Jersey, USA.

Richards, R.J. 2006. Nature is the poetry of mind, or how Schelling solved Goethe's Kantian problems. In: Friedman, M. & Nordmann, A. (eds) *The Kantian Legacy in Nineteenth-Century Science*. MIT Press, Cambridge, Massachusetts, USA.

Richards, R.J. 2007. Ernst Haeckel's alleged anti-Semitism and contributions to Nazi biology. *Biological Theory* 2, 97–103.

Rickles, D., Hawe, P. & Shiell, A. 2007. A simple guide to chaos and complexity. *Journal of Epidemiology and Community Health* 61, 933–7.

Rothman, D.J. 1997. *Beginnings Count: The Technological Imperative in American Health Care*. Oxford University Press, New York, USA.

Sandro, G., Chris, H. & George, A.K. 2009. Social epidemiology and complex system dynamic modelling as applied to health behaviour and drug use research. *International Journal of Drug Policy* 20, 209–16.

Schabas, M. 2005. *The Natural Origins of Economics*. University of Chicago Press, Chicago, Illinois, USA.

Schiermeier, Q. 2013. Renewable power: Germany's energy gamble. *Nature* 496: 156–8. Available at: www.nature.com/news/renewable-power-germany-s-energygamble-1.12755, accessed 10 February 2015.

Schwartz, W.B. 1998. *Life without Disease: The Pursuit of Medical Utopia*. University of California Press, Berkeley, California, USA.

Simms, E.-M. 2005. Goethe, Husserl, and the crisis of the European sciences. *Janus Head* 8, 160–72.

Spellberg, B., Guidos, R., Gilbert, D., Bradley, J., Boucher, H.W., Scheld, W.M., et al. 2008. The epidemic of antibiotic-resistant infections: a call to action for the medical community from the infectious diseases society of America. *Clinical Infectious Diseases* 46, 155–64.

Sterelny, K. 2012. *The Evolved Apprentice: How Evolution Made Humans Unique*. MIT Press,Boston, Massachusetts, USA.

Stuart, J. 1604. *A Counter-blaste to Tobacco*. R.B. London, UK archive.org/stream/acounterblasteto17008gut/17008.txt, accessed 31 March 2015.

Szreter, S. 1988. The importance of social intervention in Britain's mortality decline, c1850–1914. A reinterpretation of the role of public health. *Social History of Medicine* 1, 1–37.

Szreter, S. 2002. Rethinking McKeown: the relationship between public health and social change. *American Journal of Public Health* 92, 722–5.

Tansley, A.G. 1935. The use and abuse of vegetational concepts and terms. *Ecology* 16, 284–307.

Taylor, M.C. 2001. *The Moment of Complexity: Emerging Network Culture*. University of Chicago Press, Chicago, Illinois, USA.

Tett, G. 2009. *Fool's Gold: How Unrestrained Greed Corrupted a Dream, Shattered Global Markets and Unleashed a Catastrophe*. Little Brown, London, UK.

Thaler, R. & Sunstein, C. 2008. *Nudge: Improving Decisions about Health, Wealth, and Happiness*. Yale University Press, New Haven, Connecticut, USA.

Tsoukas, H. & Hatch, M.J. 2001. Complex thinking, complex practice: the case for a narrative approach to organizational complexity. *Human Relations* 54, 979–1013.

Vandenbroucke, J.P., Rooda, H.M.E. & Beukers, H. 1991. Who made John Snow a hero? *American Journal of Epidemiology* 133, 967–73.

Weber, T.P. 2007. Alfred Russel Wallace and the antivaccination movement in Victorian England. *Emerging Infectious Disease* 16, 664–8.

World Health Organization (WHO) 1986. *Ottawa Charter*. World Health Organisation, Geneva, Switzerland.

WHO 2011. *World Health Day 2011: Combat Antimicrobial Resistance*. World Health Organisation, Geneva, Switzerland.

Wildavsky, A. 1976. Doing better and feeling worse: the political pathology of health policy. *Deadalus* 106, 105–23.

Wilkinson, R.G. & Pickett, K. 2009. *The Spirit Level: Why More Equal Societies Almost Always Do Better*. Allen Lane, London, UK.

Williamson, S. 2007. *The Vaccination Controversy: The Rise, Reign and Fall of Compulsory Vaccination for Smallpox*. Liverpool University Press, Liverpool, UK.

Wilson, E.O. 1998. *Consilience. The Unity of Knowledge*. Alfred A. Knopf, New York, USA.

www.ingramcontent.com/pod-product-compliance
Lightning Source LLC
LaVergne TN
LVHW070905210926
848482LV00017B/995
9781925022407